Nursing Interventions for Infants & Children

Martha J. Craft, PhD, RN
College of Nursing
The University of Iowa
Iowa City, Iowa

Janice A. Denehy, PhD, RN
College of Nursing
The University of Iowa
Iowa City, Iowa

1990
W.B. SAUNDERS COMPANY
Harcourt Brace Jovanovich, Inc.
Philadelphia   London   Toronto   Montreal   Sydney   Tokyo

W. B. SAUNDERS COMPANY
Harcourt Brace Jovanovich, Inc.

The Curtis Center
Independence Square West
Philadelphia, PA 19106–3399

Library of Congress Cataloging-in-Publication Data

Craft, Martha.
    Nursing interventions for infants and children/Martha J. Craft,
Janice A. Denehy.

            p.   cm.

    1. Pediatric nursing..   2. Sick children—Psychology.
3. Family–Psychology.   I. Denehy, Janice Ann.   II. Title.

    [DNLM: 1. Child Psychology.   2. Family.
3. Pediatric Nursing.   WY 159 C885n]

RJ245.C7   1990

610.73′62—dc20

DNLM/DLC
                                                        89–10486

ISBN 0–7216–2129–5

Editors: Thomas Eoyang and Ilze Rader

Designer: Joan Owen

Production Manager: Linda R. Turner

Manuscript Editor: Margaret Eckman

Illustration Coordinator: Walt Verbitski

Indexer: Nancy Newman

Cover Designer: Michelle Maloney

Nursing Interventions for Infants and Children   ISBN   0–7216–2129–5

Last digit is the print number: 9   8   7   6   5   4   3   2   1

This book is dedicated to June L. Triplett, Ed.D., R.N., who devoted her career to the care of children and their families and to the education of nurses who care for them. As an educator, June influenced an entire generation of nurses, many of whom are contributing authors to this book. To her students, June was not only a teacher, but a role model, a mentor, and a friend. As graduate students, many of us were fascinated with developing technology and specialization. June widened our horizons by asking questions about the children for whom we cared, questions such as: What are the effects of hospitalization on the child? The family? What coping strategies did the child and the family use? What were the effects of the illness or hospitalization on the child's development? How might this illness alter family interaction patterns and the parent's ability to parent? At the time, such questions may have seemed simplistic in the light of burgeoning technology and the rapidly growing body of knowledge about pathological conditions and their medical treatment, yet, in retrospect, it was these questions that have opened the doors to a lifetime of concern and study and have changed our way of thinking about nursing. It was June's influence that molded our philosophy about the care of children and families.

Consistent with her holistic approach, June cared about her students not only as learners, but as individuals and as members of families. Through the years she has followed with interest the professional development of her former students. While she shared in our professional achievements, she also delighted in observing the growth and development of our families. June has supported many of us as we have combined graduate education and a career with a family. She has provided the encouragement, inspiration, and challenge to each of her students to grow personally and professionally, to apply theory not only to nursing practice but to life. Through her work with children, families, students, and colleagues, June Triplett has modeled the essence of nursing—caring and commitment.

CONTRIBUTORS

ROJANN ALPERS, M.S., R.N.
Lecturer, College of Nursing, The University of Iowa, Iowa City, Iowa.
Cerebral Edema Management

SARA ARNESON, Ph.D., R.N.
Associate Professor, School of Nursing, University of Virginia, Charlottesville, Virginia.
The Child As a Member of a Family: Overview

STEPHANIE CLATWORTHY, Ed.D., R.N.
Dean and Professor, School of Nursing, Kent State University, Kent, Ohio.
Communication through Therapeutic Play

JUDITH A. COUCOUVANIS, M.A., R.N., C.S.
Clinical Nurse Manager, Adolescent Mental Health Program, Catherine McAuley Health Center, Ann Arbor, Michigan.
Behavior Management

MARTHA J. CRAFT, Ph.D., R.N.
Associate Professor, College of Nursing, The University of Iowa, Iowa City, Iowa.
Sibling Support; Biophysical Interventions for Enhancing Homeostatic Mechanisms: Overview; Nutritional Support; Summary: The Future

JANICE A. DENEHY, Ph.D., R.N.
Assistant Professor, College of Nursing, The University of Iowa, Iowa City, Iowa.
Anticipatory Guidance; Communicating with Children through Drawings

ELIZABETH L. DOWD, M.A., C.P.N.P., R.N.
Pediatric Nurse Specialist, Visiting Nurse and Homemaker Service, Davenport, Iowa.
Home Care

JOANN ELAND, Ph.D., R.N.
Associate Professor, College of Nursing, The University of Iowa, Iowa City, Iowa.
Pain Management

SUSAN A. FAY, M.S.N., C.P.N.P., R.N.
Clinical Nurse Specialist, James Whitcomb Riley Hospital for Children, Newborn Follow-up Program, Indianapolis, Indiana.
Sleep Promotion

SUZANNE FEETHAM, Ph.D., R.N., F.A.A.N.
Director of Nursing for Education and Research, National Children's Hospital, Washington, DC.
Foreword

VICKY L. HERTIG
Lecturer, College of Nursing, The University of Iowa, Iowa City, Iowa.
Cerebral Edema Management

MARY KAY KOSTER, M.A., R.N.
Assistant Professor, School of Nursing, The University of Texas Medical Branch, Galveston, Texas.
Promotion of Self-Care

KATHY JAMISON KRAUS, M.A., R.N.
Lecturer, School of Nursing, The University of North Carolina at Greensboro, Greensboro, North Carolina.
Fostering Family Integrity

DEBRA LENERS, M.A., R.N.
Doctoral Student, School of Nursing, University of Colorado, Denver, Colorado.
Vestibular Stimulation

JO MANION, M.A., R.N.
Nurse Consultant, Dynamic Control of Longwood (Travenol), Galinburgh, Tennessee.
Preparing Children For Hospitalization, Procedures, or Surgery

JANET R. MAPEL, C.P.N.P., R.N.
Clinical Nurse Specialist, Hospital School, Division of Developmental Disabilities, The University of Iowa, Iowa City, Iowa.

WYNETTA MATSUURA, M.S., M.P.H., C.P.N.P., R.N.
Clinical Nurse Specialist, Kapiolani Women's and Children's Medical Center, Honolulu, Hawaii.
Intercultural Communication

DIANE MOLSBERRY, M.A., R.N.
Education Coordinator, Deaconess Children's Hospital, Spokane, Washington.
Communicating through Touch

JULIE C. NOVAK, D.N.Sc., C.P.N.P., R.N.
Assistant Clinical Professor, Department of Community and Family Medicine, The University of San Diego, San Diego, California.
Facilitating Fathering

ROBERT E. NOVAK, Ph.D.
Associate Professor, Department of Communicative Disorders, San Diego State University, San Diego, California.
Facilitating Fathering

ROSANNE C. PEREZ-WOODS, Ed.D., C.P.N.A., R.N.
Marcella Niehoff Chair and Professor of Maternal Child Nursing, School of Nursing, Loyola University, Chicago, Illinois.
Providing Support: A Process Model

DIANE PFLEDERER, M.A., R.N.
Director, Maternal Health Service, Saint Francis Medical Center, Peoria, Illinois.
Using Friends As a Social Support System for Children

JANA L. PRESSLER, Ph.D., R.N.
Assistant Professor of Nursing, Frances Payne Bolton School of Nursing, Case
Western Reserve University, Cleveland, Ohio.
Promoting Attachment

KATHLEEN ROSS-ALAOLMOLKI, Ph.D., R.N.
Assistant Professor, Frances Payne Bolton School of Nursing, Case Western
Reserve University, Cleveland, Ohio.
Coping with Family Loss: The Death of a Sibling

MARILYN SAVEDRA, D.N.S., R.N.
Associate Professor in Nursing, Department of Family Health Care Nursing,
School of Nursing, The University of California at San Francisco, San
Francisco, California.
Pain Management

KATHY D. SCHIBLER, M.S.N., C.P.N.P., R.N.
Formerly Lecturer, School of Nursing, Department of Pediatric, Family, and
Women's Health Nursing, Indiana University, Indianapolis, Indiana.
Sleep Promotion

MAUREEN GORDON SHOGAN, R.N.
Educational Coordinator, Deaconess Children's Hospital, Spokane, Washington.
Communicating through Touch

KATHLEEN A. SIMON, M.S., R.N.
Assistant Professor, College of Nursing, Medical University of South Carolina,
Charleston, South Carolina.
Communication through Therapeutic Play

ANN R. SLOAT, M.A., R.N.
Associate Professor, School of Nursing, The University of Hawaii at Manoa,
Honolulu, Hawaii
Intercultural Communication

PATRICIA A. SMIGIELSKI, M.S., C.P.N.P., R.N.
Clinical Nurse Specialist, Hospital School, Division of Developmental
Disabilities, The University of Iowa, Iowa City, Iowa.
Bowel and Bladder Maintenance

MARY TESLER, M.A., R.N.
Clinical Professor in Nursing, School of Nursing, University of California at San
Francisco, San Francisco, California.
Pain Management

KAREN A. THOMAS, Ph.D., R.N.
Assistant Professor, School of Nursing, The University of Washington, Seattle,
Washington.
Environmental Manipulation

MARY E. TIEDEMAN, Ph.D., R.N.
Assistant Professor, School of Nursing, Kent State University, Kent, Ohio.
Communication through Therapeutic Play

JUNE L. TRIPLETT, Ed.D., R.N.
Professor Emeritus, School of Nursing, The University of Wisconsin at
Oshkosh, Oshkosh, Wisconsin.
*Psychosocial Interventions for Maintenance of Self-Concept and Promotion of
Coping: Overview*

ALICE M. TSE, M.A., R.N.
Associate Instructor in Clinical Nursing, School of Nursing, Indiana University,
Indianapolis, Indiana.
Providing Support: A Process Model

LINDA D. VLASTUIN, M.S., R.N.
Director of Community Health Nursing, The Children's Hospital, Sewall
Rehabilitation Center, Denver Colorado; Child Health Nursing Consultant,
Alaska Department of Health and Social Services, Division of Public Health,
Anchorage, Alaska.
Home Care

REVIEWERS

CAROLYN M. BOLTER FELLER, Ph.D., R.N.
Associate Professor, Chair, Parent-Child Division, College of Nursing, Arizona State University, Tempe, Arizona

LAURA L. HAYMAN, Ph.D., F.A.A.N.
Associate Professor, Chair and Program Director, Nursing of Children, School of Nursing, University of Pennsylvania, Philadelphia, Pennsylvania

MARIE L. LOBO, Ph.D., R.N.
Assistant Professor, Department of Family and Community, College of Nursing, The Ohio State University, Columbus, Ohio

DARLENE E. McCOWN, Ph.D., P.N.P., R.N.
Associate Dean for Academic Affairs, Associate Professor, School of Nursing, University of Rochester, Rochester, New York

BEVERLY OSBAND, Ph.D., R.N.
Assistant Professor, Department of Parent and Child Nursing, School of Nursing, University of Washington, Seattle, Washington

MARION H. ROSE, Ph.D., R.N.
Professor, Department of Parent and Child Nursing, School of Nursing, University of Washington, Seattle, Washington

YVONNE M. STERLING, D.N.Sc., R.N.
Associate Professor, Parent-Child Health Nursing, School of Nursing, Louisiana State University Medical Center, New Orleans, Louisiana

FOREWORD

The integration of nursing practice and science is essential. The authors of this book make a major contribution to this integration in their discussions of nursing interventions for children and their families. This book represents the "state of the art" in nursing practice by expert clinicians who are also credentialed and have expertise in research. This impressive cadre of clinician/scientists builds on the base and impetus of the work of a smaller but significant group of clinician/scientists in maternal-child health, such as Dr. Gene Cranston-Anderson, Dr. Kathryn Barnard, Dr. Mary Neal, and Dr. Ramona Mercer.

Several criteria must be met in the advancement of nursing science and nursing practice. These include the utilization of the previous work of scientists and clinicians, the systematic testing of nursing interventions, the provision of true family-centered care based on the identification of strengths and resources of children and families, and the linkage of nursing practice and health care initiatives (or interventions) to health policy and the policymakers. The authors of this book meet these criteria.

The authors address major health policy issues identified by federal and voluntary agencies. The Office of Technology Assessment (1988) has identified seven strategies for improving the health of American children. These strategies include improving access to care, attention to child safety, and newborn screening. The health care priorities identified by nursing leaders in maternal-child health, meeting under the auspices of the Bureau of Maternal-Child Health (1987), and the Forum on the future of pediatric nursing (Christakas and Cromer, 1988) are also addressed by the authors. These priorities include comprehensive health care, knowledgeable care providers across multiple care settings, and family-centered care. The consistency of the issues addressed by the authors and the health care priorities identified by these national nursing leaders strengthen the application of the content of this book to the care of children and families.

Another important contribution of this book is that the authors provide criteria for assessing the need for nursing intervention. Through this, information is provided on instruments for assessment. These instruments not only are guides for systematic assessment but they also have evidence of reliability and validity. The interventions proposed by the authors are based on expert judgment and research followed by criteria for evaluation. The instruments for evaluation are often standardized. The efforts by nurses for systematic evaluation of nursing practice are often limited. Application of the work of these authors provides definitive direction for this important component of practice. The authors also provide explicit application of nursing diagnosis for physiological, psychosocial, and family needs throughout the text.

Family-focused care and interventions are important components of nursing addressed by many of the authors. The application of knowledge of family theory, family systems, and family interventions is central to this book. The nurse's role in the developing family is evident with guidelines for assessment and intervention to anticipate family responses, to maintain the integrity of the family system, and to establish family boundaries. Emphasis is placed on the strengths and resources of families in contrast to deficit models. While the focus of many chapters is the family, other authors integrate family theory and constructs in chapters focusing on the child.

An essential concept for determining nursing interventions is to recognize the interdependence of the child, the family, and the complex health care environment. The environment of the child and family is examined by several authors. One author examines the physical environment of the premature, others examine the social environment, including the role of friends. This attention to the interdependence of the child and family with the environment is consistent with the work of Nightingale, who described a primary role of the nurse as the mediator between the environment and the patient (Nightingale, 1969; Flaskerud and Halloran, 1980).

The complexity of the health care environment continues to increase. Because of advances in technology, there are now populations of medically vulnerable children receiving care in all health care environments and in the home. The nursing roles with these children and families are varied and require different knowledge. In this book, the authors discuss a number of nursing roles, from the direct care of children with cerebral edema to multiple session family therapy following the loss of a sibling.

The authors have provided directions and challenges for the current and future care needs and research of children and their families.

SUZANNE L. FEETHAM, PH.D., R.N., F.A.A.N.

References

Bureau of Maternal-Child Health. Proceedings, National Advisory Committee for Maternal-Child Health Nursing. Washington, D.C.: U.S. Public Health Service, 1987.

Christakas, AN, and Cromer, J. Report of forum on the future of pediatric nursing: Looking forward to the 21st century. Pediatric Nursing, 15:54–55, 1989.

Flaskerud, JH, and Halloran, E (Eds.). Areas of agreement in nursing theory development. Advanced Nursing Science, 3:1–7, 1980.

Nightingale, F. Notes in nursing (rev.). New York, Dover Press, 1969.

Office of Technology Assessment (OTA). Healthy children: Investing in the future. Washington, D.C.: U.S. Congress, 1988.

PREFACE

This book was written for nurses who are advanced practitioners, graduate students, and nursing leaders. It is you who have the opportunity and challenge to intervene in the lives of children and families in a manner that makes a difference. It is you who will build the science of nursing through study of the selection, application, and evaluation of nursing interventions. The interventions presented in this collection were chosen with the hope that they will contribute to both of these processes, and that you will add other tested interventions to this initial list.

The early part of Dr. Craft's career had been spent in nursing practice and in application of interventions that make a difference in the lives of people. When she decided to spend the last part of her career in academia, it became apparent that the concepts of nursing were emphasized rather than the development and testing of interventions. In addition, these concepts were often examined with the adult as the frame of reference, with the assumption that their application would generalize to infants and children. A colleague, Dr. Denehy, agreed that this assumption was erroneous, and their work on the book began.

The planning for *Nursing Interventions for Infants and Children* began in 1980. This book is based upon the original conceptualization of nursing by our leader and founder, Florence Nightingale. The editors believe that nursing is the art and science of intervening to put nature in a position to maintain wellness or to recover from illness. As stated by Florence Nightingale in 1860,

It is often thought that medicine is the curative process. It is no such thing; medicine is the surgery of functions, as surgery proper is that of limbs and organs. Neither can do anything but remove obstructions; neither can cure; nature alone cures. And what nursing has to do is to put the patients in the best condition for nature to act upon them ...

This book describes interventions that put infants and children in the best condition for nature to act. The selection of interventions chosen for this collection reflects the importance of psychological coping and physiological homeostasis operating within the context of a complex interaction of mind and body, which begins very early in life.

Effective coping and adequate homeostatic mechanisms begin with a foundation initiated at birth and sustained within a network of people who love and care for the infant and young child, traditionally called "the family." For this reason the first five interventions focus on the beginning years, with interventions to facilitate development of a foundation that will promote effective coping skills for the infant and child.

xiii

Such coping skills are often tested severely when accidents or illness occur. During these difficult life events, it is the responsibility of nursing to promote these coping skills, or to place the infant, child, and family in the best possible position to help themselves cope during this period of their lives.

The importance of coping is highlighted in an overview written by June Triplett, to whom this book is dedicated. The next group of interventions promote coping during illness. The last portion of the book includes interventions to enhance homeostatic mechanisms, or to assist nature in the self-healing process. We start with interventions that promote healing through appropriate stimulation, rest, comfort, and sound nutrition. The last two interventions represent the new frontiers of nursing intervention—recognition and testing. That is, they are interventions directed toward a specific biophysiological process. Nurses in acute and long-term care settings have been using such interventions for many years. However, scientists have only begun to study the significant contribution these interventions make toward the promotion of recovery, functional status, and quality of life. In the next decade the list of similar interventions to test will continue to grow.

The common theme throughout this book is that infants, children, and their families have natural psychological coping skills and physiological homeostatic mechanisms. It is the business of the nursing profession to assist them to use these resources in a positive direction toward attainment and maintenance of health through diagnosis and intervention.

Since it is our belief that interventions are driven by nursing diagnosis, each intervention is discussed within the framework of a stated diagnosis. Further, the defining characteristics being used currently with each diagnosis in the literature are those chosen by the individual authors. However, it is crucial to note that the reliability and validity of these defining characteristics for infants and children are in the process of being tested. Thus, readers need to scrutinize the defining characteristics, and it is expected that some readers will study them to determine their generalizability to infants and children.

This book is a beginning. If it stimulates thought and research that will improve the lives of infants, children, and families, one of our goals will have been met. However, a second goal is equally important: the development of nursing science through the testing of nursing interventions. The attainment of this goal is a process already begun that will continue into the next century. It is our hope that this book will make an important contribution to that process.

MARTHA J. CRAFT
JANICE A. DENEHY

ACKNOWLEDGMENTS

In the beginning there was a dream. After eight years, the dream has become a reality. This dream has involved many individuals whose cooperation and hard work have been essential in this team effort.

First, we wish to thank each of the contributing authors for their enthusiasm and commitment. Knowing the many professional and personal demands experienced by today's nurses, their gracious response to working under time constraints and their willingness to incorporate suggested changes were appreciated. We also acknowledge the helpful feedback received from the chapter reviewers; while their praise and excitement for this book energized us during the seemingly endless tedium of editing, their thoughtful suggestions for revising, reorganizing, rewording, or redoing were most helpful in polishing the finished product.

We also wish to acknowledge the enthusiastic support received from the university community, including administrators, fellow faculty members, colleagues in the clinical setting, and students. Special recognition goes to The University of Iowa, College of Nursing, for providing the technical assistance necessary to carry out this project. Nancy Goldsmith and Laura Lenz of the Research Office worked tirelessly to keep the chapters up-to-date on the word processor; knowing that we could depend upon their competent services lightened our load. Helen Van Hoozer of Instructional Design Services shared her expertise in the production of graphics.

Finally, we would like to express our gratitude to our editors, Thomas Eoyang and Ilze Rader, for believing in the importance of nursing interventions and pioneering in this important area. It is our shared hope that this book will improve the nursing care of infants and children by stimulating careful thought and rigorous study of nursing interventions—the core of nursing practice.

CONTENTS

THE CHILD AS A MEMBER OF A FAMILY

Overview

SARA W. ARNESON, Ph.D., R.N.

Most children in the United States spend their early years living within a structural system known as the family. It is among this group of individuals that most children learn how to cope with each new life event. How successful children are in dealing with maturational and situational crises will depend to a great extent on how effectively their families deal with stressful situations. This section of five chapters examines the role of family support in the promotion of children's health and discusses nursing interventions to facilitate positive family functioning. Taken together, the chapters provide a framework within which to conceptualize the impact which family members have on the health and well-being of children.

The importance of the family as the primary source of physical and psychosocial support for its members has been documented on innumerable occasions by sociologists, psychologists, and anthropologists. Despite this, pediatric nurses have not always recognized family members as critical elements in the care of ill children. For a long time, family members, especially siblings, were considered hazardous to hospitalized children. Parent visits were viewed as upsetting to both children and staff and were thus restricted to one to two hours daily. Siblings were not allowed to visit at all for fear of transmitting additional common childhood diseases to their already ill brothers or sisters. It has only been in the past 15 to 20 years that nurses have begun to recognize the value of parent and sibling contributions to the recovery of sick children.

Early studies into the importance of family support during hospitalization focused on the effects of separation from parents on young hospitalized children. One of the major concepts upon which these studies were based is the special bond which exists between parents and children. As Pressler so clearly describes, the initial parent-child attachment is crucial for an infant's healthy development and provides the basis for all subsequent relationships. While Pressler focuses exclusively on the literature related to the attachment between infants and their primary caretakers (usually mothers), Novak and Novak suggest that fathers also attach to their infants in a similar manner.

Traditionally, it has been mothers who have provided the majority of care for sick children and who have received the most attention in the pediatric literature. The concept of fathering is relatively new to the field of parent-child nursing as evidenced by the limited amount of research-based nursing literature on fathering. Yet, according to Novak and Novak, fathers are assuming increasing responsibility for child-rearing activities, including the nurturance and care of sick children. It is their observation, however, that fathers require adequate support and assistance from health professionals in order to assume this caretaking role.

The hospitalization of a child, whether planned or unexpected, generally constitutes a crisis for most families. As Chapter 4 clearly describes, a child's family is the most significant source of support and comfort during this period. Kraus comments that familiar family structures and patterns of communication will be positive forces in assisting children to cope with illness and hospitalization. Yet these familiar patterns of interaction are frequently hindered when hospitalization occurs. A great deal depends on the parents' abilities to circumvent the barriers created by hospitalization and illness.

Not surprisingly, the majority of the parents' energies and attention are focused on the sick child, often at the expense of both the parents and the other siblings at home. Craft refers to the healthy siblings as the "neglected other" family members. Until very recently, the needs and concerns of the healthy siblings were often ignored. In Chapter 3, a strong case is built for identifying siblings in need of support and providing them with nursing interventions, either directly or indirectly, so that they can marshal their own coping strategies to deal with this family crisis.

Now is a crucial time for pediatric nurses to examine their role in child health care. While a good deal of research has been conducted that supports the importance of the family in a child's physical and psychosocial health, there is still much to be learned. Family structures and relationships are continually changing. What effects will these changes have on children's health? Will techniques such as anticipatory guidance, as described by Denehy, prove to be effective in preparing parents for child rearing? What is the role of fathers in the care of sick children? How can the needs of healthy siblings best be met when a child is hospitalized? Answers to these questions will come only through the development and implementation of sound, theoretically based research studies. The findings of these studies will ultimately provide the direction for the development of nursing interventions to promote family integrity and growth during periods of crisis. The content of these five chapters forms the basis for what is known about some of the concepts basic to parent-child nursing. Hopefully, it will be used as a starting point to further advance the theoretical and practice bases of pediatric nursing.

CHAPTER 1

PROMOTING ATTACHMENT

JANA L. PRESSLER, Ph.D., R.N.

The affective ties or attachments between infants and their caregivers have been discussed since the early 1900s. First described in terms of infants' attachments to their caregivers for the express purpose of satiating hunger (Freud, 1957), the notion of attachment has risen to a dynamic, multidimensional construct that is no longer linked with food. This chapter examines what is meant by attachment and identifies the importance of attachment to nursing research and practice.

THEORETICAL FOUNDATIONS

Discrepancy in Use of the Term Attachment

In the past, the term attachment has been used by professionals representing several fields of study in reference to a wide diversity of specific and nonspecific infant and caregiver behaviors. Some of the behaviors discussed as constituting attachment and use of the term attachment by professionals (e.g., Rubin, 1967a, 1967b; Clark and Affonso, 1976; Klaus and Kennell, 1976; Peterson and Hehl, 1978; Avant, 1979; Cranley, 1981; Reisner, 1981; Tulman, 1981) are not from conceptualizations that are entirely consistent with those of attachment experts from ethology and child development (e.g., Bowlby, 1958, 1982; Ainsworth, 1973; Sroufe and Waters, 1977; Sroufe, 1979a; Campos et al., 1983; Bretherton and Waters, 1985), but instead tap constructs primarily measuring various maternal characteristics. Such ideas move away from Bowlby's (1958) primary work on infant attachment. In particular, the use of the term attachment by nurses to refer to *mothers* or the relationship between *mothers and infants* rather than exclusively to *infants* has likely evolved from the work of Rubin (1967a, 1967b), a nurse, on the maternal role as well as the work of Klaus and Kennell (1976), both pediatricians, on maternal bonding and not the ethologist Bowlby's primary work on infant attachment. The following section presents an explanation of attachment as described by current attachment experts.

Distinguishing Characteristics of Attachment

Bowlby (1958, 1982) defined attachment as a behavioral system whose primary purpose was to protect infants from predators. He viewed mother proximity as a concurrent happening or precursor to the infant's attachment to the mother and maternal protection of the infant as a subsequent function of mother proximity. He contended that behaviors such as smiling, clinging, and signaling were functionally related to each other in fostering caregiver-infant proximity. Such proximity-promoting behaviors of the infant, including crying and locomotion, were believed to be biologically elicited when the infant perceived that the caregiver was too far away. Until proximity was regained, such infant behaviors would remain active, consistent with a systems notion of a feedback loop. Consequently, Bowlby disregarded attachment as the infant's motive in reducing drives, for example, in meeting the need for food. Attachment behaviors were thought to be activated and terminated without an attachment drive. Because Bowlby (1982) eventually placed attachment in a biological context of systems theory in which attachment was viewed as a goal rather than a drive, his work of 1969 is considered an early form of an organizational view of attachment. This view conceptualizes attachment as an outcome resulting from security felt by infants to their caregivers operating in conjunction with a set of attachment behaviors for adapting to environmental stimuli. This view was later identified in the work of Ainsworth (1972) and Sroufe and Waters (1977).

Ainsworth (1972, 1973), who studied with Bowlby, makes some important distinctions about attachment. First, Ainsworth (1972) points out that Bowlby's animal-based notion, which states that the sufficient element for the development of attachment behavior is the protection from predators through the infant's close proximity with the caregiver, is not completely suitable for the human species. Instead, Ainsworth suggests that because of its significance to adaptation and its relationship to attachment behavior, the concept of exploration be added to Bowlby's definition of attachment. Therefore, according to Ainsworth, both protection and exploration, with the attachment figure functioning as a secure base, is a more accurate portrayal of attachment in the context of human adaptation. Further, as stated by Ainsworth (1972, 1973), attachment is a *product* of the nature of the infant's relating to an attachment figure and can be distinguished by the qualitative differences in the way infant attachment behaviors are organized. Attachment behavior is present intermittently, with the intensity of it varying according to the circumstances of the situation. Yet attachments bridge time and distance and cannot be conceived of as varying significantly even over extended periods of time. The existence of an attachment can be inferred from a propensity to seek proximity to and contact with an attachment figure over time and despite great obstacles. This propensity, referred to as attachment, can be assumed to have some kind of intraorganismic or "organizational" basis, whereas attachment *behavior* refers to the diversity of infant actions which promote proximity, contact, and communication with the figure or figures to whom the infant is or is becoming attached. According to Ainsworth (1973), this can be observed accurately between 11 and 13 months.

Primarily stemming from the work of Ainsworth (1972, 1973), Sroufe and Waters (1977) at the University of Minnesota Institute of Child Development generated a refined definition of attachment that is commonly subscribed to by child developmentalists today.

According to Sroufe and Waters (1977), attachment is defined as "an affective tie between infant and caregiver and to a behavioral system, flexibly operating in terms of set goals, mediated by feeling, and in interaction with other behavioral systems" (p. 1185).

With respect to humans, understanding the *affective tie* embedded in attachment as described by Sroufe and Waters (1977) is important. The affective tie takes on greater meaning than a mere differentiation of the caregiver from others: it binds the infant and caregiver together. The affective tie is represented by the expressions of positive feelings within the infant-caregiver relationship, by comfort from caregiver presence, and later by the internal representation of the caregiver.

Sroufe and Waters translate infants' affective ties with their caregivers as being evidenced by some degree of sureness in the stability of the attachment relationship, or *felt security*. Further, they contend that viewing attachment as felt security, which necessarily involves preferential treatment of the infant under stress, is central to an understanding of attachment's "organizational" nature. Attachment provides the infant with security from and affection for the caregiver. This type of security can be inferred from the infant's ability to use the caregiver as an available base from which to explore the environment. Preferential comfort from an attachment figure when the infant is distressed, especially when the distress results from separation from the caregiver, helps the infant to return to relaxed exploration. According to Sroufe and Waters (1977), when the goal of the attachment behavioral system is understood to mean felt security and not simply proximity to the caregiver or protection from predators, and when affect is integrated into the infant's behavioral system as a moderator of adaptive behavior, the infant's tendency to be more upset following certain separations and reunions can be explained. The actions of the infant in seeking proximity are flexible and contingent upon a feeling-level of security, which includes the infant's interpretation of context, familiarization, prior events, and his or her own moods.

Attachment Behaviors

Behaviors which promote contact or proximity with attachment figures, for example approaching, touching, looking, and clinging, are usually regarded within the domain of attachment behaviors. Attachment is sometimes conceptualized from a summing of attachment behaviors. Trait models of attachment (cf. Coates et al., 1972a, 1972b; Maccoby and Feldman, 1972) rely on the idea that such attachment behaviors are significantly correlated, that attachment figure differences in these behaviors are stable across time, and that a strong degree of attachment can be justifiably inferred from the performance of attachment behavior at high frequency or intensity (Waters, 1978). Yet as a result of evidence that attachment behaviors are neither strongly intercorrelated nor significantly stable across the first two years of postnatal life (Ainsworth, 1972; Sroufe and Waters, 1977), critics of the use of individual attachment behaviors as definitions of attachment have concluded that such operationalization lacks construct validity. According to Cronbach and Meehl (1955), given that the theory from which the construct has been derived is correct, measures employed must reliably represent the construct. In addition, the operationalization of the construct must also be consistent with the experimental design testing the theory in order to provide sufficient evidence of construct validity. To conclude, relying upon individual attachment behaviors as definitions of attachment is not a valid representation of the construct.

Definitions of Terms Misconstrued As Attachment

Definitions of terms similar to and oftentimes confused with attachment are presented next to show their similarities with and differences from attachment. These definitions of related terms are presented in order to help nursing professionals to better understand what attachment experts from ethology and child development mean in their discussions of attachment.

Object Relations

Sometimes the infant's attachment figure is regarded as the first object with whom the infant relates and, therefore, attachment becomes entangled with the concept of object relations. Object relations originated from psychoanalytic instinct theory. The first object relation for an infant is typically the mother or the primary caregiver providing food. According to Freud (1957), the mother serves as an object through which an infant's hunger is satisfied. He described the infant's first object relation as "anaclitic love," because he viewed the sexual instincts as being fulfilled secondarily through the self-preservation instincts (1957, p. 87). Seventeen years later, in 1931, Freud (1961) acknowledged the enduring quality of the infant-mother attachment and affirmed the importance of a person's mother as the lasting exemplar for all later love relations. More specifically, according to Ainsworth (1969), most psychoanalysts view the origin of object relations to reside in the first year of life and the infant's initial relationship with his mother to be primarily oral. Thus, in this three-way connection of the development of object relations-attachment-orality, attachment becomes entangled in object relations.

Trust

Because the quality of the maternal relationship is embedded in the notion of infant-caregiver attachment, attachment may become confused with trust. Trust originated from Erikson's (1950) reformulation of psychoanalytic theory and emphasizes ego development. According to Erikson, trust implies that the infant has learned to rely on the sameness and continuity of caregivers outside the self while also relying on the self, or inner self, to cope with urges. He insists that the amount of trust derived from even the earliest infant experience does not depend on quantities of food or love, but instead on the quality of the maternal relationship. The first task embedded in maternal care, and subsequently the first task of the infant's ego, is the firm establishment of stable trust patterns in resolving the conflict of trust versus mistrust. Erikson presented the first demonstration of trust exhibited by the infant as including "the ease of his feeding, the depth of his sleep, the relaxation of his bowels" (1950, p. 219). In this way, the quality of the maternal relationship was thought to lead to the development of infant trust of others and self.

Dependency

Attachment has been confused with some type of dependency most likely owing to the fact that infants are dependent upon their caregivers for meeting the majority of their needs and because attachments are contingent upon the emotional availability of such caregivers. Dependency originated from social learning theories. Infant dependency is generally viewed as a type of learned behavior linked to the nurturant mother, whereby the nurturance is specific neither to providing food nor to reducing tension or drives. The salient notion underlying infant dependency on the mother is the reinforcing stimulus associated with her (Gewirtz, 1956). Gewirtz emphasizes the influence of environmental factors and the strength of different stimulus events in affecting the infant's behavior. He classifies attachment as a specific form of dependency involving a functional relationship and positive stimulus control provided by a particular person (Gewirtz, 1969, 1972a, 1972b). Viewing attachment from a social learning theory of dependency, attachment becomes a trait construct having representative behaviors of the attachment trait which are intercorrelated because of their common link to reinforcing stimuli.

Bonding

Because the terms attachment and bonding have been used interchangeably at times in the literature, attachment may become easily confused with bonding. Bonding originated from behavioral research completed on sheep and goats in investigations of a sensitive period for the establishment of a tie between a mother and her offspring. On the basis of both animal and human studies, bonding has become known as "a long-lasting, affectionate attachment of a *mother toward her infant* as the result of the mother's skin-to-skin contact with her newborn during a hormonally determined sensitive period lasting for a few hours after birth" (Campos et al., 1983, p. 875).

More parsimoniously defined as early and extended maternal contact, the mother-to-infant direction of the bonding concept has been traditionally associated with the work of Klaus and Kennell (1976). However, Klaus and Kennell (1982) have since extended bonding to include fathers, and more recently consolidated bonding with infant-to-parent affectual ties.

Why an Organizational View of Attachment?

Based on its capability for predicting future social competencies, an organizational view of attachment is the most robust way to conceptualize attachment. Unlike other approaches, the organizational view seems to directly support the infant's mastery of the inanimate and social world. Research has demonstrated that an organizational conceptualization of the security of attachment significantly relates to increased social competence in terms of enthusiasm, persistence, cooperation, and overall effectiveness at two years (Matas et al., 1978). Equally impressive are the findings of greater ego resilience and curiosity at four to five years (Arend et al., 1979), decreased incidence of conflict behavior with caregivers at 12 months (Main and Weston, 1981), increased capacity to cope with separation from caregivers at 18 months (Jacobson and Wille, 1984), and enhanced peer interaction at age three years (Jacobson and Wille, 1986) as based on an organizational view of infant-caregiver attachment.

The study of attachment is important to nursing. According to Donaldson and Crowley (1977), there are several domains to be investigated in the development of nursing knowledge of attachment, one of which concerns the pattern of human behavior in interaction with the environment. Attachment can be conceptualized within this domain of knowledge development for nursing because of the patterned quality inherent in an organizational view of attachment. Further, the fact that infant security of attachment has been found to significantly influence later functioning and well-being (Sroufe, 1979a) reinforces the need for attachment to be addressed in nursing research, education, and practice.

Phases of Attachment

The process of becoming attached occupies a large part of a young child's life, during which at least three phases of the development of attachment may be distinguished. According to Ainsworth (1973), these include a phase during which social responsiveness is relatively undiscriminating; a phase of discriminating social responsiveness; and a phase marked by the emergence of active initiative in proximity-seeking, contact-seeking, and contact-maintaining behaviors.

The phase of undiscriminating social responsiveness spans roughly the first two or three months of life, during which time the infant is capable of orienting himself to salient features of his environment. Orienting behaviors include such things as visual fixation, visual tracking, and listening. Other special signaling behaviors, including smiling, crying, and vocalization, tend to elicit caregiver behavior or bring the caregiver into proximity or contact with the infant.

The transition between this phase and the subsequent phase of discriminating social responsiveness is not distinct. Discrimination between persons may be learned more rapidly and more accurately through some sense modalities than through others.

During the phase of discriminating social responsiveness, the infant continues to orient and signal but clearly discriminates between familiar figures and those who are relatively unfamiliar, responding differently to each. According to Ainsworth (1973), differential smiling, vocalization, and crying emerge first, with differential greeting and crying upon separation from caregivers coming soon thereafter. This phase ends when more active proximity-seeking and contact-maintaining behaviors set in, possibly as early as six months of age.

During the phase of active initiative in seeking proximity and contact, there is a striking increase in the infant's initiative in promoting proximity and contact. This phase typically occurs around seven months, with locomotion facilitating proximity seeking and greeting responses becoming more active and effective. It is during this phase, which coincides with the emergence of object performance, that the infant is usually first described in terms of attachment.

The Strange Situation

For research purposes, Ainsworth and her colleagues (Ainsworth et al., 1978; Ainsworth and Wittig, 1969) devised a system of analysis for assessing the quality of security of the infant-caregiver attachment relationship. Known as the Strange Situation, the structured set of observational episodes involves two brief separations and reunions between the infant (12 to 24 months) and caregiver in a laboratory setting. Attachment classifications with the mother as caregiver have been found to be stable when tested at 12 and 18 months of age (Waters, 1978).

Specifically, Ainsworth's Strange Situation consists of eight episodes, each (except the first in which the infant and caregiver are introduced to the study room for 30 seconds) three minutes in duration and organized so that the infant experiences mildly stressful situations (new room; unfamiliar adult; separation from the caregiver but in the presence of the unfamiliar adult; reunion with the caregiver; separation; return of the unfamiliar adult, and second reunion with the caregiver). Separation episodes are stopped if distress on separation lasts 30 seconds.

Primarily on the basis of proximity-seeking, avoidant, or angry-resistant responses to reunion with the caregiver, infant attachment is classified as (1) secure, (2) avoidant-insecure, or (3) resistant-insecure. A description of these attachment classifications follows.

Infants who are classified as securely attached to their mothers want either proximity and contact or interaction with their mothers, and they actively seek it, especially in the reunion episodes of the procedure. If they achieve contact, they seek to maintain it, and either resist release or protest if put down. These infants respond to the mother's return in the reunion episodes with more than casual greetings—either with a smile or a cry or a tendency to approach. There is little or no tendency to resist contact or interaction with the mother. These infants may or may not be distressed during the separation episodes, but if they are distressed, this is clearly related to the mother's absence and not merely to being alone.

Infants who are classified as avoidant-insecure conspicuously avoid proximity to or interaction with their mothers in the reunion episodes. Either the infants ignore the mother on her return, greeting her casually, if at all, or if there is approach or a less casual greeting, these infants tend to intersperse welcoming with avoidance responses—e.g., turning away, moving past, or averting gaze. There is little or no tendency to seek proximity, contact, or interact with the mother, even in the reunion episodes. If picked up, these infants display little or no tendency to cling and do not resist being released. Either the infants are not distressed

during separation or the distress seems to be a result of being left alone rather than a reaction to the mother's absence.

Infants who are classified as resistant-insecure display conspicuous contact-resisting and interaction-resisting behaviors, especially in the final reunion with the caregiver. They also show moderate to strong seeking of proximity and contact, giving the impression of being ambivalent to the mother. They show little or no tendency to ignore the mother in the reunion episodes, to turn or move away from her, or to avert their gaze. Generally, these infants tend to be more angry than infants in other attachment classifications, or they may be conspicuously passive.

Behavioral Precursors of Attachment

Precise clinical indicators suggesting the need for intervention in generating security or adaptiveness in infant attachment are not known. This predicament stems from the long-standing problem that specific behavioral manifestations of the developmental phases embedded in attachment have not been identified. Aside from waiting until the infant is 12 months old and can be evaluated for the presence of a security-of-attachment behavior pattern using a research tool (Ainsworth et al. [1978], Strange Situation attachment paradigm), the health professional must depend on speculations about the need for interventions aimed at promoting attachment security.

Since there are no clear-cut antecedents indicative of the ongoing development of secure infant attachment (namely, cause and effect), the health professional must resort to assessing the essential elements organized within an attachment relationship. These include the primary caregiver's behavior relevant to the infant's needs, and the infant's behavior, including the interactional reciprocity between infant and caregiver.

ASSESSMENT

In this section, several nursing diagnoses are identified which might assist in the assessment process. These include an alteration in parenting, infant anxiety, infant fear, and social isolation. However, the nurse should be aware of the difficulties involved in solely relying on these nursing diagnoses in evaluating the ongoing development of attachment. According to Sroufe and Waters (1977), a generally secure or insecure attachment cannot be inferred from *any particular behavior* but must be inferred from *the pattern of behavior,* with regard to context, across time. Behavior occurring in one context might be less predictive of future occurrences of that behavior in the same situation than it is of an alternate behavior in a different context. For example, the infant seeking proximity to the caregiver when distressed might more accurately predict a happy greeting by the infant upon being reunited with the caregiver after a separation rather than the infant again seeking proximity in the same situational context.

Caregiver Behavior

Some types of and qualities inherent in caregiver behavior are thought to propagate the development of infant attachment. The prediction that the security or adaptiveness of the infant's attachment to the caregiver is dependent on the caregiver's sensitivity to the infant's signals has preliminary substantiation from several studies (Ainsworth et al., 1971, 1972, 1974; Belsky et al., 1984; Grossmann et al., 1985; Maslin, 1983). According to Ainsworth et al. (1978), caregivers who are consistently more affectionate, who more frequently engage in physical contact, who are very effective in soothing their infants, who greet their infants more positively, who engage in face-to-face interaction more often, and who are generally less intrusive and better able to assess the infant's needs are more likely to have securely attached infants.

One nursing diagnosis specifically pertinent to caregiver behavior is suggestive of the need for attachment-related interventions: *Parenting, alteration in: actual or potential* (Kim et al., 1984). In this nursing diagnosis, parenting is defined as the ability of a caregiver to provide an environment that promotes the optimum growth and development of another human. Use of the defining characteristics of this diagnosis (e.g., parental verbalization of role inadequacy; lack of appropriate visual, tactile, and auditory stimulation; negative identification of characteristics of infant) might provide

data indicating actual or potential insecurity of attachment in the infant. The polar opposites of such defining characteristics, as pointed out later by Craft (see Chapter 3), might be subsequently used as general criteria for the measurement of intervention outcomes.

Difficulty arises in exclusively relying on the caregiver's behavior in diagnosing actual or potential insecurity in infant attachment. What is lacking in the caregiver might be compensated for by the infant during interactions. For example, the infant may be thriving well in terms of growth and development and appear very healthy despite inadequacies verbalized by a caregiver or demonstrated by a caregiver's parenting behaviors. Therefore, maladaptive caregiving behavior may or may not be reflected in an attachment disturbance in the infant.

Infant Behavior and Interactional Reciprocity

The prediction that security of attachment is dependent on the infant's behavior has mixed support. In 1980, Waters et al. found a positive relationship between two aspects of neonatal behavior (decreased motor maturity and less ability to regulate state) as measured by the 1973 version of the Brazelton Neonatal Behavioral Assessment Scale (BNBAS) (Brazelton, 1973) and increased resistant-insecure attachment in a group of infants from low-income families. Similarly, using a group of Japanese infants, Miyake et al. (1985) found one aspect of neonatal behavior gathered from observations that seemed to contribute to insecure or maladaptive attachment. In that study, those infants who cried more frequently during the newborn period were more likely to be resistant-insecure in their attachments in later infancy. Nonetheless, another study failed to find support for the security of attachment being dependent on infant behavior. In that investigation, when data concerning the securely attached or avoidant—insecurely attached infants were examined, no significant associations were detected between neonatal behavior on the BNBAS or nurses' ratings of neonatal behavior (Egeland and Farber, 1984; Waters et al., 1980). These discrepancies in the relationship of infant behavior and attachment might be accounted for partially by imperfections in the process of sorting out pure infant effects from the confounding effects embedded in infant behavior in response to caregiving behavior.

Three nursing diagnoses pertaining to infant behavior suggest the need for attachment-related interventions. These diagnoses are (1) *anxiety*; (2) *fear*; and (3) *social isolation* (Kim et al., 1984). Anxiety is a vaguely uneasy feeling, the source of which may be nonspecific to the individual. Examples of defining characteristics include apprehension, increased helplessness, and uncertainty. Fear is a feeling of dread related to an identifiable, self-validated source. Examples of defining characteristics include increased tension, decreased self-assurance, and fright. Social isolation is a condition of aloneness experienced by a person. Social isolation is perceived by the person experiencing it as imposed by others and as a negative or threatening state. Examples of defining characteristics include a sad, dull affect; uncommunicative or withdrawn appearance; and hostility in voice or behavior.

Once again, use of the defining characteristics might provide data indicating actual or potential insecurity of attachment in the infant (see previous discussion on the difficulties involved in using these diagnoses as sole determinants). However, in addition, the foregoing defining characteristics stated by Kim et al. as descriptions of experiences underlying the nursing diagnoses of anxiety, fear, and social isolation are not ones commonly used with respect to infants as such. There is a need for the generation and validation of appropriate defining characteristics for assessing the presence or absence of such relevant underlying experiences in preverbal infants.

Although social isolation is probably the closest representation of the three diagnoses that apply to individual infant insecurity of attachment behavior, none are consistent with an organizational understanding of attachment but, rather, represent a trait view. The chief concern with relying heavily on these nursing diagnoses in diagnosing insecurity of infant attachment is that they consider neither the situational context nor interactional reciprocity by the caregiver. Therefore, anxious, fearful, or socially isolating infant behavior patterns might or might not reflect an attachment disturbance in the infant.

The development of a nursing diagnosis which addresses infant attachment using an organizational view of felt security operating in conjunction with a set of attachment behaviors is needed to more accurately depict an infant's progression through Ainsworth's (1973) phases of becoming attached over time.

To summarize, because of a gap in the literature deriving a clinically valid attachment assessment strategy based upon the Strange Situation attachment research evaluation, at this time it is next to impossible to identify a way of predetermining which infants will actually be in need of external attachment support. But because attachment is thought to have a profound impact on infant emotional well-being (Sroufe, 1979b), it seems that the ongoing development of attachment will continue to be an appropriate area for prevention assessment and intervention.

THE INTERVENTION

As conceptualized by Bowlby (1982), attachment is not intended to be synonymous with "social bond." Likewise, attachment cannot be used in reference to describing types of play ("attachment") interactions (e.g., Censullo et al., 1985) or parental bonding (Tulman, 1985), even though such components serve important roles in infant-caregiver relationships (Bretherton, 1980). This last term, "bonding," has been confused with the term "attachment" by nurses, especially as it pertains to maternal interventions thought to directly correspond to attachment interventions. An attachment intervention program implemented by nurses which used parental bonding instead of infant attachment as an outcome measure is one example (see Schraeder, 1980). Once again, some of this confusion about attachment intervention probably stems from the interchangeable use of the terms bonding and attachment (Klaus and Kennell, 1976, 1982, 1983).

Presently, the designation of early intervention strategies focused on the infant's development of a control system that organizes attachment behavior consistently across time and across situations is only a hypothetical designation. Researchers are continuing to work on generating answers to questions posed about ways to foster secure attachment. According to Ainsworth et al. (1978, p. 152):

The most important aspect of maternal behavior commonly associated with the security–insecurity dimension of infant attachment is manifested in different specific ways in different situations, but in each it emerges as sensitive responsiveness to infant signals and communications.

Caregiver Sensitivity

Although it is difficult, if not impossible, to identify precisely the "why, what, where, how, and when" of interventions needed to facilitate infant attachment, based on an organizational view of attachment, nurses should probably begin by assessing and enhancing caregiver sensitivity to infants. The notion of "caregiver sensitivity" has been divided into three somewhat overlapping parts: (1) emotional availability (Ainsworth, 1973; Bretherton, 1985; Sroufe and Waters, 1977); (2) sensitive responses and stimulation; and (3) consistency over time (Ainsworth et al., 1978; Belsky et al., 1984; Bretherton, 1985). Although inextricably intertwined, caregiver sensitivity was separated into several constituent parts in order to more closely examine ways to integrate it in the ongoing development of infant attachment.

Enhancing Emotional Availability

Emotional availability of the caregiver refers to a relaxed and warm display of affection which is readily accessible to the infant. It includes an observable preferential treatment that might typically be exhibited while providing the infant with pleasant experiences during physical contact (Ainsworth et al., 1978; Bretherton, 1985; Sroufe and Waters, 1977). Emotional availability demands sincere and vested interest in the caregiving role and its related activities and open expression of that interest, by one means or another, to the infant. The warmth depicted in emotional availability implies an acceptance of intermittent infant attachment behavior (see earlier discussion of attachment behavior for examples) that might lead the infant to the caregiver (Ainsworth et al., 1978).

Emotional availability of the caregiver may be expanded by social support. Social support can be defined as affective and material assistance in the caregiving role, relative to the stresses experienced by the caregiver. According to Crockenberg (1981), because social support has been shown to have a strong effect on irritable infants and their mothers, social support might prove particularly critical when a family is under unusual or severe stress. For example, mobilizing social support from the infant's father, older children in the family, neighbors, friends, professionals, or a respite care service might have a significant impact if it is used in a situation where there are many stresses. Studies have not been done demonstrating the effectiveness of social support in facilitating attachment in families where mild or few stresses exist.

Sensitive Responses and Stimulation

The sensitive responses and stimulation of the caregiver are characterized by a tender, cooperative, flexible, yet contingent manner of acting in meeting infant needs (Bell and Ainsworth, 1972). Such sensitivity in responding requires that the caregiver be capable of perceiving infant experiences from an infant's point of view; viewing the infant as a distinct and separate individual; respecting activity-in-progress and, therefore, avoiding interrupting such activities especially exploratory play; and regarding infant communications and signals to be relevant guidelines for initiating caregiver behavior (Ainsworth et al., 1978). The nature of sensitive responding and stimulation suggests moderation, rather than overresponding or understimulating (Belsky et al., 1984). Sensitive caregivers cue their infants using some sense-related form (e.g., auditory, visual, tactile) before picking them up to prepare them for interaction. Caregiver sensitivity implies that infants are handled carefully and affectionately.

Findings pertaining to sensitive responsiveness of caregivers inherently suggest a number of ways caregivers might demonstrate sensitivity with their infants. Mothers who are more responsive to their infants' cries, who hold their infants more carefully, who pace their behavior with their infants' behavior contingently during face-to-face interaction, and who demonstrate gentler initiation and termination of feedings tend to have more securely attached infants (Ainsworth et al., 1978).

With regard to sensitive stimulation, Censullo et al. (1985) have shown that during mother-infant play of Caucasian dyads, mutual turn-taking cycles are normally present. Examples of caregiver-infant games which can elicit temporal patterning in social behavior are "I'm gonna getcha," "rock-a-bye-baby," "pat-a-cake," and "peek-a-boo." Such playful interactions require that the caregiver elicit the infant's attention; then, as the games change in tempo, mutual attention time is extended and the presence of positive affect is intensified. To summarize, Belsky et al. (1984) contend that sensitive care by caregivers that involves neither too much nor too little interactive stimulation promotes secure attachment of infants.

Consistency Over Time

Consistency is defined as nonfragmented caregiver behavior, predictable to the infant in interlocking his behavior with the ongoing behavior of the caregiver across various situations and over time. It suggests a set of repetitive behaviors from the caregiver that come to be socially expected by the infant (Belsky et al., 1984). A prototypical behavior representative of consistency over time is the caregiver's systematic acknowledgement of the infant upon returning from an absence from the infant.

In a study on infant crying and maternal responsiveness, Bell and Ainsworth (1972) discovered that by the end of the first year, the history of mothers' responses to infant crying reflected differences in the decline and duration of infant crying. Consistent, prompt maternal response was the most effective intervention over time in terminating infant crying. These findings were particularly enlightening in dispelling the myth that routine, quick responding to an infant's cries "spoils" a child.

Intervention Modifiers

Because so little is known generally about interventions that might facilitate attachment, it ought not be surprising that inter-

vention modification in relation to individual differences in infants, changing life circumstances, and sociocultural factors has not been addressed. Instead, what has been examined are the stability of certain individual infant factors as they relate to attachment and the stability of the nature of infant attachment patterns.

Temperamental differences in and of themselves do not appear to significantly contribute to the quality of an attachment relationship as evaluated using the Strange Situation procedure. Belsky et al. (1984) found no correlations between maternal ratings of infant temperament at three and nine months and security of attachment at 12 months. Similarly, Egeland and Farber (1984) detected no correlations between behavioral observation-generated temperament measures at three months, Carey temperament scores at six months, and security of attachment at 12 months.

Changing life circumstances have been found to have varied effects on attachment. Vaughn et al. (1979) found that family stress during the time between 12 and 18 months was associated with changes from secure to insecure attachment. Thompson et al. (1982) found that life stresses were associated with reorganizations to both secure and insecure attachments.

In conclusion, from past research studies, one can infer that interventions directed at facilitating infant attachment should be centered around developing the sensitivity of the primary caregiver to the infant's needs. The literature is unclear about how the role of a secondary caregiver, or a co-primary caregiver (e.g., father), relates to the infant's development of attachment to the primary caregiver. The primary caregiver seems to have the greatest impact on organizing the emerging attachment relationship of the infant to assure maximum attachment security attainment.

EVALUATION

Since no outcome measures have been developed at the present time, the polar opposites of the defining characteristics might be used as a guide to the development of such measurement criteria. However, changes in responses have clinical merit for evaluation as demonstrated in the following discussion.

Case Study

Six month old Julia was the first child born to John and Mary S. Although unplanned, Julia was very much wanted by both parents. Julia's father and mother were in their mid-twenties and had been happily married for three years. They were college-educated and financially secure. John was the vice president of a small construction company, and since Julia's birth, Mary had remained at home to care for her. John and Mary had a large supportive network of family and friends. However, all of them lived a great distance away.

Since discharge from the hospital on the fourth postnatal day, Julia had become moderately fussy and very active. Over the next six months she continued to require much rocking, jiggling, walking, and general handling to console. As an only child, Mary had received very little experience caring for infants, especially fussy infants. She frequently telephoned her mother to seek additional advice on ways to quiet Julia. Unfortunately, all the different methods Mary's mother suggested seemed to exacerbate and perpetuate Julia's bouts of fussiness. On taking Julia into the clinic for her six month immunizations, Mary confided to the nurse, Susan, that Julia had a tendency to fuss off and on all day long. The nurse made arrangements to make several home visits to get a clearer picture of Julia's pattern of behavior for herself.

The next morning, Susan went to Mary's home to assess Julia's fussiness. When she arrived, Julia was quietly swinging in her infant swing in one corner of the living room with a pacifier in her mouth. When Susan sat down on the couch, however, Julia looked over at Susan and stopped sucking for a minute or so. Mary seemed relieved to have some adult company, happily reporting to Susan about how she was teaching Julia to sit unassisted. When Julia began fussing, Mary told the nurse how tired she was of picking Julia up and holding her just to keep her from fussing. After Julia's fussing had noticeably intensified, Mary picked her up and consoled her. When she had only just quieted, Mary immediately returned Julia to her swing. Within what seemed like a very brief time, Julia once again began to fuss. This time Susan picked her up, consoled her by talking to her, then let her play with her keys on the couch next to her. Mary was surprised at how content Julia seemed to be playing on the couch next to Susan, a stranger she had met once or twice before at the clinic.

Susan continued to sit on the couch with Julia and listen while Mary detailed her many feelings of isolation since Julia's birth. Before having Julia, Mary had worked as the assistant office manager of a large hotel. She was used to being surrounded by adults, frequently going out to business luncheons and planning for and making daily large-scale decisions about hotel operations. She felt guilty about dearly missing her friends' company at work. Further, since marrying John, she was at the opposite end of the country from her family. She had no friends in the neighborhood because she had invested so much of her free time socializing with her co-workers at the hotel. She knew some women from her church who had offered to baby-sit for Julia, but quite frankly, Mary was embarrassed to even consider leaving a fussy baby like Julia with a baby sitter. The temptation was great, she admitted, to leave Julia with a sitter or at a day-care center and return to work. She emphasized to Susan how much she loved Julia and caring for her but didn't think she was doing a very good job with managing her fussiness. She usually allowed Julia to swing by herself most of the day because it was about the only thing that she could come up with that seemed to contain Julia's irritability.

While Mary talked, Julia remained quiet and content playing with the keys on the couch next to Susan and in close proximity to Mary. Julia was obviously very healthy and well cared for, and occasionally smiled or turned her head responsively when Mary looked over at her or spoke.

Susan acknowledged that Julia did seem to be a relatively fussy baby. Further, it would be difficult for Mary to have to contend with Julia's fussiness all of the time. She told Mary that she'd like to have additional opportunities for home visits a few days later and again the following week.

Both Julia and Mary acted much the same in subsequent home visits. When Julia began to fuss in the infant swing, Mary would wait until Julia was noticeably irritable before consoling her. Mary would hold Julia a short while until she quieted and then return her to the infant swing. Soon Julia would begin to fuss again and Mary would repeat her activities. Mary continued to verbalize her feelings of loneliness and desire for adult conversation and interaction.

From a pediatric nurse's point of view, Susan's assessment of the situation was that Mary had socially isolated herself since becoming a mother and that Julia was at an increased risk for developing an insecure attachment to Mary because of Mary's lack of understanding about Julia's socioemotional needs. Susan believed that if she could provide Mary with some acceptable adult social opportunities, Mary might be able to "free up" some energy and be more sensitive in responding to Julia's fussiness. Moreover, if Susan could support Mary's sensitive responsiveness to Julia's needs, Julia might feel more secure with Mary and be more likely to develop a secure attachment to her.

On a fourth visit to Mary's home, Susan told

Mary about her assessment and goals for Mary and Julia. She stated that maybe what Julia and Mary both needed were some outside activities. She suggested that Mary begin by taking advantage of one of the women's offers at church to baby-sit Julia and then meet her old friends at the hotel for lunch or dinner. In addition, Susan recommended the Mom and Tots Exercise and Activities program, held three times weekly at a nearby community center, so that Mary could become acquainted with some of her child-rearing neighbors. She thought the swim and play activities might give Julia a change of scenery and provide Mary with some new ideas for entertaining Julia at home. Further, Susan recommended that Mary try keeping Julia in closer proximity to her and responding immediately to Julia's fussiness rather than waiting until it became pronounced. Mary seemed pleased with Susan's suggestions and stated that she was ready to try anything to help Julia develop a happier disposition.

Three weeks later, Susan telephoned Mary to get an update on Julia. Mary reported that she had tried several different baby sitters at her church before getting one who seemed to "click" with Julia. But after finding this baby sitter, she was relieved to have some time away from Julia to socialize with her hotel friends. At first she had thought she might like to return to work and leave Julia with the baby sitter. However, it wasn't long before she decided that neither she nor Julia were ready for that yet. Mary went on to say that the Mom and Tots program had been a great idea. There she had learned all kinds of things about Julia's development and what she might anticipate at various times. The activities and new people at the program were stimulating and the other mothers there seemed to understand what it was like caring for a fussy baby. Mary stated that Julia had become a little less fussy since she started keeping her in her infant swing in closer proximity to Mary. Mary also commented that Julia was getting easier to console and that she was beginning to feel better about her handling of Julia. In fact, Mary reported that she told one of her hotel friends how rewarded she felt to be successful in soothing a baby who fusses persistently.

In her evaluation of the relationship between Julia and Mary, Susan made documentations regarding Julia's decreased fussiness in association with mother proximity. She also noted Mary's vested interest in the caregiving role and implicit expression of that interest to Julia by keeping her at her side even when Julia was fussy. Over the past several weeks, Susan believed Mary had decreased her feelings of loneliness and isolation and, as a result, had been able to increase her emotional availability to Julia. Susan concluded that it was highly likely that Julia would develop a feeling of secureness in her attachment to Mary.

RESEARCH IMPLICATIONS

According to Ellis (1982), the foremost goal of nursing as a discipline is to develop a body of knowledge and become a community of scholars. As a practice profession, the goal of nursing is to base its practice upon nursing knowledge. In order for nursing to develop an adequate body of knowledge for guiding practice, nursing must demonstrate accountability to both basic and applied research in clinical as well as laboratory settings. It is important that research and practice be understood to ensure excellence in nursing productivity, in addition to providing a foundation for the following recommendations.

Though attachment has been discussed and investigated for some time (cf. Bretherton and Waters, 1985), there are many basic dimensions within as well as associated with the construct that remain virtually unexplored. An explanation of the epigenetic sequence of attachment development, for example, has yet to be well grounded in scientific findings. Taking the process of attachment development back to its origins, how can the ontogeny of attachment be assessed? Does the timing of such onset in any way make a significant difference in the nature of the relationships that evolve?

In addition to the need to investigate new questions and describe areas related to attachment, there is also a basic need for more versatile instrumentation for attachment studies. Given that the Strange Situation is valid only as a research instrument between 12 and 18 months, evaluative means other than Ainsworth's Strange Situation procedure must be used if one intends to investigate attachment, or the precursors thereof, at other times during infancy. Tools designed to measure attachment across developmental shifts that are simultaneously valid in various contexts must be developed. Moreover, some type of simplified version which could be readily applied and evaluated within a clinical, nonlaboratory setting is urgently needed for practitioners. Such a tool could be potentially useful in providing a basis for interventions by practitioners with infants who have insecure attachments with their caregivers. Subsequently, if these investigations and tool development proceed, researchers will be better able to analyze both the constancy and change of attachment as it extends longitudinally throughout infancy, while practitioners will be able to take advantage of attachment screening tools as a normal part of assessing and addressing issues pertinent to infant well-being.

Nurses whose primary population of concern is infants must make research commitments to their clients to give greater consideration to attachment. Nurses might examine the relationships of (1) emotional availability of caregivers to infants; (2) frequencies and durations of sensitive responses to and stimulation of infants by caregivers; and (3) consistency of sensitive caregiver responses to infants across time, respectively, to security of attachment ratings of infants at 12 and 18 months using the Strange Situation tool. The investigations mentioned may lead to the identification and testing of variables amenable to change that significantly strengthen the stability of security and promote some type of desired lability of attachment across infancy.

References

Ainsworth, MDS. Object relations, dependency and attachment: A theoretical review of the infant-mother relationship. Child Development, 40:969–1025, 1969.

Ainsworth, MDS. Attachment and dependency: A comparison. In Gewirtz, JL (Ed.), Attachment and dependency. Washington, DC: Winston, 1972, pp. 97–137.

Ainsworth, MDS. The development of infant-mother attachment. In Caldwell, BM, and Ricciuti, H (Eds.), Review of child development research (Vol. 3). Chicago: The University of Chicago Press, 1973, pp. 1–94.

Ainsworth, MDS, Bell, SM, and Stayton, DJ. Individual differences in strange situation behavior of one-year-olds. In Schaffer, HR (Ed.), The origins of human social relations. New York: Academic Press, Inc., 1971, pp. 17–57.

Ainsworth, MDS, Bell, SM, and Stayton, DJ. Individual differences in the development of some attachment behaviors. Merrill-Palmer Quarterly, 18:123–143, 1972.

Ainsworth, MDS, Bell, SM, and Stayton, DJ. Infant-mother attachment and social development: "Socialization" as a product of reciprocal responsiveness to signals. In Richards, MP (Ed.), The integration of the child into a social world. London: Cambridge University Press, 1974, pp. 99–135.

Ainsworth, MDS, Blehar, MC, Waters, E, and Wall, S. Patterns of attachment: A psychological study of the Strange Situation. Hillsdale, N. J.: Lawrence Erlbaum Associates, Inc., 1978.

Ainsworth, MDS, and Wittig, B. Attachment and exploratory behavior of one-year-olds in a strange situation. In Foss, B (Ed.), Determinants of infant behav-

ior (Vol. 4). New York: Barnes and Noble Books, 1969, pp. 111–136.

Arend, R, Gove, FL, and Sroufe, LA. Continuity of individual adaptation from infancy to kindergarten: A predictive study of ego-resiliency and curiosity in preschoolers. Child Development, 50:950–959, 1979.

Avant, K. Nursing diagnosis: Maternal attachment. Advances in Nursing Science, 2:45–55, 1979.

Bell, SM, & Ainsworth, MDS. Infant crying and maternal responsiveness. Child Development, 43:1171–1190, 1972.

Belsky, J, Rovine, M, and Taylor, DG. The Pennsylvania Infant and Family Development Project, 3: The origins of individual differences in infant-mother attachment: Maternal and infant contributions. Child Development, 55:718–728, 1984.

Bowlby, J. The nature of the child's tie to his mother. International Journal of Psychoanalysis, 39:350–373, 1958.

Bowlby, J. Attachment and loss (Vol. 1). Attachment. New York: Basic Books, Inc, 1969.

Bowlby, J. By ethology out of psycho-analysis: An experiment in interbreeding. Animal Behaviour, 28:649–656, 1980.

Bowlby, J. Attachment and loss (Vol. 1). Attachment (2nd ed.). New York: Basic Books, Inc., 1982.

Brazelton, TB. Neonatal behavioral assessment scale (Clinics in Developmental Medicine, No. 88). Philadelphia: JB Lippincott Co., 1973.

Bretherton, I. Young children in stressful situations: The supporting role of attachment figures and unfamiliar caregivers. In Coelho, CV, and Ahmed, P (Eds.), Uprooting and development. New York: Plenum Publishing Corp., 1980, pp. 179–210.

Bretherton, I. Attachment theory: Retrospect and prospect. In Bretherton, I, and Waters, E (Eds.), Growing points of attachment theory and research. Monographs of the Society for Research in Child Development, 50 (1–2, Serial No. 209), 1985.

Bretherton, I, and Waters, E (Eds.). Growing points of attachment theory and research. Monographs of the Society for Research in Child Development, 50 (1–2, Serial No. 209), 1985.

Campos, JJ, Barrett, KC, Lamb, ME, Goldsmith, HH, and Stenberg, C. Socioemotional development. In Haith, MM, and Campos, JJ (Vol. Eds.), Handbook of child psychology (4th ed., Vol. 2). New York: John Wiley and Sons, Inc., 1983, pp. 783–915.

Censullo, M, Lester, B, and Hoffman, J. Rhythmic patterning in mother-newborn interaction. Nursing Research, 34:342–346, 1985.

Clark, AC, and Affonso, DD. Infant behavior and maternal attachment: Two sides to the coin. Maternal-Child Nursing Journal, 1:94–99, 1976.

Coates, B, Anderson, EP, and Hartup, WW. Interrelations in the attachment behavior of human infants. Developmental Psychology, 6:218–230, 1972a.

Coates, B, Anderson, EP, and Hartup, WW. The stability of attachment behaviors in the human infant. Developmental Psychology, 6:231–237, 1972b.

Cranley, MS. Development of a tool for the measurement of maternal attachment during pregnancy. Nursing Research, 30:281–284, 1981.

Crockenberg, SB. Infant irritability, mother responsiveness, and social support influences on the security of infant-mother attachment. Child Development, 52:857–865, 1981.

Cronbach, L, and Meehl, P. Construct validity in psychological tests. Psychological Bulletin, 52:281–302, 1955.

Donaldson, SK, and Crowley, DM. Discipline of nursing: Structure and relationship to practice. Communicating Nursing Research, 10:1–22, 1977.

Egeland, B, and Farber, EA. Infant-mother attachment: Factors related to its development and changes over time. Child Development, 55:753–771, 1984.

Ellis, R. Personal communication, May 26, 1982.

Erikson, EH. Childhood and society. New York: WW Norton and Co., Inc., 1950, pp. 219–234.

Freud, S. On narcissism: An introduction (Vol. 14). London: Hogarth, 1957, pp. 73–102. (Originally published, 1914.)

Freud, S. Female sexuality (Vol. 21). London: Hogarth, 1961, pp. 225–243. (Originally published, 1931.)

Gewirtz, JL. A program of research on the dimensions and antecedents of emotional dependence. Child Development, 27:205–221, 1956.

Gewirtz, JL. Mechanisms of social learning: Some roles of stimulation and behavior in early human development. In Goslin, DA (Ed.), Handbook of socialization theory and research. Chicago: Rand McNally and Co., 1969, pp. 57–212.

Gewirtz, JL. Attachment, dependence, and a distinction in terms of stimulus control. In Gewirtz, JL (Ed.), Attachment and dependency. Washington, DC: Winston, 1972a, pp. 139–177.

Gewirtz, JL. On the selection and use of attachment and dependence indices. In Gewirtz, JL (Ed.), Attachment and dependency. Washington, DC: Winston, 1972b, pp. 179–215.

Grossmann, K, Grossmann, KE, Spangler, G, Suess, G, and Unzner, L. Maternal sensitivity and newborns' orientation responses as related to quality of attachment in Northern Germany. In Bretherton, I, and Waters, E (Eds.), Growing points of attachment theory and research. Monographs of the Society for Research in Child Development, 50 (1–2, Serial No. 209), 1985.

Hoyer, PJ, and Jacobson, JL. The assessment of attachment in a naturally occurring strange situation. Poster presented at the Society for Research in Child Development Meeting, Toronto, 1985.

Jacobson, JL, and Wille, D. Influence of attachment and separation experience on separation distress at 18 months. Child Development, 20:477–484, 1984.

Jacobson, JL, and Wille, D. The influence of attachment pattern on developmental changes in peer interaction from the toddler to the preschool period. Child Development, 57:338–347, 1986.

Kim, MJ, McFarland, GK, and McLane, AM (Eds.). Classification of nursing diagnoses: Proceedings of the fifth national conference. St. Louis: CV Mosby Co., 1984.

Klaus, MH, and Kennell, JH. Maternal-infant bonding. St. Louis: CV Mosby Co., 1976.

Klaus, MH, and Kennell, JH. Parent-infant bonding. St. Louis: CV Mosby Co., 1982.

Klaus, MH, and Kennell, JH. Bonding: The beginnings of parent-infant attachment. St. Louis: CV Mosby Co., 1983.

Maccoby, E, and Feldman, SS. Mother-attachment and stranger reactions in the third year of life. Monographs of the Society for Research in Child Development, 37 (1, Serial No. 146), 1972.

Main, M., and Weston, DR. The quality of the toddler's relationship to mother and father: Related to conflict behavior and the readiness to establish new relationships. Child Development, 52:932–940, 1981.

Maslin, CA. Anxious and secure attachments: Antecedents and consequences in the mother-infant system. Unpublished doctoral dissertation, Indiana University, Bloomington, Ind., 1983.

Matas, L, Arend, RA, and Sroufe, LA. Continuity of adaptation in the second year: The relationship between quality of attachment and later competence. Child Development, 49:547–556, 1978.

Miyake, K, Chen, SJ, and Campos, JJ. Infant temperament, mother's mode of interaction, and attachment in Japan: An interim report. In Bretherton, I, and Waters, E (Eds.), Growing points of attachment theory and research. Monographs of the Society for Research in Child Development, 50 (1–2, Serial No. 209), 1985.

Peterson, GH, and Hehl, LE. Some determinants of maternal attachment. American Journal of Psychiatry, 135:1168–1173, 1978.

Reisner, SL. A tool to facilitate mother-infant attachment. Journal of Obstetrical and Gynecological Nursing, 10:294–297, 1981.

Rubin, R. Attainment of the maternal role, part 1: Processes. Nursing Research, 16:237–245, 1967a.

Rubin, R. Attainment of the maternal role, part 2: Models and referents. Nursing Research, 16:342–346, 1967b.

Schraeder, BD. Attachment and parenting despite lengthy intensive care. Maternal-Child Nursing Journal, 5:37–41, 1980.

Sroufe, LA. The coherence of individual development: Early care, attachment, and subsequent development. American Psychologist, 34:834–841, 1979a.

Sroufe, LA. Socioemotional development. In Osofsky, JD (Ed.), Handbook of infant development. New York: John Wiley and Sons, Inc., 1979b, pp. 462–516.

Sroufe, LA, and Waters, E. Attachment as an organizational construct. Child Development, 48:1184–1199, 1977.

Thompson, RA, Lamb, ME, and Estes, D. Stability of infant-mother attachment and its relationship to changing life circumstances in an unselected middle-class sample. Child Development, 53:144–148, 1982.

Tulman, LJ. Theories of maternal attachment. Advances in Nursing Science, 3(4):7–14, 1981.

Tulman, LJ. Mothers' and unrelated persons' initial handling of newborn infants. Nursing Research, 34:205–211, 1985.

Vaughn, B, Egeland, B, Sroufe, LA, and Waters, E. Individual differences in infant-mother attachment at twelve and eighteen months: Stability and change in families under stress. Child Development, 50:971–975, 1979.

Waters, E. The reliability and stability of individual differences in infant-mother attachment. Child Development, 49:483–494, 1978.

Waters, E, Vaughn, BE, and Egeland, BR. Individual differences in infant-mother attachment relationships at age one: Antecedents in neonatal behavior in an urban, economically disadvantaged sample. Child Development, 51:208–216, 1980.

CHAPTER 2

FACILITATING FATHERING

JULIE C. NOVAK, D.N.Sc., R.N., P.N.P.,
and ROBERT E. NOVAK, Ph.D.

HISTORICAL PERSPECTIVE

The role of the father in the home of the 1980's reflects the economics of the decade, with 70% of families functioning in a dual career model (U.S. Department of Commerce, Bureau of Census, 1985). The egalitarian approach to parenting, the increasing influence of single fathers and house husbands, a tentative societal awareness and acceptance of fathers in nurturing, and less autocratic roles are becoming realities (Giveans and Robinson, 1985). It is difficult to assess the effect of these changes on the family unit, however, without a historical perspective. In the early to middle 19th century, men and women shared responsibilities for nuclear and extended family eco-

nomic support and child rearing. Toward the end of the 19th century, with advances in economic productivity and higher incomes, more families in the United States consisted of full time housewife-mothers and full-time breadwinner-fathers. This new family constellation was "the beginning of the end of an active, involved, participating father" (Couchman, 1982, p. 11).

During the first half of this century, social scientists assumed that fathers were unimportant in child rearing when compared with mothers. The traditional American definition of fatherhood in the last half of the 20th century was molded by the social concepts and economic realities from the 1940's through the 1960's, giving the father the primary provider role for the family and allowing the mother to be free to devote herself to the care and raising of their children. The single aberration of the breadwinner stereotype was during World War II, when many women assumed traditional masculine occupations in civil and defense arenas, with their children being cared for in public child-care facilities. After World War II, mothers returned to the home while fathers entered the work force. The American father was mirrored by the television model male, home only to preside at family meals, bedtime, and weekend adventures (Giveans and Robinson, 1985).

The women's movement of the 1960's and 1970's, in combination with an economy which dictated the need for a two-salary household for many, has created a great change in the lives of many men. It was not until this time that significant research articles regarding fathers were published (Biller, 1968; Carlsmith, 1964). As recently as 1969, Pedersen and Robson collected data on father involvement from interviews with 45 mothers. In the 1970's, the father finally emerged as an object worthy of direct study, and in the past decade he has assumed an increasingly important place in social science research. It is important to note that the "typical" American family, including a father who is the wage earner and a mother who works inside the home, is now representative of fewer than 12% of American families (McLaughlin and Miller, 1986). These statistics and their implications are significant for nursing because of nursing's expanding focus on the health maintenance of the contemporary family.

Although it seems obvious that for the child, a nurturant, involved father plays a vital role in optimal development, factors promoting nurturant fathering behaviors have not been well documented. In the numerous settings in which nurses practice, they are in a position to examine the importance of the fathering role in health and illness. The purpose of this chapter is to identify developmental and interactive aspects of fathering and to propose intervention strategies which promote nurturant fathering behaviors during infancy.

THEORETICAL FOUNDATION

The early research on fathers was largely derived from studies of mothers and moth-

ering. Inferential leaps were commonly made about the effects of fathers on children from what was known about mothers. Early studies conducted by developmental psychologists focused on the married middle-class father with minimal emphasis on the diverse roles that fathers play in a complex modern society, cultural differences, and the nature of father-child relationships (Lamb and Bronson, 1980). A popular method of investigating father significance was to look at the effects of father absence (Biller, 1968; Carlsmith, 1964; Hoffman, 1971). There is still a paucity of literature concerning fathering beyond infancy.

Current literature supports the contention that fathers make unique contributions to the development of their children—beginning at birth—in areas of sex role identification, cognitive development, and general psychological and social adjustment (Marton et al., 1981). The amount and quality of social interaction an infant receives from the father are recognized as a critical factor in overall social, emotional, and physical development (Kunst-Wilson and Cronenwett, 1981). The father's progress in his own developmental trajectory has been largely ignored in the literature. Erikson (1959) has identified eight *stages* of human development hallmarked by the need to establish (1) trust in infancy, (2) autonomy as a toddler, (3) initiative as a preschooler, (4) industry as a school-aged child, (5) role identification as an adolescent, (6) intimacy as a young adult, (7) generativity in middle age, and (8) integrity in old age. Where a father is and has been in this developmental sequence may have a profound impact on his ability to enact the fathering role. Findings that older fathers in the stage of generativity are more involved with their children than younger fathers, who are still in the stage of intimacy, illustrate the importance of this issue (Weingarten, 1982).

Regarding the transition to fatherhood, Antel-May (1975, 1980) found that emotions and conflicts experienced by expectant fathers could be put into the following five categories: (1) protective feelings toward the wife, (2) anxieties concerning the role of provider, (3) fears regarding the vulnerability of the wife and child, (4) heightened dependency, and (5) nurturant emotions. Boyd (1980) found that the attitudes about parenting of first-time fathers elicited in the postpartum period correlated positively with actual paternal participation in infant caretaking activities. Little evidence exists to support the notion that fathers are biologically constrained from developing strong attachment bonds to their infants (Kunst-Wilson and Cronenwett, 1981). However, prior to 1975, mothers were frequently awarded custody in divorce cases based on the belief that mothers were the "biologically superior parent" (Novak, 1981). Nearly a half-million families in the United States are headed by single fathers (Group for the Advancement of Psychiatry, 1985).

Teenage Fathers

Although teenage fathers are not the primary focus of this chapter, it is important to highlight the specific issues they are facing. Adolescent childbearing has become an epidemic in the United States. The United States leads all developed nations in the number of pregnancies occurring among 15 to 19 year olds (Wallis, 1985). Social service agencies have long recognized the need to help teenage mothers and children. Teenage fathers, however, have been largely ignored. As recent research has begun to document the significant impact fathers have on the development of their children, teenage fathers present a particularly important challenge. Teen fathers reveal a myriad of problems. Their youth, their questionable psychological readiness for the fathering role, their lack of job skills and employment opportunities, and their low educational level defy easy solutions. Multifaceted support programs which address each of these complex problem areas must be developed (Bank Street Fatherhood Project, 1986).

Barret and Robinson (1986) found that a significant number of teenage fathers are responsible psychologically and financially, want to remain involved with the mother and infant, and expect to be included in decisions regarding child care. Redmond (1985) studied adolescent fathers and non-fathers making decisions about unexpected pregnancies and found that all subjects wanted to be told about the pregnancy. The majority favored continuing the pregnancy rather than opting for an abortion. Ninety-one percent wanted to provide emotional and financial support, and 87% wanted to participate in child care.

The Bank Street College of Education in New York coordinated a Teen Father Collaboration project in eight cities that offered vocational assistance, counseling, and classes in prenatal development and parenting. Four hundred teenage fathers participated in a recent study, and at the end of two years, 82% had daily contact with their children, 74% provided financial support, and 90% still had relationships with the mothers of their infants (Bank Street Fatherhood Project, 1986). The Bank Street model provides a framework and a resource for the design of nursing interventions specific to teenage fathers.

Paternal-Infant Attachment

It appears that early interaction between a father and his infant aids in the development of paternal-infant attachment (Greenberg and Morris, 1974; Klaus and Kennell, 1976; Parke and Tinsley, 1981). In studies of paternal-infant attachment, the responses of fathers to their infants were similar to those of mothers (Taubenheim, 1981). Cranley and Weaver (1983) state the attachment process begins during pregnancy as a result of psychological and physiological events. Expectant fathers demonstrate attachment behaviors toward their unborn infants.

Father-infant attachment is used to describe the total behavior system that demonstrates the emotional tie between the dyadic pair. Greenberg and Morris (1974, p. 520) state that there is an innate potential in fathers to demonstrate engrossment, which they describe as an absorption, preoccupation, and interest in the infant. Engrossment is characterized by seven behaviors: (1) visual awareness of the newborn; (2) tactile awareness demonstrated by the desire to hold and touch the infant; (3) awareness of the newborn's distinct features; (4) perception that the infant is perfect; (5) a strong attachment to and focus on the newborn; (6) extreme elation described as a "high"; and (7) increased sense of self-esteem. Field (1978) examined the interactions among (1) primary caregiving fathers and infants, (2) secondary caregiving fathers and infants, and (3) mothers and infants. It was found that primary caregivers, both fathers and mothers, demonstrated similar interactive behaviors, such as smiling, mimicked grimaces, and high-pitched vocalizations, with their infants. Secondary caregiving fathers demonstrated a minimum of behaviors such as holding of limbs, game playing, and poking. These behaviors, previously thought to be indigenous to fathers, may simply reflect the experience of the secondary caregiver rather than any intrinsic differences between mothers and fathers.

Toney (1983) examined the influence of early holding of the infant at the time of the infant's delivery on paternal bonding behaviors. No significant differences were found between fathers who did have contact for ten minutes with their infants during the first hour after the infant's delivery and those who did not have this contact. However, a positive relationship was noted among the variables of education, infant male gender, and bonding behaviors. Increased involvement of fathers through prenatal class attendance seems to be very important to the pregnancy and birth in that it seems to be a significant factor in determining the woman's experience of childbearing (Entwisle and Doering, 1981; May, 1982; Nicholson et al., 1983). Cranley and Weaver (1983) found that the existence of paternal-fetal attachment behaviors during pregnancy are positively correlated with both the strength of the marital relationship as perceived by the expectant father and with the physical symptoms of couvade that he experiences during pregnancy (p. 72).

Jones (1981) found that fathers were more involved with caretaking activities and demonstrated more attachment behaviors when infants were born by cesarean section or were born prematurely. Meyers (1982) found a significant difference in knowledge and caretaking at four weeks between fathers who had been taught the infant's behavioral characteristics through the Brazelton Neonatal Behavioral Assessment Scale (BNBAS) and fathers who had not. It was proposed that increased knowledge regarding behavioral states of the infant allowed fathers to receive positive reinforcement for their caretaking efforts. Jones and Lenz (1986) found that the state of the infant, as delineated by the BNBAS, emerged as a strong predictor of the relative frequency with which fathers displayed several types of interactional behavior, particularly affection toward and comforting of the infant.

Fathering Beyond Infancy

There is a paucity of literature concerning fathers of preschool and school-aged children. Radin (1981), who studied the father's role in the cognitive, academic, and intellectual development of his preschool child, found that children appear to benefit from a higher degree of paternal involvement. Verbal ability was increased, and children demonstrated a greater sense of mastery of their own fate. Stereotypical thinking about parents and parental roles was reduced. Bradley (1985) describes entry into school as a normative crisis for the family. This is a transition when family members may have to alter roles and responsibilities. Fathering at this point changes from caregiver and organizer to mediator and guide in a broader sociocultural context. Fathers report a sense of losing their infants, a fear of losing control over their children's lives, and a lessening of affectional ties. Radin and Goldsmith (1983) found the following factors influential in determining the role that fathers of school-aged children play in the socialization process: (1) the father's efforts to compensate for or to model himself after his own father's role in child care; (2) the sex of the child (higher involvement with boys); and (3) the father's educational level and occupation.

Ideally, the role of the parent should be well established prior to adolescence because the early adolescent years may be an unsettled and volatile time for the family. During this time, the adolescent is struggling with identity development, emancipation from parents, evolving secondary sex characteristics, sexuality, and determining future goals. The General Mills survey (1981) revealed that teenagers believe that parents should play an equal role in caring for children. The study also found that an increasing number of fathers choose to begin parenting later in life, allowing for more involvement in child care and more flexibility in child care roles. Martin (1985) contends that it is the emergence of the adolescent's personality in tandem with the father's maturing personality development, combined with the adolescent's approaching peak physical virility countered by the father's realization of his own mortality, that sets the stage for confrontation. Interestingly, paternal nurturance is positively correlated with enhanced masculinity in adolescent males, yet most fathers believe that strong discipline and emphasis on achievement will produce masculine sons (Martin, 1985).

Fathering in Illness

Factors Promoting Nurturant Behaviors in Neonatal Intensive Care Unit Fathers

The author (J. Novak) conducted an ethnographic study to describe development of observable nurturant behaviors in fathers of hospitalized neonates and to identify variables which seem related to the development or lack of development of these behaviors. Families of premature but physiologically stable neonates who had one to two weeks until anticipated discharge, were observed. Hispanic, Hmong, white, and black fathers were included in the sample. Two of the fathers were teenage fathers. The following were questions posed at the onset of the investigation:

1. Do fathers demonstrate nurturant behaviors in the neonatal intensive care unit (NICU)?
2. What are the observable characteristics of the father and couple when nurturant father behaviors are seen?
3. What are the observable relationships between the demonstration of these nurturant behaviors and the NICU physical environment and the staff, specifically the primary nurse?
4. What observable dyadic or triadic behavior relationships between father and nurse; father and mother; or mother, father, and nurse seem to exist when these nurturant father behaviors are or are not manifest in the NICU?

This investigation was composed of observation periods and interviews with fathers, primary nurses, and the discharge-planning coordinator. The interviews were conducted to validate investigator observations. Although this investigation was not an attempt to categorize and tally nurturant behaviors, it was important to operationally define the behaviors which were being described as nurturant and which either did or did not manifest themselves in the fathers. The observed behaviors included touching, caressing, holding, rocking the infant, eye contact, smiling, and vocalizing as well as providing routine infant care such as bathing, dressing, feeding, burping, and diapering.

From an analysis of the field notes for this investigation, it was concluded that the demonstration of nurturant behaviors by fathers of NICU infants has numerous predisposing conditions and variables. A simple statement that fathers do or do not demonstrate such behaviors simply cannot be made. The father of the NICU infant at any given moment can demonstrate the behaviors consistent with one or more of the following roles: nurturer, husband, parent, intermediary, caretaker, playmate, visitor, provider, supporter, student, sentry, and observer. From the observations of this investigator, it can be stated that some fathers demonstrate nurturant behaviors to varying degrees and at different times during the hospitalization of their infants; other fathers do not. For example, with some fathers, there was a gradual assumption over time of nurturant behaviors, which was facilitated primarily by interaction with a skilled primary nurse and the encouragement of the mothers of the infants.

From an analysis of the ethnographic study field notes, it seems that the demonstration of nurturant behaviors is related to the following factors:

1. The presence of an expert primary nurse who is able to intervene by:
   a. recognizing the powerful role that the nurse plays in the transition to parenthood
   b. empathetically, yet strongly, modeling nurturant caregiving behaviors for both parents, avoiding assumptions or misconceptions regarding cultural or ethnic stereotypes
   c. maintaining a sense of humor
   d. effectively and consistently evaluating teaching methods with return demonstrations when appropriate
   e. using any given situation to bring either or both parents to their nurturant roles
   f. teaching parents to recognize their infant's behavioral states and cues
   g. transmitting her own comfort level in the NICU setting to the parents
   h. appearing to have time for parents no matter how busy he or she might be.
2. The sociocultural background of the father and the differing values placed on

the nurturant father role by his peers or culture, which must be recognized, but overgeneralizations and stereotyping should be avoided.

3. The relationship between the parents, which can encourage nurturant fathering behaviors through the mother's positive reinforcement and offering of the infant to the father.
4. The comfort of the parents with the NICU environment.
5. The presence of other children at home for whom the father has primary caretaking responsibility.

The interviews with fathers at the completion of the study in part confirmed the conclusions which were generated from field notes on the 10 families, as did the interviews with the primary nurses and the discharge coordinator. It appeared that nurturant father behaviors were manifested when (1) the father was open to or actively pursued physical closeness with his child; (2) the mother encouraged his closeness and "surrendered" her quasi-autonomous roles of caretaker, protector, and provider for the infant; and (3) the primary nurse was there to show the parents what to do in a manner that minimized or ignored the mistakes of the parents, that recognized the uniqueness of each family, and that encouraged the father to ask questions and get to know his infant.

In summary, many of the roles required of the father of a NICU infant are new and unfamiliar, difficult to carry out, and unrehearsed, yet are called for during an unexpected medical crisis. At a time when they, too, need nurturing, fathers of high-risk infants are expected to adapt readily and be models of self-control. It is apparent from this investigation that the primary nurse is in a strategic position to assist the new father in his acquaintance with and early adjustment to his infant. Although some of the fathers observed in this study became actively involved with their children, others preferred less involvement in infant caretaking and displayed minimal nurturant behaviors. A nurse must be able to recognize these differences and support this choice. A couple's sociocultural ideology and perceptions of the father's role, as well as the family dynamics and values, need to be given primary consideration in planning nursing care. In order for the nurse to fulfill an important teaching role for the fathers of NICU infants, the nurse must meet the needs of each individual father in relation to the family system. This requires systematic and nonjudgmental assessment of paternal role development and early father-infant and father-mother-infant interactions. Although this study focuses on fathers in the NICU it has strong implications for the powerful role that nurses play in a variety of health care settings.

ASSESSMENT

Given the historical perspective and the current emphasis and social acceptance of father involvement, strategies to promote fathering would be appropriate for all fathers. Optimal times for intervention would be during the prenatal, intrapartum, and postnatal periods, times when nurses have access to families. During these periods, attitudes and expectations about fatherhood can be explored, skills needed can be identified, and strategies can be implemented that would facilitate fathering. It is also during these periods that fathers are more likely to be receptive to interventions that promote fathering. Prenatal programs should encourage paternal involvement, and obstetrical hospital policies should reflect the importance of father involvement during the intrapartum and postnatal periods.

Nursing diagnoses relating to family process and parenting may, by their defining characteristics, indicate the need to promote nuturant fathering. The birth of a child is a developmental transition that signifies a life crisis event involving the acquisition of a new role and related behaviors, as well as the addition of new responsibilities. When an infant is born prematurely or with health problems, a situational crisis occurs, adding to the demands on the father to make decisions and support the mother at a time when he, himself, needs support. Premature infants, located in special care nurseries, have specialized equipment that presents potential barriers to attachment. In such situations, nursing diagnoses of potential alteration in family process, parenting, or attachment signify the need for intervention to promote fathering.

Fathers whose infants are in intensive care nurseries usually do not have access to paternal role models. In fact, it may not be appropriate to transfer role modeling from other settings to the nursery setting where stimuli need to be carefully monitored. The inability to rehearse fathering skills necessary to role acquisition has actual or potential influence on the development of the self-confidence necessary for successful role performance.

In fathers who are coping with the transition to fatherhood, the nurse needs to consider the potential for growth of the father and the family unit by enhancing skills already present and providing anticipatory guidance for that which lies ahead (see Chapter 5).

THE INTERVENTION

Intervention strategies that promote fathering have a common theme of direct involvement of the father. Optimally, this involvement begins during pregnancy, continues by presence during the birthing process, and grows throughout childhood by participation in caretaking and involvement in every stage of development.

Nurses must individualize their intervention strategies and avoid responding to fathers in stereotypical, predetermined ways, specifically avoiding overgeneralizations regarding ethnic or cultural practices. Health histories should include a question regarding the obstetrical status of partners, recognizing the father's potential for physical symptoms of couvade, such as weight gain or loss, alterations in appetite, food cravings, excessive fatigue, and backaches. In addition, given the strong evidence to support the importance the father plays in affecting the emotional health of the mother during pregnancy and her successful adaptation to motherhood, every effort should be made to involve the father in the pregnancy and transition to parenthood. Nurses must also assist in modifying or eliminating institutional routines that arbitrarily restrict father participation.

Nurses must recognize the important role they play in teaching infant care to fathers and encourage their active participation through sensitive, nurturant role modeling and by providing time for practice. Community resources specifically for fathers must also be identified so that effective re-

ferrals can be made. Involvement of fathers in prenatal classes, particularly childbirth preparation, is widely accepted. Many classes are offered in the evening to accommodate working individuals. Involvement of the father in classes that emphasize caretaking skills, such as diapering and feeding, and parenting issues relating to role development and the sharing of parenting responsibilities assist the father in planning for this role transition. Attendance at prenatal appointments promotes attachment with the infant by allowing the father to hear the infant's heartbeat or see an image of the infant during ultrasound examination. Attending these appointments also assists the father in understanding normal physiological changes occurring in the mother and may provide a stimulus for father support during pregnancy. Nurses need to discuss planning for the infant, continuance of the couple's relationship, and resources and support that would assist during his transition stage. This would also be an ideal time for the couple to spend some time with other young families to observe the parenting process, to discuss concerns, and to actually have some hands-on experience with infant care under the guidance of experienced parents.

It is important to emphasize that parenthood is a learning process, a time when the emerging famiy is becoming acquainted, defining new roles, and developing new skills. And while it is impossible to have considered all the possible problems that may arise and develop all the needed skills, it is helpful to anticipate and discuss common concerns fathers have about their role. It is very helpful if the father has a relative, friend, or coworker who is a parent and with whom he feels free to discuss concerns.

During the prenatal period, it is important to determine the father's interest and willingness to participate in labor and delivery. Today, it is almost expected that the father will want to be involved in this process; however, nurses must assess if the father is comfortable with this participation and, if not, how much involvement would be acceptable. It is better to make this decision after the father participates in prenatal classes and makes plans with his partner. For all fathers, whether or not they actually attended the infant's birth, the opportunity to hold the infant soon after birth should be encouraged. For infants who are born prematurely or who require medical attention, fathers should get an opportunity to see or touch the infant when possible; when not feasible, information about the infant should be transmitted to the father as soon as possible.

Father participation in newborn caretaking activities, such as feeding, dressing, diapering, bathing, and soothing, should be encouraged. The father's involvement in noncaretaking activities, such as cuddling, interacting, and playing, should not be overlooked. Infant care classes and demonstrations need to be scheduled at various times to accommodate fathers as well as mothers. Flexible policies regarding father presence in the postpartum area encourage paternal attachment and participation in caretaking activities. It also gives the father time to support the mother during this stage and provides an opportunity to both parents to share their initial joys of parenthood. Offering fathers unlimited access to their newborns also allows more opportunities for fathers to rehearse caretaking skills and to become acquainted with their infant's unique behavioral characteristics. It also allows the nurse more flexibility in observing, teaching, and reinforcing skills during short postpartum hospitalizations. Nurses need to use their influence and skills to encourage fathers to become involved with their infants and participate in caretaking, and nurses should assist fathers in becoming acquainted with their newborns. Their skills in reinforcing nurturant behaviors will help fathers gain confidence in the fathering role and find interactions with their infants rewarding.

When the newborn requires constant monitoring or prolonged hospitalization, the nurse needs to spend time with the father to meet his need for information, to promote attachment, and to gradually involve the father in caretaking activities as appropriate. Reinforcing caretaking activities and support given to the mother strengthens fathering behaviors. Encouraging exploration and questioning about the infant's condition and care shows confidence in the father's ability to understand what is happening and willingness to include him in the plan of care.

After discharge, father involvement needs to be promoted during home visits and postpartum visits, as well as during vists to well child clinics. It is during this period that many changes occur as the infants establish sleeping and feeding schedules, parents return to normal schedules, and the newness of parenthood wears off. During these early postpartum weeks, there is minimal contact with health professionals to ask questions and discuss concerns. At this time, fathers as well as mothers rely on existing support systems. The availability of a nurse by phone to discuss small concerns will make this transition time less stressful for young families. Follow-up phone calls, clinic visits, or a home visit should be scheduled as indicated by the needs expressed by the parents. Involvement of the father in the resolution of concerns helps parents face problems together, develop needed skills, and utilize available resources in developing their roles as parents.

Child care classes help guide parents, not just mothers, through the developmental changes of infancy, toddlerhood, and the preschool years. They also promote the development of skills to cope with the challenges of parenthood. Such classes not only transmit information but also provide parents with an opportunity to interact with other parents and to share common concerns. Parents who share similar concerns may develop a support network outside the structured setting or begin to reach out to other parents. The involvement of fathers in classes and groups is an important component of family-centered nursing care.

Educational programs must also cover unique problems facing dual career families (Sund and Ostwald, 1985), teenage fathers (Bank Street Fatherhood Project, 1986), and those who are facing separation or divorce (Novak, 1981). In addition, effective programs must be sensitive to the developmental stage of the father and to the cultural and historical context which he brings to the fathering role. Health education programs should include opportunities that allow fathers to explore questions or unresolved issues of their own childhood, such as lack of models for father involvement or nurturance.

EVALUATION

The purpose of the intervention is to promote nurturant fathering behaviors. It is difficult to quantify the effects of the intervention by its very qualitative nature; however, if one is able to operationalize nurturant fathering behaviors, it is possible to ascertain their presence and describe their quality through increased observation and interview. Establishing baseline behavioral data assists in measuring of the effectiveness of the intervention. In measuring outcomes, the nurse needs to examine what variables influence the acquisition of nurturant fathering behaviors. Such variables are the father's age, marital status, cultural background, socioeconomic and employment status, and educational level (Marton et al., 1981). Other important variables revealed in the ethnographic study include the relationship of the father and mother, the health status of the infant, the hospital environment, and the personality and expectations of the primary nurse. The temperament of the infant also interacts with the father's personality and expectations in the development of their relationship (Ventura, 1986).

In addition to describing specific behaviors, the approach, comfort level, and enjoyment expressed by the father in caring for his infant can be used to measure the effectiveness of the intervention. Observations at intervals during the infant's hospitalization serve to document the development of the paternal role over time as the father becomes acquainted with his infant and how the health status of the infant affects the acquisition of skills necessary to the fathering role. Postdischarge follow-up at specific intervals (e.g., three, six, and 12 months) by phone and during home or clinic visits documents the permanence of behaviors and the evolution of the fathering role.

Case Study

Infant Blake was admitted to the NICU as a result of his premature delivery at 28 weeks gestation and low birth weight of 1000 gm. During his six week stay, he was treated with indomethacin for patent ductus arteriosus, ventilation for respiratory distress syndrome, theophylline for apnea and bradycardia, and supportive care for growth. Both parents were extremely anxious during Blake's hospitalization. Blake's father is a hospital pharmacist and his mother is a staff nurse in internal medicine.

Outcomes in the NICU are evaluated at three, six, and nine month intervals after discharge, at which time observations of the father-infant dyad and father-mother-infant triad are observed for nurturing behaviors, development of the infant, and sensitivity of the parents to the infant's behavioral cues and states. At 12 months, a follow-up interview is conducted with the father only.

Blake's father, Mr. M., came to the NICU follow-up clinic for the 12 month interview regarding his child's stay in the NICU and the factors that he believed facilitated his fathering of his son during the hospitalization and in the interim since discharge.

Mr. M. perceived the NICU experience as an "emotional roller coaster" with the ups and downs determined by such factors as the numbers on the child's weight card and the sporadic sounding of monitor alarms on equipment attached to Blake and other infants. Mr. M. felt that since he was a pharmacist working in the hospital and his wife was a nurse, their professional backgrounds helped them get beyond the "gadgetry and technology" sooner, enabling them to focus on their infant. He noted that it took longer for other, less medically sophisticated parents to get beyond the machinery. Mr. M. stated that he got involved with Blake's care once the infant was stable and moved to the B nursery. He felt that up until that time, Blake was so small and fragile that he was afraid of hurting him. Mr. M. stated that because he worked in the hospital, he was able to visit his son several times each day. He observed that during his child's three month stay, he was the only father to visit his child alone. He reasoned that other fathers were either working or at home taking care of older children. Mr. M. saw his primary role during the early weeks of Blake's hospitalization as being supportive to "the mom." Once he saw that his infant was going to live, he allowed himself to become more involved. Regardless of his level of involvement, however, he states that "the moms" do most of the care. He revealed that he did not attempt to bottle-feed Blake until a month after discharge from the NICU when his wife's breast milk was well established.

When asked what determined his level of comfort in the NICU besides consistent weight gain of his child and the absence of monitor alarms, he replied that it was the particular nurse who was taking care of his child. He stated that two of the nurses were "standouts" because they always "kept it light" and did not frighten the couple. "They were so supportive . . . they acknowledged problems and worked on solutions, but they focused on what was going well. They had a great sense of humor and would listen to me." He stated that having these nurses was also important to him because his wife would not listen to him and used constant dialogue with the "decision makers"—the nurses and doctors—as her method of coping. He stated that had he not been a "fairly secure person," this might have been a problem. However, he had a good relationship with his wife "which is so important when facing something like this." Mr. M. stated that the two nurses seemed to expect that he would be involved and showed him how to do everything. "They always included me and always seemed to have time for us no matter how busy they were. It wasn't just because I work here either. They did this with young dads, less educated dads, all types." He stated that some of the nurses totally focused on the mothers, and that really irritated him. "I felt lucky to have Ellen and Mary as primary nurses. In addition, Mary and Ellen stressed Blake's state of alertness so that our interactions with him would be optimal. They also showed us how to recognize the behavioral cues that signaled overstimulation, such as looking away, irritability, or splaying of his fingers. All of this teaching and modeling prepared me for an egalitarian role in raising my son."

The evaluation interview not only offered a father's perspective, but it validated some of the observations that were consistently made in the field notes of the ethnographic study. The difficult transition to the environment of the nursery, the father's fear of handling a premature infant, the important role the father plays with older siblings, the father's perception that his number one role is to take care of the mother, the observation that fathers do not actually visit alone, and the importance of the nurse's expectations, personality, and ability to teach and model for the father were emphasized.

RESEARCH IMPLICATIONS

The study of fathers and the development of the fathering role is just beginning. A majority of the fathering studies have focused on fathers during the prenatal and newborn period. At this time, it is essential to clearly delineate what is meant by fathering behaviors and to develop a conceptual framework that describes the development of fathering behaviors (Cronenwett, 1982). In a number of the early studies, father behaviors were determined by maternal report. Even through the use of paternal reports, interviews, and questionnaires, descriptions of behaviors still may not be accurate because it is likely that a father's perception of his behavior is different than the actual behavior. Therefore, behavioral reports should be supplemented with observations in natural settings over a period of time. The study of the relationship of father participation to other variables, such as attachment, child development, marital satisfaction, and mother's perception, needs to be conducted with larger samples composed of fathers representing a wide range of cultural groups, educational levels, occupational statuses, and age groups. Too often studies have been conducted on highly motivated, well-educated, middle-class white parents, making generalizations of the findings inappropriate to other populations of fathers.

How the birth of a premature or ill infant affects the development of the fathering role has yet to be studied. In the hospital setting, nursing behaviors that facilitate fathering need to be identified, tested, and incorporated into standards of care. It is also important to identify fathers at risk for paternal difficulties as early as possible to provide needed interventions. Also of interest would be how mothers and fathers complement each other's parenting behaviors.

Once fathering behaviors have been clearly articulated, it will be easier to examine how these behaviors evolve throughout childhood. Little research has been done on the role of the father in influencing the socialization and development of his offspring from birth through adolescence. Although there is considerable emphasis and excitement about early involvement of fathers with their children, how long does this involvement persist, how does it change as the child develops, and how does it vary with the sex of the child?

The impact of nursing interventions on fathering behaviors needs to be quantified to justify the time and resources allocated to this important function. Nurses also need to demonstrate that changes in hospital policies and structure do, in fact, make a difference in facilitating fathering. Nurses also need to become involved in studying changes that support fathering during the toddler, preschool, school-age, and adolescent years. Interventions to promote fathering will be strengthened by a body of literature that clearly articulates the importance of fathers in the lives of their developing children.

References

Antle-May, K. Psychological involvement in pregnancy by expectant fathers. Journal of Obstetric and Gynecologic Nursing, 4:40–42, 1975.
Antle-May, K. A typology of detachment involvement styles adopted during pregnancy by first-time fathers.

Western Journal of Nursing Research, 2:445–453, 1980.

Bank Street Fatherhood Project. Teen fathers: Partners in parenting. New York: Bank Street College of Education, 1986.

Barret, RL, and Robinson, BE. Adolescent fathers: Often forgotten parents. Pediatric Nursing, 12:273–277, 1986.

Biller, HB. A note on father absence and masculine development in lower class Negro and white boys. Child Development, 39:1003–1006, 1968.

Biller, HB. Father absence and the personality development of the male child. Developmental Psychology, 2:181–201, 1970.

Boyd, ST. Paternal involvement in the interactive behavioral assessment process. Unpublished doctoral dissertation, Texas Women's University, Denton, Texas, 1980.

Bradley, RH. Fathers and the school-age child. In Hanson, S, and Bozett, F (Eds.), Dimensions of fatherhood. Beverly Hills, Calif: Sage Publications, 1985, pp. 141–169.

Carlsmith, L. Effect of early father absence on scholastic aptitude. Harvard Educational Review, 34:3–21, 1964.

Couchman, R. The fatherhood revival. Transition, 11:11–14, 1982.

Cranley, M, and Weaver, RH. An exploration of paternal-fetal attachment behavior. Nursing Research, 32:68–72, 1983.

Cronenwett, LR. Father participation in child care: A critical review. Research in Nursing and Health, 5:63–72, 1982.

Cronenwett, LR, and Kunst-Wilson, W. Stress, social support, and the transition to fatherhood. Nursing Research, 30:196–201, 1981.

Entwisle, D, and Doering, S. The first birth. Baltimore: The Johns Hopkins University Press, 1981.

Erikson, E. Identity and the life cycle. Psychological Issues, 1:59–100, 1959.

Field, T. Interaction behaviors of primary versus secondary caretaker fathers. Developmental Psychology, 14:183–184, 1978.

General Mills American Family Report 1980–1981: Families at work. Minneapolis: Louis Harris Poll.

Giveans, DL, and Robinson, MK. Fathers and the preschool age child. In Hanson, S, and Bozett, F (Eds.), Dimensions of Fatherhood. Beverly Hills, Calif: Sage Publications, 1985, pp. 115–140.

Greenburg, M, and Morris, N. Engrossment: The newborn's impact upon the father. American Journal of Orthopsychiatry, 44:520–531, 1974.

Group for the Advancement of Psychiatry. Divorce and child custody. New York: Mental Health Materials Center, 1985.

Hanson, S, and Bozett, F (Eds.). Dimensions of Fatherhood. Beverly Hills, Calif: Sage Publications, 1985.

Hanson, S, and Bozett, F. Fatherhood and changing family roles. Family Community Health, 9:9–21, 1987.

Hoffman, ML. Father absence and conscience development. Developmental Psychology, 4:400–406, 1971.

Hott, J. Best laid plans: Pre- and postpartum comparison of self and spouse in primiparous Lamaze couples who share delivery and those who do not. Nursing Research, 29:20–27, 1980.

Jones, LC. Father to infant attachment effects of early contact and characteristics of the infant. Research in Nursing and Health, 4:193–200, 1981.

Jones, LC, and Lenz, ER. Father-newborn interaction: Effects of social competence and infant state. Nursing Research, 35:149–153,1986.

Klaus, M, and Kennell, J. Maternal infant bonding. St. Louis: CV Mosby Co., 1976.

Kunst-Wilson, W, and Cronenwett, L. Nursing care for the emerging family: Promoting paternal behavior. Research in Nursing and Health, 4:201–211, 1981.

Lamb, ME, and Bronson, SK. Fathers in the context of family influences: Past, present and future. School Psychology Review, 9:336–352, 1980.

Lamb, ME (Ed.) The role of the father in child development (2nd ed.). New York: John Wiley and Sons, Inc., 1981.

Landerholm, EJ, and Scruen, G. A comparison of mother and father interaction with their six-month-old male and female infants. Early Childhood Development and Care, 7:317–328, 1981.

Lipkin, M, & Lamb, G. The couvade syndrome: An epidemiologic study. Annals of Internal Medicine, 96:509–511, 1982.

Martin, DH. Fathers and adolescents. In Hanson, S, and Bozett, F (Eds.), Dimensions of fatherhood. Beverly Hills, Calif: Sage Publications, 1985, pp. 170–193.

Marton, P, Minde, K, and Perrotta, M. The role of the father for the infant at risk. American Journal of Orthopsychiatry, 51:672–679, 1981.

May, K. Three phases in the development of father involvement in pregnancy. Nursing Research, 31:339–342, 1982.

May, KA, and Perrin, S. Prelude: Pregnancy and birth. In Hanson, S, & Bozett, F (Eds.). Dimensions of fatherhood. Beverly Hills, Calif: Sage Publications, 1985, pp. 64–91.

McLaughlin, SD, and Melber, BD. The changing life course of American women. Seattle: The Hearst Corporation, 1986.

Meyers, BJ. Early intervention using Brazelton training with middle-class mothers and fathers of newborns. Child Development, 53:462–471, 1982.

Miller, B, and Bowen, S. Father-to-newborn attachment behavior in relation to parental class and presence at delivery. Family Relations, 31:71–78, 1982.

Moen, P. The two-provider family: Problems and potentials. In Lamb, M (Ed.), Nontraditional families: Parenting and child development. Hillsdale, N. J.: Lawrence Erlbaum Associates Inc., 1982.

Nicholson, J, Gist, N, Klein, R, and Standley, K. Outcomes of father involvement in pregnancy and birth. Birth, 10:5–9, 1983.

Novak, J. Children versus divorce. Pediatric Nursing, 8:33–39, 1981.

Parke, R. Fathers. Cambridge, Mass: Harvard University Press, 1981.

Parke, R, and Tinsley, B. The father's role in infancy: Determinants of involvement. In Lamb, ME (Ed.), The role of the father in child development (2nd ed.). New York: John Wiley and Sons, Inc., 1981.

Pedersen, F, and Robson, K. Father participation in infancy. American Journal of Orthopsychiatry. 39:467–468, 1969.

Radin, N. The role of the father in cognitive, academic, and intellectual development. In Lamb, ME (Ed.), The role of the father in child development (2nd ed.). New York: John Wiley and Sons, Inc., 1981.

Radin, N, and Goldsmith, R. Predictors of father involvement in child care. Paper presented at the biennial meeting of the Society for Research in Child Development, Detroit, 1983. Cited in Hanson, S, and

Bozett, F (Eds.), Dimensions of fatherhood. Beverly Hills, Calif: Sage Publications, 1985.

Redmond, MA. Attitudes of adolescent males toward adolescent pregnancy and fatherhood. Family Relations, 37:337–342, 1985.

Snow, M, Jacklin, C, and Maccoby, E. Sex of child differences in father-child interaction at one year of age. Child Development, 54:227–232, 1983.

Sund, K and Ostwald, SK. Dual earner families' stress levels and personal and life style related variables. Nursing Research, 34:357–361, 1985.

Taubenheim, AM. Paternal-infant bonding in the first time father. Journal of Gynecological Nursing, 10:261–265, 1981.

Toney, L. The effects of holding the newborn at delivery on paternal bonding. Nursing Research, 32:16–19, 1983.

U.S. Department of Commerce, Bureau of Census. Trends in child care arrangements of working mothers. Current Populations Reports, Special Studies, No. 117, p. 23, 1985.

Ventura, J. Parent coping: A replication. Nursing Research, 35:77–80, 1986.

Wallis, C. Children having children. Time, December 9, 78–90, 1985.

Weaver, R, and Cranley, M. An exploration of paternal-fetal attachment behavior. Nursing Research, 32:68–72, 1983.

Weingarten, K. Older men make better fathers. Denver Post, June 21, 1982.

CHAPTER 3

SIBLING SUPPORT

MARTHA J. CRAFT, Ph.D., R.N.

Children grow up in a network of individuals that includes both family and community members. The network of family members includes siblings for approximately 80% of children who are raised in the United States (Dunn, 1983). Siblings are described as individuals with at least one common parent, but the definition of siblings is actually much more complex and encompasses a large scope of genetic, demographic, developmental, environmental, and emotional variables (Webster, 1987). The impact of siblings on children is difficult to define and measure. While common sense dictates that sibling relationships have some effect upon personality and development, the effect is not always obvious. Indeed, Sutton-Smith and Rosenberg (1970) have termed siblings

the "silent variable" or a variable with an obscure influence.

The word "support" is used widely in nursing literature as an accepted and useful nursing intervention. However, nurses lack a universal, operational definition for this term. In this chapter, the term "support" will be defined in relation to sibling support as "promoting the interests of and defending as being valid and right" (Webster, 1987). The purpose of this chapter is to present the intervention of sibling support as used when another child in the family becomes ill and must be hospitalized. Siblingship as a status marker, an explanatory variable, and the siblingship role will be discussed as a theoretical framework. This framework will then be used to address the impact of illness and hospitalization on siblings and the implementation of sibling support.

THEORETICAL FOUNDATION

Siblingship As a Status Marker

Historically, siblingship has been used to preserve intact properties by inheritance customs in European law. Preservation of family properties was assured through the allocation of properties to children based upon their sibling status at the time of parental death. Siblingship was seen as the criterion for establishing inheritance and power. The theme of sibling conflict as a struggle for power recurs throughout literary history, and power seems to be the most important consideration in traditional literature (Sutton-Smith and Rosenberg, 1970). Indeed, problems surrounding sibling rivalry are discussed in most parenting books, and sibling conflict is a theme that flows through both child and adult development. It is not surprising, then, that sibling relationships have been postulated as one explanatory variable in the study of individual differences.

Siblingship As an Explanatory Variable

In order to explain the effects of siblingship on individual differences, psychologists have explored sibling status variables such as birth order, sibling spacing, and sex of the sibling. Ordinal position of siblings is thought to have some influence on personality. Studies of first-borns have been numerous, raising the question of first-born superiority. Dittes (1961) and Schachter (1964) have demonstrated that first-born children are more likely to be susceptible to social pressure. Moreover, Sears (1950) found that first-born children are more dependent, as evidenced by the need to affiliate.

Difference in years between siblings could also be important. Closely spaced siblings have been found to be more aggressive, with affection more likely with widely spaced siblings (Minnett et al., 1983). When a large gap exists between the last-born and the next sibling, the last-born's responses are more similar to those of only children than they are to the responses of first-borns or later-born children (Miller and Zimbardo, 1965).

Sex status of the sibling has also been studied as an explanatory variable. Sutton-Smith and Rosenberg (1970) noted that each sibling is affected by the sex of other siblings. Further, these effects are most obvious in the case of younger siblings. In two-child families, males with brothers have been found to have significantly higher masculinity scores and girls with sisters have been found to have significantly higher femininity scores on a measure of stated preferences. Similarly, children showed more positive responses to suggestions from siblings of the same sex than from siblings of the opposite sex (Rosenberg and Sutton-Smith, 1964). Girls as siblings have been found to be more likely to praise and teach siblings, while boys are likely to engage in neutral behavior (Minnett et al., 1983). Opposite sex siblings have been shown to have more concern with the self, suggesting that opposite sex siblings decrease the amount of sibling social relationships within the family and increase sibling self-concern (Sutton-Smith and Rosenberg, 1970). However, other researchers have found that cheating, aggression, and dominance were characteristic of sibling behavior during interactions with siblings of the same sex (Minnett et al., 1983).

The literature on the relationship of family structure variables such as birth order, sex, and spacing of siblings to intelligence, achievement, and personality suggest that sibling status variables have an influence on individual interests, preferences, style of thinking, self-esteem, conformity, and achievement as an adult (Dunn, 1983; Cicirelli, 1973, 1975, 1976, 1977, 1978; Harris, 1964; Koch, 1955a, 1955b, 1956; Marjoribanks et al., 1975; Sutton-Smith and Rosenberg, 1970; Zagonc and Markus, 1975; Wagner et al., 1979). However, the constructs of sibling spacing, birth order, and sex seem to be inadequate to explain the magnitude of differences between siblings, and the lack of direct studies of sibling interaction represents a major gap in the understanding of processes involved in the development of differences between siblings and the extent of sibling influences on development. Importantly, there is no theory to guide or interpret the sibling constellation research (Dunn, 1983; Scarr and Grajek, 1982).

In the absence of a useful theory, clinical observations of sibling interactions must be used to determine how siblings affect the environment in which a child grows and develops. The role of siblings is diverse, covering a range of scenarios from those in which siblings are harsh critics and competitors to those in which siblings are providers of solace and understanding.

The Role of Siblings

Bassard and Ball (1960) have observed that life among siblings is like living in a fishbowl, psychologically speaking. Siblings not only serve as a constant "rude awakening" for each other, but also save each other from being with their parents and other adults too much. Children tend to treat each other as equals, and children seem to prefer sibling discipline to adult discipline. Further, siblings feel they understand each other's problems better than parents do, and that adults judge children by adult standards and children judge each other by child standards. Siblings also serve the functions of (1) affection providers, (2) counselors, (3) leaders, (4) protectors, and (5) parental substitutes (Bassard and Ball, 1960).

Truly, siblings are the first peers for children. Children learn much from interactions with siblings and from observations of parental responses to sibling behavior. Socialization occurring between parents and children is different from that occurring between siblings (Baskett and Johnson, 1982).

Mauksch (1978) has identified the following four areas in which illness will make an impact on the total family: (1) economics, (2) social standing, (3) values, and (4) dynamic relationships. The power balance shifts and roles are renegotiated, sometimes unwillingly. Ill or disabled children may seem to have increased power to other siblings because most of the attention is going to them. Sibling difficulties listed by Lawson (1977) include jealousy, insecurity, and resentment. Since most children equate love with attention, it is perfectly normal for them to resent the child who receives more attention from parents because of treatments, special diets, and hospitalization. In addition, role renegotiations may include more responsibility and independence for the healthy siblings than they want. These role renegotiations can produce a continuum of responses, with the most desirable response coming from the family who rallies to the situation. On the other extreme of the continuum, the response can be family disruption (Mauksch, 1978).

ASSESSMENT

It is crucial for practicing nurses and nurse scholars to identify siblings who are in need of support, which necessitates prediction of adverse responses in siblings based upon variables that are related to sibling responses. Many variables seem to affect sibling responses. These variables have been discussed in anecdotal literature and exploratory studies. The first variable is reduction of communication between parents and siblings, leaving the sibling wondering what is wrong and what the outcome will be (Tuck, 1964; McCollum, 1975). Second, an unrealistic sense of responsibility and guilt for the hospitalized child's illness may be experienced by the magical-thinking young sibling (McCollum, 1975; Guyulay, 1978). Further, sibling fear of getting the illness can result from identification with the sick child, lack of understanding, and expectations of retribution for "bad" thoughts. Even when fears are not expressed directly, they can be seen in altered health states, depressive symptoms, and problems in school (Kruger et al., 1980; McCollum, 1975; Schoenberg et al., 1970). Siblings of children with cancer have been found to have more distress than their ill brothers and sisters in the realm of perceived social isolation. These siblings perceived their parents as overindulgent with the ill child, but demonstrated fear of expressing negative feelings. Other siblings portrayed a concern with failure. Sibling experience and the ill child's experience were found to be similar in areas of illness anxiety and vulnerability (Cairns et al., 1979).

A few studies have compared siblings who have ill brothers or sisters with siblings whose brothers or sisters are healthy. Tew and Laurence (1973) found a fourfold increase of behavioral problems in siblings of children with spina bifida. However, Gath (1965) found no difference between siblings of children with cleft palates and siblings of nonhandicapped controls. Lavigne and Ryan

(1979) compared siblings of children with hematology problems, cardiac defects, and plastic surgery with controls. Their findings showed siblings of children having plastic surgery displayed the highest degree of behavior problems. Also, a greater number of behavior problems was found among seven to 13 year old male siblings of hematology patients as compared with male siblings of healthy children. Moreover, siblings showed fewer problems than their counterparts in the control group. In summary, controlled studies have isolated variables of illness and sibling age and sex as being related significantly to adverse effects. Other variables may be significant as well.

While measures of anxiety and lowered self-esteem in children or measures of family coping seem appropriate for determining sibling response, they are limited in their applicability, since they measure singular constructs. The experiences of siblings of ill children, in contrast, is multidimensional (Craft and Oppliger, 1989; Walker, 1988).

Craft began study in the area of sibling responses several years ago with the long-term goal of developing a profile of siblings at risk so that people who work with children could target their interventions to those who need them most. The research approach was developed to remedy limitations of available research. First, sibling perception of changes in feelings and behaviors was used as the dependent measure rather than parent perception of sibling response. Second, siblings of children with acute illnesses were studied along with siblings of children who had chronic and progressive illnesses. Third, the scope of variables influencing sibling response was expanded to include variables suggested by families and variables mentioned in anecdotal literature. Last, a systematic comparison of parent and sibling reports was undertaken in all studies.

A total of 300 siblings of hospitalized children have been studied over a 10 year period. The results of three studies show that siblings who have a greater probability of experiencing a statistically significant higher number of changes during the time interval following the hospitalization of a brother or sister are (1) younger than 10 years of age; (2) emotionally close to the hospitalized child; (3) receiving only a limited explanation of the experience; (4) afraid of getting the illness themselves; (5) cared for outside their own homes; (6) perceiving their parents as acting differently toward them; and (7) brothers and sisters of progressively ill children (Craft et al., 1985; Craft, 1985).

The dependent measure used for research purposes has been a Perceived Change Scale (PCS), developed by Craft and Wyatt and refined by Craft (1986). The PCS asks siblings if they have perceived physiological and behavioral changes in the following areas during the time interval that their brother or sister has been hospitalized: (1) anger; (2) food intake; (3) sleeping difficulties; (4) difficulty in concentrating at school; (5) nervousness; (6) fights with other children; (7) nightmares; (8) nail biting; (9) withdrawal from friends and family; (10) need to be near parents (spending more time at home for siblings 10 to 17 years and increased clinging, sitting on parents' laps, or desire to sleep with parents for siblings five to nine years); (11) sadness or unhappiness; and (12) feelings of being healthy. Because of the cognitive differences in siblings ranging from five to 17 years of age, younger siblings have been administered the scale via a structured interview.

The reliability and validity data on the PCS showed the scale for siblings five to ten years of age had an alpha coefficient of .66, and the scale for siblings 11 to 17 years of age had an alpha of .80. Criterion validity was demonstrated for both scales by comparing scores for siblings of hospitalized children with scores for siblings who had brothers and sisters experiencing outpatient surgery. Concurrent validity was demonstrated using Spielberger's State-Trait Anxiety Inventory for Children (1973), with a high correlation between the PCS score for older siblings and State Anxiety (r = .82) (Craft, 1986). These data indicate that questioning siblings regarding their experiences is a valid assessment method. Factor analysis of the scales showed five factors that accounted for 67.2% of the variance. These were (1) uncertainty, (2) sorrow, (3) helplessness and frustration, (4) preoccupation, and (5) conflict (Craft and Oppliger, 1989).

Siblings who may require assistance can also be recognized by their manifestation of defining characteristics presented for two diagnoses suggesting the need for sibling support: (1) *Coping, ineffective family: compromised;* and (2) *Coping, ineffective family:*

disabling (Kim et al., 1984). The characteristics that seem most relevant include preoccupations with fear, guilt, anxiety, withdrawal, agitation, depression, aggression, and hostility and impaired restructuring of a meaningful life. It must be noted, however, that these characteristics are derived from adults and have not been tested.

THE INTERVENTION

Sibling support, or promoting the interests of siblings, is implemented through a variety of methods. Variables that affect implementation of sibling support include (1) setting, (2) developmental level of the sibling, (3) condition of the ill child, and (4) sociocultural factors.

Settings in which sibling support is given will vary a great deal. In community settings, parents may be staying at the hospital with siblings visiting frequently. In larger hospitals, one or both parents may be staying at the hospital but siblings are not visiting for a variety of reasons, including lack of sibling visitation policies. In these latter settings, nurses do not always have access to siblings and they must intervene through parents and community resources.

Making an Indirect Connection to Siblings

Nurses who intervene without access to siblings are functioning under tremendous disadvantages in both assessment and interventions. Parents are naturally anxious about their ill child and focus their emotional energy on that child, perhaps thinking that the needs of their healthy children can wait. Moreover, they may not have information on how well their other children are doing because the caretakers of their other children are not giving it to them. In addition, many caretakers are asked on short notice to care for siblings and do not know the siblings well enough to tell if they are having problems. As one neighbor noted, "She's an awfully quiet child and not eating much food, but I don't know if that's normal or not." Grandparents are placed in an especially difficult situation. They love their grandchildren but also want to protect their own children, who are already suffering

with worry over the ill child. For this reason, grandparents are sometimes careful to avoid superimposing another worry regarding the healthy children (Craft, 1985).

When assessments and the intervention of sibling support are based upon parental impressions, nurses are operating with inadequate data. Because of an inability to pick up cues from their healthy children or a lack of information, parents often do not perceive what siblings are experiencing. In spite of a great disadvantage, however, nurses without access to siblings can increase parental awareness of sibling needs, share information about common sibling responses, identify what parents can do to help, and refer siblings to community resources as indicated.

The awareness and sensitivity of parents to siblings can be increased by role-modeling awareness at admission and throughout the ill child's hospitalization. During the admission process, a patient history is taken, which should include questions regarding the number of other children in the family and their names. After these questions have been asked, nurses can inquire about siblings with questions such as, "How are they reacting to this experience?" or more specifically, "Where are they staying?" These questions can be followed by a simple statement, such as "Hospitalization of a family member is difficult for the whole family," which conveys an awareness that the children at home are also going through a period of change and potential stress. Importantly, these questions set the stage for information on sibling visitation policies, with encouragement to bring siblings to the hospital whenever possible.

Throughout the hospitalization period, nurses can foster parental awareness of sibling welfare by keeping their discussion focused on the entire family. Parents ought to be encouraged to bring pictures of their other children to the hospital. Nurses can learn the siblings' names and ask about them through daily interaction with parents. If parents have not communicated with siblings, they should be encouraged to do so, with a brief statement by the nurse about how much the call or letter will mean to family members at home.

Realistically, some parents will be too anxious to focus on the needs of their other children. In these instances, nurses will need to work to lower parental anxiety through use of communication skills (Egan, 1985) as well as by providing information (Johnson, 1972; Johnson et al., 1978; Hartfield et al., 1982; Wells, 1982) so that parents are able to appreciate what their other children might be experiencing. Parents will signal their readiness to expand their focus to the whole family by their ability to concentrate and attend to nursing questions and discussions regarding the family.

Information Sharing and Communication

The second step in sibling support is to share information regarding common sibling responses and what parents can do to help (Craft, 1979; Craft et al., 1985; Craft, 1985; Craft, 1986; Craft and Craft, 1989; Knafl, 1982; Kruger et al., 1980; Taylor, 1980). Parents should be told that siblings commonly experience changes in feelings and behavior. The most common changes are wanting to spend more time with parents, followed by a decrease in the amount of food eaten, getting nervous more often, and increased trouble concentrating (Craft, 1985; Craft, 1986). Further, the hospitalization of a brother or sister can produce enough stress to cause adverse effects in siblings. Like nurses, parents who are exhibiting a sensitivity to the needs of their other children can use the PCS or question their children about changes in their experiences since hospitalization of the ill child. The results can be used as an index of sibling response. That is, parents of siblings who report a high number of changes in feelings and behaviors should be more concerned than parents of siblings who report little change.

As mentioned previously, a few variables have been isolated through research that are significantly related to adverse effects in siblings. Identification of these variables not only assists parents in recognizing which of their children are most likely to be at risk, but also pinpoints factors that can be altered to aid siblings. For example, parents need to be encouraged to provide honest information to their other children. If there is a realistic chance that the healthy siblings can get the illness of the hospitalized child, the topic ought to be addressed openly with a discussion of how the illness can be detected and managed. However, if the chance of the healthy children getting the illness is non-existent, parents should reassure them in order to prevent the development of fear. Other variables that can be altered are provisions for child care, the nature of explanations, and patterns of parenting. Nurses should urge parents to arrange care of siblings in their own home, with relatives or close friends as baby-sitters when possible. Further, siblings should be given an open explanation regarding the events shaping their lives. This type of open communication should become an ongoing part of family life, whether the ill child is hospitalized or being seen in a clinic. Open sharing of specific information, such as lab tests, prevents the misinterpretation of such data, which can occur when it is partially overheard by siblings. Parental honesty with siblings conveys parental trust that siblings can cope with what is happening. Last, parents need to be exhorted to maintain their present parenting patterns or styles. That is, their discipline, expectations, time commitment, and affection toward all of their children should remain as consistent as possible. This consistency promotes sibling security and a sense that their importance has not changed. The normal sibling rivalry is often accelerated during hospitalization of a child, when the scarce time and attention of parents becomes especially meaningful to the children at home. It becomes essential, therefore, for parents to convey their love and appreciation of the sacrifices being made by siblings whenever they visit their children, call them, or communicate in any other fashion.

Communication with children at home is crucial, and nurses can suggest a variety of communication possibilities to parents. First, telephone calls home are meaningful even to the youngest children, since the sound of their parents' voices offers reassurance that their parents are still around and love them. In a similar vein, tape-recorded voices of both parents and siblings offer a more lengthy opportunity to communicate, even though the information exchange is delayed. Those families who own a video-cassette player and video camera may even wish to film activity at the hospital so that it can be viewed by the children at home. Equally meaningful to some children is receiving letters and cards containing reminders of appreciation and love. Younger children may especially appreciate lipstick kisses sent on postcards. In most instances, the most helpful type of communication is a visit by the siblings to the hospital, where siblings can see the ill child and their parents and learn firsthand what is happening. Hospital visitation is critical for young siblings who cannot comprehend an abstract explanation of events. Therefore, nurses should do all they can to facilitate sibling visitation, even for those families with a residence that is a long distance from the hospital.

When parents or nurses are concerned about the children at home, referral possibilities need to be explored. Visits to school counselors, social workers, and nurses are plausible options, since most school-age children spend a majority of their day in school. In fact, an ideal situation is one in which a school nurse referral would be made automatically whenever a child is hospitalized, so that school personnel would be on the alert for cues of adverse sibling responses. Other referral options include family clergy and community mental health centers.

Helping Siblings Directly

This discussion has shown how nurses can implement sibling support through indirect efforts when they do not have access to siblings. They can work to increase parental awareness, share helpful information, promote family communication, and refer siblings to community professionals. However, these nurses may have little or no opportunity to assess siblings directly or teach siblings about the nature of the illness and illness management of the hospitalized child. Fortunately, many nurses in community hospital settings, schools, and home visiting agencies do have these opportunities. These nurses can provide support directly through use of communication skills, teaching, and referral.

Unfortunately, too often siblings are truly the neglected "other" family members (Craft, 1979). Their parents may expect them to cope on their own, to be flexible enough to handle whatever comes, and, in general, to hold a "stiff upper lip." For these reasons, siblings might not share grief, anger, jealousy, or anxiety with their parents. While siblings are often hesitant to express negative feelings to parents, whom they perceive as being overwhelmed, nurses are probably perceived as "safe" listeners. This advantage offers an opportunity to incorporate communication interventions. Nurses, then, have an opportunity to become active listeners and to assist siblings to explore and clarify their concerns through the utilization of communication skills (Egan, 1985). Three other avenues for listening, exploration, and problem solving are suggested. First, use of the PCS is helpful as a listening tool, since it elicits specific information. Second, use of drawings, puppetry, and dramatic play provide a glimpse of how younger children perceive events, as is noted in Chapters 7 and 8. Last, peer sibling groups offer the ideal avenue for sibling communication of feelings, problem exploration, and clarification (Moses, 1982) (see Chapter 13). Nurses who have long-term contact with siblings can go beyond the stage of problem exploration and clarification to goal-setting and problem-solving strategies (Egan, 1985).

The use of communication skills enables nurses to identify what siblings know about the ill child's condition and illness management in order to set teaching goals. Usually, there is a need for a great deal of teaching, since siblings should know as much as the patient or parents. When parents are highly anxious, they may have given the well children little or no information. In these instances, nurses must tell siblings about the illness and reassure them that they are not likely to get the illness (when appropriate) and that they did nothing to cause the illness. From this point, an explanation of the illness follows, delivered at an appropriate developmental level.

The next teaching goal includes preparing siblings themselves as communicators. When a child is hospitalized and the parents are unavailable to community members, it is the other children in the family who are placed in the position of conveying information about the ill child and parents and even teaching others about the illness. Professionals have a responsibility to prepare siblings for this role. The content included in such a preparation should incorporate information about the anticipated illness management and suggestions for explanations to peers, teachers, and extended family members. Siblings not only function as communicators but they also can help in many other avenues. They need to know what they can do to help their family during this period. Their knowledge and assistance will offer tangible help to their family. But, as important, this knowledge will foster development or mastery of the situation. For example, a school-aged sibling can be taught to assist with dressing changes or a teenager can be taught to assist with colostomy bag changes. The content hospital nurses can teach siblings will vary with each patient. However, universal nursing goals include that siblings are (1) aware that they did not cause the illness, (2) able to realistically discuss the probability of getting the illness, (3) openly expressing positive and negative feelings, (4) learning about the illness and illness management as exhibited by the ability to correctly answer questions, (5) identifying ways to help the family, (6) discussing methods of dealing with peers and other community members, and (7) discovering methods of helping themselves to get through this difficult period. The content to meet these teaching goals is delivered when siblings visit their hospitalized brother or sister. The content can be planned and delivered systematically, or it can be delivered incidentally as the nurse is giving care and explaining the care to siblings.

Other nurses can help siblings in the school system. Anytime a child is hospitalized, school nurses can use events as teaching opportunities. For example, content on the pathophysiology can be presented in order to enhance student learning on anatomy and physiology. These occasions also lend opportunities to introduce content on coping and expressing feelings. This content will not only benefit students scholastically, but it will increase peer empathy for siblings.

Nurses who are able to interact with siblings have a more valid picture of sibling experiences and have opportunities for communication and teaching. In addition, options for referral are often greater since a core of helping professionals is located in one setting. This group of professionals have immediate knowledge of the experiences of the hospitalized child and can interpret events accurately to siblings. Once nurses have determined that referral is necessary, hospital-based psychologists, social workers, and clinical nursing specialists can be

contacted to meet with siblings when they visit the hospital.

The application of sibling support is affected by sibling accessibility, or the setting in which nurses practice. Other variables that will affect sibling support intervention are each sibling's developmental stage, condition of the hospitalized child, and socio-cultural factors.

Variables Influencing Sibling Support

Sibling Developmental Stage

In some ways, a sibling's developmental stage can be used by nurses to anticipate siblings' needs. For example, siblings who are one to two years of age will probably react more to separation from parents than separation from the ill child. Further, preschool children will require hands-on learning and concrete information, indicating that it is critical for younger children to visit the hospital in order to see their parents and the ill child. When these visits are impossible, concrete substitutes must be used, such as photographs or films. In contrast, older teenagers can handle abstract explanations of events. Similarly, during this developmental period, it can be expected that teenagers will be concerned about potential peer rejection. As one 16 year old boy stated to the author, "My biggest problem right now is what my girlfriend thinks about my brother's illness." These examples illustrate the application of developmental knowledge for predicting needs and implementing sibling support. Caution must be used, however, in assigning a developmental stage that is synonymous with chronological age, since siblings may regress both emotionally and cognitively because of the stress surrounding hospitalization of a brother or sister (Carandag et al., 1979).

Nature of Illness

The condition of the hospitalized child is a variable that will have significant impact on implementation of sibling support. Use of this variable can be illustrated by two disparate examples. First, consider the child who is flown into a pediatric intensive care unit in a comatose state from an unknown etiology. Siblings may be staying with anyone who could watch them on an emergency basis. Parents might want to explain the situation to their children at home, but they do not have any information because the doctors do not know what is happening. In contrast, consider the situation in which a child with cystic fibrosis is admitted for intravenous antibiotic therapy because of decreased pulmonary function. In the first situation, the nurse's support of the siblings will consist of managing parental anxiety, fostering parental awareness of sibling welfare, and encouraging parental communication with siblings, just to let them know the ill child is still alive and the parents care about them. If siblings are able to visit, the nurse can explain what is being done and answer all of their questions. In life-threatening situations where parental anxiety is extremely high, nurses will frequently fulfill the support and advocacy role customarily assumed by parents. In the second case, siblings could be frequent visitors to the hospital, where nurses could assess, communicate, and teach individually or in peer support groups. The condition of the hospitalized child, then, greatly affects the family organization and their ability to mobilize resources. The sensitive nurse will implement sibling support using knowledge of the ill child's condition to assist in selection of implementation strategies.

Sociocultural Variables

There are numerous sociocultural variables affecting implementation of sibling support. The three variables that will be addressed in this discussion are family structure, economic status, and coping expectations.

One of the most profound historical factors affecting children of this generation is the changing family structure. The structure of a family will affect family response to crisis. One family structure that seems especially vulnerable during periods of crisis is the single-parent family. The single parent is usually employed on a full-time basis and may not be able to take time off from the job. Moreover, this parent must deal with a hospitalized child as well as the needs of siblings. These draining responsibilities produce fatigue rapidly. Fortunately, extended family members and close friends help in some instances.

Another situation that is unique for this generation is the large number of children who are living with stepparents. Stepparents are often caring for siblings at home, while the natural mother is at the hospital with the ill child. These parents may not recognize sibling problems simply because they do not know the children well. In addition, siblings may be still developing trust in the stepparent if the change in family structure was recent. During data collection for one investigation, Craft noted that many children had experienced a change in family structure within six months of the hospitalization event (Craft, 1985). Therefore, it is not unusual for siblings to have experienced a major change in family structure close to the hospitalization of a brother or sister, meaning that two crises have occurred concurrently. This situation can alter assessment and evaluation along with implementation of sibling support. That is, nurses might assume that siblings who have a high PCS score are reacting to the hospitalization of a brother or sister, when, in fact, their most immediate concern is that their own father or mother is no longer available to provide comfort. Similarly, nurses may unknowingly approach a stepparent about sibling welfare, when the natural parent actually has the baseline data on, sensitivity to, and awareness of sibling responses. For these reasons, then, sibling support can be effectively implemented only when nurses are knowledgeable about family structure and the impact of this structure on implementation of sibling support.

Another major sociocultural variable affecting sibling support is the financial status of the family. Financial status affects decisions to make extra trips to bring siblings to the hospital, ability to pay for qualified child care when parents must be gone, and potential sacrifices faced by siblings because of the costs of the child's illness. Importantly, financial strains cause increased parental anxiety, which siblings often do not understand. This increased parental anxiety can lead to changes in parenting patterns, which are related to sibling responses (Craft, 1985).

The last sociocultural variable that will be addressed is parental coping expectations, or how parents teach their children to handle stressful events. Parental beliefs about health and illness will be related to these expectations (Wu, 1973). As one mother told the author, "In our family, we teach our children to make the best of everything. If something happens that is hard to take, we just all hang together and help one another." Another mother stated, "Our other children know that whatever happens is up to God and not ours to question. We just wait for the will of God." In the first situation, siblings might be expected to react positively toward a request for assistance with exercises for a child with cerebral palsy. In the second situation, siblings might be somewhat more passive. Unfortunately, we do not know enough about the effects of health beliefs on responses. While nurses are aware that parents try to instill values and beliefs in their children, research is needed to determine the effects of these values and beliefs on responses of children to illness.

To summarize, the sibling support intervention will be used by nurses in diverse settings, with siblings at various developmental stages. The intervention will be affected by the practice settings, the condition of the hospitalized child, and numerous sociocultural variables, as illustrated in the case study described below, in which the nurse had limited access to the siblings.

EVALUATION

Evaluation of the sibling support intervention can be accomplished by comparing sibling perception of changes prior to the intervention of sibling support with changes perceived following the intervention.

It is essential to note that sibling assessment through parent perception may not be accurate. Parent perception and sibling perception have differed in four studies done by Craft (1979, 1985, 1986; Craft et al., 1985), suggesting that communication between parents and siblings is affected by the stress surrounding the hospitalization of a child (Craft, 1985). Results of a study by Craft soon to be published show that the only variable related significantly to level of agreement between parents and siblings was sibling age. Level of agreement increased with increased parent-sibling contact for older siblings, but did not increase for younger siblings.

Importantly, use of the defining characteristics can also provide criteria for measuring intervention outcomes. That is, reversal of the defining characteristics can be a portion of data which suggests that the intervention has been effective. This approach to measurement of intervention outcome lacks precision, however. Use of the PCS to determine changes is recommended

Case Study

Four year old Danny S. had been diagnosed with acute lymphocytic leukemia for over two years. He had a sister, Amy, who was eight years old and a brother, Max, who was eleven years old. The parents' marriage was intact, and a large supportive network of relatives and friends lived close to Danny's home. His father was a farmer, and his mother did not work outside the home. Since Danny's diagnosis, his parents had taken him to two medical centers in different parts of the country for administration of experimental chemotherapeutic agents.

When the nurse, Kathy, first met this family, both parents were in the room with Danny. Within a two minute period, Danny made six requests of his parents, who jumped up immediately to get Danny what he wanted, which was never just quite right. When Kathy inquired about the welfare of Amy and Max, Mrs. S. rapidly verbalized her concerns. She stated that Amy had been staying with one relative and Max had been staying with another relative for a good portion of the last two years. The family was together only when Danny was in remission. Her husband's brother, she further noted, had experienced an illness when he was a child. Mr. S. had become jealous and still harbored much resentment and bitterness toward his brother. Mrs. S. expressed fear that her own children would develop these same feelings. She noted that her two children at home were staying away from friends, fighting, and doing poorly at school. Danny's mother talked very rapidly and jumped up to meet Danny's needs several times during this discussion. Danny's father had left the room to get his son some crayons. When Danny started screaming in rage because his father was not back, Kathy agreed to see Amy and Max when they visited on the weekend and tried to help Mrs. S. with Danny.

On Saturday, Kathy visited with Amy and Max in the recreation room, away from family members. They were both quiet and interacted briefly, but moved about the room frequently. In addition, they seemed to pick reasons to fight and argue. Kathy administered the PCS to determine their perception of changes. They both had high scores on the PCS. After completion of the scale, Amy and Max went back to Danny's room, which was full of adults. No interaction between the parents, Max, and Amy was observed. Kathy used the defining characteristics of withdrawal, aggression, and agitation and the PCS data for her diagnosis of *Ineffective coping*.

When Kathy met with Danny's mother on Monday, Mrs. S. expressed concern about the scores, but again jumped up every time Danny wanted something during the interaction. She talked constantly, and Kathy could say little. Finally, an opportunity arose for Kathy to ask permission for exploring sibling counseling possibilities in the home community. Mrs. S. gave her consent immediately and then went back to Danny.

Kathy discovered several resources in the community school system. The school social worker was contacted; she already knew of the situation and the difficulties Amy and Max were having concentrating on their studies and their withdrawal from other children. Kathy was told that their friends ridiculed them frequently, because these children could not understand why Amy and Max were always moving from family to family. Max was also in the principal's office frequently for fighting. Kathy set up a telephone conference call with the school nurse and social worker in which plans were made to deal with the first priority, to help Amy and Max deal with ridicule by the other children.

The school nurse felt that both teachers and students needed more information about new forms of leukemia treatment. Content was developed, and the school nurse presented several classes on leukemia. Next, the social worker began seeing Amy and Max weekly. Kathy continued to see them weekly at the hospital and used communication suggestions from the psychiatric clinical nursing specialist. After several discussions with Mr. and Mrs. S., Kathy was able to get them to agree on two changes. First, the parents agreed to have both Amy and Max stay at the home of an aunt for all hospitalization periods. Second, the parents set aside two hours every weekend during the visit by Amy and Max to the hospital to leave the hospital and do something fun with them. Two months later, Amy and Max were getting higher grades in school and interacting normally with other children. Mrs. S. also left the hospital to attend open house at their school.

RESEARCH IMPLICATIONS

Because the question of sibling response upon illness of children has been a neglected area of behavioral science, much work is needed. First, measurement of sibling response needs additional research. While measurement of response in older siblings is reliable and valid, further work is indicated on the scale for younger siblings (Craft, 1986). In addition, measurement instruments to assess response of siblings under five years of age should be developed. While

Craft (1985) has been working in this area for seven years, her research deals with adverse effects and high-risk siblings only, leaving untouched the potential for growth in siblings that exists with every crisis. Next, continued research is needed to examine those variables that are predictive of sibling response. Larger sample sizes are needed for multiple regression and path analysis to determine the causal flow of variables. Also, cross-validation studies are required to establish external validity of findings. Even though Craft has studied the relationship of 14 independent variables on sibling response, other variables need to be added to this list in order to account for a larger proportion of variance in sibling response. These variables include (1) family structure, (2) the number of adverse life events occurring concurrently to either siblings or siblings' caretaker, (3) parental health and illness beliefs, and (4) potential emotional or cognitive regression in siblings.

Next, longitudinal research is indicated to separate the different effects of separation and illness as well as to determine what periods are most problematic for siblings and when intervention is most helpful. Last, intervention strategies require investigation with experimental designs in order to identify those interventions that are most effective. These strategies may include the bidirectional nature of sibling relationships in which siblings motivate each other to increased levels of functioning. Such a study, conducted by Craft and her colleagues, showed that siblings can act as change agents to significantly increase functional status in children with cerebral palsy. Further, the siblings expressed increased knowledge of the condition of their brother or sister as well as increased self-esteem (Craft et al., 1989).

References

Baskett, LM, and Johnson, SM. The young child's interactions with parents versus siblings: A behavioral analysis. Child Development, 5:643–650, 1982.

Bassard, JHS, and Ball, E. The sociology of child development. New York: Harper and Row Publishers, Inc., 1960.

Cairns, NU, Clark, GM, Smith, S, and Lansky, SB. Adaptation of siblings to childhood malignancy. The Journal of Pediatrics, 9:487–492, 1979.

Carandang, MLA, Folkins, CH, Hines, PA, and Steward MS. The role of cognitive level and sibling illness in children's conceptualization of illness. American Journal of Orthopsychiatry, 49:474–481, 1979.

Cicirelli, VG. Effects of sibling structure and interaction on children's categorization style. Developmental Psychology, 9:132–139, 1973.

Cicirelli, VG. Effects of mother and older siblings on the problem-solving behavior of the older child. Developmental Psychology, 11:749–756, 1975.

Cicirelli, VG. Siblings helping siblings. In Allen, VL (Ed.), Inter-age interaction in children. New York: Academic Press, Inc., 1976.

Cicirelli, VG. Children's school grades and sibling structure. Psychological Reports, 41:1055–1058, 1977.

Cicirelli, VG. Effects of sibling presence on mother-child interaction. Developmental Psychology, 14:315–316, 1978.

Craft, M. Help for the family's neglected "other" child. MCN: American Journal of Maternal Child Nursing, 4:300–304, 1979.

Craft, M, Wyatt, N, and Sandell, B. Variables related to behavior changes in siblings of hospitalized children. In Felton, G, and Albert, M (Eds.), Nursing research: A monograph for non-nurse researchers. Iowa City, Iowa: University of Iowa Press, 1983.

Craft, M. Responses in siblings of hospitalized children. Unpublished doctoral dissertation, University of Iowa, Iowa City, Iowa, 1985.

Craft, M, Wyatt, N and Sandell, B. Feeling and behavior changes in siblings of hospitalized children. Clinical Pediatrics, 97:374–378, 1985.

Craft M. Responses in siblings of hospitalized children: Validation of self-report data. Children's Health Care, 15:6–14, 1986.

Craft, M, and Wyatt, N. Effect of visitation upon siblings of hospitalized children. Maternal-Child Nursing Journal, 15:47–59, 1986.

Craft, M, and Opplinger, B. The effects of a pediatric hospitalization of siblings as measured by the Perceived Change Scale. In review process, 1989.

Craft, M, Lakin, J, Oppliger, B, Clancy, G, and Vanderlinden, D. Siblings as change agents for increasing the functional status of children with cerebral palsy. Manuscript in preparation, 1989.

Craft, M, and Craft, J. Perceived changes in siblings of hospitalized children: A comparison of sibling and parent reports. Children's Health Care, 18:42–48, 1989.

Dittes, JE. Birth order and vulnerability to differences in acceptance. American Psychologist, 16:358–368, 1961.

Dunn, J. Sibling relationships in early childhood. Child Development, 54:787–811, 1983.

Egan, G. The skilled helper (3rd ed.). Monterey, Calif.: Brooks/Cole Publishing Co., 1985.

Gath, A. The mental health of siblings of congenitally abnormal children. Journal of Children's Psychology and Psychiatry, 13:217–225, 1965.

Guyulay, J. The dying child. New York: McGraw-Hill, Inc., 1978.

Harris, I. The promised seed: A comparative study of eminent first and later sons. Glencoe, Ill: Free Press, 1964.

Hartfield, C, Cason, C, and Cason, C. Effects of information about threatening procedures on patients' expectations and emotional distress. Nursing Research, 31:202–206, 1982.

Iles, PJ. Children with cancer: Healthy siblings' perspectives during the illness experience. Cancer Nursing, 2:371–377, 1979

Johnson, J. Effects of structuring patients' expectations on their reactions to threatening events. Nursing Research, 21:492–499, 1972.

Johnson, JE, Rice, VH, Fuller, SS, and Endress, MP. Sensory information, instruction in a coping strategy, and recovery from surgery. Research in Nursing and Health, 1:4–17, 1978.

Kim, MJ, McFarland, GV, and McLane, AM. Nursing diagnosis. St. Louis: CV Mosby Co., 1984.

Knafl, KA. Parents' views of the responses of siblings to a pediatric hospitalization. Research in Nursing and Health, 5:13–20, 1982.

Koch, HL. The relation of certain family constellation characteristics and the attitudes of children toward adults. Child Development, 26:13–40, 1955a.

Koch, HL. Some personality correlates of sex, sibling position, and sex of siblings among 5 and 6-year-old children. Genetic Psychology Monographs, 52:3–50, 1955b.

Koch, HL. Some emotional attitudes of the young child in relation to characteristics of the sibling. Child Development, 27:393–426, 1956.

Kruger, S, Shauver, M, and Jones, L. Reactions of families to the child with cystic fibrosis. Image, 12:72–76, 1980.

Lavigne, JV, and Ryan, M. Psychological adjustment of siblings of children with chronic illness. Pediatrics, 63:616–627, 1979.

Lawson, B. Chronic illness in school-aged children: Its effects on the total family. American Journal of Maternal Child Nursing, 4:32–38, 1977.

Majoribanks, K, Walberg, HJ, and Bergan, M. Mental abilities: Sibling constellations and social class correlates. British Journal of Social and Clinical Psychology, 14:109–116, 1975.

Mauksch, I. Illness and its impact on the family. Paper presented at the Changing Family Conference VII: The middle years. The University of Iowa, Iowa City, 1978.

McCollum, A. Coping with prolonged health impairment in your child. Boston: Little, Brown and Co., Inc., 1975.

Miller, N, and Zimbardo, DG. Similarity versus emotional comparison as motives for affiliation. Paper presented at the American Psychological Association meeting, Chicago, 1965.

Minnett, AM, Vandell, L, and Santrock, FW. The effects of sibling status on sibling interaction: Influence of birth order, age spacing, sex of child, and sex of sibling. Child Development, 54:1064–1072, 1983.

Moses, K. Brothers and sisters of special children: Waisman Center Inter-Actions, No. 1. Madison, Wisc.: University of Wisconsin Press, 1982.

Rosenberg, BC, and Sutton-Smith, B. Ordinal position and sex-role identification. Genetic Psychological Monographs, 70:297–328, 1964.

Scarr, S, and Grajek, S. Similarities and differences among siblings. In Lamb, ME, and Sutton-Smith, B (Eds.), Sibling relationships: Their nature and significance across the lifespan. Hillsdale, N.J.: Lawrence Erlbaum Associates, Inc., 1982.

Schachter, S. Birth order and sociometric choice. Journal of Abnormal and Social Psychology, 68:453–456, 1964.

Schoenberg, B, Case, AC, Peretz, C, and Kutscher, AH. Loss and grief: Psychological management in medical practice. New York: Columbia University Press, 1970.

Sears, RR. Ordinal position in the family as a psychological variable. American Sociological Review, 15:397–401, 1950.

Sutton-Smith, B, and Rosenberg, BC. The sibling. New York: Holt, Rinehart and Winston, Inc., 1970.

Taylor, SC. The effect of chronic childhood illness upon siblings. Maternal-Child Nursing Journal, 9:109–116, 1980.

Tew, B, and Laurence, KM. Mothers, brothers, and sisters of patients with spina bifida. Developmental Medicine and Child Neurology, 15:5–15, 1973.

Tuck, J. Impact of cystic fibrosis on family functioning. Pediatrics, 34:64–74, 1964.

Wagner, ME, Schubert, HJP, and Schubert, SP. Sibship-constellation effects on psychosocial development, creativity, and health. Advances in Child Development and Behavior, 14:57–148, 1979.

Walker, C.L. Stress and coping in siblings of childhood cancer patients. Nursing Research, 37: 208–212, 1988.

Webster's Ninth New Collegiate Dictionary. Springfield, Mass.: G & C Merriam Company, 1977.

Wells, N. The effect of relaxation on postoperative muscle tension and pain. Nursing Research, 31:236–238, 1982.

Wu, R. Behavior and illness. Englewood Cliffs, N.J.: Prentice-Hall, 1973.

Zagonc, RB, and Markus, GB. Birth order and intellectual development. Psychological Review, 82:74–88, 1975.

CHAPTER 4

FOSTERING FAMILY INTEGRITY

KATHY JAMISON KRAUS, M.A., R.N.

Most children spend their early years interacting with a person or group of persons whom they would define as "family." Although sociological definitions vary greatly, a child's family is considered to be the most significant source of physical and emotional support. Precisely because a child is so dependent upon the adult members of the family, events that disrupt or impair the ability of family members to perform their usual roles may have a very dramatic effect on the child.

Bowlby (1984) discusses the central feature of parenting as "the provision by both parents of a secure base from which a child or adolescent can make sorties into the outside world and to which he can return knowing that he will be welcomed, nourished physically and emotionally, comforted if

distressed, and reassured if frightened" (p. 276). The parental role has also been conceptualized as the fulfilling of the child's physical and emotional needs for love and security in a manner that changes in accord with the changing needs of the child (Lidz, 1970). For the purposes of this chapter, the term family will refer to that group of people who live with the child on a day to day basis and provide the child with physical, psychological, or emotional support.

The guiding premise of this chapter is that the maintenance of familiar family structure and communication patterns will be a positive factor in the child's ability to cope with illness or a change in health status. Inherent in this premise is the belief that nurses can plan and implement interventions that will specifically enhance or support family integrity and thereby promote the coping efforts of both the child and the family unit. The following discussion will examine the functions of a family from the child's perspective and the responses of families to stressful situations as a theoretical basis from which to develop nursing interventions that promote family integrity.

THEORETICAL FOUNDATION

Families define and respond to stressful situations in a variety of ways. A change in one family member, whether the change is in physical status, emotional well-being, or role within the family, inevitably has an impact on the family as a whole and can ultimately lead to a crisis situation if the family is unable to adapt to this change (Braulin et al., 1982). Baird (1979) defines crisis as an upset in steady state that occurs when events cannot be handled by the family's usual problem-solving techniques. Family members may become upset as they try various ineffective ways of coping, resulting in major disorganization if the problems cannot be solved or made tolerable.

Boss and Greenberg (1984) propose that it is the amount of ambiguity perceived by the family about whether a member is in or out of the family system that causes stress when a family member is ill or has died. They believe that uncertainty concerning family structure prevents reorganization and may often help explain a family's apparent inability to cope. Mishel (1983) has reported initial work in the development of a tool to measure what she perceives to be the four defining characteristics of uncertainty that are the major variables influencing a parent's experience with a sick child. The factors include (1) absence or vagueness of cues concerning the program of care for the child, (2) lack of clarity, (3) lack of information, and (4) inability to predict the symptoms and outcomes of the illness.

Hill (1965) states that a family's ability to deal with crisis depends on the adequacy of members' role performances as expectations shift and new patterns of interaction are worked out. He describes a conceptual framework for viewing families in crisis that has three major components. The first component is the family itself as an interacting

and transacting organization that has a specific repertoire of resources for dealing with crises and that may be more or less open to outside interventions. The second component is a precipitating event or stressor that is defined as a situation for which the family has had little or no prior preparation and is therefore viewed as problematic. The final component is the definition of the event as stressful—the component that transforms a stressor event into a crisis.

The concept of cognitive appraisal as the process used by individuals to distinguish potentially harmful from potentially beneficial events has been described by Lazarus and colleagues (1974). Primary appraisal is the initial judgment as to whether a given situation is harmful, beneficial, or irrelevant. Secondary appraisal involves the individual's perception of the range of coping alternatives that are of possible use in mastering the situation. Reappraisal of the situation is ongoing as the individual responds to changing conditions and cues that may alter his or her assessment of the situation.

While a successful experience in dealing with a crisis situation can ultimately test and strengthen a family, inability to resolve a situation can damage or destroy family structure and morale (Hill, 1965). Situations defined by the family as crises will generally result in disorganization and a temporary reduction in the ability of members to perform their usual roles (Braulin et al., 1982; Hymovich, 1976; Olsen, 1970). As the family experiments with new ways of coping, a reorganization occurs that will leave them either stronger, weaker, or dismembered (Hymovich, 1976).

Fife (1985) has developed a predictive model that utilizes role theory and is based on the belief that families that are disorganized before a crisis occurs will experience severe disruption during a crisis. She has developed a guide to assess the extent to which family roles were integrated prior to the crisis situation and proposes that family coping ability can be predicted based upon their pre-crisis level of function.

Health professionals who deal with children on a routine basis quickly become aware of the wide variation of family responses to a child's illness. "It is important to remember that there is really no such thing as being unable to cope; any behavior manifested by the parents is their way of coping with the situation" (Lewandowski, 1980, p. 84). Numerous researchers have studied the reactions of family members when a child becomes critically ill or is hospitalized (Epperson, 1977; Lansky et al., 1978; Lewandowski, 1980; Miles and Carter, 1982; Roskies et al., 1975; Skipper et al., 1968). Skipper and colleagues (1968) studied mothers of children undergoing tonsillectomy and found that the mothers suffered extreme anxiety that resulted in fearful, rigid behavior and a decreased ability to act rationally during the inital period of hospitalization. Similarly, Roskies et al. (1975) observed parents who brought their children to the emergency room of a children's medical center. Parents in this situation were preoccupied with the ramifications of their child's illness, passive in their relationship with hospital staff, and did not function well in the role of protector because much of their activity focused on making the child compliant with hospital procedures rather than supporting or comforting.

As might be expected, the unanticipated hospitalization of a child has been found to be more stressful for parents than an expected admission. Eberly et al. (1985) found that parents of children who were unexpectedly admitted to a pediatric intensive care unit had high scores in all dimensions of stress measured. Categories that were particularly stress inducing included parental role alteration, communication with staff, and response to the child's behavior and appearance.

An inductive approach was used by Miles and Carter (1982) to identify eight categories of stressors that parents experience when their child is hospitalized. These include (1) disturbing or unfamiliar sights and sounds, (2) child's appearance, (3) child's behavior, (4) child's emotional response, (5) procedures, (6) staff communication, (7) staff behaviors, and (8) parental role deprivation. Lewandowski (1980) found that parents use a variety of coping strategies to deal with the stresses imposed by the first visit to their child after open heart surgery. Some parents are initially immobilized and seem to cope by waiting and gathering their resources before initiating any contact with their child. Some use visual survey of the environment to become familiar with a new setting. Withdrawal, intellectualization, and restructuring the situation by focusing on only one

part of the child are other coping mechanisms parents use.

It is important to note at this point that hospitalization for some families may be seen as the solution to a preexisting crisis rather than a precipitating cause, particularly when the child is chronically ill (Ferraro, 1985; Roskies et al., 1975). Behaviors demonstrated by these families may vary significantly from those expected by health care professionals who are assuming the initiation of a crisis rather than its resolution.

Perhaps one of the major stressors caused by the illness or hospitalization of a child is the abrupt change required in the parental role. Knox and Hayes (1983) state that as many of the usual parenting tasks are deleted, changed, or taken over by others, the learning of new behaviors becomes extremely difficult because of the stress of the crisis situation. Parents experience fears related to the new environment and their inability to do anything to help the child as control is taken out of their hands.

Parents also may find that their expectations about their role in parenting the sick child may be incongruent with the expectations of the hospital staff (Knox and Hayes, 1983; Strauss, 1981). Parents in this situation may be labeled as "uncooperative" or may find their competence as parents questioned. Horowitz et al. (1982) claim that the authoritarian power structure within most hospitals minimizes parental authority and legitimacy as information about the child is controlled and decisions are made for the parents. One study indicated that while a majority of mothers preferred to perform many child care activities, few received any communication from hospital staff regarding activities that they were expected or would like to perform (Algren, 1985). Parents may feel threatened by the staff's ability to care skillfully and effectively for their child at a time when they may perceive themselves to have "failed" by allowing their child to become ill (Marino, 1980).

Illness or hospitalization of a child forces a family to restructure their lives and reorganize priorities. Knafl (1985) interviewed parents of hospitalized children and found that 94% felt that the sick child should become the focus of the family for the duration of the hospitalization. Other children in the family were given a secondary focus and were expected to participate more actively in family maintenance activities. A related study by Knafl et al. (1982) revealed that 11 of 13 working mothers missed work while a child was sick and spent much of their time in the hospital, while three of 13 fathers missed work by fitting visits to the hospital around existing work schedules. Siblings report that parents are in general less lenient, more preoccupied, and less likely to spend time with them (Craft et al., 1985). The effects of hospitalization on well siblings is discussed in Chapter 3.

Fathers in particular may have difficulty coping with a child's illness for many reasons (McKeever, 1981). They tend to spend less time in the hospital and, therefore, may receive less information and support from health care professionals. Many fathers cope by the use of denial and repression, remaining silent about their concerns and fears for the ill child and the family in general. Single-parent families may also be particularly vulnerable during the crisis of a sick child because they generally have fewer resources, both financial and emotional, upon which to draw (Burns, 1984). The need to continue to perform roles both at work and at home while trying to support the sick child rapidly compounds the stress and fatigue these parents experience.

The degree of marital discord and divorce caused by childhood illness is an area that has engendered much confusion and controversy. Masters et al. (1983) state that the impact on marriage is quite variable and stress that findings are difficult to interpret because there has been little effort to systematize them. Lansky et al. (1978) studied families of children with cancer and found that although marital stress levels were higher than those of the general population, the divorce rate was slightly lower. The analysis by Kalnins (1983) of qualitative studies of this topic also suggests that the divorce rate among parents of ill children was not any higher than that of the general population, that parents who did divorce rarely attributed it to the child's illness, and that many couples actually reported a strengthening of their marriage as a result of a child's illness.

ASSESSMENT

Interventions designed to maintain family integrity are indicated for use in situations where family instability would have a negative effect on the ill child. Maintenance of a familiar family structure, with members who are able to continue in their usual relationships with the child, not only supports the child's ability to cope with illness or stress but also increases the family's ability to successfully handle stressful situations.

Several nursing diagnoses (Gordon, 1982), when supported by adequate data, indicate a potential problem with family integrity. These diagnoses include (1) *Coping, ineffective family: disabling, compromised, or potential for growth,* and (2) *Parenting, alterations in: actual or potential.* A variety of data would support these diagnoses and indicate the need for specific nursing interventions. Parents or caretakers who seem to be unable to provide their usual nurturant or protective functions for an ill child may be incapacitated by stress and therefore may be ineffective in their parental roles. They often demonstrate passivity, indecisiveness, and an inability to provide comfort or support to the child. Overt conflict between parents or among any family members may signal the breakdown of usual roles and communication patterns. Although a family often attempts to present a united front to the world despite serious internal conflicts (Olsen, 1970), any discussion or behavioral evidence of family problems must be taken seriously and explored further.

Situations that precipitate a breakdown in family integrity are dependent almost entirely on the strengths and abilities of each family. The crisis-precipitating event must be one which the family perceives as stressful and for which they have no effective coping mechanisms (Hill, 1965). While a strong, well-organized family may be able to remain intact even after an event as stressful as the death of a child, another family may be paralyzed by the needs of a child who must spend a week in the hospital after an appendectomy.

Epperson (1977) studied families who were placed in severe, sudden stress situations and described a typical pattern of response. An initial period of high anxiety was characterized by physical agitation, high-pitched voice, fainting, nausea and vomiting, diarrhea, and other physical symptoms of stress. This was followed by a period of denial, which allowed the family enough hope to carry on for a time. These initial stages were followed by periods of anger and then remorse and grief. Only when the final stage of reconciliation was reached was the family able to begin mobilizing resources and coping effectively with the situation.

Fife et al. (1986) have developed an assessment tool specifically for use in evaluating the status of families of children with serious illnesses. The three areas of family functioning that the tool addresses are (1) interaction, (2) emotional adjustment, and (3) outpatient function. The tool is completed through observation and interview, and results in a numerical score that permits test-retest comparisons as the family progresses through the stressful situation.

Stein and Riessman (1980) have reported preliminary success in the development of an Impact-On-Family Scale that attempts to measure the long-term impact of chronic childhood illness on the family. Four dimensions of impact are measured, including financial, social and familial, personal strain, and mastery of the situation. Similarly, the assessment scale developed by Fife et al. (1986) is appropriate for use after a child's illness to gauge the effects of the stressful situation on family functioning.

The assessment guide that has been developed by Hymovich (1979) helps the practitioner to identify areas in which family functioning is adequate and areas where interventions are indicated. Two dimensions of family functioning are addressed: (1) developmental task attainment, and (2) the impact of major variables such as perceptions, resources, and coping abilities. A subsequently developed tool (Hymovich, 1984) helps the practitioner measure outcomes related to the impact of chronic illness on the family using three major subscales on stressors; (1) coping strategies, (2) values and attitudes, and (3) beliefs. The Coping Health Inventory for Parents (CHIP) developed by McCubbin (1984) operationally defines 45 specific coping behaviors used to identify family coping patterns.

THE INTERVENTION

Nursing interventions that are intended to support or maintain family integrity in the face of a stressful situation will vary widely in accordance with the perceived needs and strengths of the family. In this chapter, supporting the family will be defined as "promoting the interests or causes of" (Webster's Dictionary, 1987). Interventions should be initiated rapidly once a problem has been identified, with the goal of maintaining the family members in their usual roles to the extent possible or helping them to achieve satisfactory new roles.

Exploration of Existing Resources

Other appropriate actions at this point would be ones that would reduce extraneous stressors such as hunger, prolonged sleeplessness, lack of clean clothes, or financial concerns. The simple act of making family members feel physically comfortable may increase their ability to cope effectively with the situation at hand. A thorough examination of the situation would begin with a discussion of the family's perception of the situation and precipitating events. Exploration of their understanding and beliefs about the situation will help the nurse understand if and why these events precipitated a crisis in the family (Baird, 1979). The nurse may also observe family members for overt physical symptoms of stress such as tearfulness, nausea and vomiting, and distractibility.

The degree of disruption of the family should be explored, both by questioning and by observing family interactions. Situational stressors, such as the perceived need for parents to return to work, lack of transportation, or siblings at home needing care, may increase the family's level of stress, while the availability of social supports, such as grandparents, neighbors, or baby sitters, may help minimize family disruption (Baird, 1979; Braulin et al., 1982).

By definition, a crisis occurs when events cannot be handled with usual problem-solving or coping techniques (Baird, 1979). The usual coping patterns of the family can be a positive resource. They may be revealed through discussion of both the present situation and similar past situations. It is often necessary for the nurse to find similarities between the present event and past events, which then can be used by the family as they identify possible methods of dealing with the present crisis. During this process, it is important for the nurse to encourage verbalization of emotional responses and to foster hope in the family that the situation has positive aspects. Even when a negative outcome is inevitable, family members can sometimes focus on comforting aspects of the situation, such as the child's lack of pain (Baird, 1979; Braulin et al., 1982). Lewandowski (1980) stresses the importance of respecting whatever coping mechanisms the family is using. Rushing or pushing them into behaviors that the nurse thinks should be used may ultimately hinder the family's ability to develop coping patterns that best fit their style.

Family members often require help in dealing with their feelings and recognizing their normality. Epperson (1977) has documented some of the emotions families experience during stressful situations and has suggested ways of responding. During initial periods of high anxiety and stress, brief, accurate information should be given, and the family should be allowed ample time to talk and ask questions. This is often followed by a period of denial that is a necessary and adaptive defense mechanism. This defense should not be stripped away, but should be injected with reality as necessary. Feelings of anger toward the ill child or health care workers often cause a great deal of guilt within the parents, who need to be reassured that such feelings are normal and acceptable.

Providing Information

The provision of information about their child's status and support for parents early in the stressful period has been validated frequently in the literature as an essential nursing intervention. Hymovich (1976) has identified three basic tasks that parents must accomplish in order to successfully deal with a child's illness. First, parents must understand and manage the medical aspects of the illness. The nurse can help them accomplish this task by providing specific information about the illness and proposed treatment protocols, by directing them to appropriate resource agencies, and by giving the parents guidance and support as they learn. Second, parents must help their child understand and cope with his or her illness. Nurses can provide invaluable assistance by

helping parents understand how children of different ages respond to illness and hospitalization and by teaching parents adaptive ways to respond to the ill child's behaviors. Finally, parents of ill children must meet the needs of other family members, a task that becomes considerably more difficult as the length of illness increases.

Skipper et al. (1968) provided parents of tonsillectomy patients with a special nurse at the time of admission who focused on communicating information about the child's procedure and supporting the mother. They found that the amount of anxiety and stress perceived by these mothers was significantly less than that of the mothers who had no special nurses. Children of the prepared mothers were less fearful than those whose mothers were less prepared. In a similar study, Wolfer and Visintainer (1975) found that parents who received systematic psychological preparation and continued supportive care had lower self-ratings of anxiety and were more satisfied with their child's care than a control group who received no specific preparation.

Role Maintenance

Changes in usual family and parenting roles are stressful for all family members and indicate the need for nursing interventions directed specifically toward helping parents maintain their usual roles as much as is possible. Horowitz et al. (1982) claim that although institutions are increasingly allowing parents and families to perform more of their usual caretaking functions, those who do not conform to "good parent" stereotypes or who question the system may quickly find themselves in a battle with the nursing staff for control of the child's care. Marino (1980) states that nurses can deal with conscious or unconscious competition between parents and staff by recognizing that competition exists and by helping parents deal with normal feelings, such as insecurity about ill children and ambivalence about their ability to care competently for them.

Family members can be supported in their usual roles whether they "room in" with the child or visit on an inconsistent basis. An initial conference with parents is helpful in ascertaining what the preferences and capabilities of the parents are. While parents are frequently asked to "help" the nursing staff care for their child, it may be more effective to approach the child's care as a joint venture in which the responsibility is shared. Parents must be made to feel that their parenting expertise is valued and that their ability to comfort and interact with their child is a skill that cannot be duplicated.

Although the mother is often the parent who receives the bulk of staff support, it is crucial to recognize the major role that the father plays in the family constellation. Many fathers undertake the double role of continuing to work while trying to maintain some type of normal home life for other family members when a child is ill. Special efforts may need to be made to keep the father up to date about his child's condition or to provide him with access to physicians and other caretakers during the times he can visit. Because men tend to be less verbal about their anxieties, fears, and concerns, providing emotional support to the father requires a perceptive, thoughtful nurse who recognizes his special needs (McKeever, 1981).

The needs of siblings are addressed in Chapter 3, but in the context of this discussion it needs to be emphasized that their reactions to a stressful situation will have a significant impact on the rest of the family. Parents are faced immediately with the difficult task of balancing the needs of the ill child against those of the rest of the family and often require support in making difficult decisions. It may be hard for parents to appreciate the long-term implications of family disruption at a time when they are overly concerned about the welfare of one particular family member. The nurse may need to stress the importance of finding time for various family members to be alone together away from the stresses of the sick child and the hospital environment. Planning for a substitute caretaker to stay for an evening while the parents go out together or spend time with siblings may facilitate or enhance family communication and integrity.

It is possible for family members to maintain contact and continuity of roles even if geographical or other problems prevent frequent contact. The use of telephone calls, tape recordings of daily events, cards, letters, or photographs may help maintain relationships between the ill child and other family members when face-to-face contact is impossible.

Variables Related to Outcome of Interventions

Prior discussion has emphasized that families are complex systems that demonstrate unique responses to stressful or challenging situations. A number of variables affect the ability of the nurse to intervene successfully in any given situation.

In order for crisis or stress reduction interventions to succeed, the nurse must have accurately assessed the situation as stressful or crisis producing for the family. Hill (1965) emphasizes that the entire family's definition of the event as stressful, regardless of the perception of the primary caretaker, is the component that transforms a stressor into a crisis. If the nurse expects or assumes family problems where none exist, interventions may be inappropriate at the least and at the worst, counterproductive (Ferraro and Longo, 1985). Similarly, situations that seem minor or inconsequential to the nurse may overwhelm a poorly organized family.

Family structure and repertoire of coping mechanisms will affect their ability to deal successfully with a crisis. Nursing interventions must become more or less structured and directive as dictated by the needs of each individual family. A poorly organized family with few coping skills might require more direct assistance and have less success in dealing with crisis than a better organized, more resilient family. Knafl (1985) found that families in which all members participated actively in responding to the stressful situation had little need for outside help or support, while those that had less participation required more extensive help.

Knox and Hayes (1983) have identified several variables that they feel have a positive impact on the family's ability to adapt to the hospitalization of a child. Among these variables are the nurse's ability to trust the caregivers and to engage in open, honest communication with them. Hall and Weaver (1974) claim that families may use crises as growth-producing events if they are able to attain cognitive mastery of the situation. These findings emphasize the need for the nurse to provide honest, consistent information to families and to be available to help them gain an understanding of the situation.

The availability of situational supports is a variable widely mentioned in the literature (Baird, 1979; Braulin et al., 1982; Hall and Weaver, 1974; Knox and Hayes, 1983). The provision of such basics as food, money, and a place to sleep will greatly enhance the amount of physical and emotional energy that are available to solve problems. A related variable is the number of situational stressors that are competing for family energies. They may include such distractions as other children at home with no caretaker, lack of transportation, and concern about job responsibilities. It must never be assumed that the hospitalization of the child is the only crisis facing the family.

Nurses have enormous power to provide or enhance situational supports through the use of agency resources, but often neglect to do so. Nurses may intervene to reduce stressors by helping the family solve problems and draw upon available resources, as well as by referral to appropriate social service and community agencies.

EVALUATION

The ultimate goal of nursing intervention in a stressful or crisis situation is the facilitation of the family's adaptation and the return of their ability to function at a pre-crisis level or higher. Measurement of this goal is often difficult because assessment of pre-crisis function is rarely possible. However, evaluation of family functioning after intervention can be done through observation of reversal of the behaviors that supported the nursing diagnoses; self-report by the family that "things have returned to normal"; or through the use of tools designed to measure family coping skills, level of functioning, and utilization of resources. While such tools are designed to assess family coping style, perceptions, and strengths, when used over a period of time they may also yield data that show growth in the area of family functioning. Evaluation data will assist nurses in knowing what intervention strategies do, in fact, make a difference in fostering family integrity, and will provide the profession with a knowledge base upon which to make decisions about how to most

effectively support families through a crisis situation.

Case Study

John Parker was a one year old white male with a cleft lip and palate who had recently been admitted to the hospital with a diagnosis of sepsis thought to be related to recurrent otitis media. John had been hospitalized at age six weeks for repair of his lip, and his parents were planning to have John's palate repaired at about age 18 months. Prior to the current admission, John had been hospitalized several times with upper respiratory infections.

Mrs. Parker was a 35 year old woman who had quit her job as a teacher when John was born with a defect. She was an active member of La Leche League and seemed to derive a great deal of satisfaction from participation in their programs. Mr. Parker was employed as a salesman for a local manufacturing firm. Three other children, ages five, eight, and ten years, completed the family unit, which had seemed relatively stable and secure during John's previous hospitalizations.

After John had been in the hospital for several days, the primary nurse realized that although Mrs. Parker had rarely left John's bedside, neither her husband nor any of the other children had been in to visit. Mrs. Parker stated that the rest of her family had become used to her absences during John's hospitalizations and that her husband had too much to do at home to worry about coming in to visit.

After several days of antibiotics, John's condition had not improved. Mrs. Parker became increasingly distracted and sleepless, talking incessantly to anyone who would listen. She hovered over John's bed, monitoring his status constantly, and reported the slightest variations in his condition to his nurse. She continued to have almost no contact with her husband or children, communicating with them entirely through brief telephone conversations.

Despite Mrs. Parker's denial that there were any family problems, the primary nurse concluded that the integrity of the family was at risk and that specific interventions were indicated. This assessment was based both on her observation of Mrs. Parker's behavior and her knowledge of this family's interaction patterns during past hospitalizations. She decided that her first priority must be to decrease Mrs. Parker's level of physical stress and thereby increase her ability to look at the situation calmly and rationally. Special provisions were made for a staff member whom Mrs. Parker trusted to stay in the room with John while she made quick trips home to shower, nap, and change clothes. Although she refused to go home for the night, she did agree to sleep in a quiet room down the hall where she could rest more peacefully.

As John's condition improved and Mrs. Parker began to get more rest, the primary nurse talked to her about the needs of the rest of her family. Mrs. Parker revealed that she harbored a great deal of guilt about John's defect and felt that she was the only person who could really meet his needs. She recognized that the rest of her family also had needs that were not being met, but she could not bring herself to "abandon" her youngest child when he was so ill. As the discussions progressed, Mrs. Parker and the primary nurse talked about ways in which she could begin delegating some of John's care to other family members or trusted adults. They also discussed the potential effects that her intense emotional and time commitment to John and his problems could have upon her relationship with her husband. In addition, they discussed the need to begin including Mr. Parker in the day-to-day experiences of John's hospitalization.

For the remainder of the hospitalization, the nursing staff made a consistent effort to collaborate with Mrs. Parker in giving John's care. Their goal was to respect her expertise, yet demonstrate that they could care for John competently during the times she chose to go home. The nurses made special efforts to arrange visiting times for Mr. Parker and John's siblings that would be pleasant and positive and subsequently noted that the frequency of their visits increased.

When John was discharged, the primary nurse made two referrals in an effort to provide ongoing support for this family, which would continue to experience stress related to John's medical condition. One referral was to a local chapter of a cleft lip and palate parent support group. The other referral was to the local family counseling center, where Mr. and Mrs. Parker could gain insight into and understanding of their responses to their son's problems. The nurse also began work on a long-term plan of care that she hoped would anticipate and help prevent similar family problems during subsequent hospitalizations.

RESEARCH IMPLICATIONS

The profound impact of childhood illness upon families has long been recognized, and initial efforts have been made to document the extent of the impact. Continued study of the responses of families to stressful situations, both immediate and long term, is needed to strengthen the theoretical base upon which interventions are planned and evaluated.

Of particular importance is the need to study the impact of illness upon the family in relation to specific stressors rather than disease categories. Assessing the impact of known variables such as family structure, length of hospital stay, or illness outcome, regardless of the causative disease, would allow research results to be contrasted, compared, and generalized to larger populations.

Much of the research to date has focused on the development of assessment tools to measure the initial impact of illness on family members. These efforts should be further refined in reliability and validity and be expanded to be useful in measuring family impact and outcomes during different stages of illness, hospitalization, and recovery.

The greatest need for nursing research is in areas that define or measure the effectiveness of specific nursing interventions. Few interventions have actually been proposed or tested in a systematic manner. The development of measurable outcome criteria, both short term and long term, is an essential step in the examination of the efficacy of nursing interventions. As the impact of illness upon the family becomes an increasingly well-defined phenomenon, much work remains to be done in documenting and validating the contributions nurses make in maintaining family integrity.

References

Algren, CL. Role perception of mothers who have hospitalized children. Children's Health Care, 14:6–9, 1985.

Baird, SF. Crisis intervention strategies. In Johnson, SH (Ed.), High risk parenting: Nursing assessment and strategies for the family at risk. Philadelphia: JB Lippincott Co., 1979.

Boss, P, and Greenberg, J. Family boundary ambiguity: A new variable in family stress theory. Family Process, 23:535–546, 1984.

Bowlby, J. Caring for the young: Influences on development. In Cohen, RS, Cohler, BJ, and Weissman, SH (Eds.), Parenthood: A psychodynamic perspective. New York: The Guilford Press, 1984.

Braulin, JL, Rook, J, and Sills, GM. Families in crisis: The impact of trauma. Critical Care Quarterly, 5:38–46, 1982.

Burns, CE. The hospitalization experience and single-parent families. Nursing Clinics of North America, 19:285–293, 1984.

Craft, MJ, Wyatt, N, and Sandell, B. Behavior and feeling changes in siblings of hospitalized children. Clinical Pediatrics, 24:374–378, 1985.

Eberly, TW, Miles, MS, Carter, MC, Hennessey, J, and Riddle, I. Parental stress after the unexpected admission of a child to the intensive care unit. Critical Care Quarterly, 8:57–65, 1985.

Epperson, MM. Families in sudden crisis: Process and intervention in a critical care center. Social Work in Health Care, 2:265–273, 1977.

Ferraro, AR, and Longo, DC. Nursing care of the family with a chronically ill, hospitalized child: An alternative approach. Image, 17:77–81, 1985.

Fife, BL. A model for predicting the adaptation of families to medical crisis: An analysis of role integration. Image, 17:108–112, 1985.

Fife, BL, Huhman, M, and Keck, J. Development of a clinical assessment scale: Evaluation of the psychosocial impact of childhood illness on the family. Issues in Comprehensive Pediatric Nursing, 9:11–31, 1986.

Gordon, M. Nursing diagnosis: Process and application. New York: McGraw-Hill, Inc., 1982.

Hall, JE, and Weaver, BR. Crisis: A conceptual approach to family nursing. In Hall, JE, and Weaver, BR (Eds.), Nursing of families in crisis. Philadelphia: JB Lippincott Co., 1974.

Hill, R. Generic features of families under stress. In Parad, HJ (Ed.), Crisis intervention: Selected readings. New York: Family Service Association of America, 1965.

Horowitz, JA, Hughes, CB, and Perdue, BJ. Parenting reassessed: A nursing perspective. Englewood Cliffs, N.J.: Prentice-Hall, Inc., 1982.

Hymovich, DP. Parents of sick children: Their needs and tasks. Pediatric Nursing, 2:9–13, 1976.

Hymovich, DP. Assessment of the chronically ill child and family. In Hymovich, DP, and Barnard, MU (Eds.), Family health care: General perspectives (Vol. 1). New York: McGraw-Hill, Inc., 1979.

Hymovich, DP. Development of the chronicity impact and coping instrument: Parent questionnaire (CICI;PQ). Nursing Research, 33:218–222, 1984.

Kalnins, IV. Cross-illness comparison of separation and divorce among parents having a child with a life threatening illness. Children's Health Care, 12:72–77, 1983.

Knafl, KA. How families manage a pediatric hospitalization. Western Journal of Nursing Research, 7:151–176, 1985.

Knafl, KA, Deatrick, JA, and Kodadek, S. How parents manage jobs and a child's hospitalization. American Journal of Maternal-Child Nursing, 7:125–128, 1982.

Knox, JE, and Hayes, VE. Hospitalization of a chronically ill child: A stressful time for parents. Issues in Comprehensive Pediatric Nursing, 6:217–226, 1983.

Lansky, SB, Cairnes, NU, Hassanein, R, Wehr, J, and Lowman, JT. Childhood cancer: Parental discord and divorce. Pediatrics, 62:184–188, 1978.

Lazarus, RS, Averill, JR, and Opton, EM. The psychology of coping: Issues of research and assessment. In Coehlo, GV, Hamburg, DA, and Adams, JE (Eds.), Coping and adaptation. New York: Basic Books, Inc., 1974.

Lewandowski, LA. Stresses and coping styles of parents of children undergoing open heart surgery. Critical Care Quarterly, 3:75–84, 1980.

Lidz, T. The family as developmental setting. In Anthony, JE, and Koupernik, C (Eds.), The child in his family (Vol. 1). New York: Wiley Interscience, 1970.

Marino, BL. When nurses compete with parents. Children's Health Care, 8:94–98, 1980.

Masters, JC, Cerreto, MC, and Mendlowitz, DR. The role of the family in coping with childhood chronic illness. In Burish, TG, and Bradley, LA (Eds.), Coping with chronic disease. New York: Academic Press, Inc., 1983.

McCubbin, M. Nursing assessment of parental coping with cystic fibrosis. Western Journal of Nursing Research, 6:407–418, 1984.

McKeever, PT. Fathering the chronically ill child. MCN: American Journal of Maternal Child Nursing, 6:124–128, 1981.

Miles, MS, and Carter, MC. Sources of parental stress in pediatric intensive care units. Children's Health Care, 11:65–69, 1982.

Miles, MS, Carter, MC, Spicher, C, and Hassanein, RS. Maternal and paternal stress reactions when a child is hospitalized in a pediatric intensive care unit. Issues in Comprehensive Pediatric Nursing, 7:333–342, 1984.

Mishel, MH. Parent's perception of uncertainty concerning their hospitalized child. Nursing Research, 32:324–330, 1983.

Olsen, EH. The impact of serious illness on the family system. Postgraduate Medicine, 47:169–174, 1970.

Roskies, E, Bedard, P, Gauvreau-Guilbault, H, and LaFortune, D. Emergency hospitalization of young children. Medical Care, 13:570–581, 1975.

Skipper, JK, Leonard, RC, and Rhymes, J. Child hospitalization and social interaction: An experimental study of mothers' feelings of stress, adaptation, and satisfaction. Medical Care, 6:496–506, 1968.

Stein, RE, and Riessman, CK. The development of an impact-on-family scale: Preliminary findings. Medical Care, 18:465–472, 1980.

Strauss, SS. Abuse and neglect of parents by professionals. MCN: American Journal of Maternal Child Nursing, 6:157–160, 1981.

Webster's Ninth New Collegiate Dictionary. Springfield, Mass.: Merriam-Webster, Inc., 1987.

Wolfer, JA, and Visintainer, MA. Pediatric surgical patients' and parents' stress responses and adjustment. Nursing Research, 24:244–255, 1975.

CHAPTER 5

ANTICIPATORY GUIDANCE

Janice A. Denehy, Ph.D., R.N.

Anticipatory guidance is an intervention used by nurses who work with children and families. It has been described as the giving of information or counseling to a client prior to an anticipated event. In the child care setting, anticipatory guidance might include interpretation of normal developmental patterns in children, anticipated behavioral responses of the child or the family to the specific developmental milestone, and child-rearing methods appropriate to the situation. Anticipatory guidance may also cover communication skills, coping strategies, and problem-solving techniques; it is a tool to promote parenting. It is also a method of promoting optimum health and development of children. When parents have received information about what lies ahead, their ability to cope with expected developmental changes is enhanced. Anticipatory guidance also can be given directly to children and adolescents to help them cope with expected developmental changes, such as the onset of puberty.

The purpose of this chapter is to examine anticipatory guidance as an intervention to promote parenting, to assess the indications for its use, to propose a variety of ways anticipatory guidance can be implemented, and to examine the difficulty of evaluating the outcome of this widely used nursing intervention.

The purposes of anticipatory guidance are (1) to promote a better understanding of the normal growth and development of children; (2) to provide parents with an opportunity to physically, emotionally, and cognitively prepare for expected developmental changes of childhood; (3) to encourage parents to develop, observe, and rehearse skills needed to parent; (4) to assist parents in developing coping strategies needed to deal with the realities of everyday living with developing children; and (5) to help parents enjoy their children and receive satisfaction in their parental role.

For many nurses, anticipatory guidance is a checklist of developmental milestones, safety hazards, and parental concerns expected at a specific chronological time in the life of children. The task at hand is to assess the developmental level of the child, relate the findings to the developmental tasks occurring at that time, and then inform parents about what lies ahead on the developmental road map. Appropriate coping methods and child-rearing skills may also be included as part of anticipatory guidance. While this information is important and may be helpful to many parents in understanding their children and in the development of parenting skills, some professionals question the efficiency and effectiveness of this form of client education directed to individual families. Information directed to parent groups or other aggregates is another method of providing anticipatory guidance. The use of print or visual media can also serve as a vehicle to transmit anticipatory information. More recently, promoting problem-solving skills has been identified as a means of enhancing parenting. It is hoped that parents will be able to transfer these skills to the wide range of challenges they face as their children develop.

THEORETICAL FOUNDATION

Anticipatory guidance is an intervention that developed as a preventive measure to reduce the anxiety associated with life change or crisis. According to Aguilera and Messick (1982), "The Chinese characters that represent the word 'crisis' mean both danger and opportunity" (p. 1). Caplan (1964) views a crisis as a transitional period in the life of an individual which presents the opportunity for growth, as well as a time of increased vulnerability to mental disorder. The outcome, whether it be increased health and maturity or a diminished capacity to cope with life's problems, is dependent upon the way the crisis is handled.

A crisis is provoked by a stressor, defined by Hill (1965) as an event or "situation for which the family has had little or no prior preparation and must therefore be viewed as problematic" (p. 34). Crisis-precipitating events are different for every given family, as are the methods the family uses to cope with the stressful event. The origin of crises is either from within the family unit or from outside the family unit. According to Le-Masters (1965), the impact of a crisis on a family is dependent upon the following variables: "(1) the nature of the crisis event, (2) the state of organization or disorganization of the family at the point of impact, (3) the resources of the family, and (4) its previous experience with crisis" (p. 111).

Two distinct types of crises have been identified in the literature: (1) the situational or accidental crisis and (2) the developmental or maturational crisis (Erikson, 1963; Aguilera and Messick, 1982; Hymovich and Barnard, 1979b). Situational crises are sudden and unpredictable in nature, such as the onset of an acute illness or a vehicle accident. Although Caplan (1964) states that, like accidents, situational crises "can often be statistically predicted" (p. 35), it is difficult to provide the necessary preventive interventions to persons or populations identified at risk.

Developmental crises, on the other hand, are associated with developmental changes or transitions that occur throughout the life span. These changes cause disequilibrium because existing coping mechanisms prove to be inadequate in dealing with new situations. Because the nature and timing of developmental changes are relatively predictable, intervention prior to the anticipated change serves to minimize the stress associated with the change. Anticipatory guidance is a widely used method of preparing parents for the many developmental changes or crises that occur as their children mature. This chapter focuses on preparing parents through anticipatory guidance for the developmental crises of childhood. For a discussion of preparatory interventions for situational crises, see Chapter 6.

Anticipatory guidance is an intervention that developed in maternal-child care clinics as a method of preventive health care. In a classic guide for practicing physicians and child health conference personnel, anticipatory guidance is described as "teaching the mother what to expect *before* she begins to worry or make mistakes" (American Public Health Association, 1955, p. 47). It further states, "The time to prevent a problem is before it becomes a problem" (p. 47). This brief description of anticipatory guidance and its purpose is followed by a listing of problems and concerns to be anticipated during the prenatal period, after the birth of the infant, and during selected special situations, such as separation. Recommendations of what to do should these problems arise are also included. Other authors have added to and refined the list of concerns and problems parents experience during the childbearing and child-rearing process, often developing specific categories of concerns for each developmental level (Mitchell, 1977; Pernice and Mott, 1985; Vanderzanden, 1979; Casey et al., 1979). Such summaries and lists have been the basis for socializing health care practitioners about the content and methodology of anticipatory guidance, as well as providing structure and scheduling for anticipatory guidance offered to parents.

Developmental assessment and appropriate anticipatory guidance have become an accepted part of well-child care (Chamberlin, 1983; Reisinger and Bires, 1980; Vanderzanden, 1979; Schulman and Hanley, 1987). Numerous studies have attempted to quantify the amount of time spent by health professionals, particularly physicians and nurse practitioners, in counseling and health teaching during clinic visits. Although the results vary, one study of pediatricians indicated that the average time for a well-child visit was ten minutes, 90 seconds of which was spent giving anticipatory guidance (Reisinger and Bires, 1980). The time spent giving anticipatory guidance varied with the age of the child; the greatest length of time (one minute and 37 seconds) was spent with mothers of infants under five months of age, and the least time (seven seconds) was spent with adolescents. Reisinger and Bires (1980) report that nearly half of the anticipatory guidance given to infants under one year was devoted to potential feeding problems. Very little time was spent addressing safety, sex education, growth, and behavior. Rogers (1980) reported that a quality assurance chart audit conducted by the American Academy of Pediatrics showed that pediatricians put a low priority on counseling; a

follow-up indicated that the lack of documentation of counseling activity was frequently an omission of care, not just an omission of recording. Foye et al. (1977) compared the content and emphasis of well-child visits of pediatricians and pediatric nurse practitioners. Their findings indicate that nurse practitioners offered comparable child health supervision but spent significantly more time than pediatricians discussing child development and behavior. In addition, they reported these discussions were in greater depth, nurses made more specific recommendations, and offered more maternal support. Nurse visits in this study were longer than pediatrician visits, averaging 25.5 minutes as compared with 17.6 minutes for pediatricians.

The value of routine well-child care and its frequency are being questioned, particularly in light of the lack of empirical evidence that preventive health care for children and their families is beneficial (Hoekelman, 1975, 1980). In a study designed to determine the effects of educating mothers about child development, Chamberlin et al. (1979) found that maternal knowledge of growth and development was greater among those who received care from pediatricians who made an effort to teach this information. This group of mothers reported that they made more positive contacts with their children and felt that they received more help in their child-rearing efforts than did mothers who received care from pediatricians who made little effort to teach. However, there were no significant differences in the developmental status of the two groups of children at 18 months. In fact, mothers who received teaching reported more behavioral problems.

Broussard (1976) studied the effect of televised anticipatory guidance on first-time mothers' perceptions of their newborns, measured by the Neonatal Perception Inventories. Although mothers in all groups had more positive perceptions at one month, the change was significant for those mothers who had received televised anticipatory guidance. Hoekelman (1975) compared the adequacy of well-child care given by pediatricians and pediatric nurse practitioners on a three-visit versus a six-visit schedule during the first year of life. No differences were found on the outcome measures of maternal knowledge, maternal satisfaction, maternal compliance, and health supervision. Hoe-kelman concludes that infant care delivered by the nurse practitioner is as effective as that given by the physician during the first year of life and that abbreviated care schedules by either professional do not reduce the adequacy of care (p. 325).

Brazelton (1975) presents a challenge to health care providers to become involved in the child's entire well-being. He states that a case of colic is more demanding on a physician's resources than a strep throat and much more exciting to manage (p. 533). He also states that information needed to plan anticipatory guidance includes a familiarity with both the child's family and environment. A trusting relationship must be established with the child's caretaker. By identifying coping strengths of parents and basing practice on normal growth and development, parent-child relationships and the developmental potential of children can be facilitated.

Brazelton (1984) has developed a tool to describe the behavioral capabilities of newborns, the Brazelton Neonatal Behavioral Assessment Scale (BNBAS). The BNBAS is a tool designed to help parents "get to know" their infants, to promote parent-child interactions, and to enhance family functioning. Clinically, the BNBAS can be used to teach parents about the capabilities of infants and to acquaint them with unique characteristics of their neonate. It also can be used to promote more realistic expectations of infant behavior and to plan child care activities unique to their infant's behavioral cues. Researchers have found that mothers had more positive perceptions of their infants (Hall, 1980), were more responsive to them (Anderson, 1981), and spent more time talking to and playing with them (Liptak et al., 1983) after observing the administration of the BNBAS or after receiving information about their infant gained through the BNBAS. Myers (1982) used the BNBAS as a method of teaching both parents about infant behavior by helping parents administer the scale items. The results showed parents had increased knowledge of infant behavior at one month and fathers participated more in the care of their infants after such teaching. However, only modest gains were seen in satisfaction and self-confidence, and no gains were found in behavioral treatment. Belsky (1982) states the purpose of early

intervention is to optimize functioning. Professionals need to develop cost-effective, acceptable methods of providing this service to those who need it most. In addition, interventions need to be delivered at a time when receptivity to information is increased, for instance, when individuals are about to become parents or when a couple's child is approaching a major developmental milestone.

The use of information about temperament to customize anticipatory guidance given to parents of eight month old infants is described by Little (1983). The temperament of each infant was assessed using the Revised Infant Temperament Questionnaire by Carey and McDevitt (1978) prior to the scheduled well-child visit. During the visit, information about their infant's temperament on the nine behavior clusters (activity, regularity, approach and withdrawal, adaptability, threshold, intensity, mood, distractibility, and persistence) was shared with parents. Emphasizing the positive, the examiner related temperamental characteristics to behaviors and child-rearing techniques unique to the child's temperament. Little (1983) reports a very enthusiastic response on the part of participating parents and has decided to continue the use of temperament in planning anticipatory guidance. A follow-up survey of parents revealed that nearly 90% had a better understanding of their children, 87% believed the time spent was worthwhile, and 57% changed their approach to child rearing.

Other practitioners recommend beginning anticipatory guidance for parents during the prenatal period. Vanderzanden (1979) believes that mothers are better able to incorporate information regarding infant care during the prenatal period before they are subjected to the stresses of postpartum fatigue and sleepless nights. She also conducted a two-week follow-up visit based only on the information needs of the mother and reported a 1% failure rate (20% is the expected rate) as evidence of high interest in and need for such a visit (p. 28). Berger and Rose (1983) describe the importance of pediatricians becoming involved with parents prenatally to provide anticipatory guidance for concerns that may occur during the immediate postpartum period, such as initiating breast-feeding and circumcision, and to provide continuity of care that will continue after birth. They recommend seeing the mother prior to 37 weeks gestation, for after that time the attention of the mother is focused on labor and delivery. The authors also state that the prenatal period is an ideal time to involve the father in pediatric care and in planning for the infant.

The importance of anticipatory guidance for adolescents and their parents has received considerable attention in the literature. While knowledge about a subject does not necessarily change attitudes or behavior, Hanley (1984) states that physicians serve as an important resource to adolescents who are gathering information about health-related psychosocial concerns during this period of identity formation. Anticipatory guidance for adolescents should focus on the major health concerns of this developmental period, which have been organized around the acronym SPACES (smoking; pot and peer pressure; alcohol; chaperons, curfew, parent power, and dating; exercise, diet, and personal responsibility; and sex) (p. 222). Kimball and Campbell (1979) emphasize the responsibilities of health professionals providing guidance to adolescents. These responsibilities include developing unique communication skills necessary to form a trusting relationship, maintaining confidentiality, gathering information about the adolescent from a variety of sources, and assessing how major developmental changes of adolescence are affecting the individual adolescent.

Anticipatory guidance can also be delivered to groups of parents or children. Although the outcomes and attendance of parent education programs have been disappointing, Roberts (1981) reports that analyzing the problem can help reconceptualize present approaches to an approach based on adult education principles, a careful needs assessment, and the use of a model to clarify parent education needs. The two-dimensional model developed by Roberts is based on four levels of parent education needs, which are coupled with four levels of professional response. This model centers around a needs assessment that would clarify the information needed by the client and the appropriate professional response to the need. An anticipatory guidance program described by Oberst (1971) outlines the complementary approach of office counseling with structured group classes offered in the

pediatric office during the evening hours. Topics included in the classes rotate over a two- to three-year period and cover development from infancy through adolescence for parents and discussion classes specifically designed for adolescents. Although no evaluation of the program is reported, Oberst states that such a program is an important contribution to the community and to the health of its families.

The anticipatory guidance protocols described up to this point have been content oriented, focusing on the provision of specific information about anticipated developmental crises. Pridham et al. (1977, 1979) describe a conceptualization of anticipatory care as a paradigm of problem solving—a process-oriented approach to anticipatory guidance. The focus of this model is the preparation of clients for future stressors through the identification and development of problem-solving skills—skills that can be transferred to a variety of developmental stressors expected during the life span. Although the model is still in the development phase, components of the problem-solving process have been described and examined (Pridham and Hansen, 1980). Because this model is more precise than other conceptualizations of anticipatory guidance, it provides structure for practice and outcome measurement.

In summary, anticipatory guidance is counseling or information given to parents in anticipation of a developmental crisis. It is often a structured part of care given in an ambulatory setting to parents of well children of all ages and stages to promote a better understanding of normal child development. The goal of anticipatory guidance is to assist the parents to mobilize their coping resources and plan for the anticipated event. Although anticipatory guidance is a widely accepted and frequently used intervention with families, there is surprisingly little information in the literature about this intervention. From the literature reviewed, it is evident that anticipatory guidance encompasses diverse information delivered by any number of different methods at any time along the developmental continuum. Particularly evident is the lack of data validating the effectiveness of this important component of well-child care.

ASSESSMENT

Children and families regularly face a predictable array of developmental crises as they proceed through the various stages of development. Approaching developmental milestones, such as the toilet training of a toddler, the birth of a sibling, the beginning school for a child, or the onset of menarche for an adolescent, are considered developmental crises in the lives of the individuals and families involved. Because anticipatory guidance by definition and purpose is designed to promote parental understanding of child development and parenting skills that lead to optimum growth and development, anticipatory guidance would seem to be indicated for *all parents* at any time along the developmental continuum. Although most nurses believe that all parents can benefit from anticipatory guidance, careful assessment will assist the nurse in identifying those parents who are ready for and able to benefit from this nursing intervention. The use of nursing diagnoses will help differentiate between families who are in the process of experiencing problems that would impair their ability to anticipate future developmental phenomena and families who, because of their strengths and interests, are ready to think, plan, and look forward to the future. Indications for use of the intervention are based on nursing diagnoses.

In ambulatory settings, coping families who have the potential for growth are ideal candidates for anticipatory guidance. Characteristics that define this group (Kim et al., 1984) include demonstrating effective management of the child's present developmental needs and showing a readiness and desire for information that could lead to enhanced growth and development of the child and the family unit. Families who exhibit ineffective coping may also benefit from information about child development, parenting, and coping strategies to increase their effectiveness as parents. However, in these families, the focus may of necessity be on dealing with present problems instead of anticipating future developmental needs. Detailed assessment may indicate that the energy of these families may be consumed by dealing with multiple crises compounded by the lack of support systems. By minimizing or eliminating the stresses experienced by families who are having difficulty coping, energy needed to parent can be conserved and focused on promoting the development of their children (Bishop, 1976).

Differentiation between actual and potential alterations in parenting will assist in identifying which parents might be recipients of anticipatory guidance. While parents who are actually experiencing difficulty in nurturing or creating an environment conducive to growth may require intensive counseling or referral, parents potentially at risk for difficulties in parenting would be identified as clients to receive anticipatory guidance. Advance information about anticipated developmental crises and appropriate parenting skills in groups at risk, such as adolescent parents or parents of premature infants, would serve as a preventive measure. Frequent follow-up may be indicated to reinforce strengths and develop parenting skills.

Parents who exhibit characteristics of anxiety or verbally express anxiety or fear about parenting would benefit from anticipatory guidance. This is an intervention that is intended to minimize the anxiety associated with changes expected as children develop. It can also assist parents in developing parenting skills that may reduce their feelings of inadequacy about their effectiveness. Through better understanding of their children and the development of parenting skills, previously anxious or fearful parents can anticipate the future without dread. Anticipatory guidance may also be a valuable intervention to improve the self-concept and self-esteem of parents. By increasing parental knowledge and promoting parenting skills, confidence in being able to successfully perform role expectations is nurtured. Parental questions or statements relating to self-esteem and role performance may indicate the need for anticipatory guidance.

Last, but certainly not least, a frequently used nursing diagnosis in ambulatory settings is *Knowledge deficit*, identified by a lack of information about (1) child development, (2) promoting growth and development, and (3) methods of dealing with and communicating with children. Many adults have had little or no preparation for their role as parents. Their understanding of growth and development and what to expect of children is often minimal or unrealistic. Some of today's parents have grown up in small families, and therefore have not had the opportunity to care for younger siblings or observe the parenting process. Mobile families seldom have grandparents or other extended family nearby to seek information about child rearing. However, most parents take their parental role seriously and want to do a good job. They are anxious to learn about children and parenting and want parenthood to be a rewarding experience. These characteristics indicate the use of the intervention anticipatory guidance by nurses who work with children and families in any setting.

THE INTERVENTION

Nurses are often in the position to offer anticipatory guidance in any health care setting that serves children and families. Although anticipatory guidance is often associated with ambulatory health care settings, it is also an important component of nursing care given in the community, as well as in hospital inpatient areas. Anticipatory guidance as a nursing intervention can be implemented using a number of different strategies. The choice of intervention method is based on the assessed needs of the child, family, or target group; the time frame in which the nurse has to work; and the skills and knowledge base of the nurse. Skillful use of nursing assessment and diagnosis, in-depth knowledge of growth and development, the ability to apply teaching-learning principles, and effective communication skills will enhance the effectiveness of the nurse implementing anticipatory guidance.

Anticipatory guidance is a teaching-learning process where the nurse-provider plans a strategy to meet the information needs of the client-recipient. When the recipient is a parent, strategies need to be planned with the unique characteristics of the adult learner in mind. This demands that the information provided be relevant, practical, and readily applicable to the learner's life experience or dilemma (Redman, 1984). In addition, when possible, the parents need to be involved in planning learning objectives, selecting strategies that complement their learning style, and outlining evaluation methods (Van Hoozer et al., 1987). Discussion, opportunities for question-and-answer sessions, problem-solving activities, and practical application through hands-on experience or role-playing are appropriate strategies for adult learners. Parents also seem to benefit from hearing others who have similar interests, concerns, or problems share their personal experiences with the challenges of parenthood.

Individual-Directed Anticipatory Guidance

Anticipatory guidance is frequently given on a one-to-one basis, nurse to client, and consists of information given to parents about upcoming developmental tasks and what can be done to deal effectively with these anticipated developmental changes. For example, anticipatory guidance for parents of a nine month old child might focus on changes that can be anticipated with the child's increasing mobility, the importance of home safety, and child-rearing skills. At this time there are also other anticipated changes, such as teething and changing eating behaviors, which may be viewed as problematic by parents. Information given to parents is usually specific to the developmental task yet emphasizes the wide range of normal times and behavioral manifestations that are associated with any developmental task.

Anticipatory guidance given to individual parents should be based on a careful assessment of the child's developmental level, as assessed through such tools as the Denver Prescreening Development Questionnaire or the Denver Developmental Screening Test. It can also be based on individual characteristics of the child as determined by the BNBAS, the Nursing Child Sleep Activity Record (Barnard, 1979), or temperament scales. It is also important to base anticipatory guidance on interests and concerns expressed by parents, as determined by answers to questions such as, "Tell me, how are things going?" Such open-ended questions give parents an opportunity and permission to share concerns that are important to them, yet ones they may feel seem trivial to health professionals. This technique demands listening skills as well as the ability to further assess how parents are feeling about the child and the job they are doing as parents. It is also an opportunity to analyze how parents handle problematic situations. Nurses can assist parents in problem solving by determining what parenting strategies they have tried and by exploring the parents' perceptions of why certain strategies were or were not successful in achieving the desired results. Assessment may reveal the need to provide information on realistic expectations relating to child behavior or information on specific parenting techniques. It may also identify strengths parents possess which can be reinforced and used to assist parents in revising existing child-rearing techniques and in promoting parental self-esteem.

Advantages of using the one-to-one approach to anticipatory guidance is that the intervention can be customized to the individual family. It gives parents an opportunity to express personal concerns and receive guidance that is individualized. One-to-one anticipatory guidance provides the nurse the opportunity to do an in-depth assessment of the child's development and the parents' skills and concerns in promoting the development of the child. Anticipatory guidance can then be based on a synthesis of the assessment data from both the parents and the child. When continuity of nursing care and careful documentation are present, nurses are able to build on information previously gathered, to follow up on the effectiveness of guidance given in previous encounters, and to nurture a long-term, trusting relationship with a family.

One criticism of the one-to-one method of giving anticipatory guidance is that it is likely that communication is one-way, from nurse to client, and the nurse is in the active information-giving role and the client is in a passive recipient role. Other disadvantages of this method are also evident to nurses who work in busy settings. There may not be enough time to make an in-depth assessment of the family, particularly when competing priorities are present, such as a physical complaint or concern or a distressed or active child who requires parental comfort or supervision. The content of anticipatory guidance may be based on the developmental level of the child rather than the interest or readiness of the parents. Nurses feel a responsibility to present information they believe is important and would be helpful to parents, especially if there will be no contact with the family again or if the next scheduled visit is in the distant future. In such instances, information presented may not relate to major concerns or parental readiness and may overload parents. Other concerns about one-to-one anticipatory guidance are its cost-effectiveness and lack of evidence of its efficacy as a preventive measure. Because one-to-one anticipatory guidance is geared to specific developmental changes, new information is continually needed as the child moves through successive developmental stages.

Group-Directed Anticipatory Guidance

Another method of giving anticipatory guidance is via group presentations. This methodology has been popular to present content in such areas as infant care, preparation for the birth of a sibling, and adoptive parenthood. Presentations to groups have the advantage of reaching a large audience at one time. They also give parents an opportunity to meet and interact with other parents who share similar concerns. Such sharing serves to illuminate the similarities and differences of children, and in addition, parents may receive new ideas about parenting from others.

Group parenting classes can be structured around specific topics, such as toilet training or discipline, or a specific age group, such as infants or toddlers, or classes may be less structured and develop out of the needs expressed by attending parents. In any case, advance planning and preparation is required of nurses in assessing the need for such a class, planning the format, picking the time and place, publicizing the event, and planning for its implementation and evaluation. If the class is to be structured, appropriate content, sequencing, and method of delivery need to be planned according to the identifying characteristics of the target audience. Knowledge of growth and development, child-rearing skills, and educational methodology is necessary to this planning. Communication skills are important in delivering content, facilitating group discussion, and fielding and dealing with difficult or sensitive questions and opinions that may arise. Nurses, by virtue of their broad educational and experiential base, are often an excellent choice to present or coordinate anticipatory guidance for groups in the hospital, office, clinic, or community setting. The scope of educational programs presented by nurses is limited only by their creativity, courage, and time. Involvement in providing anticipatory guidance to groups of parents is also possible through voluntary, civic, neighborhood, or church organizations.

An advantage of group presentation of anticipatory guidance is the delivery of content to a large number of people at one time. It also gives parents the opportunity to meet and interact with other parents who have similar concerns in a supportive environment. When parents hear that other parents are experiencing similar joys and trials, they are better able to put their parenting experience into perspective. Nurses conducting group anticipatory guidance establish credibility as professionals who care and are knowledgeable about the growth and development of children and families.

Disadvantages of group presentations include the possible difficulty of addressing individual needs of group members, especially if the group is large. Question-and-answer periods or group discussion can serve to meet individual concerns in a group; however, some individuals are not comfortable communicating or sharing ideas with others in group settings or with strangers. In order for a structured group to be effective, it needs to be relatively homogeneous, focusing on a common concern, age group, or specific goal. Too frequently, parent groups are poorly attended, and those parents who attend are often those least likely to need information about children and parenting. A group to whom anticipatory guidance is commonly directed is postpartum mothers. Although this group could benefit from anticipatory guidance, shorter postpartum hospitalizations, sometimes less than 24 hours, make ambitious formal teaching programs unrealistic, especially at a time when new mothers are recovering from labor and delivery, getting acquainted with their infants, and preparing for discharge. New mothers might be better served by anticipatory guidance programs prenatally, in the home or community after delivery, or by one-to-one or media-based anticipatory guidance during hospitalization. Anticipatory guidance to groups requires a commitment of time and energy from nurses, time for which they may

not be compensated, and frequently means taking time away from their families during evening hours. A lack of resources often prevents even the best-planned and -executed programs from continuing on a long-term basis.

Media-Based Anticipatory Guidance

Another way to provide anticipatory guidance is through the use of media. This strategy may be used alone or to supplement one-to-one or group anticipatory guidance. The use of printed material, such as pamphlets, handouts, or books, allows parents to have a ready reference to information as they need it. Many nurses give printed materials to parents as a part of well-child care. Some of this printed information is produced by nurses specifically for the setting; others may be purchased or complimentary from child care product manufacturers. Well-child clinics, child care providers, and libraries often publish lists of parenting books.

A recent exploration by graduate students of the author revealed that many of the books included on such lists are not available in bookstores or libraries; no information about the major theme or content of the book is included; and many of the books are lengthy, require at least a high-school education to understand, and would only appeal to motivated, already knowledgeable middle-class parents. The graduate students evaluating the parenting literature identified the need for books that are attractive and appropriate for adolescent parents, parents with less than a high-school education, and parents of lower socioeconomic groups. Also helpful would be the inclusion of a brief annotation to assist parents in choosing from the many books available. Nurses who recommend readings to parents need to be informed about the availability of those titles recommended and the appropriateness of the material for the intended reader.

Movies or videotapes can also be used as a vehicle to present anticipatory guidance. Careful selection or production of media can greatly enhance the effectiveness of information for parents. Because parents have been socialized to visual media, this method may be well received. Advantages include the fact that videotapes can be checked out and watched at the convenience of the parents. In outpatient clinics or other settings, viewing areas can be used before and after appointments or during hospitalization. The videotaping of parenting classes could be a beginning in the development of a videotape library in a health care setting or for a local library. Nursing and other organizations are now offering a wide range of films and videotapes for purchase or rental that can be used for individuals or groups in providing anticipatory guidance.

Visual and print media should be viewed as complementary to, not replacements for, direct interaction with parents to provide anticipatory guidance. It is easy to give parents a pamphlet on oral hygiene at an appointed chronological time, but this is no substitute for two-way interactions about the importance of dental health throughout childhood based on assessments of the family and concerns expressed by parents. Disadvantages of media-based anticipatory guidance include the cost of purchasing materials, the cost of equipment needed to view visual media, and the difficulty of supervising and maintaining equipment. For media produced in-house, considerable time, talent, and funds are required to produce attractive programs that are able to be used over a long period of time and serve the informational needs of diverse parent groups.

Anticipatory Guidance: A Problem-Solving Process

A final approach to anticipatory guidance is focusing on the problem-solving process engaged in by health professionals and clients in anticipatory care rather than on specific content. This process is being developed and tested by Pridham and associates (1977, 1979, 1980). Although specific content is used in implementing the problem-solving model, the major focus is the problem-solving process, not the problem to be solved. The goal of this process is to prepare families to solve problems or accomplish goals relating to particular anticipatable stressors (Pridham, et al., 1977).

Seven phases of the problem-solving methodology have been identified and are currently being tested. They are as follows (p. 1080):

1. Scanning—discovering problems or goals important to the patient.

2. Formulating—exploring, specifying, and naming identified problems or goals.

3. Appraising—mutual decision of client and professional about importance, readiness, and willingness to work on identified task.

4. Developing willingness or readiness to solve problems—when either the client or professional is ready to work on a task, but the other party is not yet ready or willing to do so, work must be directed on developing the readiness of the other party.

5. Planning—decisions about the who, what, and how of the problem-solving process.

6. Implementing—the professional may provide leadership in (a) orienting, (b) guiding, (c) developing rules and strategies, and (d) practicing skills needed to solve a problem.

7. Evaluating—appraising if the intervention enabled the client to cope with or solve the identified problem.

The use of the problem-solving model is a more structured and sophisticated method of providing anticipatory care. Although it appears to be a departure from current methodologies, many nurses incorporate one or more aspects of the process in their planning of anticipatory guidance. The major difference is focus on process rather than content. The advantage of this model is that it is an attempt to delineate nursing practice and make it empirically observable. It also deals with the realization that it is not feasible for nurses or other professionals to be available to give anticipatory guidance for all of the numerous challenges present during each developmental stage. Such an approach will assist professionals in promoting parental problem-solving skills, skills that will serve them in dealing with the many crises of parenthood.

In summary, anticipatory guidance is information given to parents prior to an anticipated developmental crisis that is designed to assist in parental coping. This information can be delivered on a one-to-one basis or in structured or unstructured group settings. In addition, anticipatory guidance can be given through print or visual media. Although anticipatory guidance is likely to be content centered, it can also be process oriented. The use of a variety of strategies in presenting anticipatory guidance helps create and maintain interest and motivation among recipients; a variety of approaches also serves to maximize the advantages of each approach while counteracting the disadvantages of other approaches. Nurses, because of their holistic approach to the health of children and families, can be active in assessing the need for and implementing anticipatory guidance.

EVALUATION

One of the greatest challenges in nursing today is measuring the outcome of interventions in quantifiable terms that are readily communicated to others. Such outcome measures are essential to determine the efficacy of nursing care and to validate the value contributed to patient care. As cost containment becomes a concern of all health professionals, efforts and resources will be allocated to those activities with proven results. Such empirical data is needed for the intervention of anticipatory guidance.

As previously stated, anticipatory guidance is an intervention that may be offered to any parent at anytime during the development of their offspring. Content and method of delivery are determined by individual practitioners, based on the assessed needs of the individual family or target group. Variables such as the time available, the preparation and philosophy of the health professional, and the readiness of the client may determine the nature of the intervention. Since there is little standardization, measurement of effectiveness is difficult. In addition, outcomes may not be realized for a long time after the intervention, during which time it is impossible to control or identify numerous intervening variables. Longitudinal follow-up studies are expensive and require a serious commitment of time and energy by researchers. A high dropout rate of subjects frequently limits generalizing the findings. However, because health professionals intuitively believe that anticipatory guidance is desirable, they continue to provide this intervention without empirical validation of its effectiveness.

A beginning step in measuring the effec-

tiveness of anticipatory guidance would be meticulous documentation of content presented to parents or groups, how this information related to assessed needs and concerns of the parents or group, the methods used (including such information as resources recommended and handouts given), and an evaluation of the parent's or group's interest in and understanding of the information presented. Also important is documentation of the parents' or group's strengths, problems, and ideas for future follow-up. The time spent with the parents or group should also be recorded. On follow-up visits or classes, determination of the value of anticipatory guidance from the prior visit or class would provide a beginning base for evaluating outcomes and planning subsequent interventions.

To determine the effectiveness of anticipatory guidance, it is essential to look to the stated purposes for this intervention. Although all practitioners may not agree on the purposes stated in the introduction of this chapter and not all anticipatory guidance programs are designed to meet all of the stated purposes, these statements of purpose provide some structure for outcome measurement. However, examination of each purpose reveals the nonspecific nature of the goals for this intervention. The first purpose, increased knowledge about growth and development of children, is the one that can most readily be quantified via pretest and posttest measures. Measurement of this outcome would be most appropriate for group anticipatory guidance where the intervention is consistent for all subjects in the treatment group.

The other stated purposes are difficult to measure empirically. Although some attempts have been made to address these purposes by asking parents after the fact if they were better prepared, coped more effectively, and enjoyed their parenting role more after anticipatory guidance, this information is often anecdotal and not very helpful in revising programs or making decisions about program retention. It is also not very powerful in justifying the time or money spent for providing anticipatory guidance as an integral part of child health supervision.

As evident from the review of the literature, few practitioners or researchers have attempted to measure the outcomes of anticipatory guidance. In fact, there is no consensus of what an appropriate outcome measure is for this intervention. It is time for nurses to put their creativity to the test and design some research studies that describe what difference anticipatory guidance makes in the development of healthy children and nurturing parents and how this intervention can be most effectively and efficiently implemented.

Case Study

Mrs. L. came into the pediatric clinic with her 11 month old daughter, Dawn, who had a fever of 102° F. and had been irritable for the last two days. A medical diagnosis of otitis media was made. While Mrs. L. was dressing Dawn, the nurse brought Mrs. L. a prescription and gave instructions for taking the medication. After receiving the instructions, Mrs. L. sat exhausted in a chair. She explained that she had been up most of the previous night because Dawn was crying. She had just found out last week that she was pregnant—a pregnancy not planned at this time because she had been hoping to go back to work in a few months so the family could afford to buy a house. Mrs. L. told the nurse that things seemed to be falling apart at home. Her 3½ year old son, David, had been acting terribly lately, unable to get along with Dawn. She explained that she hadn't felt they had any problems with sibling rivalry because the two children had gotten along beautifully until recently. David had attended sibling preparation class prior to Dawn's birth and had been very helpful and loving with Dawn. Mrs. L. and her husband made sure David had his own special time each day and before bedtime.

Since Dawn had become more mobile, she had been following David around the house like a shadow. She was particularly intrigued by his toys, wanting to put everything in her mouth. Mrs. L. said that she had tried to explain to David that Dawn was too young to understand how to play with his toys when she interrupted his play. Then David would scream when she came near, and Dawn would scream when she was removed from David's toys. Mrs. L. told the nurse she was too tired to deal with the situation and wondered how she would ever be able to handle a third child.

Synthesis of assessment data led to a nursing diagnosis of fatigue based on statements made by Mrs. L., her pregnancy, and the sleepless night spent comforting an irritable, sick child. Realizing that Mrs. L. would be able to get more rest and uninterrupted sleep as Dawn got better, the nurse decided to explore ways Mrs. L. could plan for additional rest during her pregnancy to give her energy to cope with the demands of parenthood. Because of her fatigue, Mrs. L. wasn't able to be very productive in planning rest periods; she did, however, identify this as an important area to think about with her husband.

Because this family appeared to have been coping effectively prior to the recent stress of illness, a diagnosis of *Potential alteration in parenting* was made. As Dawn entered a new developmental stage, toddlerhood, her new behaviors necessitated new strategies on the part of her caretakers. These changes were stressful to the parents, especially when the behaviors were anxiety provoking and expectations were unrealistic. Identifying characteristics included difficulty dealing with sibling interactions and unrealistic expectations of sibling behavior. These stresses were compounded by fatigue in the mother because of pregnancy and Dawn's illness, which caused sleepless nights for Dawn's mother.

Interventions included a recognition of the mother's feelings about her children and her concerns about having another child. Because of the mother's fatigue, one-to-one anticipatory guidance about sibling rivalry was given briefly. The mother was encouraged to identify strengths in the children's relationship and to think about ways for them to each meet their developmentally related play needs. Dawn was scheduled for a two-week follow-up visit at which time the nurse planned to follow up on identifying methods with Mrs. L. to provide rest and to enhance sibling relationships.

When Mrs. L. returned to the clinic to have Dawn's ears checked, she appeared more relaxed and optimistic. She stated that she was better able to cope with her children when she wasn't so tired. Although her housekeeping was slipping, she was feeling better and was considering a preschool two mornings a week for David. David would benefit from interaction with peers, and she needed the time to give Dawn some individual attention. Although David and Dawn continued to squabble, Mrs. L. was beginning to realize that this behavior was normal, not due to her failure as a parent. Mrs. L. expressed continued concern about her pregnancy and the added demands it would make on her as a parent. However, she added that things appeared less overwhelming this week. With some encouragement, Mrs. L. was able to make her rest needs a priority; and with minimal assistance from the nurse, Mrs. L. outlined a plan with scheduled rest periods for her and the children.

In addition to notes about Dawn's physical condition, the nurse carefully documented her observations about Mrs. L.'s concerns and the anticipatory guidance given. Upon Mrs. L.'s return visit, observations of the outcomes were documented in the chart, with particular emphasis on the problem-solving approach used by Mrs. L. in planning a solution to the problem she identified in the earlier visit. At that time, the nurse also recorded her ideas about strategies that appeared to suit the learning style of this family, their strengths, and areas in which surveillance and additional anticipatory guidance were indicated during future clinic visits. A duplicate copy of this information was placed in the chart of the sibling for cross-reference.

RESEARCH IMPLICATIONS

The need for research on the intervention of anticipatory guidance has been illustrated throughout this chapter. Outcome measures need to be specified and related to the purposes of this important nursing intervention. Research should focus on the following three areas: (1) the effect of anticipatory guidance on the child, (2) the effect of anticipatory guidance on the parents, and (3) the process and strategies of anticipatory guidance.

Research analyzing the impact of anticipatory guidance on children clarifies how intervention enhances development, promotes mental and physical health, and improves parent-child relationships. Through the use of longitudinal designs, it may be possible to determine the effect of anticipatory guidance on development and health. The use of existing tools, such as the BNBAS or temperament scales, may make it possible to determine how advance knowledge of individual characteristics can be used to enhance parental perceptions, relationships, and skills and what effect this enhancement has on the child. It is challenging to measure the effect of anticipatory guidance on children, for instruments need to be developed that measure behaviors that are difficult to observe and measure. As with many developmental phenomena, interactions from many variables, such as genetic endowment, temperament, parental expectations and past experiences, socioeconomic status, and culture, influence the development of the child.

Identifying the benefits of anticipatory guidance for parents also needs to be considered. Outcome measures need to be determined, operationalized, and made measurable. Strategies to describe knowledge and parenting styles and competencies would provide a basis to determine if interventions could influence these variables. Using existing measures of role satisfaction and self-esteem might provide some insight into the benefits of anticipatory guidance for parents. Present concerns about parental satisfaction

with anticipatory guidance could be extended to parental analysis of the intervention, including suggestions for content and methodology. Both short-term and long-term outcomes need to be delineated and measured. The research needed is time-consuming, expensive, and demanding of talent and commitment. Through collaboration with professionals in related disciplines, a team approach to studying the outcomes of anticipatory guidance on children, parents, and the parent-child system will provide the strength and breadth needed to tackle this difficult challenge.

Evaluating the process of identifying the need for anticipatory guidance and the actual intervention strategies also provides fertile ground for research. The model being developed by Pridham and associates (1979) is an exciting step forward in attempting to validate the process involved in anticipatory guidance. These researchers have not only identified the problems and limitations of measuring outcomes, but have developed a model that provides structure where little structure previously existed. They also appear to have developed a long-range program of research as they carefully examine each component of the model before proceeding with the next step of the research program. The model developed by Roberts (1981) also helps to clarify the level of educational need of the client and its relationship to intervention. Such models provide a beginning basis for the testing of nursing interventions.

Additional questions to be answered include the following: Are families able to identify needs to promote family functioning, or is the professional best suited to perform this task? What is the most efficient and effective method of assessing needs? What methods, such as one-to-one, group, or media, are most effective in providing anticipatory guidance? What is the optimal timing? How many sessions are appropriate? Which individuals or groups receive the most benefit? Are certain methods more effective for certain clients or specific topics? Is follow-up needed? If so, what type and how long? The answers to these questions would provide direction for practitioners in planning and implementing anticipatory guidance for families.

It is likely that some nurses have been conducting informal studies on anticipatory guidance. Others possess vast knowledge gained through years of practice. This valuable information needs to be communicated to others in the profession via nursing journals and meetings of nursing organizations so nurses do not keep reinventing the wheel. These informal nursing studies, hunches, and practical experiences need to be shared, discussed, and analyzed. In time this information may generate hypotheses that develop into more formal, structured, and rigorous research studies. Nursing needs an empirical basis for one of its most frequently used interventions—anticipatory guidance. Data provided by carefully designed and executed research studies will ensure that health care resources, both human and fiscal, are invested wisely in promoting the health and development of children and families.

References

American Public Health Association. Health supervision of young children. New York: The American Public Health Association, Inc., 1955.

Aguilera, DC, and Messick, JM. Crisis intervention: Theory and methodology (4th ed.). St. Louis: CV Mosby Co., 1982.

Anderson, CJ. Enhancing reciprocity between mother and neonate. Nursing Research, 30:89–93, 1981.

Barnard, K. Nursing child assessment training (NCAT): Sleep activity manual. Seattle: The University of Washington, School of Nursing, 1979.

Belsky, J. A principled approach to intervention with families in the newborn period. Journal of Community Psychology, 10:66–73, 1982.

Berger, LR, and Rose, E. The prenatal pediatric visit revisited. Clinical Pediatrics, 22:287–289, 1983.

Bishop, B. A guide to assessing parenting capabilities. American Journal of Nursing, 76:1784–1787, 1976.

Brazelton, TB. Anticipatory guidance. Pediatric Clinics of North America, 22:533–544, 1975.

Brazelton, TB. Neonatal behavioral assessment scale (Clinics in Developmental Medicine, No. 88, 2nd ed.). Philadelphia: JB Lippincott Co., 1984.

Broussard, ER. Evaluation of televised anticipatory guidance to primipara. Community Mental Health Journal, 7:203–209, 1976.

Caplan, G. Principles of preventive psychiatry. New York: Basic Books, Inc., 1964.

Carey, WB, and McDevitt, SC. Revision of the infant temperament questionnaire. Pediatrics, 61:735–739, 1978.

Casey, P, Sharp, M, and Loda, F. Child-health supervision for children under 2 years of age: A review of its content and effectiveness. The Journal of Pediatrics, 95:1–9, 1979.

Chamberlin, RW. Well child care. In Thornton, SM, and Frankenburg (Eds.), Child health care communications. New Brunswick, N.J.: Johnson & Johnson, 1983.

Chamberlin, RW, Szumowski, EK, and Zastowny, TR. An evaluation of efforts to educate mothers about child development in pediatric office practices. American Journal of Public Health, 69:875–886, 1979.

Erikson, E. Childhood and society (2nd ed.). New York: WW Norton and Co., Inc., 1963.

Foye, H, Chamberlin, RW, and Charney, E. Content and emphasis of well-child visits. American Journal of Diseases of Children, 131:794–797, 1977.

Hall, LA. Effect of teaching on primiparas' perceptions of their newborns. Nursing Research, 29:317–322, 1980.

Hanley, KK. The adolescent visit: An opportunity for anticipatory guidance. Journal of the Florida Medical Association, 71:221–224, 1984.

Hill, R. Generic features of families under stress. In Pared, HJ (Ed.), Crisis intervention: Selected readings. New York: Family Service Association of America, 1965.

Hoekelman, RA. What constitutes adequate well-baby care? Pediatrics, 55:313–326, 1975.

Hoekelman, RA. Got a minute? (commentary). Pediatrics, 66:1013–1014, 1980.

Hoekelman, RA. Well-child visits revisited. American Journal of Diseases in Children, 137:17–20, 1983.

Hymovich, DP, and Barnard, MU (Eds.). Family health care: Volume 1, General perspectives (2nd ed.). New York: McGraw-Hill, Inc., 1979a.

Hymovich, DP, and Barnard, MU (Eds.). Family health care: Volume 2, Developmental and situational crises (2nd ed.). New York: McGraw-Hill, Inc., 1979b.

Kim, MJ, McFarland, GK, and McLane, AM (Eds.). Pocket guide to nursing diagnoses. St. Louis: CV Mosby Co., 1984.

Kimball, AJ, and Campbell, MM. Psychologic aspects of adolescent patient health care. Clinical Pediatrics, 18:15–24, 1979.

LeMasters, EE. Parenthood as crisis. In Pared, HJ (Ed.), Crisis intervention: Selected readings. New York: Family Service Association of America, 1965.

Liptak, GS, Keller, BB, Feldman, AW, and Chamberlin, RW. Enhancing infant development of parent-practitioner interaction with the Brazelton Neonatal Assessment Scale. Pediatrics, 72:71–78, 1983.

Little, DL. Parent acceptance of routine use of the Carey and McDevitt Infant Temperament Questionnaire. Pediatrics, 71:104–106, 1983.

Mitchell, RG (Ed.). Child health in the community. Edinburgh: Churchill Livingstone, 1977.

Myers, BJ. Early intervention using Brazelton training with middle-class mothers and fathers of newborns. Child Development, 53:462–471, 1982.

Oberst, BB. The continuum of guided growth: An anticipatory guidance program for a pediatric and adolescent office practice. Clinical Pediatrics, 10:615–618, 1971.

Pernice, J, and Mott, SR. Anticipatory guidance. In Mott, SR, Fazekas, NF, and James, SR (Eds.), Nursing care of children and families. Menlo Park, Calif.: Addison-Wesley Publishing Co., Inc., 1985.

Pridham, KF, and Hansen, MF. An observation methodology for the study of interactive clinical problem-solving behavior in primary care settings. Medical Care, 18:360–375, 1980.

Pridham, KF, Hansen, MF, and Conrad, HH. Anticipatory care as problem solving in family medicine and nursing. The Journal of Family Practice, 4:1077–1081, 1977.

Pridham, KF, Hansen, MF, and Conrad, HH. Anticipatory problem solving: Models for clinical practice and research. Sociology of Health and Illness, 1:177–194, 1979.

Redman, BK. The process of patient education (5th ed.). St. Louis: CV Mosby Co., 1984.

Reisinger, KS, and Bires, JA. Anticipatory guidance in pediatric practice. Pediatrics. 66:889–892, 1980.

Roberts, FB. A model for parent education. Image, 13:86–89, 1981.

Rogers, K. The case against routine visits. In Smith, D, and Hoekelman, R (Eds.), Controversies in child health and pediatrics. New York: McGraw-Hill, Inc., 1980.

Schulman, JL, and Hanley, KK. Anticipatory guidance: An idea whose time has come. Baltimore: Williams & Wilkins, 1987.

Vanderzanden, EC. Anticipatory guidance for the first two months of life. Journal of Nurse Midwifery, 24:28–34, 1979.

Van Hoozer, HL, Bratton, BD, Ostmoe, PM, Weinholtz, D, Craft, MJ, Gjerde, CL, and Albanese, MA. The teaching process: Theory and practice in nursing. Norwalk, Conn.: Appleton-Century-Crofts, 1987.

SECTION II

THE CHILD EXPERIENCING ALTERED HEALTH STATUS

PART 1

Psychosocial Interventions for Maintenance of Self-Concept and Promotion of Coping

Overview

JUNE L. TRIPLETT, Ed.D., R.N.

The chapters which follow provide the practicing nurse with a wide range of ideas for helping children experiencing alterations in their health status. The unspoken goals for this section are twofold: to help children (1) cope effectively with these alterations and their consequences, and (2) view themselves as competent and worthwhile individuals. To achieve these goals, the authors discuss a variety of concepts which are useful at various points in the nursing process. For example, Denehy states that drawings of children may give the nurse clues as to how children perceive their situation (*assessment*). Providing an opportunity for children to draw pictures may be a useful *intervention* for children whose verbal skills are limited, and a series of drawings over time can provide *evaluative* evidence of the progress of children in understanding what is happening to them. Several chapters discuss intervention concepts which are potentially useful in a variety of situations, while others deal with more specific concerns, such as childhood loss and grief or disruptive behaviors.

Although the focus of Chapter 6 is on preparing children for hospitalization, procedures, or surgery, it serves as a useful base for the other chapters in that preparation for other changes is also crucial. For Manion, preparation includes providing information, enhancing coping skills, and offering emotional support. The first of these, providing information, is dealt with extensively by Manion and is further elaborated by Tiedeman, Simon, and Clatworthy as they talk about using the language of play to teach about the realities of illness and treatments. The chapter by Koster on self-care also focuses on providing information and teaching new skills to reduce a child's self-care deficit. These authors share a common belief that as children gain knowledge and competence their ability to cope also increases. Several authors speak specifically to teaching a variety of coping skills as a first step in enhancing the self-view of children as competent and worthwhile. This is particularly evident in Coucouvanis' discussion of disruptive behavior. She views inappropriate behavior as a manifestation of ineffective coping skills in which children rely on acting out rather than verbally expressing themselves. Teaching such children how to express feelings verbally helps them learn a more effective coping strategy which can be generalized to other situations.

Providing information to children which will strengthen their coping skills and enhance their self-concepts is a challenge even under ordinary circumstances, but is much more difficult when the child and caregiver are from different cultures. The chapter by Sloat and Matsuura provides insights as to potential differences among cultural groups which can interfere with health care delivery and the child's full recovery.

The chapters by Pflederer, by Tse and Perez-Woods, and by Molsberry and Shogan have a common theme of providing support to children with alterations in their health status, although other chapters also speak to its importance. Tse and Perez-Woods believe that support consists of physical and psychological interventions which provide the child with new resources, maintain existing resources, and stimulate the development of potential resources. They examine a variety of support sources, whereas Pflederer focuses on the child's peers and how children learn new ways of coping as they interact with each other. As the number of children's friends increases in adolescence, their range of coping strategies also expands. When a child is stigmatized by an illness, peers not only provide support but can also influence the child's self-concept.

Support is often conveyed through the judicious use of touch—by offering a hand to squeeze during a traumatic procedure, by giving a hug to the youngster who tried to comply, or by simply placing a hand on the shoulder of a crying adolescent. Molsberry and Shogan expand on the effective use of touch to convey support as well as its use in stimulating energy fields.

Support is a key word in Ross-Alaolmolki's discussion of minimizing the effects of grief by facilitating the grief process. Although children are often taught to be resilient in the face of change, this resilience can be strengthened by a supportive family milieu and an extended support system which encourages the child's coping efforts and enhances those efforts by reinforcing the child's positive values.

As medical technology becomes more complex and medical payment plans place increasing limitations on hospital care, more chronically ill children are being treated at home. Dowd and Vlastuin discuss the challenges which family members face when caring for a sick child at home. It is likely that in the future, families will be expected to provide increasingly sophisticated care for their sick children. Their abilities to do this effectively will depend to a great extent on the preparation and support they receive from health professionals.

The suggestions for needed research included in each chapter are thought-provoking, exciting, and almost overwhelming. More information is desperately needed about assessing children's perceptions of various health disruptions and determining the types of interventions which are most effective in each of many different situations. Because the research implications are so broad and varied, it is difficult to isolate a common thread of inquiry, but the goal remains constant. Answers are needed which will enable nurses to help children with alterations in their health status to cope effectively with the consequences of these disruptions and to feel valued and competent in doing so.

CHAPTER 6

PREPARING CHILDREN FOR HOSPITALIZATION, PROCEDURES, OR SURGERY

JO MANION, M.A., R.N.

A child facing hospitalization, medical procedures, or the need for surgery is in a vulnerable position. The situation is probably unlike any he or she has previously experienced. Separation from familiar surroundings and loved ones is part of the event. In addition, the new and strange experiences may be painful, upsetting, and confusing. It is no wonder that research in recent years has focused extensively on methods and techniques for preparing children and their families for these experiences.

Preparation for hospitalization, procedures, or surgery as defined for this discussion consists of the activities and interactions engaged in by a child and parents, on a purposeful basis, before the event occurs. The purpose of this preparation is to psychologically ready the child and parents for the impending event and subsequent emotional changes. Preparation is a process rather than an event in itself (Azarnoff and Woody, 1981; Thompson and Stanford, 1981). The purpose of this chapter is to review preparation methods available and suggest implementation strategies likely to be successful. A discussion of preparation as a coping mechanism in response to a stressful event will provide the theoretical framework. From this framework, the impact of preparation on the child and family will be explored.

THEORETICAL FOUNDATION

Stress and Coping

As defined by Selye (1974), stress is a nonspecific response of the body to any demand made upon it. Selye points out that the individual impact of stressors depends on the person's perception of the stressors, the conditioning factors brought to the situation, and the coping mechanisms used to adapt. These three variables are closely interrelated. One concept of coping, for example, explains that the way individuals define or perceive a situation influences the way in which they cope (Lazarus, 1966; Lazarus and Launier, 1978). An assumption of this approach is that coping is not only affected by but, to a large part, is also determined by personal attributes of the individual. Thus, an individual evaluates an event as harmful or potentially harmful according to that person's understanding of the situation, its power to produce harm, and the resources available to the individual for dealing with the event. Therefore, the individual's appraisal determines whether a situation will result in a stress response.

Although coping is generally defined as a response by the individual to stress, an important component includes the responses of others in the situation, which may enhance the person's coping response (Miles and Carter, 1985). A goal of nursing intervention when related to a child requiring hospitalization or a medical procedure is to foster mastery of the experience. Elimination of pain and avoidance of emotional distress are not feasible goals. However, effective nursing intervention can result in the child and parents accurately perceiving the event and coping with the situation in a positive way.

Preparation As an Intervention

Preparation, as implied by its definition, is an intervention that can address the three variables identified by Selye (1974), namely, the individual's perceptions, conditioning from previous events, and coping mechanisms. During the preparation activities, the child's and parents' perceptions of the event can be explored. Previous experiences or events affecting the individual's present situation may be identified, and finally, the previous patterns of coping can be explored and modified or strengthened.

That psychological ill effects of hospitalization, surgery, and other procedures can be prevented or minimized is accepted widely today by health care professionals (King and Ziegler, 1981; Thompson, 1985). A review of the literature in 1965 (Vernon et al.) noted that discussion of preparation efforts focused on three major themes: (1) information imparted to the child, (2) encouragement of emotional expression, and (3) establishment of trusting relationships with the hospital staff. This review revealed a limited number of actual studies pertaining to the psychological preparation of children for hospitalization. Since 1965, there has been a proliferation of research that explores the use of preparation interventions with children and parents in a variety of settings. The research has primarily focused on the content or composition of the intervention and the method used to deliver the intervention.

Information as Preparation

Providing accurate information about impending events is a primary means of preparing an individual for those events. Vernon et al. (1965) identified two reasons why an accurate understanding of one's circumstances is beneficial. First, vague and ill-defined threats are more upsetting than threats which are known and understood. Second, unexpected stress is more upsetting than expected stress. Several research studies have demonstrated the effectiveness of providing preparatory information. The information can consist of either procedural or sensory information or both. Procedural information refers to a description of what will happen: the routines and occurrences. Sensory information includes what the person will see, smell, hear, and feel.

Minde and Maler (1968) studied 149 school-aged children hospitalized for medical conditions and found that giving them information about their diseases resulted in less anxiety. Children in the experimental group were visited for 30 to 45 minutes by a child psychiatrist on their second and third days of hospitalization to discuss their illness, treatment, and the fears commonly experienced by hospitalized children. Children in the control group received no such visits. A significant decline in the experimental group's self-ratings of anxiety occurred after the intervention. It was interesting, however, that although the children rated themselves as less anxious, the nurses' ratings of the children's anxious behaviors remained unchanged over the same period of time.

Fifty-two children hospitalized for rheumatic fever were studied by Rie et al. (1968). The children, eight to 11 years old, were assigned to one of two treatment conditions, one labeled a tutorial group and the second a psychotherapy group. Each treatment consisted of a series of three small group meetings. In the tutorial meetings, children were taught about onset, treatment, and follow-up care for their disease. Those in the psychotherapy meetings explored the variety of concerns and fantasies they might have about being hospitalized and ill, but no specific information about rheumatic fever was offered.

Subjects in both experimental groups evidenced a significant increase in knowledge about the disease immediately after the interventions. Not only did the knowledge level increase but in the tutorial group there was also a significantly lower anxiety score after the intervention, as measured by the Children's Manifest Anxiety Scale (Castaneda et al., 1956).

The preparation of children for hospitalization and surgical procedures by presenting basic information has been studied by Thomson (1972). Following their admission, children six to ten years of age were given a preoperative explanation by an operating room nurse on the afternoon prior to surgery. Procedural explanations were adapted to the interests and attention spans of the children. The control group received no visit or instruction from the operating room nurse. Each child's anxiety was rated by nurses at five times prior to and following surgery based on specific behavioral manifestations. Children receiving the intervention were consistently rated as less anxious than those in the control group.

Roberts et al. (1981) demonstrated the effectiveness of a slide-tape program on increasing children's knowledge about medical terminology and procedures. All of these studies provide support for the premise that information results in increased knowledge about one's condition. Other studies have demonstrated an inverse relationship between knowledge and upset behavior. Lende (1971) found a child's knowledge about a surgical procedure was significantly related to the child's behavior. High levels of knowledge were associated with low upset. A study by Siaw et al. (1986) found that children who had the best understanding of medical instruments also reported having the least amount of anxiety about medically related procedures.

The effects of information on the child's knowledge and the relationship between the knowledge and the level of upset was examined in a study by Melamed et al. (1983). Children in one group viewed a hospital-related film and were found to have a significantly greater knowledge of hospital procedures than did children in the second group who viewed a control film. The increased knowledge was associated with less intense reactions to the hospital and to anesthesia induction by mask and resulted in a shorter hospital stay. The authors also found previous hospital experience was associated with increased knowledge.

Recent studies have suggested that the particular kind of information included in explanations is a significant variable affecting beneficial results of preparation. Johnson et al. (1975, 1976) proposed that the discrepancy between what a person expects and what is actually experienced during an event is related to the intensity of the emotional response. They concluded that the provision of accurate sensory information would reduce this discrepancy and the upset it produces.

To examine this supposition, 84 children, six to 11 years of age, who were scheduled for orthopedic cast removal were assigned to one of three groups. Children in the sensory information group listened to a 2½ minute tape recording describing the sounds (including the actual noise of the saw), smells, sights, and tactile sensations associated with the procedure. The procedure information group heard a tape outlining the procedure of removing a cast, and the third group heard no tape.

Prior to cast removal, the children were asked how afraid they were about having the cast removed. This report of fear correlated to distress scores taken during the procedure. The children who were fearful prior to cast removal were helped to cope only by the sensory information. Children reporting no fright prior to the procedure benefited by either the sensory or the procedural information.

The sensory tape did not describe intensity of sensation to be expected, nor did it make any suggestions about how to behave during the procedure. The children who heard the sensory tape had the lowest average distress score, and children hearing the procedural tape had lower distress scores than did the control group. Studies by Abrams (1982) and Eland (1981) also compared the benefits of sensory and procedural information. Unlike Johnson et al., they did not find a significant difference between the two methods.

In summary, the literature reviewed clearly supports the contention that accurate information about coming events is a means of preparing for those events. The particular kind of information included also affects the results, with accurate, complete information having the most positive result.

Enhancing Coping Skills as Preparation

In addition to informational content, either procedural or sensory, other studies have explored the benefit of including information on coping skills to use during the stressful event. These studies are based on the belief that children can control their emotional and behavioral responses through the use of specific cognitive techniques. Thompson (1985), in his review of the literature, identifies these skills as relaxation techniques, the use of distracting imagery, and comforting self-talk.

The effectiveness of filmed modeling has also been investigated by several studies and adds to the knowledge available about preparation interventions that use coping skills. Most filmed interventions have consisted of exposure to rehearsal models exhibiting either a coping model (initially anxious model who overcomes anxiety) or a mastery model (one who demonstrates no fear).

Vernon (1973) observed children experiencing anesthesia induction. Half of the subjects saw a film showing children of various ages responding calmly to anesthesia induction by mask. The control group saw no film and exhibited more fear at the time of induction. In another study, by Vernon and Bailey (1974), a film depicting a mastery model (a series of children receiving injections with no apparent fear or pain) was shown. The experimental group viewing this film experienced the greatest upset. Vernon suggested that modeling which presents inaccurate or distorted information may actually increase upset as compared with no preparation at all.

Sixty children between four and 12 years of age were shown films prior to undergoing elective surgery in a study by Melamed and Siegel (1975). Half the group saw a peer-modeling film of a child being hospitalized and having surgery. The control group saw a medically unrelated film. Self-report and behavioral and physiological measures of anxiety revealed a significant reduction of preoperative and postoperative fear in the experimental group.

Ferguson (1979) evaluated both a preadmission home visit and a peer-modeling film. She measured anxiety by electromyography readings during administration of the Hospital Fears Rating Scale. She found anxiety was most effectively relieved for younger children by viewing the film. In older children, the two interventions were equally effective.

Meng (1980) reported less anxiety in children after pre-admission preparation using a filmed coping model. In 1982, Meng and Zastowny reported on a stress inoculation program which incorporated the use of filmed modeling and group preparation. Information on stress and coping skills was introduced, and then a film showed a mother and child applying these techniques at certain hospital stress points. The parent was given a booklet for use at home to review the techniques. Results revealed that peak anxiety levels occurred on the day of admission. Children who had received the stress training exhibited less stress and coped significantly better at hospital stress points and during the posthospitalization period than children without the training.

Evaluations of the effectiveness of coping techniques have revealed other interesting findings. Nocella and Kaplan (1982) reported that relaxation and positive self-talk were effective for the experienced dental patient. Klorman et al. (1980) found that experienced dental patients were unaffected by filmed modeling interventions. Siegel and Peterson (1980, 1981) found both coping skills and sensory information to be more effective than emotional support alone. The beneficial effects of their interventions persisted a week later during subsequent treatment.

To summarize, information on coping skills that can be used during the stressful event has been shown to be beneficial. Studies have demonstrated that children can control their emotional and behavioral responses through the use of specific, learned coping techniques.

Emotional Support as Preparation

In addition to procedural and sensory information and coping skills instruction, preparation interventions can include a significant element of emotional support. Support, as defined by Webster's Ninth New Collegiate Dictionary (1987), is "to promote the interests or cause of." Emotional support occurs as a result of the child or parents having extended contact with a health care professional during the intervention. The research suggests that emotional support is at least somewhat effective in preparing children for hospitalization, surgery, or other procedures (Schwartz et al., 1983).

In a study by Fassler (1980), both experimental groups, one receiving information and emotional support and one receiving emotional support alone, were significantly less upset than the control group. The emotional support provided consisted of the presence of a supportive adult reading the child a story, talking with the child, and engaging in play with the child. In the first experimental group, these activities included information about the hospital experience and surgery. Anxiety and upset were measured by the use of the Manifest Anxiety Test based on the standard Children's Manifest Anxiety Scale and the Callahan Anxiety Pictures Test. In a study by Minde and Maler (1968), both the information and emotional support groups reported less anxiety than the control group. Lende (1971), however, found no difference in the behavior of patients undergoing tonsillectomies between groups receiving attention but no information and groups receiving information by reading a preparatory book, by discussion, or by playing through the experience. Other studies do not clearly demonstrate the effect of emotional support through the provision of attention (Nocella and Kaplan, 1982; Siegel and Peterson, 1980, 1981) over other techniques.

Stress Point Preparation

A comprehensive method of preparing children and parents that combines the elements of procedural and sensory information, rehearsal of behavior, and support at designated times of threat has become known as stress point preparation (McGrath, 1979; Visintainer and Wolfer, 1975; Wolfer and Visintainer, 1975, 1979). The stress points during the hospitalization were the blood test, medication injection, transportation to surgery, induction of anesthesia, and postoperative fluid intake. Children receiving this systematic preparation were more cooperative and less upset than the control group, as measured by the Manifest Upset Scale and the Cooperation Scale, which were completed by a nurse observer. In addition, the amount of recovery room medication given, observations of the ease of postoperative fluid intake, and the time to first postoperative voiding were indirect measures used. Posthospital adjustment was measured by the Posthospital Behavior Questionnaire. These children's parents were more satisfied and less anxious, as measured by an Information Questionnaire, an Anxiety Questionnaire, and a Satisfaction Questionnaire.

The stress point preparation was found to be more effective on the behavioral ratings used than single-session preparation which included the same information but in a single 45 minute session after admission. It was also more effective than the intervention of consistent supportive care in which a nurse offered parents and children support and reassurance at the same stress points but with no systematic presentation of information.

McGrath (1979) evaluated stress point preparation and found that systematic group preparation was more effective than individual, one-to-one preparation. In addition to the measures used by Visintainer and Wolfer (1975), she recorded pulse rates. The parents were also better informed and more satisfied.

The implication for nursing practice of pediatric group instruction incorporates the advantage of a structured time for teaching, a chance to identify with others in a similar situation, and the gaining of peer support through this identification. This is an especially positive implication since a strong argument against individual preparation programs has been that they are time consuming, costly, and an impractical use of staff time.

Although there are contradictions in the research findings conducted on preparation of children for hospitalization or procedures, the findings are very helpful in determining strategies to use. The major methods of preparation studied have included provision of information, enhancement of coping skills, provision of emotional support, and stress point preparation.

ASSESSMENT

Children or parents requiring preparation can be recognized through use of established nursing diagnoses. Three diagnoses indicating the need for preparation are (1) Anxiety, (2) Knowledge deficit, and (3) Ineffective coping. The defining characteristics of these three diagnoses provide data indicating the need for nursing intervention. Resolution of these characteristics can also be a portion of data which suggests the intervention has been successful.

Most authors suggest that there are behavioral or physiological manifestations which indicate the need for preparation interventions. The validity of observer-related behavioral upset was questioned when Ferguson (1979) found that the observer's ratings of anxiety and distress in the child did not correlate with the child's self-reported anxiety levels. She suggested—and is supported by other authors (Minde and Maler, 1968)—that children's outward behavior may not be an accurate assessment of their anxiety.

Rather than using behavioral cues, a more effective approach may be to assess the presence of a situation requiring preparation intervention as suggested by Zurlinden (1985). He has developed a model for assessing children and their state of crisis. His goal in developing the model was to increase the number of children who experience growth as a result of hospitalization. As shown in Figure 6–1, the model is a matrix with three axes: (1) the child's age, (2) hazards of hospitalization, and (3) balancing factors. The nurse assesses the information for the applicable cubes.

The child's age is on the first axis and is divided according to the age groupings identified by Petrillo and Sanger (1980). The categories infants (up to 12 months), toddlers (13 months to young three year olds), older three year olds to seven year olds, seven to 13 year olds, and adolescents (13 to 18 years old). The second axis includes the five hazards of hospitalization as identified by Visintainer and Wolfer (1975). These are (1) harm or injury (such as physical discomfort, pain, mutilation, or death); (2) the unknown (such as new and strange things in the hospital environment and the behavior of hospital workers); (3) separation (from routines, parents, peers, and trusted adults); (4) uncertain limits (such as an unclear definition of acceptable and expected behavior while in the hospital); and (5) loss of control (including either loss of competence or loss of the ability to make decisions). The third axis identifies balancing factors as described by Aguilera and Messick (1981). These factors determine whether the hazard will become a crisis for the child, and the axis includes the child's perceptions of the event, social supports, and coping skills. Using this model, the nurse assesses the child's age-appropriate balancing factors for the five hazards and determines the need for nursing intervention.

Questions to answer when using this model for assessment include the following: Is the child's developmental age comparable to the chronological age? What are the events that will occur for this child and family? What are the hazards that exist? What is the child's level of understanding and perception of events? What are the child's social supports, including parents, siblings, pets, relatives, or other significant caretakers? What are the previous experiences related to illness and hospitalization? How does the child normally cope with new and different events? Application of this model to specific children and families can provide a way to accurately assess the situation. Based on findings from this model and these questions, the nurse can develop interventions which better meet the needs of the child and family.

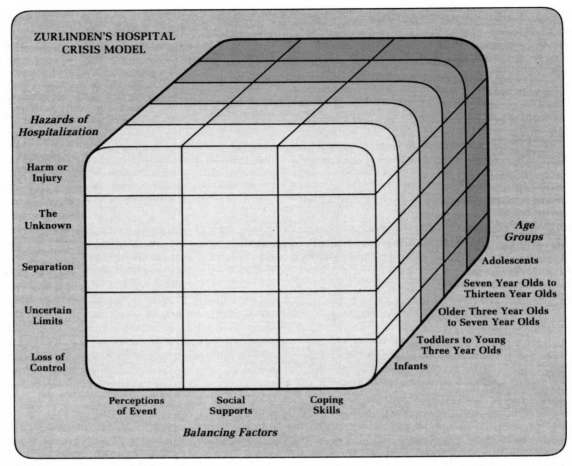

Figure 6–1. Zurlinden's hospital crisis model. (From Zurlinden, J. K. Minimizing the impact of hospitalization for children and their families. MCN: American Journal of Maternal Child Nursing, 10:179, 1985.)

THE INTERVENTION

Effective preparation includes the elements of emotional support; facilitation of emotional expression; and the provision of information, both procedural and sensory (Thompson and Stanford, 1981). Preparation strategies can be implemented in various ways. In addition to planning of the actual intervention, the appropriate content must be determined and the method and timing for delivering the preparation need to be considered. Significant variables affecting these decisions include (1) age and developmental level of the child, (2) involvement of family, (3) timing, (4) physiological status of the child, (5) psychological status and individual differences of the child, (6) setting, (7) sociocultural factors, and (8) past experience with illness and hospitalization.

Preparation strategies, as with many elements of preventive care, tend to be more praised than practiced. The principles of intervention should be incorporated into planned preparation sessions as well as into the routine of nursing care. Smith (1976) found that nurses spend an extremely brief time (1½ minutes) with a child during each encounter and that most contacts nurses made with children were intended expressly for carrying out nursing procedures affecting physiological status rather than interacting socially with the children or promoting positive, effective relationships with them. All nursing care activities should be viewed as teaching situations. Children can use these opportunities to handle the supplies and equipment, hear explanations, and ask questions. Incorporating play activities with the child into the nursing routine will provide more data for planning future interventions. Group teaching and play activities are effective and more efficient for the busy staff nurse with a heavy assignment than individual activities (Luciano and Shumsky, 1975). Group activities are also attractive to the child and have been shown to be effective (McGrath, 1979).

Creative reorganization of nursing care routines and practices can result in more effective preparation strategies. Looking at the nursing unit through a child's eyes can reveal frightening or stressful situations needing change. Admission, which is a routine procedure for hospital staff, is stressful for the child and parents (Meng, 1980; Rasmussen and Murphy, 1977). Although routine, many times admissions are an interruption in the work flow of a busy nurse's schedule. One creative solution to this problem is the formation of an admission room or assignment of an admission nurse (Koss and Teter, 1980). When a newly admitted family arrives, the admitting nurse is responsible for the admission assessment, orientation, and initial teaching of the child and family. The relationship between the child, family, and hospital staff then begins on a more relaxed and positive note. A system of primary nursing and adequate staffing may preclude the necessity for these measures.

Parents are trying to cope with the disruption and anxieties of a hospitalization along with their children. Establishing rapport with parents is essential, as is assessment of the parents' level of knowledge and understanding. Patience with repeated questions is crucial since anxiety decreases the accuracy with which children and parents will perceive information. As their anxiety decreases, they will be less likely to misinterpret verbal communication. Parents should be encouraged to act as a liaison between the nursing staff and their child and to remain with their child during and after treatments and procedures.

Specific preparation sessions are necessary for scheduled surgery or procedures. Based on assessment data, planning for the intervention includes taking into consideration the child's age, knowledge, and level of understanding; choosing appropriate methods of explanation; and using available teaching aids. The person responsible for these sessions needs accurate information about what will happen and what the child is likely to experience. All teaching materials should be gathered and an undistracting room chosen. A time when the child is alert and comfortable should be selected for preparation.

A planned outline is developed for each session, including content that is relatively standardized and agreed upon by the nursing and child life staff. Checklists or guidelines on the Kardex or care plan are effective methods for ensuring inclusion of appropriate content (Luciano, 1974; Treloar, 1978). The actual information shared and the approaches found to be well received by the child and family can be recorded for easy communication to other staff members.

Content

The need to present honest information to the child and parents regarding hospitalization and procedures is widely accepted. Stanford (1985) gives specific guidelines to use when choosing language to talk with children about painful or stressful events. He suggests that the words used are as important as the content they convey. Vivid descriptions of the colors, sounds, sensations, shapes, and sizes that the child will encounter are helpful to the child. For example, a child not expecting the computerized axial tomography scanner to be so large can feel overwhelmed when confronted with the actual equipment.

Simple comparisons can be used, but they must be familiar to the child for him or her to incorporate the information. Describing a noise as being like that of a chain saw will not be helpful to a child who has never heard one before. A noise can be described as being like a vacuum cleaner or a spot described as being as big as a nickel. One must also be careful with metaphorical language, for children take such language literally and may believe there are actually pipes inside their bodies if told about their "plumbing system."

Words that children cannot understand should not be used. Medical terms such as injection and intravenous should be explained the first time they are used. Words with many syllables or words expressing unfamiliar concepts such as numb or relax should be avoided. Further, words that can be misinterpreted can upset children. Some obvious examples of these are short, deaden, stretcher, and dye. Other words with dual meanings like drapes and stool are simply confusing.

Telling a child the reason for hospitalization or a procedure is important because it helps dispel the fantasies and fears of the child. Reasons should be stated in positive and reassuring ways. For example, the child can be told that restraints are to help him hold still, and NPO helps the stomach rest during the operation. It is easy to inadvertently use negative suggestions. "You'll be really brave; you'll be glad when it's over" implies that the child will need courage. Telling a child the x-rays won't hurt needlessly introduces the possibility of pain. The child probably never thought an x-ray would hurt! An alternative is to tell the child, "You won't feel anything unusual."

Emotionally charged words such as *cut*, *pull*, and *stick* are distressing to a child. Instead, such terms as *making an opening*, *ease out*, and *gently slide* can be used. Imperative language such as "You must be very still so I can get the I.V. in" is generally unhelpful. A more positive way of stating the same idea would be "This is a time to hold still" or "You'll be able to hold your arm still." In a study comparing empathic and directive approaches in preparing children for venipuncture, Fernald and Corry (1981) found a child-centered supportive approach was more effective. The alternative, a directive approach of informing the child the procedure will occur but telling the child to be big and brave, not to cry, and to sit still actually produced more crying and upset behavior.

In an effort to be open and honest in talking with children, many professionals have inadvertently been dishonest (Stanford, 1985). For example, telling a child that he or she will feel pain during a procedure or that it will feel like a bee sting or mosquito bite may not be accurate. The perception of pain is affected by many variables. What is painful for one person may not be painful for another. Pain and discomfort can also be modified by time and external events. An approach that maintains trust and avoids negative suggestions is needed. The characteristics of this approach are (1) understanding that no one else knows how a procedure will feel for the child, (2) outlining the range of possibilities to the child, (3) ascertaining

how the child would like the procedure to feel, and (4) asking the child if it would be all right if the procedure didn't hurt much at all (McHugh et al., 1982; Stanford, 1985).

Methods

There is no single technique or method of preparation that is most effective. Instead, experienced practitioners have found a combination of methods to be most helpful. The following discussion outlines common methods currently available.

Person-to-Person Interaction

Almost without exception, effective preparation techniques have included interaction between the child and an adult. To be thorough and effective, the process should involve a variety of individuals. Logically, preparation begins with the physicians when the need for a procedure, surgery, or hospitalization becomes evident. The role of the physician should be active (Mellish, 1969), incorporating many of the principles discussed previously. Other members of the health care team can then become involved almost immediately. Preparation can be done by a nurse child life worker, or other individual who has a knowledge of medical procedures, child development, and the emotional needs of children and their families.

In order to develop the relationship of trust, which has been reported as an effective means of providing emotional support, it is recommended that a single individual be responsible for most of the preparation (Thompson and Stanford, 1981; Visintainer and Wolfer, 1975; Wolfer and Visintainer, 1975, 1979). A system of primary nursing ensures a consistent nurse-family involvement as well as coordination of other professionals as needed.

Play

Play, structured and unstructured, hospital-related and non–hospital-related, has been advocated widely as a preparation technique (Chan, 1980; D'Antonio, 1984; Dorsky, 1984; Ellerton et al., 1985; Hansen and Evans, 1981; Knudsen, 1975; Letts et al., 1983; Meer, 1985; Schwartz et al., 1983). The purposes for play include (1) imparting information, (2) reinforcing information, (3) assessing the child's understanding of information, (4) encouraging emotional expression, and (5) increasing the child's comfort and independence. Although play is widely accepted as a natural activity for children, the effectiveness of play for preparation for hospitalization, surgery, or medical procedures has not been a major focus in recent research. A few studies, as discussed in the following paragraphs, have attempted to address the effects of play and puppetry as preparations as well as the sharing of information with a child to determine which intervention was responsible for the resulting decrease in the child's anxiety.

Cassell (1965) found that children prepared for cardiac catheterization by use of play with miniature models, puppets, and toy medical instruments were rated as less upset during the catheterization procedure. These children also exhibited greater willingness to return to the hospital later. Schulz et al. (1981) evaluated the effect of a presentation followed by the opportunity to play with the medical equipment models. A significant reduction in the anxiety of the children was noted following the intervention. Investigators have found that the opportunity to play, even when unaccompanied by medical information, may be nearly as effective in reducing a child's upset as the combination of medical information and play (Schwartz et al., 1983).

Puppetry as a therapeutic tool is another technique of interest and has been evaluated in several studies (Cassell, 1965; Letts et al., 1983; Schulz et al., 1981). Alger et al. (1985) believe puppetry is valuable because it is active, immediate, and engages a child both verbally and physically. Many children can express their feelings more easily through the medium of a third "person" such as a puppet than they can directly with a person. Puppetry or the use of a puppet show for teaching must be carefully assessed, however. In some instances, volunteers rather than experienced puppeteers operate the puppets, and they may not be as responsive to the cues of the children in the audience. In other instances, the children can be so interested in the puppet show that the message is entirely missed.

Play, related or unrelated to the hospital and procedural events, is universally accepted as the work of the child. Play in the hospital brings a sense of normality to an otherwise confusing and overwhelming environment. Materials used for play should be considered only as supplements to the preparation process. A caring, knowledgeable individual is essential for providing security and responses to the questions, fantasies, and misconceptions that may surface.

Written Material

Written material in the form of books or pamphlets is widely used for preparation. These books and pamphlets can supplement verbal information and can be referred to repeatedly as needed. Many books are available to acquaint the child with the hospital setting. Altshuler (1974) offers helpful guidelines for book selection: (1) Does the book meet the special needs of the individual child for the type of illness, the specific institution, and the age and types of characters with whom to identify? (2) Does the book present a realistic picture of the hospital experience? (3) Is the story well told, with illustrations of high artistic quality that appeal to children?

Selection of written material should be done carefully for several reasons. Written material can inadvertently perpetuate myths about hospitalization and increase fear and anxiety in the child (Stanford, 1985). Pictures showing injections in the arm with no pain, ice cream tasting good after a tonsillectomy with no pain when swallowing, or a child happily waving good-bye to parents promote an unrealistic picture of the hospital. Material using fantasy figures, such as dragons and witches, is not only difficult for the child to relate to but is also hardly reassuring. A story that lets the child identify with another child who is having the same procedure performed is more helpful than stories about mice, monkeys, or frogs.

Written information given to parents prior to the event can be helpful and should include (1) simple booklets to read to prepare their child; (2) specific information on what their child is likely to experience; and (3) general hospital information, including a description of the admission procedure, travel directions, telephone numbers, and instructions on what to bring to the hospital (Zweig, 1986). These booklets should be prepared by the health professionals on staff and tailored to the specific setting. Input from involved department staff as well as review by parents and children is helpful in the development of this material. Material must be reviewed periodically to ensure information is up to date. Written information and pictures can help parents to explain to their child what the child will see, hear, and experience during the hospital stay. The role of the parents and specific information about the procedure or surgery to be done should be included.

Guidelines for talking with children, including an emphasis on the importance of initiating such conversations, are important. Many parents cannot offer articulate, accurate information unless or until someone has helped them. Their hesitancy to talk with their children can result in a total lack of information being given to their children. When parents avoid talking about health care information, their children may perceive the message that the topic is too terrible to discuss.

Audiovisual Materials

Well-designed, accurate films, slide-tape programs, and auditory tapes in combination with contact of a supportive adult are effective methods of preparation (Abrams, 1982; Demarest et al., 1984; Ferguson, 1979; Johnson et. al., 1975). However, these audiovisual materials may not be as helpful for patients with previous experience (Klorman et al., 1980) and may actually be harmful if inaccurate (Vernon and Bailey, 1974).

Children who actively experience events such as using a blood pressure cuff, riding a bed, wearing a mask, or using a stethoscope following a slide-tape presentation have less anxiety than children who just view the audiovisual material (Demarest et al., 1984). Information alone can result in increased anxiety if the child doesn't have the opportunity to discuss, draw pictures of, or play out the information (Fassler, 1980; Melamed and Siegel, 1975).

Slide-tape programs produced for the specific setting are inexpensive, utilize both visual and auditory senses, and are easily updated or modified. Although the content on videotapes is fixed, they are easy to use in almost any setting and, with expansion of the home video market, may become more

widely used for preparation of children at home prior to hospitalization.

Accuracy of the audiovisual information is essential. Any differences between what is viewed and what will occur need to be explained to the child. The material should be viewed only with an adult present to respond to questions and correct misunderstandings and fantasies. The child's reactions to the material can be closely observed and the film or program stopped if necessary. Activities such as discussion and play following the program will facilitate learning.

Music therapy techniques have been suggested as a method for helping children cope with surgery (Siegel, 1983). Tapes of a child's favorite music have been found to be an effective stress reduction technique (Claire and Erickson, 1986). Siegel (1983) found the use of music relaxation techniques during the preoperative and postoperative period resulted in patients requesting less pain medication.

Pictures and Diagrams

Pictures and diagrams can be used in a variety of ways (see Chapter 8). Young children can be shown pictures of familiar hospital scenes and events and asked to tell a story about the pictures. This approach elicits information about the child's response to the hospitalization and provides an opportunity to dispel existing misconceptions (Mandleco, 1976).

Preschool children as well as school-aged children may have difficulty in verbally expressing and describing their perceptions accurately. Asking children to draw pictures about what is happening can also give the professional cues about the perceptions of children (Porter, 1974).

A wide variability in the levels of knowledge about body organs and illness exists in children (Smith, 1977). Petrillo and Sanger (1980) recommend the use of outlined body diagrams in sharing anatomical information with children. These can also be used to assess the child's understanding of his or her disease or the impending procedure.

Variables Affecting Preparation Strategies

Timing

Optimal timing of the preparation will depend upon both events and the age and developmental level of a child. Preparation should be planned to precede a scheduled hospitalization or procedure. Preschoolers' magical thinking and fantasies require preparation beginning closer to the actual event. Because their conception of time centers around activities of daily living, they should be told about procedures occurring "just before lunch," or "after your nap." School-age children and adolescents have a good grasp of time and perceive the future and the past. They can begin preparation as soon as the procedure is scheduled (Melamed et al., 1976; Mellish, 1969).

Azarnoff and Woody (1981), in a survey of 1427 hospitals providing inpatient pediatric care, reported only one third offered preparation on a regular basis. Of those hospitals that offered preparation on a regular basis, 64% offered preadmission preparation. Purposes of these programs included (1) familiarization of the child and parents with the hospital environment and procedures; (2) reduction of anxiety, fears, and misconceptions; (3) provision of information; and (4) offering of comfort and support (Atkins, 1981; Gross et al., 1976; Meng, 1980; Trouten, 1981). Although less widely utilized, preadmission programs can be an effective method for preparing for the event (Sauer, 1968; Schreier and Kaplan, 1983). A preadmission tour familiarizes children and parents with the environment, personnel, and equipment. It provides an opportunity for questions to be asked and answered in a relatively unthreatening environment and, perhaps most important, it allows children to return home, thereby dispelling fears that once inside a hospital, children never leave.

There are many instances when hospitalization or the need for medical procedures arises unexpectedly. In such instances, explanations and support must be given on an ongoing basis even after the event has occurred (Betz, 1982; Dorsky, 1984). Postprocedural sessions are also important even when there has been prior preparation. After the event, the child can explore his feelings and perceptions, and reinforcement can be given for coping techniques used. Parents will be better able to help their child cope with fears and fantasies if included in these sessions. Documenting the emotional and behavioral responses of children will facilitate communication with other staff members.

Timing is also a significant factor, because often the same procedure is repeated as a continuing part of therapy or a child may require repeated hospitalizations and the intervention should be performed when it will help the child most. The child may have more information as a result of these previous experiences, but that does not mean the child is better prepared. In fact, anxiety can escalate with the anticipation of a previously encountered stressful or painful event (Betz, 1982; Crocker, 1980; Johnson and Salazar, 1979; Melamed et al., 1983; Thomson, 1972).

In this situation, the child becomes both a learner and a teacher in the preparation sessions. The child is the one with the experience and will "teach" the listener about what concerns him most. The nurse can be an active listener and clear up misconceptions and fantasies. Review and support of coping mechanisms can be given.

Intervention prior to rehospitalization can reduce fear and anxiety for both the child and family (Johnson and Salazar, 1979). Exploring previous experiences, reviewing coping strategies, and just suggesting that it doesn't have to feel the same way the next time can be helpful (Stanford, 1985).

Age and Developmental Level

The process of preparing a child for hospitalization or a specific event is influenced by the age and developmental level of the child. Zurlinden (1985) notes that the hazards of hospitalization and the available balancing factors are both related directly to the age of the child. The major developmental tasks can influence the child's responses to a stressful event (Bavin, 1983). The degree of regression exhibited by the child may also influence the choice of language and methods for preparation. Petrillo and Sanger (1980) group children according to age and offer specific guidelines for preparation interventions for each age group. It is generally accepted that children of different age groups react differently to preparation and to the methods used (Melamed et al., 1983; Meng, 1980; Schwartz et al., 1983).

If age and developmental level are not considered, inappropriate language may be used because adults often estimate the level of understanding in children inaccurately (Hansen and Evans, 1981; Smith, 1977; Stanford, 1985). Both Pidgeon (1977) and Pontious (1982) have reviewed characteristics of thinking in children and the implications for health teaching.

The way the child perceives the world, thinks, reasons, and uses language is qualitatively different in each of the following age groups: sensorimotor (birth to two years), preoperational (two to seven years), concrete operational (seven to 12 years), and adolescent (12 years and on) according to Piaget and Inhelder (1969). For example, children before the age of two learn about the world through their senses. Thought and reasoning are just emerging, and language is mostly imitative. As a result, verbal explanations are virtually meaningless, and preparation efforts must be focused on the parents.

Preoperational children, from two to seven years, see the world strictly from their own viewpoint and cannot accept the view of another. They are capable of seeing only one aspect of an object at a time. For example, taking medicine to take away head pain makes no sense to them, because the medicine goes into the stomach, not the head. Also, two concepts are involved, the medicine and the pain, and that is more than these children can handle.

Children in the concrete operational stage view the world more objectively and realistically. These children are aware of reversibility, can classify objects and experiences, and have a grasp of the concept of time. Words represent reality, and these children understand the use of language for communication. However, they do not yet thoroughly comprehend words with multiple meanings or words for things they have not yet experienced.

In addition to age affecting the way children think, reason, and use language, the fears of children vary with age. Miller (1979) found fears change with age and may parallel cognitive and perceptual development. Fears become better articulated, and more varied and realistic as children grow from one to 12 years of age. Broome (1986) found a child's fear of a medical experience is related to the occurrence of more negative behavior during the experience.

Involvement of the Family

Family relationships and structure are influencing variables to consider when planning intervention strategies. Families differ according to their development as a unit (Petrillo and Sanger, 1980). A young family that has been established for less than three years is still settling marital and parental roles and is more likely to use health professionals for advice and support. A family established for four to ten years has routinized patterns and roles and is less susceptible to outside influence. The older family, established for ten to 20 years, has set patterns and may find it more difficult to adjust to the hospitalization of a child.

Especially vulnerable during periods of crisis are the single-parent family and the newly blended family. A large number of children today are living with a single parent, living alternately with each parent, or living with stepparents. These factors will affect balancing factors which children can use to deal with stressful events.

Involvement of at least one parent in preparation interventions is important. Skipper and Leonard (1968) found that mothers who were given information about the hospital setting were less anxious, and in turn their children were less anxious, than families in the control group. The involvement of parents is even more important for the child under five since a child in this age group is indirectly supported through his parents (King and Ziegler, 1981; Vardara, 1978). Behaviors and attitudes of the patient and family in the hospital setting were found to be mutually interdependent (Dziurbejko and Larkin, 1968). Each responds to the other, and events affecting one also affect the other. In addition, some children are more inclined to participate actively in preparation sessions if parents are present (Crocker, 1980).

Parents with little or no past hospitalization experience are poorly equipped to prepare their child for impending hospitalization (Meng, 1980). Without basic information and support, parents may inadvertently misinform, withhold information from, or nonverbally communicate anxiety to a child. Parents who have not been prepared for the hospitalization of their child react with fear and anxiety (Freiberg, 1972). The most common source of their anxiety is fear about procedures and lack of information.

When a child is ill or requires hospitalization, stress exists for the entire family. The well siblings and parents are affected in various ways. Important tasks for the parents include understanding and managing their child's illness and assisting their child in understanding and coping (Hymovich, 1976; Smitherman, 1979). Performing these tasks requires information and emotional support. A common way parents cope is by asking questions, talking with other parents, and being vigilant about their child's care (Miles and Carter, 1985).

In addition to information and support, parents also need to be given a role by the nurse. Algren (1985) studied mothers of hospitalized children and found few mothers had received information regarding their role in caring for their child. Most parents want to take an active role in their child's care but do not know what information can be shared or the best methods to share it.

A major factor influencing a child's reaction to stress is the child's social supports (Aguilera and Messick, 1981; Zurlinden, 1985). It is imperative for the nurse to know who is the primary caretaker for the child and to assess that person's desire for participation in the child's care. Other significant supports, such as siblings, other relatives, pets, and unrelated caretakers and baby sitters, should also be considered. Information regarding the primary caretaker and his or her preferences for participation must be documented on the nursing Kardex or care plan for communication to involved staff (see Chapter 4).

Physiological Status

The physiological status of the child will have an impact on the effectiveness of preparation and should be considered in planning and timing preparation. A child who is disoriented, in severe pain, or seriously ill will have difficulty comprehending information. Explanations should still be given, using the basic guidelines suggested previously, although the child may be a passive participant. Shorter, more frequent preparation sessions are recommended and, if at all possible, when the child is rested and afebrile and when pain is at a minimum.

Communication with the child during emergency or unanticipated procedures or hospitalization is important, because silence communicates fear and increases anxiety (Thompson and Stanford, 1981). The fact that the situation is already occurring doesn't mean the child has no need to know what is happening and why. Postprocedural sessions can also give information, encourage emotional expression, and provide support (Betz, 1982).

Psychological Status

Preparation interventions are affected by the personality, psychological status, and coping styles of children. Individual coping styles vary from child to child (LaMontagne, 1984a, 1984b) and can be assessed by questioning the parents or child and in some instances by observing the child's reactions to situations (Tarnow and Gutstein, 1983).

To be most effective, interventions should be based on the individual child's coping style. The three styles identified are active, avoidant, and active-avoidant (LaMontagne, 1984a, 1984b). Children exhibiting active coping characteristics are overly alert to the emotional or threatening aspects of the event. They have detailed information on all aspects and are ready to discuss them. Because of this heightened awareness of the situation, active copers might experience increased stress. These children need further clarification of information as well as reassurance about the recovery course.

Children who are avoidant copers show denial of emotional or threatening aspects of the impending event. There is a hesitancy or unwillingness to discuss their thoughts and concerns. It is most helpful to provide reassurance and support rather than detailed information, which can be overwhelming to these children. Explanations should reinforce what the children already know and introduce new information only selectively.

Children who show both of these styles are called active-avoidant copers. The information they seek is usually general and limited to the procedure. Because they tend to deny or avoid the unpleasant aspects of a situation, they can benefit from anxiety-reducing techniques such as relaxation and positive-thinking exercises.

Setting

Children may face the event of a medical procedure in a variety of settings, including the school, clinic, physician's or dentist's office, emergency room, or hospital. Preparation should precede any procedure, including those in ambulatory settings and day-surgery units. In a study by Azarnoff and Woody (1981) of 1427 hospitals, it was found that preparation was usually random, occasional, and insufficient. This finding is interesting in light of the belief of most health professionals that preparation should be a continual process. It should begin at home and continue in the school and community, and should be reinforced before a procedure occurs. Ambulatory settings and day-surgery units can incorporate the principles of preparation. Well-designed audiovisual media can supplement other methods of preparation and offer a consistent and simple way of providing information (Abrams, 1982). Play materials can be available in waiting areas and can also be used in explaining procedures to a child (Meer, 1985). The office nurse can play a significant role in preparation of the child (Robison, 1979). Nurses in every setting that provides services for children can implement the techniques recommended.

Beckemeyer and Bahr (1980) outlined an effective method of helping toddlers and preschoolers cope during suturing of minor lacerations. Pain and anxiety were reduced by slowly dripping a local anesthetic onto the area near the wound prior to injection of that area; offering age-appropriate explanations; answering questions; encouraging self-control rather than physical restraint; reinforcing positive behavior; and using existing support systems, such as parents. These basic principles can be incorporated into any emergency room, clinic, or physician's office and will actually save time and reduce stress for all involved.

Concerned professionals are advocating the introduction of well children to the possibility of hospitalization through various programs (Abbott et al., 1970; Hardgrove-Aldrich, 1975; Pomarico et al., 1979; Thompson and Stanford, 1981; Zweig, 1976). These programs usually include a hospital tour with an emphasis on explanations of services offered should the need for hospitalization arise. In some communities, health professionals visit in the school setting and talk with children about the role of the hospital in the community, demonstrate equipment, show pictures, and answer questions. These programs are based on the assumption that increased knowledge will help children cope. The effectiveness of such programs is yet to be documented through research.

Socioeconomic Factors

Socioeconomic factors influence the type of preparation the child receives. La-Montagne (1984b) found children in high-income families were more likely to believe they had some control over events happening to them. Their parents were more likely to attend preadmission programs or seek out information with which to prepare their child (Meng, 1980; Schmeltz and White, 1982; Schreier and Kaplan, 1983). High-income parents are generally better educated and tend to have more support systems and resources available to them with which to handle the crisis arising from the illness or hospitalization of a child. Thus, children of low-income families may need special attention to ensure effective preparation.

To summarize, the key elements of preparation include the provision of information, emotional expression, and support. The choice of preparation strategies used by the nurse will be influenced by the variables of age and developmental level, family and social supports, timing, the child's physiological and psychological status, the setting, and socioeconomic factors. The case study example of Beth Ann illustrates an effective preparation strategy.

EVALUATION

Methods used for measuring intervention effectiveness contain the same measures used to identify the need for preparation. Numerous tools and behavioral measurements have been used, but no single tool offers a complete answer. These tools and measurements include the Hospital Picture Test (Mandleco, 1976); the Manifest Upset Scale and the Cooperation Scale (Schwartz et al., 1983; Wolfer and Visintainer, 1975, 1979); the Palmar Sweat Test (Winter et al., 1963); the Children's Manifest Anxiety Scale (Castaneda et al., 1956); the Callahan Anxiety Pictures Test (Callahan, 1978); the Posthospital Behavior Questionnaire (Vernon et al., 1966); the Hospital Fears Rating Scale (Scherer and Nakamura, 1968); electromyographic measures of muscle tension (Ferguson, 1979); use of analgesic medication, early postoperative voiding, and pulse rates (Wolfer and Visintainer, 1975, 1979); and self-reports of anxiety levels.

Case Study

Eight year old Beth Ann had been diagnosed with cystic fibrosis at the age of three after repeated respiratory problems. She and her three year old brother, Kevin, lived with her parents. Her maternal grandparents lived in the same city and were actively supportive and involved with the family. Her father, who suffers from Crohn's disease, had experienced repeated hospitalizations and had negative feelings about hospitals.

Although Beth Ann's parents had faithfully complied with all treatment regimens, her disease had progressively worsened, requiring repeated hospitalizations over the years. Beth Ann had experienced previous intravenous antibiotic therapy but not surgery. Her parents and the hospital staff had always shared information openly with Beth Ann. As a result of her active coping style, she knew a great deal about her disease and its treatment.

During the latest hospitalization, Beth Ann's condition worsened, with her secretions becoming extremely thick and tenacious. By that Friday evening, traditional methods were providing no relief and the physician elected to perform a bronchial washing the following day. At the time, this was a new procedure at the hospital, and the staff was uninformed about what to expect. Beth Ann had never experienced surgery or a procedure like this and was very anxious. Both Beth Ann and her parents verbalized fears that Beth Ann was going to die during the procedure. They knew she had breathing problems and believed the risk of anesthesia was enormous. A nursing diagnosis of *Ineffective coping related to lack of information* was made.

The nurse working with Beth Ann and her parents talked with the attending physician and contacted another hospital in the state to determine how the procedure would be done. The nurse then gathered the necessary materials and explained to Beth Ann what would be done and described what sights, sounds, smells, and feelings she might experience in the operating room. Beth Ann's parents were present and all three openly asked questions.

The following day and the time for the scheduled procedure arrived. Although Beth Ann and her parents were anxious, they were optimistic and seemed supportive of each other. The information and their understanding of the procedure helped relieve their anxiety. The procedure went well, and Beth Ann awoke tired and uncomfortable. Two mornings later, the nurse collected the materials for medical play, including syringes and needles. Selecting a time when interruptions would be minimal, she approached Beth Ann to talk with her about the procedure and how Beth Ann felt about the procedure.

Beth Ann indicated an interest in giving the doll an injection and, after watching the nurse, carefully prepared the syringe. With the syringe ready, she accepted the doll and jabbed the needle through the nose of the doll with enough force to jam the needle into the table beneath. Although the nurse was surprised, she did not react outwardly but instead asked Beth Ann if she would like to prepare another injection. Beth Ann continued to jab the doll through the nose, although with less force each time. Her anger and hostility seemed to fade, and after the thirteenth injection in the nose, she began injecting the doll in the leg with more gentleness and only after explaining in detail what she was going to do.

The nurse's quiet observation, "I notice you put the needle in her nose" opened the conversation to strong feelings and the misconceptions Beth Ann had that her disease was a "breathing disease." Additional information and clarification were given and reinforced. As subsequent bronchial washings were scheduled, Beth Ann no longer feared the trip to surgery but instead required reassurance that she could cope with the discomfort that followed.

RESEARCH IMPLICATIONS

Although there has recently been a significant emphasis on research relating to preparation techniques for children facing hospitalization or medical procedures, additional work is needed. Less than half of the research reviewed included children 12 years or older. Further, in several studies, the effects of the interventions were difficult to evaluate because age groups were mixed. Research is needed which limits ages in the sample to obtain clear information regarding age-specific interventions.

The research has focused almost exclusively on children admitted for surgical procedures. The child with a medical diagnosis was seldom evaluated, and the child with a chronic condition not considered at all. Effective preparation strategies for children who undergo repeated procedures or who have had previous negative experiences need to be identified.

The majority of the research focuses on preparation which occurs after admission to the hospital. Because of that, several questions remain neglected: (1) Is preadmission preparation effective? (2) Is there merit in preparation efforts being focused on the parents? (3) What are the effective methods for preparing parents?

The studies on modeling indicate that inaccurate or distorted information can actually increase the child's distress. Therefore, study is needed to determine if there are other interventions currently accepted that may be harmful. For example, what is the effect of written information, films, and programs that use frightening or fantasy-producing characters such as dragons, headhunters, or frogs in an effort to appeal to the child? Health professionals need to know the potential effect of various interventions.

And finally, the most effective, yet cost-efficient interventions that are practical and realistic in today's health care environment must be identified. A demonstration of effectiveness of preadmission home visits by the nurse in the prospective reimbursement climate is, unfortunately, not applicable for many institutions. However, a demonstration that preparation of children and parents will result in shorter hospital stays and decreased utilization of other scarce hospital resources would be a tremendous asset for the nurse manager working to justify preparation programs on cost issues.

References

Abbott, N, Hansen, P, and Lewis, K. Dress rehearsal for the hospital. American Journal of Nursing, 70:2360–2367, 1970.

Abrams, L. Resistance behaviors and teaching media for children in day surgery. AORN Journal, 35:244–258, 1982.

Aguilera, D, and Messick, JM. Crisis intervention: Theory and methodology (4th ed.). St. Louis: CV Mosby Co., 1981.

Alger, I, Linn, S., and Beardslee, W. Puppetry as a therapeutic tool for hospitalized children. Hospital and Community Psychiatry, 36:129–130, 1985.

Algren, C. Role perception of mothers who have hospitalized children. Children's Health Care, 14:6–9, 1985.

Altshuler, A. Books that help children deal with a hospital experience. (U.S. Department of Health, Education, and Welfare Pub. No. 74–5402). Washington, DC: U.S. Government Printing Office, 1974.

Atkins, DM. Evaluation of a preadmission preparation program: Goals clarification as the first step. Children's Health Care, 10:48–52, 1981.

Azarnoff, P, and Woody, P. Preparation of children for hospitalization in acute care hospitals in the United States. Pediatrics, 68:361–368, 1981.

Bavin, R. Pediatric cardiac preoperative teaching. Focus on Critical Care, 10:36–43, 1983.

Beckemeyer, P, and Bahr, JE. Helping toddlers and preschoolers cope while suturing their minor lacerations. MCN: American Journal of Maternal Child Nursing, 5:326–330, 1980.

Betz, CL. After the operation: Postprocedural sessions to allay anxiety. MCN: American Journal of Maternal Child Nursing, 7:260–263, 1982.

Broome, ME. The relationship between children's fears and behavior during a painful event. Children's Health Care, 14:142–146, 1986.

Callahan, R. Rest manual for the Callahan anxiety pictures. Los Angeles: Sunset Distributors, 1978.

Cassell, S. Effect of brief puppet therapy upon the emotional responses of children undergoing cardiac catheterization. Journal of Consulting Psychology, 29:1–8, 1965.

Castaneda, A, McCandless, R, and Palermo, D. The children's form of the manifest anxiety scale. Child Development, 27:317–326, 1956.

Chan, JM. Preparation for procedures and surgery through play. Pediatrician, 9:210–219, 1980.

Claire, JB, and Erickson, S. Reducing distress in pediatric patients undergoing cardiac catheterization. Children's Health Care, 14:146–152, 1986.

Crocker, E. Preparation for elective surgery: Does it make a difference? Journal of the Association for Care of Children's Health, 9:3–11, 1980.

D'Antonio, IJ. Therapeutic use of play in hospitals. Nursing Clinics of North America, 19:351–359, 1984.

Demarest, DS, Hooke, JF, and Erickson, MT. Preoperative intervention for the reduction of anxiety in pediatric surgery patients. Children's Health Care, 12:179–183, 1984.

Dorsky, LT. Using dolls to prepare children for surgery. Patient Education Newsletter, 7:4–5, 1984.

Dziurbejko, M, and Larkin, J. Including the family in preoperative teaching. American Journal of Nursing, 68:1892–1894, 1968.

Eland, JM. Minimizing pain associated with prekindergarten intramuscular injections. Issues in Comprehensive Pediatric Nursing, 5:361–372, 1981.

Ellerton, ML, Caty, S, and Ritchie, JA. Helping young children master intrusive procedures through play. Children's Health Care, 13:167–173, 1985.

Fassler, D. Reducing preoperative anxiety in children: Information versus emotional support. Patient Counseling and Health Education, 2:130–134, 1980.

Ferguson, B. Preparing young children for hospitalization: A comparison of two methods. Pediatrics, 64:656–664, 1979.

Fernald, CD, and Corry, JJ. Empathic versus directive preparation of children for needles. Children's Health Care, 10:44–46, 1981.

Freiberg, KH. How parents react when their child is hospitalized. American Journal of Nursing, 72:1270–1272, 1972.

Gross, C, Hedenkamp, E, Lovelace, B, and Meissner, AM. Preparation of children for cardiac surgery using a team approach. Journal of the Association for the Care of Children's Health, 4:12–16, 1976.

Hansen, BD, and Evans, ML. Preparing a child for procedures. MCN: American Journal of Maternal Child Nursing, 6:392–397, 1981.

Hardgrove-Aldrich, C. Preparing nonpatient children for hospitalization. Unpublished manuscript, University of California, San Francisco, 1975.

Hymovich, D. Parents of sick children: Their needs and tasks. Pediatric Nursing, 2:9–23, 1976.

Johnson, JE, Kirchhoff, KT, and Endress, MP. Altering children's distress behavior during orthopedic cast removal. Nursing Research, 24:404–410, 1975.

Johnson, JE, Kirchhoff, KT, and Endress, MP. Easing children's fright during health care procedures. MCN: American Journal of Maternal Child Nursing, 1:206–210, 1976.

Johnson, M, and Salazar, M. Preadmission program for rehospitalized children. American Journal of Nursing, 79:1420–1423, 1979.

Kim, MJ, McFarland, GV, and McLande, FM. Nursing diagnoses. St. Louis: CV Mosby Co., 1984.

King, J, and Ziegler, S. The effects of hospitalization on children's behavior: A review of the literature. Children's Health Care, 10:20–28, 1981.

Klorman, R, Hilpert, PL, Michael, R, LaGana, C, and Sveen, OB. Effects of coping and mastering modeling on experienced and inexperienced pedodontic patients' disruptiveness. Behavior Therapy, 11:156–168, 1980.

Knudsen, K. Play therapy: Preparing the young child for surgery. Nursing Clinics of North America, 10:679–686, 1975.

Koss, T, and Teter, M. Welcoming a family when a child is hospitalized. MCN: American Journal of Maternal Child Nursing, 5:51–54, 1980.

LaMontagne, LL. Children's locus of control beliefs as predictors of their preoperative coping behavior. Nursing Research, 33:76–85, 1984a.

LaMontagne, LL. Three coping strategies used by school-age children. Pediatric Nursing, 10:25–28, 1984b.

Lazarus, RS. Psychological stress and the coping process. New York: McGraw-Hill, Inc., 1966.

Lazarus, RS, and Launier, R. Stress-related transactions between person and environment. In Pervin, LA, and Lewis, M, (Eds.), Perspectives in interactional psychology. New York: Plenum Publishing Corp., 1978, pp. 281–327.

Lende, EW. The effect of preparation on children's response to tonsillectomy and adenoidectomy surgery. Unpublished doctoral dissertation, University of Cincinnati, 1971.

Letts, M, Stevens, L, Coleman, J., and Kettner, R. Puppetry and doll play as an adjunct to pediatric orthopedics. Journal of Pediatric Orthopedics, 3:605–609, 1983.

Luciano, K. The who, when, where, what, and how of preparing children for surgery. Nursing 74, 4:64–65, 1974.

Luciano, K, and Shumsky, C. Pediatric procedures: The explanation should always come first. Nursing 75, 5:49–52, 1975.

Mandleco, BH. Monitoring children's reactions when they are hospitalized for percutaneous renal biopsy. MCN: American Journal of Maternal Child Nursing, 1:288–292, 1976.

McCaffery, M. Children's responses to rectal temperatures: An exploratory study. Nursing Research, 20:32–45, 1971.

McGrath, MM. Group preparation of pediatric surgical patients. Image, 11:52–63, 1979.

McHugh, NH, Christman, NJ, and Johnson, JE. Preparatory information: What helps and why. American Journal of Nursing, 82:780–782, 1982.

Meer, PA. Using play therapy in outpatient settings. American Journal of Maternal-Child Nursing, 10:378–380, 1985.

Melamed, BG, and Siegel, L. Reduction of anxiety in children facing hospitalization and surgery by use of filmed modelling. Journal of Consulting and Clinical Psychology, 43:511–521, 1975.

Melamed, BG, Meyer, R, Gee, C, and Soule, L. The influence of time and type of preparation on children's adjustment to hospitalization. Journal of Pediatric Psychology, 1:31–37, 1976.

Melamed, BG, Dearborn, M, and Hermecz, DA. Necessary considerations for surgery preparation: Age and previous experience. Psychosomatic Medicine, 45:517–525, 1983.

Mellish, RW. Preparation of a child for hospitalization and surgery. Pediatric Clinics of North America, 16:543–553, 1969.

Meng, AL. Parents' and children's reactions toward impending hospitalization for surgery. Maternal-Child Nursing Journal, 9:83–90, 1980.

Meng, AL, and Zastowny, T. Preparation for hospitalization: A stress inoculation training program for parents and children. Maternal-Child Nursing Journal, 11:87–94, 1982.

Miles, MS, and Carter, MC. Coping strategies used by parents during their child's hospitalization in an intensive care unit. Children's Health Care, 14:14–21, 1985.

Miller, SR. Children's fears: A review of the literature with implications for nursing research and practice. Nursing Research, 28:217–223, 1979.

Minde, K, and Maler, L. Psychiatric counseling on a pediatric medical ward: A controlled evaluation. Journal of Pediatrics, 72:452–460, 1968.

Nocella, J, and Kaplan, RM. Training children to cope with dental treatment. Journal of Pediatric Psychology, 7:175–178, 1982.

Petrillo, M, and Sanger, S. Emotional care of hospitalized children: An environmental approach (2nd ed.). Philadelphia: JB Lippincott Co., 1980.

Piaget, J, and Inhelder, B. Psychology of the child. New York: Basic Books, Inc., 1969.

Pidgeon, VA. Characteristics of children's thinking and implications for health teaching. Maternal-Child Nursing Journal, 6:1–8, 1977.

Pomarico, C, Marsh, K, and Doubrava, P. Hospital orientation for children. AORN Journal, 29:864–871, 1979.

Pontious, SL. Practical Piaget: Helping children understand. American Journal of Nursing, 82:114–117, 1982.

Porter, CS. Grade-school children's perceptions of their internal body parts. Nursing Research, 23:384–391, 1974.

Rasmussen, M, and Murphy, C. Hospital admission through a child's eyes. Pediatric Nursing, 3:43–46, 1977.

Rie, HE, Boverman, H, Grossman, BJ, and Ozoa, N. Immediate and long-term effects of intervention early in prolonged hospitalization. Pediatrics, 41:755–764. 1968.

Roberts, MC, Wurtele, SK, Boone, RR, Ginther, LJ, and Elkins, PD. Reductions of medical fears by use of modeling: A preventive application in a general population of children. Journal of Pediatric Psychology, 6:293–300, 1981.

Robison, SJ. A nurse's role in preparing children for surgery. AORN Journal, 30:619–623, 1979.

Sauer, JE. Preadmission orientation: Effect on patient manageability. Hospital Topics, 46:79–83, 1968.

Scherer, MW, and Nakamura, CY. A fear survey schedule for children: A factor analytic comparison with manifest anxiety. Behavior Research and Therapy, 6:173–182, 1968.

Schmeltz, K, and White, G. A survey of parent groups:

Prehospital admission. Maternal-Child Nursing Journal, *11*:75–86, 1982.

Schreier, A, and Kaplan, D. The effectiveness of a preoperation preparation program in reducing anxiety in children. Children's Health Care, *11*:142–147, 1983.

Schulz, JB, Raschke, D, Dedrick, C, and Thompson, M. The effects of a preoperational puppet show on anxiety levels of hospitalized children. Journal of the Association for Care of Children's Health, *9*:118–121, 1981.

Schwartz, BH, Albino, JE, and Tedesco, LA. Effects of psychological preparation on children hospitalized for dental operations. Journal of Pediatrics, *102*:634–638, 1983.

Selye, H. Stress without distress. New York: JB Lippincott Co., 1974.

Siaw, SN, Stephens, LR, and Holmes, SS. Knowledge about medical instruments and reported anxiety in pediatric surgery patients. Children's Health Care, *14*:134–141, 1986.

Siegel, LJ, and Peterson, L. Stress reduction in young dental patients through coping skills and sensory information. Journal of Consulting and Clinical Psychology, *48*:785–787, 1980.

Siegel, LJ, and Peterson, L. Maintenance effects of coping skills and sensory information on young children's responses to repeated dental procedures. Behavior Therapy, *12*:530–535, 1981.

Siegel, SL. The use of music as treatment in pain perception with postsurgical patients in a pediatric hospital. Unpublished Master's thesis, University of Miami, Miami, 1983.

Skipper, JK, and Leonard, RC. Children, stress and hospitalization: A field experiment. Journal of Health and Social Behavior, *9*:272–287, 1968.

Smith, E. Are you really communicating? American Journal of Nursing, *77*:1966–1968, 1977.

Smith, JC. Spending time with the hospitalized child. American Journal of Maternal-Child Nursing, *2*:164, 1976.

Smitherman, CH. Parents of hospitalized children have needs, too. American Journal of Nursing, *79*:1423–1424, 1979.

Speilberger, CO State-trait anxiety inventory for children: Preliminary manual. Palo Alto, Calif.: Consulting Psychologists Press, Inc., 1973.

Stanford, G. Beyond honesty: Choosing language for talking to children about pain and procedures. Paper presented at the 20th Annual Conference of the Association for the Care of Children's Health, Boston, 1985.

Tarnow, JD, and Gutstein, SE. Children's preparatory behavior for elective surgery. Journal of the American Academy of Child Psychiatry, *22*:365–369, 1983.

Thompson, RH. Psychosocial research on pediatric hospitalization and health care: A review of the literature. Springfield, Ill.: Charles C Thomas, Publisher, 1985.

Thompson, RH, and Stanford, G. Child life in hospitals: Theory and practice. Springfield, Ill.: Charles C Thomas, Publisher, 1981.

Thomson, E. Preop visits: For the nurse or for the patient? AORN Journal, *16*:75–81, 1972.

Treloar, DM. Ready, set—no: Something is missing from pediatric preoperation preparation. American Journal of Maternal-Child Nursing, *3*:5051, 1978.

Trouten, F. Psychological preparation of children for surgery. Dimensions in Health Service, *58*:9–13, 1981.

Vardara, JA. Preadmission anxiety and mother-child relationships. Journal of the Association for the Care of Children's Health, *7*:8–15, 1978.

Vernon, DTA. Use of modeling to modify children's responses to a natural, potentially stressful situation. Journal of Applied Psychology, *58*:351–356, 1973.

Vernon, DTA, and Bailey, WC. The use of motion pictures in the psychological preparation of children for induction of anesthesia. Anesthesiology, *40*:68–72, 1974.

Vernon, DTA, Foley, JM, Sipowicz, RR, and Schulman, JL. The psychological responses of children to hospitalization and illness: A review of the literature. Springfield, Ill.: Charles C Thomas, Publisher, 1965.

Vernon, DTA, Schulman, JL, and Foley, JM. Changes in children's behavior after hospitalizaton. American Journal of Diseases of Children, *111*:581–593, 1966.

Visintainer, MA, and Wolfer, JA. Psychological preparation for surgical pediatric patients: The effect on children's and parents' stress responses and adjustments. Pediatrics, *56*:187–202, 1975.

Webster's Ninth New Collegiate Dictionary. Springfield, Mass.: Merriam-Webster, Inc., 1987.

Winter, WO, Ferreira, JR, and Ransom, R. Two measures of anxiety: A validation. Journal of Consulting Psychology, *27*:520–524, 1963.

Wolfer, JA, and Visintainer, MA. Pediatric surgical patients' and parents' stress responses and adjustment. Nursing Research, *24*:244–255, 1975.

Wolfer, JA, and Visintainer, MA. Prehospital psychological preparation for tonsillectomy patients: Effects on children's and parents' adjustments. Pediatrics, *64*:646–655, 1979.

Zurlinden, JK. Minimizing the impact of hospitalization for children and their families. American Journal of Maternal-Child Nursing, *10*:178–182, 1985.

Zweig, CD. Reducing stress when a child is admitted to the hospital. American Journal of Maternal-Child Nursing, *11*:24–26, 1986.

Zweig, IK. A new way to get acquainted with the hospital: Pediatric open house for well children. American Journal of Maternal-Child Nursing, *1*:217–219, 1976.

CHAPTER **7**

COMMUNICATION THROUGH THERAPEUTIC PLAY

MARY E. TIEDEMAN, Ph.D., R.N.,
KATHLEEN A. SIMON, M.S., R.N., and
STEPHANIE CLATWORTHY, Ed.D., R.N.

Play is an essential component of childhood. For children, play is fun and a self-motivating activity. Children use it to develop into social beings (Christie and Johnsen, 1983), to learn about themselves and others (Erikson, 1963, 1964), and to communicate feelings they are unable or unwilling to communicate verbally (DelPo and Frick, 1988; Fraiberg, 1959). Although play and all of its functions are not completely understood, existing knowledge indicates that it promotes growth and development and is crucial for the mental health of children (Athey, 1984; Begue, 1972; David, 1973; Dimock, 1960; Ellis 1973; Piaget, 1962; Pelligrini, 1985).

Play has been described in various ways in an attempt to convey an understanding of its importance in the life of children. Hartley and Goldenson (1963) noted that play is not only a response to life for children but is also their life if they are to be vital, growing, creative individuals.

Play has also been called the work of children. Play is very serious business because it confirms what children know about their world and allows them to guess the rest (Sutton-Smith, 1971). It is the laboratory in which children learn to master their environment, and it provides children with the opportunity and means to learn about themselves and their environment. Play allows them to take an active role, master an experience, and gain an increased sense of competence. Thus, these experiences allow children to confirm what they know about the world and to experiment with the unknown to integrate their existence (Bolig, 1984; Chance, 1979; Erikson, 1963, 1964, 1972; Piaget, 1972; Sutton-Smith, 1971).

Play has been further described as the language of childhood; it is the talk of children, and toys are its words. Thus, play is a vehicle for self-expression and provides a means of communication between the child world and the adult world (Athey, 1984; Ginott, 1961; Woltman, 1960). According to Hartley (1971), to read the language of play is to read the hearts and minds of children.

THEORETICAL FOUNDATION

Meaning of Play

Play can take many forms. Garvey (1977) compiled a list of characteristics of play; these characteristics help distinguish activities that can be considered play from those activities that cannot be considered play. Characteristics of play include the following:

1. Play is pleasurable, enjoyable. Even when not actually accompanied by signs of mirth, it is still positively valued by the player.

2. Play has no extrinsic goals. Its motivations are intrinsic and serve no other objectives. It is more an enjoyment of means than an effort devoted to some particular end.

3. Play is spontaneous and voluntary. It is not obligatory, but is freely chosen by the player.

4. Play involves some active engagement on the part of the player.

5. Play is systematically related to activities that are not play.

Play serves a variety of functions that enhance the growth and development of children (Athey, 1984; Chance, 1979). It promotes physical skills. With biological maturation of the nervous and musculoskeletal systems, children gain ever increasing gross and fine motor skills. Play provides the motivation to exercise the body and continue the development and refinement of physical abilities. However, children do not play to develop their bodies, but for the pure pleasure inherent in their play. It is through play that new skills, made possible by biological maturation, are discovered and refined (Athey, 1984; Chance, 1979; Thompson and Stanford, 1981).

Play promotes the development of cognitive and intellectual skills (Athey, 1984; Chance 1979; Pelligrini, 1985). According to Piaget (1962, 1970, 1972), young children learn about the world around them through their own actions and explorations. During their play, children are continually taking in or assimilating new information. Later, they will alter their old patterns of thinking to allow for the further assimilation of information through a process of accommodation.

Play also has an important role in social development (Athey, 1984; Chance, 1979; Christie and Johnsen, 1983). Much of the play of young children (birth to two years) is isolated and independent of other children. Although these children are engaged in play with adults, their interactions with their infant peers are limited. With time and opportunity, children from ages two to three years will begin to play next to each other in parallel play. Soon the interaction between children increases to the point of cooperative play around four years of age. Through play, children learn how to function and interact with other individuals (Caplan and Caplan, 1973: Piaget, 1970).

Play is seen by Erikson (1940) as a function of the ego in an attempt to synchronize the bodily and social processes with the self. It takes time for children to organize their experiences to fit concepts and categories so familiar to adults. In play, children can manipulate the smaller world of toys and materials. If given the time and opportunity to play in their own way, children are able to adapt themselves to and learn to cope with the complexities of their world (Erikson, 1963, 1964; Hyde, 1971). According to Erikson (1963), to play is the most natural, self-healing measure that children can take. Thus, the positive features of all play foster the emotional growth and development of children.

Categories of Play

Although play has been described as a necessary component of life for children, there is no one authoritative definition of play. The literature describes play as pleasurable, spontaneous, self-motivating, actively engaging, internally controlled, and creative (Garvey, 1977; Neumann, 1971). Therefore, all play promotes health and development and is beneficial in nature.

Three broad categories of play have been identified by Clatworthy (1982). These categories are (1) spontaneous play, (2) diversional play, and (3) therapeutic play. Spontaneous play is initiated and conducted independently by the child, either alone or with other children. It is usually conducted without adults and is easily encouraged by having play materials in the environment. It fosters physical, cognitive, social, and emotional growth and development. Spontaneous play fosters the organization of life skills to the degree that children operate in reality. However, if children have misconceptions about their environment or reality, spontaneous play will not clarify or resolve their confusions.

Diversional play may be initiated by the child or by an adult; however, it is generally initiated by an adult to provide children with a respite from their reality. Diversional play allows a release from coping with the immediate environment and life experiences and facilitates a return to a level of coping that is comfortable for and well developed by the individual child. Diversional play is usually structured according to developmental level. It may be done individually or with groups of children, and an adult may be present in the environment for supervision. Sending a child on a bike ride to help pass the time while waiting for dinner is one example of diversional play prescribed by parents. Encouraging children to go to the playroom in the hospital is another form of diversional play that can be prescribed by a nurse. These children are free to use the play-time in any way they choose. Diversional play can be provided by parents, nurses, child life workers, or other adults. While adults may play with the children for companionship, the purpose of diversional play is not to establish therapeutic communication.

In contrast, therapeutic play uses play specifically as a language for children to communicate their thoughts and feelings, and it is goal directed with a specific purpose established by the nurse following input from the child. Therapeutic play uses the language of play to assist children in becoming knowledgeable about their reality by facilitating the exploration of their perceptions and allowing for the intake of new information. It fosters the development of skills conducive to optimal growth, development, and well-being by giving children the opportunity to try out new coping strategies in the play arena with the support and play language management provided by the nurse. Therapeutic play may be nondirective, totally directed by the child; directive, prescribed by the nurse; or a combination of directive and nondirective (Axline, 1969; Guenery, 1984; McCue, 1988). Whether directive or nondirective, the use of therapeutic play requires a relationship between the nurse and the child.

The focus of this chapter is on therapeutic play as a nursing intervention with children. Therapeutic play is a relationship between the child and the nurse which is built around the child's responses (Oremland, 1988). Therefore, this chapter is not intended as a comprehensive how-to chapter with conclusive strategies for using therapeutic play as a nursing intervention. Rather, it is the intention of the authors to acquaint the readers with this intervention modality and perhaps stimulate them to seek the further knowledge and skills needed to implement it and test its effectiveness through research.

Conceptual Framework

In the course of their development, children experience life events which may produce stress and require coping. The literature identifies a variety of events which may produce stress. These include desirable events, such as outstanding personal achievement or going to school; undesirable events, such as illness and hospitalization; events that involve gains, such as the birth of a sibling or having grandparents come to live with the family; and events that involve losses, such as the death of a parent or change of residence (Coddington, 1972; Monoghan et al., 1979; Rutter, 1981; Varma, 1973). The behavioral and emotional responses of children to these events are a concern of professionals interested in promoting the mental health and optimal development of children. The belief that the stress resulting from these events can be mediated by the use of appropriate interventions is accepted by professionals working with children (Crocker, 1981; Fore and Poster, 1981).

Whether or not a given event is stressful depends on the perceptions of the individual experiencing the event (Lazarus and Launier, 1978). Through the process of cognitive appraisal, the event is evaluated in relation to its significance for the well-being of the individual and to the available coping resources and options. An event is stressful when the individual perceives that the demands of the event tax or exceed the resources. This perception may lead to emotions such as fear and anxiety (Lazarus and Launier, 1978).

The perceptions of children are dependent on cognitive development, which does not reach maturity until adolescence or beyond. Because of cognitive immaturity and the limited experience of children with stressful events, children are more likely than adults to perceive that demands tax or exceed their resources.

When stress is experienced, the child's resources must be mobilized, because automatic, routine responses are not sufficient to meet the demands of the situation (Lazarus and Launier, 1978). The resources of children for coping with life events are less developed than those of adults, since coping behaviors are learned (Aguilera and Messick, 1986) and are related to the amount of experience with stressful events, particularly the same stressful event. Children frequently have no previous experience with a given stressful event, such as illness and hospitalization, and they may have had limited experience with other stressful events.

Therapeutic play is an appropriate and effective intervention for assisting children in various life situations to mobilize their resources. Children have limited language skills and are less able to express their feelings verbally. Thus, play is a natural outlet for this purpose, as it provides children with the opportunity and means for telling others about themselves: their feelings, fears, misunderstandings, and concerns (Axline, 1955, 1969; Barton, 1962; Clatworthy, 1981; Dimock, 1960; Ellis, 1973; Geist and Bost, 1965; Haller et al., 1967; Plank, 1971; Potheir, 1967). Therapeutic play can help children mobilize resources by assisting them to review their current coping skills or develop new coping skills and by altering their perceptions of the situation.

Therapeutic play can also be used preventively before an anticipated or planned stressful event, such as hospitalization or elective surgery, to enable children to better understand what will happen and to play out their fears prior to the stressful event. Thus, coping abilities are facilitated based on a realistic perception of the event rather than an imagined perception. By playing out the anticipated situation, children may be helped to avoid stress and promote their sense of well-being.

Hospitalization is an event which is generally stressful for children (Astin, 1977; Barton, 1968; Clatworthy, 1981; Farquhar, 1983; Tiedeman, 1988). Hospitalization forces a passive role on children, whereas play allows them to take an active role, thus allowing them to master the experience and gain an increased sense of independence (Kunzman, 1972; Peller, 1952; Petrillo, 1968; Petrillo and Sanger, 1980). Knudsen (1975) noted that through play, misconceptions can be corrected and new and foreign experiences can be mastered. Play negates the difficulties that may arise from a lack of information and understanding of illness and hospitalization. Through play, children are able to explore and experiment with new objects, sensations, activities, and feelings in a nonthreatening way and to expand the concept of self (Kunzman, 1972; Welch, 1977).

Play helps children cope with the fears and anxieties associated with stressful situations such as hospitalization (Welch, 1977). Hospitalized children can play out uncomfortable feelings and bring some aspects of normality to an otherwise confusing and overwhelming environment (Azarnoff, 1974; Nickerson, 1974). Further, the establishment of a pleasant association with an unpleasant situation strengthens the sense of control and brings a greater sense of continuity with the outside world. The developmental tasks that children need to master can be incorporated into their hospital experience. As children express their feelings and cope with stressful events, they can develop skills which prepare them for adult roles and further their development. Therefore, play has an even greater importance than it usually has when children are experiencing hospitalization or other stressful events (Jolly, 1968).

The importance of therapeutic play is based on the acceptance of the importance and meaning of play in the lives of children. Individuals who use this intervention modality differ in their philosophies and in their theories of personality dynamics; however, similarities remain. All those who use therapeutic play approach it with the basic human values of faith, acceptance, and trust, which they attempt to communicate to the child. The child-centered philosophy of therapeutic play is concerned with the kind of relationship that enables children to grow emotionally, to gain faith in themselves and their feelings, and to achieve feelings of security and worthiness (Moustakas, 1953).

Children have reasons for what they do, and they may not be able to express verbally many thoughts which are important to them. They are striving to make sense of their world and must be accepted for what they are in order to be free and spontaneous in their play (Smith, 1977). Within a trusting relationship, an environment can be created where children feel free to express their thoughts and feelings. As thoughts and feelings are expressed, children can identify, face, and master them and work out the effects of difficult experiences, such as hospitalization, at their own pace (Ellis, 1973; Peller, 1978; Plank, 1971; Oremland, 1988).

Therapeutic Play Modalities

A description of various therapeutic play modalities provides the basis for a better understanding of therapeutic play. The use of play as a therapeutic modality began as an application of psychotherapy to children and adolescents. Axline (1955) was one of the first to use play as a language. She developed a psychoanalytic, or nondirective, mode of therapy, whereby she provided the environment and allowed the child to lead the way, as a means for children to discover themselves and their strengths. This nondirective approach was based on the assumption that children have within themselves the ability to solve their own problems satisfactorily and a growth impulse which makes developmentally appro-

priate behavior more satisfying than other behavior (Axline, 1969).

The nondirective approach to therapeutic play provides children with toys and a friendly, understanding, accepting nurse. Children select the toys they will play with and the manner in which they will play with them. The nurse is sensitive to and accepting of the feelings expressed through both play and verbalizations and reflects these feelings back to the children to assist them in understanding these feelings more fully (Axline, 1969; Oremland, 1988). The nondirective approach requires regular play sessions over a period of time to allow children the full opportunity to learn about themselves and to learn new, more supportive behavior (Axline, 1969; Clatworthy, 1982). Nursing situations often provide very short periods of time to interact; however, this approach is essential to a strong relationship.

Nondirective therapy is usually done more satisfactorily with an individual child, although it may be done with groups of two to three children. The group should include the same children in each session. Group therapy adds to the therapeutic experience the ongoing evaluation of behavior by peers and the impact of the children upon one another, thus adding to the therapy the reality of interacting with other children, the consideration of the reactions of other children, and the development of consideration for the feelings of other children. When problems center around social adjustment, group therapy may even be more effective than individual treatment (Axline, 1969).

The nondirective process works well when there is sufficient time (Axline, 1969) and children are interacting with their environment (Clatworthy, 1982). However, some children are withdrawn or overwhelmed by their environment, and for these children, more directive approaches to therapy may be appropriate. With the directive approach, the nurse selects the play modality and content and "reaches in" and "grabs hold" of children to pull them forward. Use of puppets (Woltmann, 1960, 1972), bibliotherapy or storytelling (Gardner, 1971, 1972), and art (Nickerson, 1974) are but a few of the specific directive modalities. Directive therapy allows the nurse therapist to interact more aggressively, which may more readily facilitate effective coping in a limited period of time.

Therapeutic Play Categories

Whether directive or nondirective, therapeutic play encompasses three basic categories of play: role or fantasy play, expressive play, and aggressive play (Clatworthy, 1982). Role play allows children to take on various roles and to play out their feelings and concerns in fantasy, thus providing an escape from reality, distance from the self, and safety for expressing feelings. Role or fantasy play supports the acting out of life stresses, such as family stress, separation, and hospitalization, and enhances the ability to learn new forms of behavior (Curry, 1988; Fein, 1984; Nickerson, 1974).

Expressive play allows for the expression of feelings and concerns without words (Nickerson, 1974). Art is one expressive modality. Drawings are viewed as graphic means of communication (Machover, 1953; Nickerson, 1974) with qualitative characteristics which reveal something personal (DiLeo, 1970, 1973) and reflect the subjective experience of the artist (Taylor and Williams, 1980). Children often reveal in drawings what they cannot put into words (Clatworthy, 1980, 1986; Koppitz, 1968), and drawings are less susceptible to the influence of defense mechanisms than speech (DiLeo, 1970). Drawings have been found to enhance the expression of an individual's deepest fantasies, wishes, and fears (Eichenbaum and Dunn, 1971). A complete discussion of communication through drawings is given in Chapter 8.

Aggressive play consists of activities such as throwing balls at targets, hitting punching bags, pounding and smashing clay or Play-doh, and knocking over building blocks. Such activities provide children with a method of releasing and communicating feelings of anger and frustration without hurting themselves or others, thereby protecting children from the guilt they would feel if these feelings were expressed in a more direct manner. Aggressive play affords children the opportunity to release feelings of anger and frustration in a safe and acceptable manner and provides the opportunity for regrouping of inner resources to foster coping and learning (Clatworthy, 1982).

In summary, therapeutic play offers children a nonverbal, alternative means of expressing and dealing with tension, anxiety, frustration, anger, loneliness, fear, and confusion. It allows the nurse to gain insight into the feelings, perceptions, and needs of children in stressful situations and to use the language of play to assist them in coping. Thus, therapeutic play can facilitate the growth, development, and well-being of children in stressful situations.

ASSESSMENT

Assessing children's anxieties and fears is difficult and requires verification and validation by a professional nurse. Because children cannot always verbalize what they are feeling, asking them if they are afraid or anxious may only bring responses such as "I'm Ok," "I'm not afraid," or "It's all right." If asked directly, they may be able to tell you that they have the "iggly squigglies" inside, but they do not have the cognitive or language skills to say they are experiencing fear, anger, or anxiety.

Children are more likely to express their feelings in actions or behavior (Burns and Kaufman, 1970). Horney (1950) delineated three major patterns of behavior observed in individuals experiencing stress or threat: (1) moving with people by being weak and compliant, (2) moving against people by being aggressive and competitive and by seeking to control others, and (3) moving away from others by being withdrawn and detached. Behaviors suggestive of Horney's (1950) three patterns in children's responses to threat may be indicated by behaviors such as complying with painful procedures without protest, striking out against others physically and verbally, or being quiet and withdrawn. Such behaviors need further assessment in order to validate their meanings, identify the underlying causes, and plan appropriate interventions. Therapeutic play is one method of assessment. The nurse observes the play and identifies themes and patterns which provide clues to the child's thoughts, feelings, and perceptions (Clatworthy, 1982; Oremland, 1988).

Art is another method which may be used to assess children's responses to a situation (McLeary, 1979; Nickerson, 1974). The nurse may ask a child to draw a picture of his or her family or a person in the hospital. The topic for the picture is selected in accordance with the specific situation. Such an approach is based on the use of drawings as a projective technique (Hammer, 1958) and assumes that the nurse can learn about the feelings of children through the drawings.

The Child Drawing Hospital* (CDH) (Clatworthy, 1986) is one example of using art as an assessment technique. It was developed specifically to assess anxiety levels of children in relation to hospitalization. Children are asked to draw a picture of a person in the hospital. The CDH is evaluated using criteria related to the size, shape, position, and facial expression of the person; color use and selection; use of paper; quality of strokes; hospital equipment depicted; and developmental level of the child. Additional criteria include the depiction in the drawing of exaggeration, de-emphasis, distortion, and omission of parts; mutilation; transparency; mixed profiles; and shading. The drawing is also evaluated using the overall response of the scorer to the drawing: that is, an assessment of whether the picture is bright and happy, sad and constricted, or bizarre and distorted (Clatworthy, 1980, 1986; Clatworthy et al., 1985). Drawings may be used in other situations with similar criteria applied in evaluating and interpreting the pictures.

Children's pictures reflect their inner beliefs and perceptions of the world (DiLeo, 1970) and therefore should be respected. When adults do not understand, they often make the mistake of saying such things as "What is that?" or "It looks like a house to me." Such remarks tend to hinder further communication between the child and adult. A method of gaining further insight into the content of the picture and the child's response to the situation is by asking the child to tell a story about the picture. Having children tell stories about their pictures allows them to express their feelings and perceptions in fantasy and provides some distance from the self, thereby making it easier and safer to express their feelings. Their stories can be used for the concept of bibliotherapy as used by Gardner (1971, 1972).

Bibliotherapy or storytelling (Gardner, 1971, 1972) may also be used to assess a child's response to a situation. The nurse selects a story which focuses on a specific need, such as dealing with separation or having a bad day. The story is read and the child encouraged to interact with the nurse regarding the feelings of the character in the story. This provides a mechanism for expressing feelings via the character in the story, thereby making it easier for the child to express his or her feelings. Another approach is to ask the child to tell a story, perhaps about a given subject relative to his or her concerns or situation. The stories can be enhanced by puppets or dress-up clothes for a drama production.

Communication via puppets (Woltmann, 1960, 1972) is another technique for assessing children's responses to a situation. The child and nurse may interact by having the puppets carry on a conversation, with the nurse directing the conversation to focus on feelings and concerns. As with storytelling, communication via puppets makes it possible for children to express their feelings indirectly in fantasy. Puppets may also be used to talk directly to children. Since puppets "speak the language of children," it is all right for children to tell puppets their feelings.

Various assessment strategies provide the nurse with data to support nursing diagnoses. The defining characteristics of each diagnosis assist in the categorization of data; however, these defining characteristics serve only as guidelines. The defining characteristics, as identified by Gordon (1987), focus on verbal, behavioral, and physiological signs and symptoms and may be incomplete or at times inappropriate for use with children. For example, children may express anxiety by the characteristics of their drawings but may not verbalize apprehension, fear, or concern directly.

Nursing diagnoses from the functional health patterns of self-perception–self-concept and coping-stress tolerance may be particularly amenable to further assessment and intervention with therapeutic play. Two appropriate nursing diagnoses which arise from the self-perception–self-concept pattern are *Fear* and *Anxiety*. Fear is the appropriate diagnosis when the source of the perceived threat or danger to the self can be identified. For example, children may state directly or reveal through their play a fear of needles. Fear produces a feeling of dread. Anxiety is the appropriate diagnosis when the source of the vague, uneasy feelings is

---

*For more information on the Child Drawing Hospital write to: Stephanie Clatworthy, Ed.D., R.N. Professor and Dean, School of Nursing, Kent State University, Kent, OH 44242.

nonspecific or unknown (Gordon, 1987). An appropriate nursing diagnosis from the coping-stress tolerance pattern is *Ineffective coping*. Ineffective coping occurs when the adaptive behaviors and problem-solving abilities of an individual are not sufficient to meet the demands of a situation. Ineffective coping leads to anxiety, fear, and anger (Gordon, 1987). Although fear, anxiety, and ineffective coping are the primary diagnoses where therapeutic play can be utilized, it is also possible to use therapeutic play in dealing with other nursing diagnoses. These diagnoses include *Body image disturbance, Self-esteem disturbance, Powerlessness,* and *Anticipatory anxiety*.

THE INTERVENTION

The use of play as a therapeutic modality requires a sound theoretical knowledge base related to play, communication, psychotherapy, and mental health needs. Therapeutic play is goal directed and is therefore based on assessment and identified nursing diagnoses. The specific modalities used require preparation and planning prior to implementation of therapeutic play as an intervention with children.

Preparation for Therapeutic Play

In preparing for therapeutic play, the play media are selected in accordance with the real or perceived needs and the developmental level of the children. However, there are some general guidelines for selecting the play materials. Play media should allow for role or fantasy play, expressive play, and aggressive play (Axline, 1969; Clatworthy, 1982; Moustakas, 1953). Table 7–1 lists toys used in therapeutic play. Materials for role play include family dolls and various puppets. The availability of dolls representing the appropriate racial groups is desirable for children in the concrete stage of cognitive development. Animal families are also useful for role play because they provide an escape from the child's reality and distance from the self. Children who are not ready to "play out" their feelings using family dolls may be able to do so using an animal family. Baby bottles and baby dolls which can be fed, cuddled, and bathed are also useful

because they allow children to "play out" regressive behavior and feelings related to their need to be taken care of by a caring person.

With hospitalized children, play media for role play may include materials related to the hospital, specific treatments, and diagnostic procedures (Clatworthy, 1982; McCue, 1988). Such materials, as listed in Table 7–2, include hospital gowns and pajamas, blood pressure cuffs, stethoscopes, bandages, tape, laboratory coats, surgical attire, and hospital equipment such as beds, intravenous poles, and stretchers. When the real equipment is not available or use of it is not feasible, make-believe or miniature equipment will serve the purpose. Dolls which can be dressed as patient, nurse, and doctor help facilitate role play of the perceived reality of children within the hospital situation. To facilitate role playing and examination of feelings, syringes with needles and water for injections can be most helpful. Individual supervision of this activity is essential.

Materials for expressive play include crayons, paints, finger paints, paper, scissors, and paste. Art requires little physical energy, which makes it useful in therapeutic communication and intervention with children who are hospitalized or confined to their beds. Crayons, paints, and paper are familiar to children, and hence they may be more willing to engage in play with these materials.

Play media also need to facilitate aggressive play. Aggressive play can be done with the use of punching bags, balls, targets, vehicles, Play-doh, clay, and other materials that can be used to push, throw, and punch without harm to the environment or to others.

When selecting toys for the individual child, several factors need to be taken into consideration. Toys should be appropriate for the age and developmental level of the child, although toys appropriate for children of a younger age and developmental level may be more effective if the child is experiencing stress-related regression. The use of toys appropriate for children of an older age and developmental level may frustrate the child and hinder the therapeutic process. Further, the toys selected need to be safe and children must be able to use them in the given environment. For example, a child

Table 7–1. TOYS FOR USE IN THERAPEUTIC PLAY

Role or Fantasy Play	Expressive Play	Aggressive Play
Family dolls	Crayons	Punching bags
Mother	Paints	Balls
Father	Finger paints	Targets
Brother	Paper	Cars and trucks
Sister	Paste	Play-doh
Baby	Scissors	Clay
Grandparents		Beanbag
Baby doll		Paddleballs
Baby bottle		Blocks
Animal families		
Puppets		
Family puppets		
Animal puppets		
Soft, cuddly, e.g., dog,		
bunny		
Angry, aggressive, e.g.,		
lion, bear		
Doll house with furniture		

with intravenous lines which could be dislodged would not be given a paddleball, and wooden building blocks would be difficult to use if a child is confined to bed.

Considerations other than the play materials are needed when preparing for therapeutic play. One such consideration is the knowledge and skills of the nurse using therapeutic play. The nurse with expertise in child development, communication, psychotherapy, and the use of play as a therapeutic modality will be best prepared to use this intervention (DelPo and Frick, 1988). It is also necessary for the nurse to have full knowledge of the child's situation and previous experience with medical encounters (Oremland, 1988). It is the belief of the authors that a professional nurse with an advanced education that included supervised practice in the use of therapeutic play will best meet these criteria.

Table 7–2. TOYS FOR USE IN HOSPITAL
ROLE PLAY

Hospital gowns and pajamas
Blood pressure cuff
Stethoscope
Bandages
Tape
Needles and syringes
Laboratory coats
Surgical attire
Hospital equipment
  Intravenous poles
  Stretchers
  Beds
Doctor and nurse dolls

Establishing a Therapeutic Environment

The establishment of a warm, caring relationship with a feeling of permissiveness which gives children a chance to express their feelings is necessary for the implementation of therapeutic play. To establish such a relationship, the nurse must be accepting and avoid expressing approval and disapproval. It is important for the nurse to listen to the feelings expressed (Axline, 1969; Moustakas, 1953). It is also important to remember that words and actions may be defending mechanisms; the feelings behind the words and actions are expressed in a variety of ways and are most likely to be the true message being communicated. The repetitive nature of an action, words, or play should be noted to aid in the identification of feelings (Oremland, 1988). As in all communication, validation, reflection, and mutual exploration are essential. This process allows for a diagnostic conclusion and appropriate nursing intervention.

To engage in therapeutic play with children, it is necessary for the nurse to develop a contract that sets limits with each child (Axline, 1969; Clatworthy, 1982; Moustakas, 1953). This contract should include what is expected of the child, the time that will be spent in play, what can be done with the toys, and whether the child may leave the play area. Expectations of the child may include no hurting of self or others and no damage to the toys. It is best to establish only those limitations which are necessary to anchor the play sessions to the world of reality and to avoid confusion, guilt feelings, and insecurity (Axline, 1969). The establishment of a contract with limits provides some guidelines for children, thus fostering a feeling of trust and security and facilitating an environment conducive to the expression of feelings (Axline, 1969; Moustakas, 1953). The contract needs to be comfortable for the child and the nurse and must be open to renegotiation.

Essential to the therapeutic process and the contract is the nurse validating with children that it is "OK" to talk about feelings which all children have (Axline, 1969; Moustakas, 1953). The nurse may say, "Feelings are what make us happy and sad. Sometimes feelings get all jumbled up and make us feel bad and do things we do not want to do. We are going to use toys and play to help you talk about your feelings."

It should be clear to the child that it is safe to share feelings with the nurse and that what is shared in the play will be private (Axline, 1969). Should feelings, needs, or concerns be revealed that need to be shared with parents or other health professionals, the nurse is advised to share this need with the child and incorporate the child into the collaboration with the parents or other health professionals. In this way, it is hoped that the trusting relationship and mutual respect will be maintained.

Therapeutic play not only requires a special relationship with the nurse but also a special relationship with the toys. This relationship formation is necessary to promote optimal effectiveness of therapeutic play. Therefore, the toys should not be left with the child between play sessions because the special relationship with the toys will not occur when the nurse is not present to observe the child's use of toys.

Supervision of role play is essential and is another reason for not leaving the toys with the child between play sessions. An example will serve to illustrate what can occur when role play is carried out without supervision. Three boys, ages six, eight, and nine years, had been admitted for circumcision the following morning. They had been provided with a blood pressure cuff and scrub suits for dress-up play. All three boys were in one bed cubicle with the curtain pulled around them. The following was overhead by the nurse:

First boy:	"You have to have this because I said so."
Second boy:	"But what are you going to do?"
Third boy:	"We're going to cut it off. I've told you not to play with it."

At this point the nurse enters the scene:

Nurse:	"Gosh, you boys are playing hospital. May I play too?"
First boy:	"Yes. This boy has to go to OR and have it cut off."
Nurse:	"Are you going to the OR?"
Boys (in unison):	"Yes."
Nurse:	"Why are you going to the OR?"
First boy:	"We have to have that 'cision' thing done."
Nurse:	"Oh, you mean a circumcision?"
First boy:	"Yes."
Nurse:	"I wonder what that means. Let's pretend you two are doctors, he's the patient, and I'm the nurse."

Through the interaction of play, misconceptions were clarified and the boys were facilitated in learning about their circumcisions. If the role play had continued unsupervised, these misconceptions could have remained, and there may have been increased fear and anxiety.

Stages of Therapeutic Play

The implementation of the process of therapeutic play involves the three stages of a therapeutic relationship: (1) assessment, (2) intervention, and (3) termination. During the assessment stage, the nurse and the child are assessing one another. Most children will explore the environment, the toys, and the nature of the contract. They may test and explore the contract by asking questions such as, "Can I really play with the toys any way I want?" or "Will you really stay with me?" Limits may be tested by attempting to leave the play area or verbally threatening harm to the self or the nurse. During this stage, children may give brief glimpses of their feelings, which then need to be reflected and verified by the nurse.

When a nondirective approach is used during the assessment stage, children are provided with all the play equipment. Most children rapidly explore all the toys, and the majority begin to interact in a given area of play. When using a directive approach to assessment, the nurse selects the play medium. For example, the nurse may use art or puppet play to foster the expression of feelings.

During the intervention stage, therapeutic play continues to focus on perceptions and feelings. The most painful feelings are demonstrated by a series of repeated play activities which begin to create a pattern and help identify and resolve feelings. The following example illustrates the play activities and interaction during the intervention stage using a nondirective approach in which the child selected the play medium and content of the sessions.

A six year old girl whose parents had recently divorced was engaged in regular play sessions with the nurse. At her first session with the nurse, the child drew a picture that showed a big yellow ball almost totally filled with red. During succeeding play sessions, she continued to draw large yellow objects but with decreasing amounts of red in them. By her fifth play session, she drew a yellow ball with only a small red dot. At this point, the nurse sought to further clarify and validate the meaning behind the drawings. The nurse described her observations of the child's drawings and asked, "Can you tell me about it?" The child responded with, "Oh, that's easy. When you first came, I had lots of hurt inside me. I'm still sad but the hurt is going away."

The directive approach may also be used during the intervention stage of therapeutic play to focus the expression of feelings and perceptions, to provide information, and to clarify the child's misconceptions. The following example illustrates directive role playing.

A five year old boy was admitted with a fractured arm that was due to a fall off a bicycle. He sat quietly in his bed and only nodded yes or no when questions were asked of him. The plan was to apply a cast in the operating room within six hours. The nurse arranged for a play session with dolls and hospital equipment to help the boy understand what would happen when he went to surgery. She allowed him to explore all the materials for a while and then asked, "Are you ready to talk about what will happen?" The boy nodded yes, and the nurse began to describe where the cast would be placed using a doll. She indicated that only the arm would be put in a cast and continued to describe the procedure. She then asked the boy if he would like to "be the doctor" and put a cast on the doll. He applied the cast and while it was drying the nurse used an old cast to show him how hard a cast becomes. She removed the tape which held it together so the boy could see the doll's arm, then taped the cast back on, pointing out that now he couldn't see the arm but it was still there. The boy took the old cast on and off ten times before he was certain the arm was always under the cast.

The closure or end of the play session follows the process of resolution or termination, the final stage in any therapeutic relationship. As children communicate feelings within the therapeutic relationship, they are able to deal with and resolve those feelings. This resolution may be indicated by a willingness to discontinue the play sessions. The initial contract between the nurse and child indicated the duration and number of the play sessions. Knowing that the play sessions will end after so many sessions or at discharge helps children move toward resolution and termination because they know that time is limited and they need to deal with their feelings within that time. At the end of the contracted time, the nurse and child may renegotiate for more play sessions if conflicts have not been resolved or if new needs have been identified.

During the final stage, children may return to behaviors similar to those exhibited during the first play session or if it is a one-time play session, they may return to behaviors exhibited during the first five to ten minutes of play. During this stage, children will explore many things but nothing in depth. It is a way of bringing closure to the feelings and self that were exposed. At this time, the nurse must reaffirm what has been said regarding feelings and self and provide support for the child. The following example illustrates the termination stage of the therapeutic relationship.

A six year old girl from Thailand had been adopted by a family in the United States. Until the age of five, she had been raised by her grandmother in Thailand. At that time, her grandmother became very ill and was dying. She could no longer care for the child.

The adoptive mother was concerned because the child never cried or talked about her grandmother. Although she was not doing badly in school, it was believed she could do better. She had night terrors and difficulty getting along with other children.

During each play session, she would play with family dolls and draw one picture. During the first session, she drew a picture of a family. On one page, she drew her American family, but she did not include herself. On a second page, she drew a picture of herself. She immediately wadded up both pictures and threw them in the trash saying, "That's not right."

The nurse decided to use bibliotherapy to facilitate the child's expression of loss and transition. The story selected was "Heidi," about a girl who had to leave her grandfather on the mountain and go to the city to live with her aunt Clara. The first time the story was read, the child was quiet and attentive but could not interact with the nurse regarding Heidi's feelings. At the second play session, the story was read again at the request of the child. Again she was quiet and could not interact.

During the third play session, the nurse began to read the story again. The child took the book away from her and said, "This time I'll tell the story. Once upon a time there was a little girl who lived in Thailand with her grandmother." She proceeded to tell how hard it was to leave and come to a new country. When she finished the story, she immediately got up and went to the doll house, then to the trucks, and then to the blocks. She then drew a picture of her family which showed all members of her present family on one page. The child then announced to the nurse that she would not be returning because she was "OK." Follow-up

with the mother revealed that her night terrors had ceased, her grades had improved, and she had made a best friend.

Therapeutic Play with Hospitalized Children

Because of the basic mental wellness of most hospitalized children and the degree of stress hospitalization creates, the majority of children readily engage in therapeutic play and move from one step of the process to the next. However, some children are so stressed that they cannot readily engage in the process, and for other children, hospital stays are of short duration or procedures are scheduled with little lead time. For these children, more directive approaches are appropriate.

Therapeutic play for hospitalized children is based on the same theoretical principles as therapeutic play in other settings; however, some adaptation of the methods may be needed. Because of the nature of the hospital environment, it may be necessary to conduct play sessions in a variety of settings, such as the playroom, the child's bed, the child's room, a conference room, or wherever some space and privacy are available. Thus, equipment should be somewhat portable. Portable doll houses with the toys inside, a suitcase, or large canvas bags are containers which may be used to transport the toys. These authors have found it useful to use small tackle boxes for the storage and transportation of needles, syringes, and other small hospital equipment. The use of a tackle box has the advantage of providing an easy way to account for each needle and syringe, thereby avoiding accidentally leaving such an item at a child's bedside.

Privacy is an important consideration which takes on additional significance in the hospital where the child may perceive that no one can be trusted and that no place, not even bed, is safe. In such a situation, it is imperative that therapeutic play time be protected and that no treatments, doctors, or other distressing interruptions are allowed.

Children in the hospital generally have some degree of physical illness and physical discomfort. In addition, the illness may require restrictions of activity and mobility. Therapeutic play must be adapted based on these considerations. Examples of such adaptations include hanging a punching bag on the overhead frame for a child in traction and using portable toys so that the play activities may be taken to the child. Strategies for hospitalized children must be based on the realities of their physical health. The establishment of a therapeutic relationship within the hospital may also require a greater degree of structure and more limits to provide children with the needed security. Because of the nature of hospitalization and the different developmental levels and needs of children, the nurse must be able to use both directive and nondirective approaches based on the needs of each child.

Clinical observations of hospitalized children engaged in therapeutic play reveal some patterns. It is frequently observed that children eagerly "attack" hospital play. Syringes are "stabbed" everywhere, water is drawn up and "shot" into dolls, animals, and the environment. Stethoscopes are explored and hung around the neck, and blood pressure cuffs are blown up to abnormally high levels. Verbalizations reveal anger, loss of control, fear, and pain. A child may say to a patient, "Shut-up—you have to have this no matter what." When asked why, the child has no response. By role playing, these children are expressing their feelings and revealing their knowledge of the situation. As the nurse assesses the child's knowledge, he or she uses role play to fill in reality.

This acting out play helps children deal with their immediate and somewhat overwhelming concerns regarding hospitalization. Once the acting out play has been expressed, children are able to go on to their other fears of separation, death, and guilt. Often this takes two to three sessions to uncover. Anger at the health care system and at parents is rarely processed by children prior to this hospital play. Children must first deal with their more immediate concerns regarding hospitalization and separation before they can cope with their anger at their parents and the health care system related to their hospitalization. Once hospitalization and illness are dealt with, children proceed to family issues and everyday relationships with friends, school, and life.

Another frequently found play behavior is evidenced by children who initially ignore the hospital toys but engage readily in play with family dolls or other play media—what some children call regular play. These chil-

dren should not be pushed to engage in hospital play unless there is some urgency to accomplish this because of scheduled procedures. When left on their own time, children will usually engage in hospital play by the second or third session.

Through therapeutic play, a nurse who is educated in the use of this intervention modality may help hospitalized children to understand their hospitalization and treatment and to develop new coping behaviors. Thus, therapeutic play may support children in their development and assist them in attaining optimal levels of well-being.

EVALUATION

The goals and outcome criteria for therapeutic play are directly related to the identified nursing diagnoses and the conceptual framework. The goals are increased effectiveness in coping, decreased fear, and decreased anxiety. Outcome criteria for determining goal attainment flow directly from assessment data and may be evaluated through behavioral observation, art, stories, and play: the modalities utilized for the initial assessment. Reversal of defining characteristics indicates that the intervention has been effective. The process of the evaluation of goal attainment based on outcome criteria is an ongoing process.

The following case studies illustrate the nondirective and directive approaches to therapeutic play.

Case Studies

ANDREW, NONDIRECTIVE

Andrew was a ten year old boy who had been hospitalized for a possible kidney transplant to relieve chronic renal failure. His renal failure was the result of repeated urinary tract infections, and he had been on dialysis three times a week for the past ten months.

Andrew was one of five children in a single-parent family. His father had died a year ago. The family lived 300 miles away from the hospital, and his mother could only visit every other weekend. She called every other day.

Andrew was small for his age. He spent most of the morning in bed and the remainder of the day in his room. He expressed frustration over the imposed fluid restriction. He had recently begun experiencing nighttime enuresis.

Andrew was referred to a nurse-play therapist by his primary nurse who felt frustrated by his behavior. The primary nurse was concerned that with the potential for long-term hospitalization his behavior could only get worse. Because of his long-term hospitalization and his ability to interact, a nondirective approach was selected. Family dolls, puppets, paint, crayons, paper, an assortment of cars, and punching toys were provided for Andrew in the playroom. Hospital equipment, including needles, syringes, and dress-up clothes were also provided. A contract was established between Andrew and the nurse-play therapist in which they agreed to meet for play sessions one hour a week for six weeks, or longer if he was still hospitalized. Andrew was encouraged to talk about his feelings regarding long-term hospitalization during these sessions.

The nursing diagnoses for Andrew included *Anxiety, Fear, Ineffective coping, Powerlessness,* and *Self-concept disturbance* related to his small size and perceived inability to play sports. Andrew directed his play sessions to his hospitalization and illness, his sense of helplessness, and his self-image. Although he expressed concerns about what a ten year old boy would do in the play sessions, he readily began to play "hospital." For three weeks, he played out a variety of surgeries in which each patient went to surgery and died. He adamantly insisted that no one survived. Any attempts by the nurse to explore his feelings about surgery were met by the statement, "There will be no problems." He was stoic about his status but repeatedly asked questions about what happened to a person who died. During the third session, he began to play out a funeral but stopped abruptly and began to play with the puppets, claiming they were his two brothers.

During these sessions, Andrew also conveyed much about his self-image. During the second play session, he drew a picture of himself. The picture showed a very small, constricted person who he stated was "at bat." He stated, "I'm not very good at any sports. I only play with Brent [his brother] because he lets me do what I want." He continued by saying, "Brent is my favorite brother and he's going to give me his kidney." He also expressed the feeling that "it is not fun to be sick so much."

During the fourth session, Andrew once again played out surgery with the patient dying. He had become more verbally angry at the doctor and accused him of doing something wrong. The nurse stated, "Some people are afraid the doctor will make a mistake and they will die. Are you afraid that you will die?" He stated emphatically,

"No, but my dad died." Andrew had revealed his anger and unresolved guilt about his father, who had died during surgery which would have allowed him to be a kidney donor for Andrew. He was also dealing with his own reality. Andrew stated that his father's death still made him sad and that it had made things very hard for his mother. His feelings were validated, and via the therapeutic play, he was able to talk about this fear and guilt.

The following week, Andrew again played the surgeon, but this time the patient survived. Andrew stated that "the kidney was a good one" and that "it would work better than dialysis." This session occurred before Andrew had surgery.

During the sixth session, Andrew drew another picture. Although the facial expression still showed frustration and tension, the larger size of the figure demonstrated a greater sense of self.

Andrew was discharged following the sixth play session. At that time, the nighttime enuresis had stopped, and Andrew had become more social. This increased sociability demonstrated more effective coping, as did his increased willingness to verbalize his concerns. As demonstrated by his drawing, his self-concept was improving. The anxiety and fear surrounding the surgery had also been resolved.

SHARI, DIRECTIVE

Shari was a five year old who was admitted to the hospital for observation following a fall from the diving board at the local pool. At 3:00 p.m. when she was admitted, she was happy and cheerful and readily engaged in spontaneous and diversional play. She was eating and drinking without difficulty.

At 3:00 p.m. the following day, it was reported to the nurse-play therapist that Shari had an elevated blood pressure; a rapid pulse; cold, clammy skin; and projectile vomiting. The neurosurgeon had been called, and Shari was scheduled for surgery to rule out intracranial bleeding. The nurse found Shari curled up in a corner of the bed and talking in a high, squeaky voice.

As a result of Shari's withdrawal and the short period of time before surgery was scheduled, a directive approach was selected. Shari was picked up and carried to the playroom where puppets were incorporated into play. The following interaction took place between Shari and the nurse through the use of puppets.

Bunny puppet (Nurse):	"Oh, I'm so afraid. I went to the pool to have a good time, and then my mother brought me to the hospital and left me all night long. Have you ever been alone before?"
Owl puppet (Shari):	"No."
Bunny (Nurse):	"Then what are you doing in the hospital?"

Owl (Shari) (in a quiet voice):	"My mommy brought me to the hospital too. I'm afraid she'll never come back again."
Bunny (Nurse):	"Oh, no. Moms always come back. Does your mom work?"
Owl (Shari):	"Yes."
Bunny (Nurse):	"Well, see. She's still at work. I feel less scared when I tell someone I'm afraid. Are you less scared now that you've told me, Mr. Owl?"
Owl (Shari):	"I don't know."
Bunny (Nurse):	"When I'm scared, I have the iggly squigglies in my tummy. Have you ever had the iggly squigglies?"
Owl (Shari):	"Yes."
Bunny (Nurse):	"Do you have the iggly squigglies now?"
Owl (Shari):	"Yes."
Bunny (Nurse):	"Let's reach down and pull them out. Each iggly squiggly we pull out will be one part of what you're afraid of. Reach down and pull one out. What do we have?"

This process continued, revealing fear of abandonment, lack of understanding of frequent blood pressure measurements, and guilt (she had not been behaving at the pool). A blood pressure cuff and stethoscope were provided for Shari to play with.

This session took place in approximately ten minutes, with the nurse being very directive with Shari's feelings and with the play. At the end of the session, Shari was upright and alert and speaking in a normal tone of voice. Her skin temperature was normal, and her vital signs were within normal limits. The neurosurgeon arrived and concurred with the nursing diagnosis of *Acute anxiety.* Surgery was canceled, and Shari was discharged at 6:00 p.m. Without the intervention of therapeutic play, Shari may have undergone unnecessary surgery.

RESEARCH IMPLICATIONS

Any hospitalization creates stress for children. The stressful nature of hospitalization has been supported by a number of studies (Astin, 1977; Clatworthy, 1981; Visintainer and Wolfer, 1975; Wolfer and Visintainer, 1975a, 1975b). The literature provides some empirical support for the use of therapeutic play with hospitalized children. The findings of a study by Cassell (1965) revealed that children, ages three to 11 years, who received puppet therapy demonstrated less emotional disturbance while undergoing cardiac catheterization than did children who did not receive puppet therapy. The children who received puppet therapy also expressed more willingness to return to the hospital for further treatment.

Schultz et al. (1981) investigated the effects of a preoperative puppet show on the anxiety levels of two to seven year old children. The children in the experimental group demonstrated a decrease in anxiety, whereas the children in the control group demonstrated an increase in anxiety.

Clatworthy (1981) examined the effects of therapeutic play on the anxiety of hospitalized five to 11 year old children. At discharge from the hospital, the children who did not receive therapeutic play demonstrated higher anxiety than did the children who received therapeutic play.

One study examined the effects of various preparation procedures on the anxiety levels of hospitalized three to nine year old children. Children who had been prepared using hospital equipment and role play demonstrated less anxiety than children who had not been prepared (Demarest et al., 1984).

The study of therapeutic play as a nursing intervention has been limited. The previous studies have focused largely on school-age children and preparation for procedures. There is a need to explore the effects of therapeutic play with various groups of hospitalized children, such as children experiencing same-day surgery, children with chronic illnesses, and children with potentially terminal diagnoses. With the ever-decreasing length of hospitalization for some children and the increasing length of hospitalization or the repeated hospitalizations for other children, there is a need to investigate the effectiveness of therapeutic play with each of these groups of children. It is important in a time of decreased resources to identify by systematic study those groups that may most benefit from this therapeutic modality.

The effectiveness of therapeutic play with children experiencing other stressful situations, such as parental divorce, sibling or parental hospitalization and illness, sibling death, or parental death, needs to be explored. Children experiencing such events are likely to be experiencing emotions that are difficult to express. It would seem logical that therapeutic play could be useful in assisting them in learning to cope with the situation and to continue to grow and develop. At this time, there is no research in this area. Research needs to be conducted to identify the effectiveness of therapeutic play as a preventive measure to assist children to learn in advance of hospitalization and to prevent stress.

The studies supporting the effectiveness of therapeutic play are few. There are difficulties related to methodology and research design which may have discouraged research and influenced findings. The study of this intervention is costly and time-consuming because one needs measures before and after the intervention if one is to document effectiveness. In addition, much research to date has measured the anxiety of children using adult reports of behavior or verbal measures of anxiety. The reliability and validity of such measures is questionable. Researchers, therefore, must continue to develop new measures.

The continued study of therapeutic play through quasi-experimental designs is required, as only through the use of a control group can one demonstrate that an intervention produced a change. However, there is a need to systematically describe the process, identifying the use of specific play modalities by various groups of children. This will allow for the replication of research studies and will enhance the body of knowledge related to therapeutic play.

As stated earlier, there is a great need for the continued development of measurement tools for children that will address both emotional and behavioral outcomes. Children need to be the source of the data because adults, for example, parents, teachers, and nurses, do not perceive the situation in the same way as the children. The area of projective, psychometric techniques may provide a basis for the development of more tools. The usefulness of verbal questionnaires with children needs to be evaluated.

In summary, there is a great need for further study of the use and effects of therapeutic play. There appears to be a great benefit in the use of this therapeutic modality; however, our beliefs in the rightness of this intervention must be supported by empirical evidence if the body of nursing knowledge in this area is to increase.

References

Aguilera, DC, and Messick, JM. Crisis intervention: Theory and methodology (5th ed.). St. Louis: CV Mosby Co., 1986.

Astin, EW. Self reported fears of hospitalized and non-hospitalized children aged 10 to 12. Maternal-Child Nursing Journal, 6:17–24, 1977.

Athey, I. Contributions of play to development. In Yawkey, TD, and Pelligrini, AD (Eds.), Child's play: Developmental and applied. Hillsdale, N.J.: Lawrence Erlbaum Associates, Inc., 1984, pp. 9–27.

Axline, VM. Play therapy procedures and results. American Journal of Orthopsychiatry, 25:618–677, 1955.

Axline, VM. Play therapy. New York: Ballantine Books, 1969.

Azarnoff, P. Mediating the trauma of serious illness and hospitalization in childhood. Children Today, 3:12–17, 1974.

Barton, PH. Play as a tool of nursing. Nursing Outlook, 10:162–164, 1962.

Barton, PH. The relationship between fantasy and overt stress reactions of children to hospitalization. Dissertation Abstracts, 29:809A, 1968. (University Microfilms No. 68–12, 979.)

Begue, MTA. Play: The hospitalized child's best friend. Hospital Topics, 51:45–48, 1972.

Bolig, R. Play in hospital settings. In Yawkey, TD, and Pelligrini, AD (Eds.), Child's play: Developmental and applied. Hillsdale, N.J.: Lawrence Erlbaum Associates, Inc., 1984, pp. 323–345.

Burns, RC, and Kaufman, SH. Kinetic family drawings (K-F-D): An introduction to understanding children through kinetic drawings. New York: Brunner/Mazel, Inc., 1970.

Caplan, F, and Caplan, T. The power of play. Garden City, N.J.: Anchor Press/Doubleday, 1973.

Cassell, S. Effect of brief puppet therapy upon the emotional responses of children undergoing cardiac catheterization. Journal of Consulting Psychology, 29:1–8, 1965.

Chance, P. Pediatric round table 3: Learning through play. Piscataway, N.J.: Johnson and Johnson, 1979.

Christie, J, and Johnsen, P. The role of play in social-intellectual development. Review of Educational Research, 53:93–116, 1983.

Clatworthy, S. Children's drawing-hospital: PSCS score evaluation. Paper presented at the meeting of the Association for the Care of Children's Health, Dallas, 1980.

Clatworthy, S. Therapeutic play: Effects on hospitalized children. Children's Health Care: Journal of the Association for the Care of Children's Health, 9:108–113, 1981.

Clatworthy, S. Play: The language of children. Paper presented at Nursing Clinic Day, Children's Hospital, Detroit, Mich., 1982.

Clatworthy, S. Child drawing hospital. Unpublished manuscript, Kent State University, Kent, Ohio, 1986.

Clatworthy, S, Simon, K, and Tiedeman, M. The development of the child drawing hospital: An instrument designed to measure the emotional status of hospitalized school-age children. Paper presented at the meeting of the Association for the Care of Children's Health, Boston, 1985.

Coddington, RD. The significance of life events as etiologic factors in diseases of children: Part I—A survey of professional workers. Journal of Psychosomatic Research, 16:7–8, 1972.

Crocker, E. Introduction. In Crocker, E (Ed.), Association for the care of children's health: Preparing children and families for health care. Washington, DC: 1981, p. 1.

Curry, NE. Enhancing dramatic play potential in hospitalized children. Children's Health Care: Journal of the Association for the Care of Children's Health, 16:142–149, 1988.

David, N. Play: A nursing diagnostic tool. Maternal Child Nursing Journal, 2:49–56, 1973.

DelPo, EG, and Frick, SB. Directed and nondirected play as therapeutic modalities. Children's Health Care: Journal of the Association for the Care of Children's Health, 16:261–267, 1988.

Demarest, DS, Hooke, JF, and Erickson, MT. Preoperative interventions for the reduction of anxiety in pediatric surgery patients. Children's Health Care: Journal of the Association for the Care of Children's Health, 12:179–183, 1984.

DiLeo, JH. Young children and their drawings. New York: Brunner/Mazel, Inc., 1970.

DiLeo, JH. Children's drawings as diagnostic aids. New York: Brunner/Mazel, Inc., 1973.

Dimock, HG. The child in hospital. Philadelphia: FA Davis Co., 1960.

Eichenbaum, IW, and Dunn, NA. Projective drawings by children under repeated dental stress. Journal of Dentistry for Children, 38:164–174, 1971.

Ellis, MJ. Why people play. Englewood Cliffs, N.J.: Prentice-Hall, Inc., 1973.

Erikson, EH. Studies in the interpretation of play: Clinical observations of play disruptions in young children. Genetic Psychology Monograph, 22:557–671, 1940.

Erikson, EH. Childhood and society. New York: WW Norton and Co., Inc., 1963.

Erikson, EH. The meaning of play. In Haworth, MR (Ed.), Child psychotherapy: Practice and theory. New York: Basic Books, Inc., 1964.

Erikson, EH. Play and actuality. In Piers, MW (Ed.), Play and development. New York: WW Norton and Co., Inc., 1972, pp. 127–167.

Farquhar, SE. A study in the relationship of anxiety in children in a school setting and children in a hospital setting, ages 5–11. Unpublished master's thesis, Wayne State University, Detroit, Mich., 1983.

Fein, GG. The self-building potential of pretend play or "I got a fish all by myself." In Yawkey, TD and Pelligrini, AD (Eds.), Child's play: Developmental and applied. Hillsdale, N.J.: Lawrence Erlbaum Associates, Inc., 1984, pp. 125–141.

Fore, C, and Poster, EC. Meeting the psychosocial needs of children and families in health care. Washington, DC: Association for the Care of Children's Health, 1981.

Fraiberg, S. The magic years. New York: Scribner, 1959.

Gardner, RA. Therapeutic communication with children: The mutual storytelling technique. New York: Science House, 1971.

Gardner, RA. Mutual storytelling techniques in the treatment of anger and inhibition problems. International Journal of Child Psychotherapy, 1:34–64, 1972.

Garvey, C. Play. Cambridge, Mass.: Harvard University Press, 1977.

Geist, H, and Bost, C. A child goes to the hospital. Springfield, Ill.: Charles C Thomas, 1965.

Ginott, HG. Group psychotherapy with children: Theory and practice of play therapy. New York: McGraw-Hill, Inc., 1961.

Gordon, M. Manual of nursing diagnoses, 1986–1987. New York: McGraw-Hill, Inc., 1987.

Guenery, LF. Play therapy in counseling settings. In Yawkey, TD, and Pelligrini, AD (Eds.), Child's play: Developmental and applied. Hillsdale, N.J.: Lawrence Erlbaum Associates, Inc., 1984, pp. 291–321.

Haller, JA, Talbert, JL, and Dombo, RH (Eds.). The hospitalized child and his family. Baltimore: The Johns Hopkins University Press, 1967.

Hammer, EF. The clinical application of projective drawings. Springfield, Ill.: Charles C Thomas, 1958.

Hartley, R. Play: The essential ingredient. Childhood Education, 48:80–84, 1971.

Hartley, RE, and Goldenson, RM. The complete book of children's play. New York: Crowell, 1963.

Horney, K. Neuroscience and human growth. New York: WW Norton and Co., Inc., 1950.

Hyde, D. Play therapy: The troubled child's self-encounter. American Journal of Nursing, 71:1366–1370, 1971.

Jolly, H. Play and the sick child. Lancet, 2:1286–1370, 1968.

Knudsen, K. Play therapy: Preparing the young child for surgery. Nursing Clinics of North America, 10:679–686, 1975.

Koppitz, EM. Psychological evaluation of children's human figure drawings. New York: Grune and Stratton, Inc., 1968.

Kunzman, L. Some factors influencing a young child's mastery of hospitalization. Nursing Clinics of North America, 7:13–26, 1972.

Lazarus, RS, and Launier, R. Stress-related transactions between person and environment. In Pervin, LS, and Lewis, M (Eds.), Perspectives in interactional psychology. New York: Plenum Publishing Corp., pp. 287–327.

Machover, K. Human figure drawings of children. Journal of Projective Techniques, 17:85–98, 1953.

McCue, K. Medical play: An expanded perspective. Children's Health Care: Journal of the Association for the Care of Children's Health, 16:157–168, 1988.

McLeary, KA. Children's art as an assessment tool. Pediatric Nursing, 5:9–14, 1979.

Monoghan, JH, Robinson, JO, and Dodge, JA. The children's life events inventory. Journal of Psychosomatic Research, 23:63–68, 1979.

Moustakas, CE. Children in play therapy. New York: McGraw-Hill, Inc., 1953.

Neumann, E. The elements of play. New York: MSS Information, 1971.

Nickerson, ET. Helping children: Readings in the practice of working therapeutically with children. Lexington, Mass.: Xerox College Publications, 1974.

Oremland, EK. Mastering developmental and critical experiences through play and other expressive behaviors in childhood. Children's Health Care: Journal of the Association for the Care of Children's Health, 16:150–161, 1988.

Peller, L. Models of children's play. Mental Hygiene, 36:66–83, 1952.

Peller, L. Theories of play and a survey of development. In Plank, E (Ed.), On development and education of young children. New York: Philosophical Library, 1978, pp. 128–193.

Pelligrini, A. The relationship between symbolic play and literate behavior: A review and critique of the empirical literature. Review of Educational Research, 55:107–121, 1985.

Petrillo, M. Preventing hospital trauma in pediatric patients. American Journal of Nursing, 68:1469–1473, 1968.

Petrillo, M, and Sanger, S. Emotional care of hospitalized children: An environmental approach (2nd ed.). Philadelphia: JB Lippincott Co., 1980.

Piaget, J. Play, dreams, and imitation in childhood. London: Routledge and Kegan Paul, Inc., 1962.

Piaget, J. The psychology of the child. New York: Basic Books, Inc., 1970.

Piaget, J. Some aspects of operations. In Piers, MW (Ed.), Play and development. New York: WW Norton and Co., Inc., 1972, pp. 15–27.

Plank, EN. Working with children in hospitals: A guide for the professional team. Cleveland: Case Western Reserve University, 1971.

Potheir, P. Resolving conflict through play fantasy. Journal of Psychiatric Nursing, 5:141–149, 1967.

Rutter, M. Stress, coping, and development: Some issues and some questions. Journal of Child Psychology and Psychiatry, 22:323–356, 1981.

Schulz, JB, Raschke, D, Dedrick, C, and Thompson, M. The effects of a preoperational puppet show on the anxiety levels of hospitalized children. Children's Health Care: Journal of the Association for the Care of Children's Health, 9:118–121, 1981.

Smith, LF. An experiment with play therapy. American Journal of Nursing, 77:1963–1965, 1977.

Sutton-Smith, B. Child play: Very serious business. Psychology Today, 5:67–69, 1971.

Taylor, MM, and Williams, MA. Use of therapeutic play in the ambulatory pediatric hematology clinic. Cancer Nursing, 3:433–437, 1980.

Thompson, RH, and Stanford, G. Child life in hospitals: Theory and practice. Springfield, Ill.: Charles C Thomas, 1981.

Tiedeman, ME. An examination of the anxiety responses of 5- to 11-year-old children during and after hospitalization. Doctoral dissertation, Wayne State University, Detroit, 1988.

Varma, VP. Stresses in children. London: University of London Press, 1973.

Visintainer, MA, and Wolfer, JA. Psychological preparation for surgical pediatric patients and their parents: The effect on children's and parents' stress responses and adjustments. Pediatrics, 56:187–202, 1975.

Welch, C. The nurse's role in play. Nursing Care, 10:14–15, 1977.

Wolfer, JA, and Visintainer, MA. Pediatric surgical patients' and parents' stress responses and adjustment. Nursing Research, 24:244–255, 1975a.

Wolfer, JA, and Visintainer, MA. Prehospital psychological preparation for tonsillectomy patients: Effects on children's and parents' adjustment. Pediatrics, 64:646–655, 1975b.

Woltmann, AG. Spontaneous puppetry by children as a projective method. In Rabin, A, and Haworth, M (Eds.), Projective techniques with children. New York: Grune and Stratton, Inc., 1960, pp. 305–312.

Woltmann, AG. Puppetry as a tool in child psychotherapy. International Journal of Child Psychotherapy, 1:84–96, 1972.

CHAPTER 8

COMMUNICATING WITH CHILDREN THROUGH DRAWINGS

JANICE A. DENEHY, Ph.D., R.N.

The drawings of children became the focus of interest among psychologists interested in child development during the latter part of the 19th century. A number of clinical studies done from that time through the 1920's provided the theoretical foundation for the use of children's drawings (Mortensen, 1984). Over the last 60 years, numerous researchers have added to the literature on the use of drawings as a way to assess development and intelligence and as a projective tool to analyze the psychological state and feelings of children (Goodenough, 1926; Machover, 1949; Harris, 1963; Koppitz, 1968; DiLeo, 1970; DiLeo, 1973; Burns, 1982; and Koppitz, 1984). Currently, there is an increasing interest on the part of health professionals in the use of drawings as a means to communicate with children with altered health states. Drawings are a natural medium of expression for young children. Through their drawings, one can see the world from the perspective of a child. Drawing is also a recreational activity for children, an activity from which the child receives enjoyment from the kinesthetic activity of manipulating media and the joy of creating a truly unique product. Drawings are used as an assessment tool to determine a child's developmental or knowledge level. Drawing can also be a therapeutic activity in which the child is free to put into pictures that which he or she may not be able to put into words because of a lack of vocabulary or because of the anxiety the subject provokes (Siemon, 1982; Lewis and Green, 1983).

Health professionals use drawings to gain a greater understanding of their young clients by using a communication channel that is attractive to and developmentally appropriate for children. This technique is helpful when working with children experiencing stress—the stress of illness and hospitalization or family stresses such as divorce, abuse, or death. Because young children do not always have the vocabulary or insight to put their feelings and concerns into words, drawings are used to provide children with a familiar medium of expression that does not not require the use of words. The challenge to the professional is to derive meaning from the drawings. In order to interpret the message that children may be communicating through their drawings, it is essential to have an understanding of the normal developmental progression of children's drawings. In addition, the professional needs to carefully plan, implement, and evaluate this intervention to avoid the possibility of inaccurately interpreting or reading too much meaning into the drawings of children.

The purpose of this chapter is to examine the use of drawings as a method of communication with children, to describe the developmental stages of drawings during childhood, to assess the indications for the use of drawings, to propose a variety of ways this intervention can be implemented, and to discuss methods to measure the outcome of this intervention.

THEORETICAL FOUNDATION

As one examines the literature on communication, it is evident that there is not a well-defined, organized body of knowledge (Samovar and Rintye, 1979). What is revealed is a collection of studies from a wide range of disciplines, including education, psychology, anthropology, and philosophy. Nursing, like other disciplines, has selected those communication principles and theories which are useful to its practice domain.

The basic elements of human communication consist of the sender, the message, and the receiver (Berlo, 1960). The sender encodes or translates the message into a medium or channel for transmission to the receiver. The receiver, upon receiving the encoded message, decodes the message from the sender. Examining this model, one can identify a number of points where a breakdown in communication is possible. In children, developmental level and speech may present a potential barrier to effective communication. Cultural and language differences may inhibit communication. The readiness, attention, and frame of reference of the receiver also influence communication. In addition, the choice of communication channel or medium has an impact on communication. Because young children are just beginning to develop language skills, one needs to rely on other methods of communication to supplement or substitute for the spoken word. Nonverbal cues and behavior also communicate a child's feelings and needs.

An essential component of communication is feedback from the receiver to the sender to validate that communication has, in fact, occurred and that the receiver has correctly decoded the intended message. This is especially important with children because their skills in encoding messages may be limited by cognitive development and lack of vocabulary and further confounded when the receiver has a different frame of reference. Providing feedback becomes more complicated when the receiver attempts to couple verbal messages with nonverbal cues and behavior.

To communicate effectively with children, one must gather data from as many sources as possible. Drawing is a medium that is attractive to children and that has the potential to become a powerful channel of communication. However, in order for the nurse to encode messages that are communicated through this modality, it is important to understand the development of drawings during childhood and review the literature on interpreting the drawings of children.

Developmental Stages of Children's Drawings

Although authors label and divide the developmental stages of children's drawings differently, most seem to be describing the same phenomena (Lowenfeld, 1947; Harris, 1963; Kellogg, 1969; DiLeo, 1970). In fact, many characteristics of children's drawings have been noted through the ages and across cultures (Harris, 1963; DiLeo, 1970; Koppitz, 1984). Some variation has been noted, especially today, when children are encouraged or taught to use the correct shape and color when drawing. For most children, however, there is a universal progression of skills that is linked with cognitive and psychomotor development (DiLeo, 1970).

The Kinesthetic or Scribbling Stage

The first stage seen in the drawings of children is described as the kinesthetic or scribbling stage, which commences sometime after the child's first birthday and lasts until about the age of three years. During this stage, a child's response to paper and crayon (or any other writing implement) is avid scribbling with emphasis on movement and activity (DiLeo, 1970). The focus of this kinesthetic activity is on motion, expression, and enjoyment, not on content or form. Scribbling begins as a spontaneous behavior; however, it may also be an imitative behavior, modeling the often observed behavior of adults writing or drawing. Scribbling begins as a continuous zigzag motion, mostly horizontal in nature. As the child nears three years of age, movements become more vertical and circular shapes appear as neuromuscular development progresses and hand-eye coordination improves (Kellogg, 1969).

DiLeo (1970) states that scribblers do not seem to be communicating through the content of their drawings. However, children communicate much about themselves in the manner the activity is approached and performed—the process. The approach to drawing, whether it is intellectual, hesitant, joyful, or hostile, tells the observer about the child's personality and temperament. The quality of the stroke used to scribble also communicates information about the child; is there freedom to explore and create or does the child display inhibitions and fear-

fulness? Of greatest interest and meaning is a collection of drawings over time which illustrate the cognitive and personality development of a child. Even during their early years, much can be learned about children as they communicate through drawings.

The Transition Stage

At about three years of age, the child will discover, quite accidentally, that the round, circle-shaped scribble looks like a human head (DiLeo, 1970). Although it is likely that each child will in time independently discover this, many children have this resemblance pointed out to them at home or in day-care settings by well-meaning parents and other caregivers. Once children have made this link, they begin to see their power to create their own designs, to be creative. The change from scribbling to the representational mode of drawing is very gradual and uniquely individual. During this transition phase, from about three to four years of age, drawings become more deliberate and more intellectual (Kellogg, 1969; Mortensen, 1984). The focus on activity and the joy of movement is redirected to a more purposeful endeavor. Children become more conscious of what is communicated through drawings, even though this awareness may not be evident to them or they may not be able to articulate in words the full meaning or description of their artistic creation. It is important not to force children to attach labels to their drawings by asking, "What is it?" While such labeling may please adults, it inhibits creativity and spontaneity in children. This is a time when the children need to be free to create and explore the world through drawings.

The Representational Stage

Around the age of four years, with much variation for individual differences so characteristic of any developmental task, the drawings of children become representational in nature: that is, they take on meaning for the child. Drawings represent the mental image the child has of the object drawn, often complete with emotional shadings of that object. At this time, the object drawn often tells more about the artist than it does about the object, capturing the inner reality of the artist. In contrast, many adults attempt to capture the optical reality of an object in their drawings, attempting to reproduce or draw the object as it is.

Piaget (1966) sees the growth of children's drawings as parallel to the growth of cognition and logical thought. Drawings help to indicate the status of the development of mental constructs; however, they are often colored by prelogical feelings and experience. During this stage, children draw things as they perceive them, reflecting their own emotional reality. However, it is during this time that children enter school and are encouraged to draw things as they really are: an optical reproduction of reality. During their early years, children vacillate between drawing from the heart—the emotional reality of life, free flowing, flamboyant, and producing enjoyment at the sense of creativity—and drawing from the head—drawings that are more realistic, easy to explain, and pleasing to others. In each case, drawing is a method of communication, telling those who "listen" more about the child than can be heard through words alone.

The Reproduction Stage

Somewhere between the ages of eight and 12 years, one begins to note an increasing tendency to create drawings that attempt to capture or reproduce optical reality. It becomes more difficult for children to be spontaneous and allow themselves to become a part of their drawings; consequently, it becomes harder to ascribe meaning to drawings. This inhibition is furthered by a self-consciousness about what others may think of their drawings. These drawings contain considerable detail and attention to correct proportion (Siemon, 1982). During this stage, a concern about skill and the ability to reproduce optical reality becomes predominant; this concern for accurateness produces frustration and discouragement. It is during adolescence that most children cease drawing for enjoyment. After the age of ten to 12 years, limited improvement is seen in the drawing skills of most children. This phenomenon also seems to be related to the increase in verbal skills and the ability to express thoughts and feelings graphically through writing (DiLeo, 1970, p. 142). In addition, at about the age of ten years, when

the brain becomes more lateralized, children come into conflict over the best method to draw—logically and analytically or creatively with symbolic representation (Mortensen, 1984). In a society where there is considerable emphasis on analytic and verbal ability, development of nonverbal, intuitive ways of relating is devalued.

After puberty, drawing is no longer a natural activity. Only the artistically gifted child will persist in the further development of drawing skills (DiLeo, 1970). In fact, there is little difference seen in drawing skills at this age and adult drawing skills. The artistic interests and endeavors of young adolescents are likely to move in other directions using a wide assortment of media other than paper and pen.

Human Figure Drawings

Young children tend to draw that which is most important to them—namely, people, particularly parents and other family members (Harris, 1963; DiLeo, 1973; Mortensen, 1984; Koppitz, 1984). Other than people, children are likely to draw animals, such as the family pet; houses; and trees. According to DiLeo (1973), drawings are influenced by what is remembered at the time, colored by feelings, and are based on some, but not all, of what the child knows about the object.

During the transition stage, the beginning of human figure drawings (HFD) is observed as the child draws a circle to represent the head. The head is the focus of communication between the parent and child beginning in infancy when the mother aligns herself en face with her infant during the attachment process. The face becomes a symbol of nurturance and survival to the young infant. Likewise, the infant is fascinated by the eyes of the caregivers. Eye contact is also a prime determinant in the attachment process (Avant, 1979). The eyes, often drawn like goggles, are the first characteristics drawn on the circle representing the head. Soon after, the mouth and nose are added. The mouth and eyes are predominant in communication with the young child, who is rapidly acquiring language skills and vocabulary. The primacy of the head is indicated by its large size, which becomes more evident as the child adds small stick-like arms and legs (Fig. 8–1). Even though the meaning of this form is disputed, it has been described as a tadpole or cephalopod person (DiLeo, 1970; Mortensen, 1984).

When the child is about four to five years of age, the trunk, drawn considerably smaller than the head, is added. This may take the form of a stick, box, or circle attached to the bottom of the head. As the child matures, the trunk becomes larger in proportion to the head. A number of children have been noted to add the bellybutton at age four (Fig. 8–2), but by five to six years, children no longer add this feature (DiLeo, 1970; Mortensen, 1984). After the trunk has been added, extremities drawn as sticks will come from either the head or the trunk. Hands and feet are often omitted but may be drawn as small circles or spider-like stick fingers.

Young children are likely to differentiate the sex of human figures in their drawings by the addition of hair—specifically, more hair for the female figure. As the child matures, more details are added to the drawings which reveal the sex of the person drawn, such as dresses, skirts, and jewelry for females and pants and ties for males. More recent observations, however, indicate that changing cultural trends are reflected in children's drawings; children began to draw females wearing pants and males with long

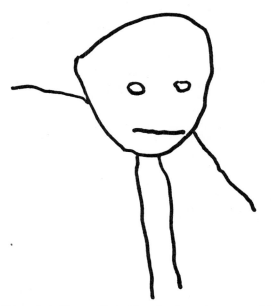

Figure 8–1. Human figure drawing by a three year old boy.

hair and jewelry (Koppitz, 1984; Mortensen, 1984).

Preschool and school-aged children do not usually include genitalia in HFDs (DiLeo, 1970). Koppitz (1968) reported that the few children she encountered who included genitalia in their drawings were clinical patients who were deeply disturbed or overly aggressive. She concludes that this characteristic is an indicator of anxiety, poor impulse control, and psychopathology. This characteristic seems to be true across time and culture, even in cultures where there are fewer cultural taboos regarding sexuality than are seen in Western cultures.

Mortensen (1984) had hypothesized that in Denmark, a country with a relatively free and open attitude regarding both sexuality and the discussion of sexuality with children, there may be more freedom to include genitalia in drawings. However, in the 540 drawings she collected from children five to 13 years old, there was no increase in the number of genitalia included in the drawings. In the few instances where they were included, there were associated disturbances, confirming the findings of earlier studies. Children who have experienced sexual abuse, lived in sexually stimulating environments, or who have had pathology or surgery relating to the urinary or reproductive system are more likely to include genitalia in their drawings. When this is observed in drawings or is a predominant theme in other forms of communication, it is a cue to take time to listen to what the child is communicating, note how and when this communication occurs, and try to understand the significance of what is being communicated. For some children, this may be a way of communicating interest in sexual matters; for others, it may be a way of revealing an abusive incident without actually "telling" verbally that which the child has promised or has been under threat to keep secret. A few children will use sexual explicitness for the associated shock value or attention-getting gains.

Somewhere between the ages of seven and ten years, the drawing of the human head evolves from a full front view to a complete profile. The drawing of a profile figure is necessary to illustrate action, movement, and direction and may occur earlier in boys because of the activity-orientated nature of their drawings (DiLeo, 1970). The develop-

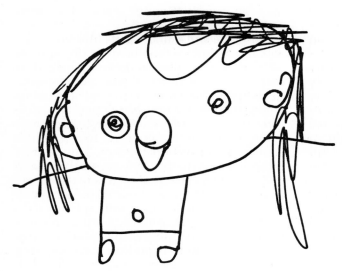

Figure 8–2. Human figure drawing by a four and a half year old girl.

ment of profile drawing illustrates the change from intellectual realism to visual realism and occurs in two distinct stages: (1) the profile of the face is drawn, but two eyes and a complete smile remain—the mixed or full face profile and (2) a complete profile is drawn with only one eye and a half mouth, illustrating the transition from transparency to opacity. A complete profile is usually seen after ten years of age; however, many never achieve this level of sophistication. After facial profile drawings begin to develop, attempts to draw the body and extremities in profile to accentuate movement, direction, or attention is evident.

DiLeo (1970, p. 20) believes the HFDs of young children are not an image of self, but a reflection of a significant adult of the same sex. He reports children at this age are more interested in adults than self, and this interest is reflected in their drawings. Children's drawings will reflect their wishes, fears, and conflicts and are likely to be drawn in terms of their own self-concepts (Koppitz, 1968; Machover, 1949). It is not until children are old enough to draw the family that they will specifically draw themselves in the family constellation. An exception to this may be the anxious or poorly adjusted child, who is more focused on self because of energy expended in coping with life's demands. When a child draws a self-portrait, it is likely to be an idealized self-image: older, more mature, more beautiful, and powerful (Koppitz, 1968, 1984).

Researchers have found differences between the drawings of girls and boys. Goodenough (1926) noted that boys emphasize feet and draw longer extremities. They also draw a profile view earlier, a characteristic needed to depict activity. Harris (1963) found that girls scored higher on drawings because they included more detail in their drawings. He speculated that this characteristic might be due to more mature intellectual development in prepubescent girls and the cultural emphasis for females on quiet activity, fine motor skills, and detail. Koppitz (1968) found males included more action in their drawings, including anger, hostility, and aggression. The drawings of school-age females showed more emphasis on hair; facial features, especially eyes and lips; and dress. Harris (1963) hypothesized that this may be due to a greater sex role identification for females. Koppitz (1984) found in her later study that males appeared to be including more emphasis on hair, clothing, and appearance.

Koppitz (1984) also noted an emerging difference in the drawings of black children. Prior to 1960, black children drew HFDs with white features; however, after the civil rights movement, a change in attitudes began to be reflected in the drawings of black children. During the 1970's, the Afro hair style became a status symbol and was evident in drawings. However, few black children depicted human figures with dark skin; racial identity was instead revealed in the treatment of hair and facial features (pp. 74–75).

The significance of a dominant color in children's drawings is based on numerous observations made in clinical settings (Lewis and Green, 1983). The trends observed by these authors reflect others reported in the literature. A predominance of red usually indicates hostility and aggression and may be observed during or following periods of stress or emotional difficulty. Blue is likely to be indicative of a child who is more stable, self-confident, and self-sufficient. It is characteristic of a child who is gaining mastery and self-control. When yellow dominates the drawings of a child, one is likely to observe a child who is outgoing and emotional, yet who is likely to be dependent upon adults for approval. Such a child often displays attention-getting behaviors. The preponderance of green in drawing may indicate maturity and self-reliance; these children often approach life in a cool, restrained manner. The dominant use of dark colors, such as purple or black, may be a cry for help or an indication of unhappiness or depression. The use of black or dark tones is often seen during times of emotional crisis. It should be added that when using color to analyze the mood or feelings of a child, it is important to look for trends that occur in subsequent drawings over time, in theme or predominant color, rather than making a judgment based on one drawing.

ASSESSMENT

Using drawings as a communication tool is particularly appropriate for preschool and school-aged children because drawings are a meaningful mode of expression during these developmental periods (Goodnow, 1977). Also antecedent to the use of this intervention are the child's cognitive and psychomotor abilities essential to comprehend and participate in drawing.

Children with the nursing diagnosis of *Impaired verbal communication* resulting from developmental, cultural, or psychological factors would be good subjects for the use of drawing as a communication intervention. Drawings in this instance would provide children with a method to express themselves when it is difficult to find words

to describe thoughts or fears. The use of drawings is also helpful for children experiencing stress that may be reflected in a nursing diagnosis of *Altered family process* or *Dysfunctional parenting*. Alterations in family process or parenting due to situational or maturational crises have an effect on all family members. Children may not be able to identify the crisis or its impact on family functioning. However, they sense the effect, because of the diversion of parental attention and energy from parenting to crisis management. Young children may become fearful when they see their parents upset or having difficulty coping; they often fear for their place in the family or the continued existence of the family unit. Drawing provides an opportunity to express these fears in a supportive milieu.

Children with the nursing diagnosis of *Ineffective individual coping* manifested by inability to perform at a level consistent with the developmental level in the family, neighborhood, or school environment, would also be ideal candidates for the use of drawings. Drawings are one way to communicate emotions and perceptions that interfere with optimum functioning and continued development. Drawings may also be useful in communicating with children who are experiencing difficulty in coping with the stresses of hospitalization, invasive procedures, or a disfiguring illness. Drawings give the nurse another method of reaching these children traumatized by the effects of hospitalization, illness, and treatment which may help in understanding how young children internalize these stressful experiences. This is also true with children for whom the nursing diagnosis of *Alteration in self-concept, body image, or self-esteem* has been determined.

Drawings have been used with children who have experienced sexual abuse, a nursing diagnosis of *Rape trauma syndrome*. Abused children have been severely traumatized, physically and emotionally, often by persons they trust; fear and confusion are characteristic. Through drawings, abused children are given an opportunity to express feelings and recreate events that are very painful for them.

A recurring theme evident in the defining characteristics of the preceding nursing diagnoses is fear. While fear is manifested in many traumatic events, it is also inherent in any new or strange situation children face. This includes any encounter with health care providers or the health care system where new routines and unexpected procedures are the norm. Because children's recollections of visits to health care providers are often associated with discomfort or pain, such as immunizations, illnesses, or emergency room visits to receive sutures or treat fractures, it is likely that fear of pain or the unknown will impede children's communication with health professionals. Drawings are a method of helping children express these fears as well as their perceptions of health care.

THE INTERVENTION

Drawing is a method to view the world through the eyes of a child. This method of communication is particularly well suited for the young child who may not have the language skills to communicate verbally or for the child who is undergoing a stressful event. For the child who is experiencing family-related stress, drawings are a medium to express feelings about the family in a way that is less stressful than the spoken language. It may also be a way to help a child gain insight into his or her feelings. For the ill or hospitalized child facing a fearful or strange situation, drawing provides a way to communicate fears and perceptions of what is happening.

Setting the Stage for Drawing

For the nurse using drawing as an intervention, four things will be needed: (1) plain paper and writing implements; (2) a smooth, flat surface for drawing; (3) a relatively quiet space that is free from interruptions; and (4) time to spend with the child during the intervention. The choice of medium is at the discretion of the nurse and is dependent on the purpose of the intervention and the developmental level of the child. Choices include crayons, pencil, pen, markers, and paint. An ample supply of plain paper 8½ × 11 inches or larger is essential. Provision of a flat surface for children who are immobilized by traction or in a prone position becomes a challenge. For children who are

ambulatory, a table or surface appropriate to their height is desirable. An area and time where no disruptions are anticipated should be sought. This is important to avoid the possibility of a person interrupting the drawing session by asking about or commenting on the child's drawing or disturbing the session for procedures, examinations, mealtime, or visitation. Children are more likely to be more open in their drawings when others are not present, especially school-aged children, who are concerned about what others think of their drawings and are easily influenced by what other children are drawing. Although some recommend leaving the child alone during the drawing session and returning later to discuss the drawing, the author recommends the nurse stay with the child during the session. The nurse's presence communicates caring and helps the child stay on task. It also provides the opportunity to observe the process of drawing; for example, the nurse can observe how the child undertakes the task—hesitantly, aggressively, or with confidence. When present, the nurse is also able to hear verbal comments made by the child during the activity, which may be valuable in communicating about the drawing after its completion. The nurse can keep busy with some other activity, such as writing, if the child is self-conscious. No time limits should be placed on the activity.

When drawing is used as an intervention, either a directive or nondirective approach can be used in facilitating this activity. Regardless of the approach, DiLeo (1970) found that in 20 years of collecting drawings from children, few refused to participate; those who were hesitant usually responded positively when given encouragement. When using a directive approach, the nurse provides materials and gives the child directions on what to draw, such as, "Draw me a picture of your family." The instructions can be general or specific, including time parameters when applicable. When the directive approach is used, the nurse is attempting to elicit specific information relating to specified topical areas, such as feelings, perception, or development. When a nondirective approach is used, the child is offered a wider range of materials and told to draw whatever he or she chooses. While this approach may be used to gain specific information, it is more likely to be used as a recreational, diversional, or therapeutic activity. Whatever the approach, the nurse needs to plan the intervention strategy best suited to realize the outcome goals. The nursing diagnosis, the personality and developmental level of the child, and the knowledge base and skills of the practitioner all must be taken into account when planning the intervention.

After the child has completed the drawing, the nurse facilitates communication about the drawing by saying, "Tell me about your drawing." Encouraging the child to tell a little about each member included in a family drawing or the interactions depicted among family members will assist the nurse in understanding that which is being communicated through the drawing. The information the child shared about the drawing, the conditions under which the drawing was made, the date, and the child's name and age should be recorded and attached to the picture. The nurse should also include impressions about how the child approached the task and executed the process, because this often provides insights about the child's personality and temperament. The recorded summary is important when comparing drawings done over time, conducting research on drawings, or validating the interpretation of drawings. This information, when gathered on a number of drawings and viewed retrospectively, often leads to new insights about what is being communicated through drawings.

While it is a good idea to keep the drawings of children as a record and to observe trends over time, there are times when a child is reluctant to give his or her creation to the nurse. In these cases, it is important to honor the child's request to keep the drawing. Many times the child will draw another picture to give to the examiner or may share the drawing long enough to get a photocopy to be kept in the records. An exception to this rule of allowing a child who wants a drawing to keep it may be in cases of abuse where the drawing may serve as evidence necessary to case management or prosecution.

Assessment of Developmental Level

Although it is not an intervention strategy, the Goodenough (1926) Draw a Person Test,

modified by Harris (1963), is often used to assess intellectual development and provide a baseline of the drawing ability of children between the ages of four and ten years. The results of this test are based on the number of items and details included in the drawing of a person. Although there has been considerable discussion of this test over the years, validity and reliability studies indicate that it remains a relatively consistent, culture-free way of assessing cognitive maturity (DiLeo, 1970, p. 224). However, it should not be used as an intelligence test in the absence of other accepted measures. Data gathered on this test only supplement information about the developmental level of the child and provide a beginning in establishing communication through drawing.

Human Figure and Family Drawings

A frequently used directive technique is to ask the child to draw a person, the HFD. As mentioned previously, DiLeo (1970) believes that HFDs done by young children represent a significant adult, not self. On the other hand, Machover (1949) describes the human figure as drawn by young children as an expression of self. Perhaps the best person to describe the identification and significance of the figure drawn is the child, who can be asked a question such as, "Tell me about the person you have drawn." Koppitz (1984) asks the child if the person is someone he or she knows or made up; how old the person is; and what the person is thinking, doing, and feeling. However, it is important not to force the child to attach a label or meaning to a drawing.

Numerous authors describe the significance of various characteristics in HFDs. While the themes are similar, some authors attribute more meaning to specific characteristics than others. Human figure drawings are commonly used as a projective technique to reveal information about a child's personality, relationships, attitudes, and values that is not freely communicated in words (Harris, 1963; Koppitz, 1968, 1984). From a child's perspective, HFDs communicate reality. Decoding the reality communicated via drawings requires knowledge, skill, and practice. For example, heavy pressure with a crayon or pen suggests tension, anxiety, or

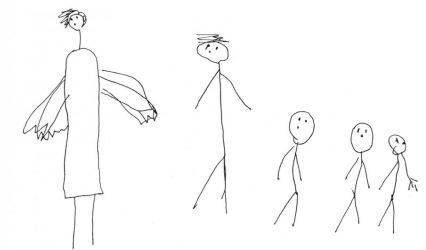

Figure 8–3. Human figure drawing by a five year old boy.

aggressiveness while light pressure may indicate timid, insecure, or hesitant characteristics. Enlarged body parts and details suggest importance attached to or preoccupation with that part of the body, while omission of body parts may indicate denial. Shading, particularly over an area just drawn, may show anxiety or the desire to conceal what was revealed in the drawing. However, as the child gets older, shading is a technique used to add dimension and depth to the object drawn (Koppitz, 1984).

Loney (1971) found that disturbed school-aged children and adolescents often were not responsive to the request to draw a person for diagnostic purposes. She discovered, however, that these school-aged and adolescent children, particularly males, were very responsive when requested to draw a car. She found that information about personality characteristics and life stresses can also be communicated from the drawing of a car. For example, normal children will describe the car as a family vehicle, a way to go to family activities, and easy to handle; on the other hand, an impulsive child may draw a car with powerful engines and flames with little or no regard to the steering mechanism or the ability to control the car. Children with low self-esteem are likely to describe their cars in a negative way—old, beat-up, rusty, and dirty. This strategy would also be appropriate for older children who sense the purpose of HFDs in a therapeutic setting or feel they are "too old" for their use. Koppitz (1984) stated that adolescents are also more likely to draw cartoons,

space ships, monsters, and television characters and will avoid drawing a human figure.

The drawing of the family is a projective technique that communicates information about how a child views himself within the family constellation (Fig. 8–3). When family drawings are used, particular attention is paid to who is included or excluded, the order of the persons drawn, the position of the family members within the drawing (particularly the child doing the drawing), the size of the various family members, and the characteristics of each person drawn. A good understanding of the child's family constellation and history helps put the drawing into perspective. For example, a child who has experienced divorce of parents or the death of a family member may exclude the member who is no longer in the household. The child who has two family units because of divorce and remarriage of a parent has a decision about which family unit or members to include or omit. Such inclusions and exclusions communicate the child's feelings about family relationships and conflicts. Children in a family unit are frequently drawn in ordinal position with the first-born closest to the parents. Alteration in this order, particularly as it relates to the child who is doing the drawing, warrants attention because it often communicates who feels close to or distant from whom. Size of the family members is also related to ordinal position, with the parents being drawn larger than the children. The dominant parent may be drawn taller or larger than a passive or nonparticipating parent. Characteristics included in the drawing communicate information about family members and relationships. Colorful drawings with hearts and flowers communicate happiness or the wish for happiness, while darker colors with storm clouds may indicate sadness, confusion, or depression. Sunshine or light beaming down on a family shows warmth or the desire for love. Sibling rivalry is often evident in drawings because the child is free to safely express hostility or ambivalent feelings about a sibling. This is shown in Figure 8–4, in which an older sister has portrayed her attractive younger sister with a large nose, crossed eyes, a wart, and straight hair.

Burns (1982) has extended the use of family drawings by developing Kinetic Family Drawings (K-F-Ds) in which children are asked to draw everyone in their family, including themselves, doing something. The focus of these drawings is not only the family unit but also the activity and interaction of each family member. Kinetic Family Drawings describe a child's perspective of family dynamics and his or her place in the family matrix. Burns states, "K-F-Ds have a special language telling us a great deal about family interactions, if we speak the language" (1982, p. 3) and continues by saying they are a rich source of personal and interpersonal information. To decode children's communication through drawings, one might ask oneself the following questions:

Whom do I see? What is happening?
What do I notice about physical intimacy or distance?
Is the drawing warm or cold, pleasant or unpleasant?
Are the people touching or shut off from one another?
Who is facing whom? Who is interacting and how?
Are family members isolated or encapsulated by lines?
What is the affect of the family members?
Do I feel love and involvement?
What would happen if the drawing came to life?

Burns and Kaufman (1972) have described the interpretation of K-F-Ds, including action, style, and symbols present in drawings, as observed in their research and practice. For example, playing ball may indicate competition between family members, while compartmentalizing family members with lines shows isolation, fear, or dislike. Beds in K-F-Ds are rare and usually associated with sexual or depressive themes. The choice of family activities, household items, and other objects may reflect areas of concern and conflict for the child.

Burns (1982) has quantified the most frequently occurring themes in K-F-Ds, devised a schema to quantify the characteristics observed in the drawings, and developed a grid to measure the size and placement of family members. The use of this research tool provides data to observe the growth and changes in family dynamics and the development of self over time (Burns, 1982). An important fact to note is that when a child is asked to draw a single person, the result will be more detailed and more representative of the child's developmental level than would be seen in the human figures drawn in a K-F-D in which the focus of the child's attention has been redirected to the entire family constellation and activity (Burns, 1982, p. 17). Kinetic Family Drawings have been used with children in different countries and cultures with similar and promising results (p. 65).

Drawings of Children Experiencing Stress

Drawings of children experiencing stress may be disorganized and portray a regres-

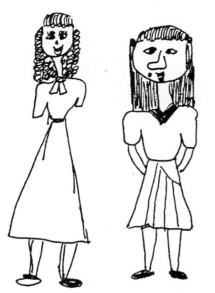

Figure 8–4. Drawing by a ten year old girl of herself and her eight year old sister.

sion from previous levels of skill. When evaluating the effect of stress on a child through drawings, it is helpful to have examples of the child's previous drawings to provide a baseline of the skills and developmental level of the child. From the information communicated through drawings, one can see the impact of stress upon the child as well as the effects of treatment over time. Sturner and Rothbaum (1980) studied the effect of preparation for stressful procedures during hospital admission as revealed through HFDs. Changes in drawings done at the time of admission and after a stressful procedure, a venipuncture, were greater for those children who were not given preparation.

Wohl and Kaufman (1985) used drawings to study children from violent homes. The drawings communicated feelings of helplessness, anxiety, fear, and depression these children experienced. The drawings also revealed damage to the child's developing personality. Children from violent homes use a lot of energy to protect themselves and their siblings physically and emotionally. Communication within the family has broken down, and support from adult parents is unpredictable at best. Communication through drawing allows the child a safe medium to express feelings in a therapeutic setting as well as providing information about the effects of violence on the child.

A creative use of drawings is employed by Lamb and Dodge (1985) in a workbook designed to help children work through the grief associated with the death of a sibling. The workbook provides blank pages for the child to record his feelings over time about the death through pictures or a diary. Such a record assists the child in expressing feelings of sadness and guilt. The author also encourages the child to draw and document positive memories of the good times and special things about the sibling. This technique could also be applicable to hospitalized children, as well as children encountering stressful life situations such as chronic illness or family disorganization.

The Child Drawing Hospital (CDH) is a projective technique designed to assist children in communicating their perceptions of and anxieties about hospitalization (Clatworthy, 1986). The child is asked to draw a picture of a person in the hospital. The child is then encouraged to tell a story about the picture, providing a safe method to communicate fantasies, perceptions, and feelings about the hospital experience (see Chapter 7). This technique could be adapted to other situations and settings to facilitate communication with children.

Drawings have been an effective way to communicate with sexually abused children (Burgess et al., 1981; Miller, 1985; Kelley, 1985). Drawings provide a safe way for children to describe what has happened and discuss their feelings about the incident. Young children do not have the vocabulary to communicate about sexual activity (Kelley, 1985). Therefore, they should not be expected to be able to express what has happened to them verbally. For many children, verbalizing is too painful or embarrassing. If the abuse has been perpetrated by a family member or friend or has occurred over a long period, the child has likely been threatened or has promised not to tell about the abuse. Drawings provide a way to distance the information from the child, providing a safe way of disclosing abuse to a trusted caretaker or health professional. This disclosure may take place in a single clear depiction of the incident or may occur gradually over time.

When child abuse is suspected, the child might be encouraged to draw a family; when abuse has been established, the child could be requested to "draw a picture of what happened," or "draw a picture of what you remember" (Kelley, 1985, p. 426). The trauma of sexual abuse or rape is often revealed in disorganized drawings that illustrate regression from previous levels of drawing (Burgess et al., 1981). The inclusion of genitalia in drawings indicates the possibility of sexual abuse. Drawings of abused children may depict the self with no arms or hands, reflecting powerlessness and vulnerability (Kelley, 1984), and no legs or feet, showing lack of stability and security. Drawings of the perpetrator may be large in size with exaggerated arms and hands, a symbol of power, force, and aggression. Drawings may also disclose rooms in the house or places where the abuse has occurred. Accurate and detailed records of the dialogue between the nurse and child about the drawing should be made to assist the child in coping with the trauma of abuse. This information may also be used in identification and prosecution of the perpetrator.

Summary

Drawings collected over a period of time and interpreted in the context of the child's life experience best represent the child's world. An isolated drawing may or may not be representative of reality to the child. Also considered is the verbal description of the drawing. The following vignette illustrates how important each factor is in attributing meaning to the drawings of children.

The parents of a shy kindergartener noticed that the drawings their daughter brought home from school were done in black and brown and were mostly scribbles in contrast to the neat, recognizable drawings previously done at home. The mother telephoned the teacher about this observation, concerned that her daughter was having difficulty adjusting to school. The teacher noted that this trend continued and discussed it with the school psychologist. The psychologist suggested that the teacher ask the child to describe her drawings and her choice of colors. The youngster explained that the more aggressive children pushed ahead of her and got the "good colors," leaving only black. By the time she got a crayon and attended to drawing, she did not have enough time to complete a picture. Consequently, she hurriedly scribbled a picture in order to have something to hand in.

In the above scenario, at first glance it would seem that the child's drawings expressed depression, confusion, and regression from a previous developmental level, and that would justify concern. However, getting input from the child about her drawings explained that this was not the case and that manipulation of the drawing environment would likely produce a dramatic change in the quality of the child's drawings.

EVALUATION

The purpose of the use of drawings as an intervention is to enhance communication with the child. Criteria for evaluating the outcome of this intervention, therefore, relate to effective or improved communication. In order to determine if this goal has been accomplished, individual baseline data is needed to indicate communication level and skills and to identify problems in communication. From this baseline data, a plan of nursing action is indicated to meet stated measurable objectives.

Because communication is a uniquely personal experience between individuals, each situation must be evaluated individually. Change and movement toward objectives need to be recorded. When working with children, establishing a trusting relationship is the basis for good communication. This relationship is built slowly over time. Often the failure of the intervention is the result of an unrealistic expectation about the rapidity and yield of results. In the zeal for measurable outcomes, care must be taken not to read meaning into a drawing that is not there. It is a mistake to believe that all drawings reveal a child's personality and self-concept or are indicative of problems (Koppitz, 1984), any more than that all verbal communication is a profound indicator. However, one can begin to identify developmental trends as well as underlying tendencies and problems from drawings, especially as they are repeated over time. Information gained from children through their drawings must be evaluated in relationship to the context of their total situation and in combination with other data. Drawing is but one source of information from children and must be weighed accordingly.

Evaluation of the communication occurring through the drawings is interpreted by the child, the nurse, and others who are knowledgeable about children's drawings. Like any other communication skill, developing expertise in communication through drawing takes study, practice, and time. While it may be appropriate to refer children with serious disturbances to specialists, nurses can use drawings with hospitalized children and children who are experiencing stressors common in today's society. During the learning process, nurses need to validate what they see in drawings with other professionals and compare it with other relevant data. With time and experience, nurses will feel more comfortable with their judgments in their specialized areas of practice, yet will continue to grow as their observations are validated by others. Most important, the child needs to be given an opportunity to share his or her perception of what has been drawn and of what is going on in the picture.

Nurses also learn about children by observing the process of drawing. Personality characteristics of a child may be exhibited in a timid, aggressive, confident, self-deprecating, or joyful approach to drawing. Temperament may also be expressed in approach; for instance, the child may find it difficult to stay on task or may be easily distracted. The approach the child takes is also indicative of comfort with the environment or examiner. A newly hospitalized child may be fearful because of the many strange procedures and persons in that unfamiliar environment and may therefore be hesitant to participate in a relaxed manner during the initial intervention. However, on subsequent contacts, as the child develops a relationship with the nurse and becomes more familiar with the hospital environment, the child's approach is likely to become more relaxed and the drawings more representative of the child's abilities and feelings. Burns (1982, pp. 256–268) has summarized the findings of numerous authors who have described the significance of the form and substance of children's drawings. This reference is a helpful beginning for nurses who want to increase their understanding of children's drawings and use this intervention with children.

Case Study

Seated on the bench in the waiting room with her four siblings was eight year old Amanda, waiting for her younger brother to be seen in the child health clinic. Amanda's family had visited the clinic last summer when this migrant family was working in the area and visiting nearby relatives. This year, her mother was about to give birth to another child. Amanda and her older sister cared for the younger siblings while their parents worked in the fields and were very attentive to their needs. The children were clean, well nourished, and very well behaved. The way the family interacted with one another gave evidence of a caring, close-knit family. Because the family moved frequently, neither of the older children attended school regularly. Amanda sat quietly, yet seemed anxious to communicate, to have some attention. The nurse provided the children with paper and crayons and suggested that they each draw a picture of their family.

Amanda's picture included each family member, excluding herself, in correct ordinal position standing next to the old converted school bus where the family lived. She told about each family member and their life traveling around in the bus. In the upper corner of the paper was a picture of a girl, smaller than the other children in the picture, surrounded by a fence. When

asked about the girl in the corner, Amanda replied, "These are the bus people," pointing to her family standing by the bus, "and this is Amanda," pointing to the child isolated from the family. The nurse gave Amanda another piece of paper and asked Amanda to draw a picture of herself. Amanda spent over 15 minutes engrossed in her drawing. The colorful drawing she created portrayed a smiling girl standing by a house with flowers blooming in the front yard and the sun shining down on the house and the child. Totally surrounding the house and the girl was a tall fence with no gate. When asked to tell a story about the picture, Amanda told of her desire to live in a house with flowers, a house that could not move so she could make friends and go to school. She also described the many rooms in the house, where there was room to play, sleep, and have lots of things. When asked about the fence, she stated that the fence would not let her move away and would keep her there forever. When she left the clinic, Amanda refused to leave the picture; in fact, she asked for more paper to take home.

On two subsequent interactions with the family that summer, Amanda seemed to radiate a special closeness with the nurse, desiring to be physically close to her and to have some special attention. She asked for paper to do more drawings, which all reflected the same theme. Amanda's drawings communicated her feelings of isolation, poor self-esteem, and desire for stability, feelings she did not share with her family. Although Amanda participated willingly in the family process, she did not identify with the family she called "the bus people." She seemed anxious to share her fantasy of living in a house surrounded by flowers and flooded by sunlight—symbols of happiness and warmth. The fence ensured security and stability for Amanda and her desire for this lifestyle. The message communicated through Amanda's drawings gave the nurse a greater insight into the feelings and family dynamics of a little girl reaching out for someone to share her feelings and dreams.

RESEARCH IMPLICATIONS

There is a large body of literature on development and use of children's drawings in therapeutic settings. Only recently have nurses begun to incorporate drawings into their practice as a means of learning more about children. Drawings have great potential as a method of communication with children. As nurses gain a greater understanding of how this important communication tool can be used, the application of this intervention will spread to many settings and serve diverse populations of children. The challenge is to develop a method to systematically study the validity of what is communicated through drawings. Because of the individual nature of the communication process and each child's life situation, anecdotal records complete with children's drawings need to be kept over time. This longitudinal approach to data collection will yield data rich with information about development, the effects of stressors on the child as reflected in drawings, and the validity of the interpretations made about drawings. Drawings also have the potential to graphically represent the effectiveness of treatment regimens, such as interventions used to reduce stress or improve the self-concept of a child.

The case study method is a research approach that would be appropriate when using drawings over time with a specific child (Stake, 1978). Many times the problems associated with stress, such as chronic illness, child abuse, or family dysfunction, are long-term problems with effects that persist over time. Changes are more difficult to observe when they occur slowly over weeks, months, or even years. Collecting extensive baseline data, including drawings, provides a yardstick to measure these subtle changes. Through the case study approach, periodic collection of data will help paint the total picture, which may not come into focus for quite some time. By including drawings in this data bank, one has a different point of reference for what is going on in a child's life.

Collections of drawings by specific populations of children, for example children with congenital heart disease or diabetes, may reveal certain commonalities about self-concept or perceptions each group of children share about how their condition interacts with family life or school. The use of instruments such as the CDH will assist children in communicating their perceptions and fears about hospitalization, information that could be useful in modifying procedures and environments to be less threatening to children. The principles of this instrument could be modified to communicate with children in settings other than the hospital.

In order to develop the knowledge base of nursing, nurses must communicate with their peers about the use of drawings with children, the effectiveness of this intervention, and recommendations for revisions and further use of drawings in the clinical setting. Nurses need to try interventions reported by others and create new strategies and applications for existing interventions. Research must become an integral part of the practice setting, a tool to enhance and further nursing practice. Drawing is but one area that needs continued research effort, but it is a significant area, for drawing provides another avenue of communication between the nurse and the child, a very special link to children who are not yet sophisticated verbally, but have so much to tell.

References

Avant, K. Nursing diagnosis: Maternal attachment. Advances in Nursing Science, 2:45–55, 1979.

Berlo, DK. The process of communication: An introduction to theory and practice. New York: Holt, Rinehart and Winston, Inc., 1960.

Burgess, AW, McCausland, MP, and Wolbert, WA. Children's drawings as indicators of sexual trauma. Perspectives in Psychiatric Care, 19:50–58, 1981.

Burns, RC. Self-growth in families: Kinetic family drawings (K-F-D)—Research and application. New York: Brunner/Mazel, Inc., 1982.

Burns, RC, and Kaufman, SH. Actions, styles and symbols in kinetic family drawings (K-F-D): An interpretative manual. New York: Brunner/Mazel, Inc., 1972.

Clatworthy, S. Child drawing hospital. Unpublished manuscript, Kent State University, Kent, Ohio, 1986.

DiLeo, JH. Young children and their drawings. New York: Brunner/Mazel, Inc., 1970.

DiLeo, JH. Children's drawings as diagnostic aids. New York: Brunner/Mazel, Inc., 1973.

Goodenough, FL. Measure of intelligence by drawings. New York: World Book Co., 1926.

Goodnow, J. Children's drawing. Cambridge, Mass.: Harvard University Press, 1977.

Harris, DB. Children's drawings as measures of intellectual maturity. New York: Harcourt, Brace and World, Inc., 1963.

Kelley, SJ. The use of art therapy with the sexually abused child. Journal of Psychosocial Nursing and Mental Health Services, 22:12–18, 1984.

Kelley, SJ. Drawings: Critical communications for sexually abused children. Pediatric Nursing, 11:421–426, 1985.

Kellogg, R. Analyzing children's art. Palo Alto, Calif.: National Press, Inc., 1969.

Koppitz, EM. Psychological evaluation of children's human figure drawings. New York: Grune and Stratton, Inc., 1968.

Koppitz, EM. Psychological evaluation of human figure drawings by middle school pupils. Orlando, Fla.: Grune and Stratton, Inc., 1984.

Lamb, JM, and Dodge, N. Sharing with thumpy: My story of love and grief by (child's name). Springfield, Ill.: Prairie Lark Press, 1985.

Lewis, D, and Green, J. Your child's drawings . . . Their hidden meaning. London: Hutchinson, 1983.

Loney, J. A car test to reflect personality. Des Moines Sunday Register, September 26, 1971.

Lowenfeld, V. Creative and mental growth. New York: Macmillan Publishing Co., 1947.

Machover, K. Personality projection in the drawing of the human figure. Springfield, Ill.: Charles C Thomas, 1949.

Miller, EL. Interviewing the sexually abused child. MCN: American Journal of Maternal Child Nursing, 10:103–105, 1985.

Mortensen, KV. Children's human figure drawings (Vol. 1). Denmark: Dansk Psykologisk Foorlag, 1984.

Piaget, J. The language and thought of the child. Cleveland: Meridian Books, World Publishing Co., 1966.

Samovar, LA, and Rintye, ED. Small group communication: A reader (3rd ed.). Dubuque, Iowa: Wm C Brown Group, 1979.

Siemon, M. Using DiLeo's and Koppitz's models for assessing children's drawings. In Babich, KS (Ed.), A workbook: Assessing the mental health of children. Boulder, Colo.: Western Interstate Commission for Higher Education, 1982.

Stake, RE. The case study method in social inquiry. Educational Research, 7:5–8, 1978.

Sturner, R., and Rothbaum, F. The effects of stress on children's human figure drawings. Journal of Clinical Psychology, 36:324–331, 1980.

Wohl, A, and Kaufman, B. Silent screams and hidden cries. New York: Brunner/Mazel, Inc., 1985.

CHAPTER 9

COMMUNICATING THROUGH TOUCH

DIANE MOLSBERRY, M.A., R.N., and
MAUREEN GORDON SHOGAN, B.S.N., R.N.C.

It is a fact that much of health care in society is becoming increasingly technical in nature. Technology has given health care providers new tools with which to assess, diagnose, and treat clients. It is even predicted that by the middle of the 21st century, computerized body organs may be readily available (Kaiser, 1986, 1988). It is also predicted that as society and health care become more "high-tech," human beings will also realize the need and desire to engage in more "high-touch" activities. Low-tech "mind technologies," including the arts of teaching, of listening, and of touching, will become as critically important and vital to human lives as high-technology (Kaiser, 1986, 1988).

The profession of nursing is ahead of many other health care professions in real-izing the importance of these mind technologies to the well-being of clients. Touch is an integral component of the science of nursing that is basic and pervasive in the nurse-consumer relationship (Weiss, 1979). Indeed, nursing is one of the few health care professions which "carries out a major portion of its function through touching patients" (Johnson, 1965, p. 59). Barnett (1972) surveyed 900 health personnel who were caring for 540 patients in two hospitals and found that registered nurses touch patients almost twice as frequently as other health care personnel.

Nurses caring for infants and children utilize touch with their young patients daily and, at times, almost unthinkingly. Generally speaking, touch is defined by Webster's

Ninth New Collegiate Dictionary as the act of "bringing a bodily part into contact with, especially so as to perceive through the tactile sense." Most often, the body part is skin, and it is brought into contact with an object or another person (Dossey, 1983). Medical dictionaries refer to touch in the context of palpation or exploration (Dorland, 1967; Taber, 1981). Medical touch is described by Gorski et al. (1984), as that touch which is vital to the care and survival of the ill patient and is routinely used in the daily care given by nurses (p. 86). While assessing, nurses palpate, feel, and touch their young patients. Nurses use medical touch while performing any number of procedures and treatments, but nurses also use social, communicative touch, especially with infants and young children. Nurses pat, stroke, hold, or rock a child who is distressed, be it distress that has resulted from physical discomfort, fear, or separation from parents and loved ones. The conceptual inability of infants and young children to understand their altered health status, various medical procedures, care settings, and separation necessitated by their treatment also leads nurses to instinctively utilize touch in an attempt to help ease the fears of their clients.

While nursing utilizes touch as defined above, touch is also viewed as a form of nonverbal communication (Wolf et al., 1979; Murray and Zentner, 1975; Campbell, 1984; Jasmin and Trygstad, 1979; Barnett, 1972; Weiss, 1979). Review of recent nursing literature reveals numerous references to the use of therapeutic touch. An exciting but controversial topic, this form of touch is utilized to achieve outcomes other than those achieved through assessment and verbal communication. Based on concepts of the body as an energy field, therapeutic touch arises from, but is different than, the ancient art of laying on of hands. Therapeutic touch is a conscious, intentional act utilizing the art of interpersonal energy transfer to promote healing through (1) interbody contact between the nurse and the client and family, (2) interbody contact between the patient and patient's family, and (3) contact between the patient and other health personnel (Krieger, 1976; Krieger et al., 1979; Clark and Clark, 1984; Weiss, 1979).

Although medical touch is frequently used in routine caregiving, the purpose of this chapter is to discuss touch as a purposeful intervention used to communicate with infants and children who are experiencing altered health states.

THEORETICAL FOUNDATION

Psychophysiological Basis of Touch

The haptic system is that body system which pertains to sensations of touch. Within the central nervous system (CNS), all humans have the capacity to take in and sort out sensory messages received as a result of personal contact with other humans. Afferent impulses are received in the CNS from these five different surface receptors: (1) free nerve endings, (2) Meissner's corpuscles, (3) expanded tip tactile receptors, (4) hair end organs, and (5) Pacini's corpuscles. Stimulation of these receptors results in impulse transmission to the CNS via afferent nerve fiber pathways. These pathways differ in size, degree of myelinization, and structure of synapses. Differences in specialization of nervous pathways permit the CNS to fully evaluate and discriminate between the different types of input it receives (Weiss, 1979; Guyton, 1986).

Touch is the earliest sense to develop in the fetus (Montagu, 1978; Hynd and Willis, 1988) and is closely followed by the sense of proprioception. A classic study by Hooker (1952) demonstrated that beginning at just 7½ weeks gestation and continuing for the next seven weeks, the entire surface of the human embryo becomes sensitive to touch. As evidenced by reflexive activity of the embryo in response to touch, the sense of touch begins developing at the lips and ends at the legs and feet. At birth, the haptic nerves are prominent on the soles of the feet, the palms of the hands, the back, the genital area, and the mouth. The infant is most sensitive to touch in these areas. Further, until three months of age, the infant is most sensitive to pressure on the right side of the body (Turkewitz, 1974).

The myelinization process first begins in the fourth month of fetal life (Guyton, 1986; Hynd and Willis, 1988). Evidence suggests that nerve tracts become functional at the time they first become myelinated (Guyton, 1986; Hynd and Willis, 1988; Langworthy, 1933). According to Kolb (1959), the sensory pathways involving kinesthetic and tactile activities are the first to complete myelinization in the infant. At birth, the pathway mediating tactile sensation is myelinated in the spinal cord and brain stem to the level of the thalamus (Guyton, 1986; Hynd and Willis, 1988). Nerve tracts involving auditory and visual senses are next to complete myelinization. Myelinization is not totally complete until between 15 and 20 years of age (Guyton, 1986; Hynd and Willis, 1988). Functions developing early in embryological development logically appear to be more fundamental and essential to the survival of the organism (Montagu, 1978; Fanslow, 1983). Touch appears to be a very basic function, serving as a cornerstone for other, higher-order functions (Weiss, 1979).

Hebb (1949) theorized that cell assemblages, or diffuse structures made up of cells within the cortex and diencephalon, are formed within each individual by sensory stimulations, such as touch, which are repetitive in nature. Relationships develop between these early cell assemblages and later sensory stimuli experienced by the individual. The significance and subjective meaning of later sensory experiences are all based upon those early groupings of experiences which form a core to be drawn on and built upon throughout life. Thus, cell assemblages provide the basis for the eventual meaning an individual assigns to any given tactile experience. In relating this theory to the sensation of touch, consider a mother gently stroking her infant's back. This act generates specific neuromuscular sensations in the infant, which the infant subjectively interprets. Later, the mother may pat her infant's back in a rhythmic fashion. The neuromuscular sensations are related to those which were experienced earlier. The understanding the infant has of this sensation is based on the summation of both experiences. The interpretation of any similar sensations experienced later will be related to the early experiences. This theory may explain why touch has such varied meanings among individuals and in different cultures. It also provides a theoretical basis for the technique of anchoring, utilized in neurolinguistic programming (NLP) and discussed later in this chapter.

In addition, cell assemblages were viewed as a receptor hierarchy by Schloper (1962). In this hierarchy, individuals must first learn via tactile stimulation before being able to learn through other modalities (Weiss, 1979). Based on the aforementioned studies, Weiss (1979) summarizes:

> Development of perceptions and conceptions which provide each individual with meaning can depend on the initial tactile stimulations to which one was exposed,... The nature of the significant touch experiences which facilitate development in the child and which later reinforce maintenance of health in the adult are extremely important, for the actual occurrence of each tactile act carries physiologic impact with psychosocial meaning (p. 77).

Dossey (1983) states that "concrete impingements on the skin generate a cascade of biochemical events whose reverberations in the body are more complex than might be imagined" (p. 2). To illustrate, of rabbits that were fed a diet rich in fat and cholesterol, those who were touched demonstrated a 60% lower incidence of atherosclerotic lesions than those who were not touched. The touch intervention was not a planned part of this study. It was the habit of the researcher caring for this particular group to hold and touch them at feeding time (Nerem et al., 1980). In addition to biochemical events, complex neuroendocrinological pathways involved in endorphin and enkephalin production are also stimulated by touch (Dossey, 1983).

Developmental Aspects of Touch

Nurses need not wait until a child is born to begin to effectively utilize touch as an intervention. An obstetrician named Rene Van deCarr has developed classes for parents entitled Prenatal University. Van deCarr (1986) instructs mothers to begin stroking and touching their unborn fetuses beginning at 28 weeks gestation. Mothers are told to say the words pat, pat as they are patting their fetuses, as well as squeeze, tap, stroke, rub, and shake as they are performing each of those types of touch. Ultrasound scanning has shown that the fetus responds with movements specific to each intervention. Van deCarr also reports that the newborn responds with a particular movement even if the mother only says the word that goes with the particular mode of touch.

Surrounded by amniotic fluid in utero, the fetus is constantly influenced by the rhythmic beat of the mother's heart and the warmth and movement of the amniotic fluid

(Frank, 1957). With the onset of labor and uterine contractions, a series of massive cutaneous reactions begins which assists in activating vital body systems (Barnett, 1972). For the full-term fetus, the action of labor contractions and compression of the uterus on the body prepare the infant for firm touch stimuli.

The sense of touch is well developed at birth, as demonstrated by the following: (1) the quieting of an infant to firm, gentle touch; (2) the generalized Moro's reaction to painful stimuli; and (3) the elicitation of the rooting and sucking reflex by simple touch of the perioral region (Pillitteri, 1981). Firm touch is generally best received by the newborn infant since light touch has been found to cause discomfort (Coursin, 1972).

Preterm infants differ significantly from term infants in their behavioral responses to touch. Als et al. (1979) have developed a conceptualization of the stages of very early behavioral organization, the synactive model of newborn behavioral organization. According to this model, the subsystems of an organism stabilize and become integrated with one another, allowing for the differentiation and emergence of subsystems. These newly developed subsystems feed back into the integrated system (Als et al., 1982, p. 43).

The premature infant, given time and provided with devices such as nesting material, water beds, beanbag beds, and sheepskins, all of which simulate the intrauterine environment, gradually develops the fully integrated and functional response to touch seen in the term infant (Scott and Richards, 1979; Korner, 1984; Blackburn, 1983).

Rubin (1963) described mothers progressively touching their newborns in a systematic fashion beginning with fingertip touch. Mothers advanced to palm touch over a period of days. Klaus et al. (1970) found identical progression but at a much faster rate, advancing from fingertip to palm touch within four to eight minutes. This profound time difference may be because, in 1963, babies were clothed when introduced to their mothers after they had recovered from delivery. In Klaus et al.'s study, the babies were all undressed and introduced to their families soon after delivery.

In the same study by Klaus et al., the touch sequence of mothers of premature infants was also observed. In the mothers of full-term infants, maternal fingertip touch decreased from 52% to 26% of total observation time and maternal palm touch increased from 28% to 62% within the first three to nine minutes of interaction. In contrast, the mothers of premature infants spent only 26% of total observation time in fingertip touch and 23% of the time in palm contact after the third visit (which averaged five days after delivery). All of the premature babies were in Isolettes during this interaction, which may have had an effect upon the experience.

Evidence which supports the importance of touch to development is increasing. Studies of infants and children have shown that touch is crucial to early physical and mental growth (Frank, 1957). Indeed, lack of touch has been linked to failure-to-thrive syndrome and even death (Harlow, 1962; Patton and Gardner, 1963; Yarrow, 1961; Ribble, 1965; Province and Lipton, 1962). Claims have been made that early tactile contact, or the lack of it, influences attachment, sociability, growth rate, adaptability, exploratory behavior, learning, activity level, ability to withstand stress, and immunological development in many young mammals (Gottfried, 1984, p. 114).

Sameroff and colleagues (1987) examined four year olds to determine whether a low measure of intelligence was best explained as a function of low socioeconomic status or as a confounding variable of environmental risk factors that are more often found in low socioeconomic status groups. A set of ten environmental variables that are correlates but not equivalents of socioeconomic status were examined. One variable examined was Mother Interactive Behaviors, which included the spontaneous behaviors of smiling at, vocalizing to, and touching the child. The high-risk group (those with low intelligence quotients) included the 25% of least spontaneous mothers (Sameroff et al., 1987, p. 345).

It must be noted that in many if not most studies, touch does not operate as an isolated variable. Touch, often referred to as cutaneous stimulation, operates simultaneously with vestibular stimulation and social communication. Thus, it is difficult to separate out these factors when analyzing the effectiveness of some interventions. As will be shown later, many interventions in the neonatal period which involve touch also relate to vestibular stimulation (see Chapter 18).

Infants are dependent on caregivers for the provision of much-needed touch, but they may also develop alternate sources of tactile contact, such as a special blanket or cuddly toy (Blackburn, 1983). By the time American children reach adolescence, touching between them and their parents is minimal as dependency lessens (Montagu, 1978; McAnarney, 1984). Never again in the life cycle does the amount of touch people receive parallel that which is received in infancy. It must be noted, however, that illness, hospitalization, or stress frequently results in regression (Barnett, 1972). With regression, an individual's utilization and need for a basic form of communication such as touch frequently increases (Barnett, 1972; Bibler, 1970; Mercer 1966).

Communicative Aspects of Touch

In order to communicate, one must be capable of both receiving incoming signals and transmitting messages. Further, for a message to be understood, signals must be phrased in terms that are understandable to others (Barnett, 1972). These signals can be detected by even young infants, who have the capability of perceiving touch and utilizing it as a form of communication. Tactile stimulation also serves as the basis for deriving meaning from other stimuli (Frank, 1957).

Weiss (1978, 1979) describes four major characteristics of touch as (1) duration, (2) location, (3) intensity, and (4) sensation. These characteristics have the power to affect the pain/pleasure balance of the body, the body's perceptual ability for sensory discrimination, and body image.

As children grow, they gradually begin to associate sounds, such as words and vocal intonations, and sight with touch. Thus, the use of auditory and visual communication are added to or may even replace touch (Frank, 1957). Indeed, the true meaning of many verbal symbols depends upon prior tactual experience to give symbols their meaning (Barnett, 1972). Touch has the potential to be the most meaningful form of communication, particularly when communicating feelings and attitudes (Johnson, 1965).

Communication techniques promulgated in the field of NLP provide a basis for practical application of the above findings. One technique espoused by NLP is that of anchoring, defined as "the process of associating an internal response with some external trigger [similar to classical conditioning] so that the response may be quickly, and sometimes covertly reaccessed" (Dilts, 1983, p. 61). Anchoring is not a new phenomenon or technique. It is a naturally occurring phenomenon and is believed by some authors to be the basis for all of our learning (Grinder and Bandler, 1979; Grinder, 1986a; Knowles, 1984; King et al., 1983).

Grinder (1986a) states that "our world is full of natural anchors" (p. 41). Anchors may be visual, auditory, or tactile-kinesthetic in nature or may be any combination which elicits specific feelings associated, consciously or unconsciously, with past experiences. For example, if one's face is stroked lightly, one may experience a sense of well-being linked to similar touch experienced during loving moments in childhood. Other examples of anchors abound. They exist in every health care setting and in almost every interaction. Nurses need to consider that a patient may respond on the basis of preestablished anchors of which both nurse and patient may or may not be aware (Grinder, 1986a; King et al., 1983). Nurses also need to recognize and utilize, if possible, preexisting anchors which may be of benefit to patients. Conversely, negative anchors need to be avoided or, if possible, dealt with and changed. A description of a technique for establishing a positive anchor is given later in this chapter.

Neurolinguistic programming also provides a means of establishing congruency and thus enhancing the effectiveness of communication between individuals. Individuals think about and process any experience using sensory system representations. Some think and process information in the form of pictures, others in terms of sounds, while still others process and think of input in primarily kinesthetic or feeling terms (Bandler, 1985; Grinder and Bandler, 1979). By utilizing findings from the fields of communication, psychology, and education and by studying expert communicators, NLP has identified specific behaviors displayed by individuals when utilizing a given representational system to process information. These behaviors include predicates used in speech, speed of speech, breathing patterns, eye movements, and body movements. Individuals who tend to think and process information in kinesthetic or feeling terms are more likely to want or need to use touch as a means of communicating or learning (Grinder and Bandler, 1979; Bandler, 1985; Grinder, 1986b; Knowles, 1984; King et al., 1983).

Therapeutic Touch

Therapeutic touch remains controversial, but it is presented so that the reader can assess it and make individual decisions regarding its application to nursing practice. It has been defined as the art of interpersonal energy transfer for the purpose of healing (Krieger et al., 1979). Direct anatomical and physiological evidence substantiating the mechanisms of action of therapeutic touch is not readily identifiable. However, some suggestive evidence exists in research into the mechanisms of acupuncture and endorphin and enkephalin production (Boguslawski, 1980). Chapter 20 also discusses this mechanism.

The theoretical framework which underlies the use of therapeutic touch as a nursing intervention includes the following three assumptions: (1) each human is an energy field; (2) humans and the environment (referring to everything outside of a person, including other people) are constantly exchanging energy with each other; and (3) universal order is a force innate to all energy fields (Boguslawski, 1979, p. 9).

It is believed that people have seven energy fields. However, four major fields, or levels, are most directly related to health, illness, and the healing process. These are the physical level or the body; the ethereal level, which extends 1½ to 2 inches beyond the physical level and is closely related to it; the psychodynamic level; and the mental level or brain activity. These levels are thought to be interactive with the environment rather than discrete (Boguslawski, 1979).

Communication between different energy levels, a human's energy field, and the environment takes place via special channels referred to as chakras. On the physical level, the energies of these chakras relate to the central nervous system and major nerve plexus of the body. There are seven major chakras: (1) the crown; (2) the brow; (3) the throat; (4) the heart; (5) the spleen; (6) the navel; and (7) the root, located at the base of the spine (Boguslawski, 1979).

In health, energy flows freely between humans and the environment and can be replenished at will. In disease, the free flow of energy is blocked by physical, emotional, or mental factors. Those who utilize therapeutic touch seek to restore a free flow of energy, thus facilitating the ability individuals have to heal themselves (Krieger et al., 1979; Boguslawski, 1979).

While these concepts are well accepted in Eastern philosophies, they are only gradually being accepted by science in the Western world. Research in the areas of extrasensory perception; biofeedback; and Kirlian photography, a specialized photographic technique believed to capture energy fields on film, is generating indirect support for the aforementioned concepts and for the concept of the transference of energy between two human fields, according to Boguslawski (1980).

In the Eastern view, *prana*, or life energy, is related to respiration and is intrinsic in what we know as oxygen. Because hemoglobin is essential for the transportation of oxygen, Krieger (1973), who has done extensive work with therapeutic touch, reasoned that the hemoglobin value in the ill individual would be the best measure of the energy exchange thought to take place in therapeutic touch. In two separate studies, Krieger (1973, 1975) found that the hemoglobin levels of subjects in the experimental groups who were treated with therapeutic touch were significantly higher following treatment than those in the control groups. Other studies have demonstrated that therapeutic touch can decrease physiological tension and promote a state of generalized relaxation in ill people (Krieger et al., 1979). Heidt (1981) found therapeutic touch significantly decreased acute anxiety in patients hospitalized in a cardiovascular unit. However, Randolph (1984) failed to support a hypothesis that a group of college students exposed to stressful stimuli and then treated with therapeutic touch would remain more relaxed than the group not treated with therapeutic touch.

In summary, touch is one of the senses by which humans perceive the world. Consisting of stimulation of the skin by an object or another person, it is a form of nonverbal communication and may be described in terms of four qualities: duration, location, intensity, and sensation (Weiss, 1978, 1979). Touch is necessary for normal psychophysiological functioning and normal growth and development. Touch is used by nurses to communicate, comfort, and facilitate healing and may be used as an intervention by itself, or may be included as a part of other nursing activities.

ASSESSMENT

Antecedent conditions common to all nursing diagnoses in which touch may be a useful intervention include medical diagnoses of a life-threatening or chronic illness or disease state, prolonged periods of immobilization, hospitalization, the necessity of being in an intensive care setting, isolation, separation from loved ones and peers, and family stressors rendering coping and caretaking by the family ineffective.

Identification of common antecedent conditions and use of the defining characteristics of the diagnoses described indicate the need for touch. Of the antecedents and diagnoses discussed, all have in common the need for an intervention which communicates caring. Touch may be a needed intervention for infants and children diagnosed with any number of nursing diagnoses. Indeed, so pervasive is the use of touch to nursing practice that it may be the one nursing intervention universal to almost all diagnostic categories! Nursing diagnoses for which touch may be an especially effective form of communication and comfort and which may aid in the healing of young children include but are not limited to (1) *Anxiety*; (2) *Fear*; (3) *Alterations in comfort or pain*; (4) *Impaired verbal communication*; (5) *Ineffective family or individual coping*; (6) *Alterations in parenting*; (7) *Grieving*; (8) *Spiritual distress*; (9) *Disturbances in self-concept*; (10) *Self-esteem disturbance*; (11) *Social isolation*; (12) *Diversional activity deficit*; (13) *Decreased activity tolerance*; (14) *Sensory deprivation or sensory overload*; and (15) *Nutritional alterations, decreased* (Gordon, 1982).

In looking at defining characteristics of nursing diagnoses where touch may be useful, it is helpful to group the diagnoses according to Gordon's functional health patterns (Gordon, 1982). Note that a majority of these diagnoses arise from the following categories of functional health patterns: (1) self-perception–self-concept patterns; (2) role relationship patterns; (3) coping-stress tolerance patterns; (4) cognitive perceptual patterns; and (5) activity and exercise patterns (Gordon, 1982). Specific data for each individual patient and each specific nursing diagnosis will vary, of course. Table 9–1 summarizes these categories and their defining characteristics.

When one is identifying the need for touch, it is also helpful to identify those who prefer a kinesthetic-tactile mode of communication, which is usually preferred by children. Behavioral cues which are indicators of the representational system utilized by an individual to process information are given in Table 9–2. Although all modes are utilized by any one person, most individuals have a preference for one of the three modes when they experience stress. When not stressed, people are more flexible and more easily process information using a combination of all three representational systems.

Consider young children. When communicating or thinking, they often look down toward the handed side. They do not look another person in the eye very often. Rarely are they still; they shuffle or tap their feet or fingers and speak slowly. As discussed earlier in this chapter, individuals who utilize the tactile-kinesthetic representational system heavily are much more likely to want or need to use touch as a means of communicating or learning.

THE INTERVENTION

Touch is a nonverbal communication measure often utilized to comfort; to teach; to convey trust, caring, and reassurance, and to facilitate orientation of an individual. To achieve these communication outcomes, touch may be done in many ways, including hand to hand; hand to shoulder, arm, or extremity; hand to head; and, finally, hand to trunk as done with hugging or holding. However, specific guidelines as to when, where, and specifically with whom touch should be used to communicate can only be inferred from the literature, and nurses must rely on their instincts in order to know when

Table 9–1. Summary of Functional Health Patterns with Related Defining Characteristics*

Gordon's Functional Health Pattern Categories	Defining Characteristics
Self-perception and self-concept patterns	Affective changes Behavioral changes
Role relationship patterns	Changes in usual communication patterns Rigid communication and behavioral patterns Inability to meet family needs
Coping/stress tolerance patterns	Fear Anxiety Hostility Anger Weeping Despair or other signs of grief
Cognitive perceptual patterns Alterations in comfort/pain	Verbalizations Indications on pain assessment tools specific to children Physiological and behavioral indicators of pain Other

Sensory deficit/overload	Disorientation
	Confusion
	Irritability
	Anxiety
	Sleeplessness
	Time-out or disengagement cues of the premature infant:
	  Apnea
	  Mottling
	  Gaze aversion
	  Gagging and spitting up
	  Hiccups
	  Sneezing
	  Yawning
	  Arching head, arms, neck, back
	  Finger splaying
	  Frowning
	Air "sitting"
	"Stop sign"
	Sagging cheeks or chin
	Tongue thrusting

Alterations in consciousness related to increased intracranial pressure	Coma
Activity-exercise pattern Decreased activity tolerance	Dyspnea Tachypnea Tachycardia Fatigue
Impaired mobility	Immobility Traction
Diversional activity deficit	Isolation Hospitalization
Self-care deficit	Age/developmental level Situational characteristics

*From Gordon, M. Nursing diagnosis: Process and application. New York: McGraw-Hill Book Co., 1982.

to utilize touch as part of their repertoire of interventions.

The general act of touching, be it hand to hand, hand to shoulder, hand to arm, or hand to face, can indeed be very comforting and effective. Temple (1979) very effectively summarizes:

The loving touch communicates more to the sick child than scores of words. If there is a common fear of the . . . ill child, it is the fear of being abandoned. Being in touch with a caring adult can remind them of our commitment not to run away and our wish to remain very near at hand no matter what they have to experience.

When considering the use of touch as an intervention, the parents or other caregivers must be seen as an extension of that patient. Appropriate use of touch with parents can be as necessary and beneficial to the child

Table 9–2. IDENTIFYING PREFERRED MODES OF COMMUNICATION*

	Eyes	Body Movement	Voice Speed	Processing Speed	Predicates
Visual	↑ ↑	still	fastest ⟶		see, foggy, look, picture, focus, reveal, watch, notice, clear, appears, observe, behold, view, witness
Auditory	← →	metronome (ex: tapping or swinging of foot or pencil)			listen, talk, said, speak, hear, rhyme, sounds like gripe, attend, give ear to, get
Kinesthetic		lots of movement (ex: wiggling, squirming, total body movement)	slowest ⟶		grasp, handle, feel, grab, hold it, action words, "I don't get it," sting, knockout, thrill, tingle, itch, sore spot, thin-skinned, sharpen

*From Grinder, M: The educational conveyer belt. Battle Ground, Wash.: Michael Grinder, Inc., 1986a.

as actually touching the child. Touch is an important way of showing caring, providing support, eliciting trust, and of calming a parent. A parent who is supported will be better able to provide for the needs of his or her child (Miles and Carter, 1982a, 1982b; Carter et al., 1985).

Holding

Holding is one touch strategy which nurses may use or teach others to use effectively. Holding may be done by touching a specific body part or by holding the entire child. For example, comforting a crying infant may be facilitated by firmly but gently placing a hand on the infant's body. For those infants who can be picked up, the change in movement from the lateral to ventral plane may quiet the infant. During this maneuver, it is important to make the infant feel warm and secure by holding him or her firmly and snugly, because temperature and muscle tension are important components of touch and must be considered when holding or hugging an infant or child (Fig. 9–1). These two factors contribute to the communication of comfort, security, and trust to the infant or child who is held (Scipien et al., 1975; Triplett and Arneson, 1979). Holding a painful body part may also be helpful in reducing or controlling that pain (Mc-

Caffery, 1979). Chapter 20 gives a thorough discussion of other interventions for pain.

Nesting

While it may not be possible to hold a premature or critically ill infant, surround-

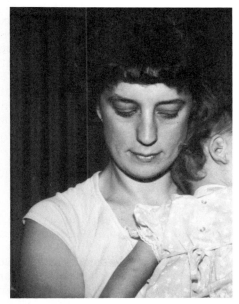

Figure 9–1. Holding is one touch technique that communicates comfort and security. (Courtesy of Deaconess Community Hospital, Spokane, Wash.)

ing the infant with blanket rolls or placing the infant in a flexed position may be comforting and beneficial; this type of position is often called nesting (Blackburn, 1983). For the premature infant, nesting has been shown to contribute to earlier maturation of midline behavior; that is, hands are more likely to be held in the midline of the body rather than extended back by the head. Nesting also provides the tactile stimulation the premature would have received had he remained in utero. Without nesting or other tactile stimuli, the premature infant may gradually move to a corner or door of the Isolette, seeking a boundary much like that he or she would have had in utero. Other interventions hypothesized to simulate the sensations of the uterine environment include waterbeds, beanbag beds, and sheepskins (Scott and Richards, 1979; Korner, 1984).

Swaddling

The time-honored practice of swaddling infants provides cutaneous sensation while simultaneously limiting movement and is effective as a comforting measure (Moss and Solomons, 1979). Swaddling is done by wrapping an infant snugly in a blanket or other wrap so as to keep arms and legs close to the body and prevent their unlimited movement. Keeping an infant's arms flexed yet close to the body allows for self-consolation via hand to face or hand to mouth contact and movement and is reminiscent of the infant's experience in the womb. The effectiveness of swaddling may be attributed in part to the warmth and tension provided by the swaddling materials (Hazinski, 1984), two factors which contribute to the effectiveness of holding.

"Kangarooing"

Another strategy which simulates the intrauterine environment and provides tactile stimulation in a manner similar to swaddling was found by Anderson et al. (1986) in Bogotá, Colombia. There, preterm infants as small as 1200 grams go home to be cared for by their mothers, where they are constantly cradled skin to skin between their mothers' breasts. Morbidity and mortality decreased when these infants were sent home to be exposed to the constant warmth, skin sensation, movement, and maternal heartbeat.

Similarly, many commercial infant frontpacks are available in North America. From parents' reports, numerous parents have found their use to be comforting for their infants. No studies are reported which objectively describe benefits of these pouches; this is an area of needed research.

Massaging

General massage may help to promote relaxation by decreasing anxiety and channeling energy, thereby helping the young patient to achieve control. Massage also helps to interrupt the fear-tension-pain syndrome identified by Dick-Read (1959). In addition, the stimulus provided by touch and massage may serve as a distraction from pain or from an anxiety-producing situation.

Localized massage of a painful area may help to relieve pain. Unless contraindicated, the painful area itself may be massaged, or massage may be done in the same area on the contralateral side of the body or between the area of pain and the brain (McCaffery, 1979). Caution needs to be taken when considering use of this intervention on the preterm infant. Beaver (1987) found that in a small sample of preterm infants who were born at 33 weeks' gestation, stroking the leg at the same time that a heelstick was performed created a greater drop in transcutaneous PO_2 than a group in which a heelstick only was performed. This may be due to excessive stimulation, which the preterm infant is unable to tolerate.

When contemplating the use of massage, the nurse should consider whether and specifically how this technique is used by the primary caretakers. It is helpful to perform massage in the same manner as primary caretakers, thereby taking full advantage of any anchoring effect this strategy may have. Observation of parent-child interaction or data gathering during the admission history may provide this data.

Massage may be done either firmly or lightly, depending on the preference and the response of the child. In practice, the authors have found that using firm fingertip and thumb pressure in a kneading type of action and moving in a circular or upward and outward motion is the most effective in providing relief of pain or discomfort in a localized area. When the goal of massage is to relax the infant or child, using more of the hand, including the ball of the hand, is very effective. Moving slowly in an upward and outward or circular motion seems to work best. Massaging the back of the child in this manner is a time-honored and effective technique facilitating relaxation.

Rubbing

Rubbing is another touch strategy which may be utilized with infants and young children. Rubbing is similar to massage; however, rubbing lacks the kneading type of action of massage. Instead, rubbing consists of a back and forth action, utilizing in most instances a large portion of the hand or the pads of the fingers. Like massage, rubbing may be effectively utilized for relief of pain (McCaffery, 1979). Rubbing may also serve to calm an infant or child and to help relieve anxiety. Frequently, rubbing an infant's back in synchrony to the infant's breathing—that is, rubbing upward as the infant inhales and downward as he or she exhales—will help to achieve a calm, relaxed state (Grinder, 1986b).

Stroking

Stroking is similar to rubbing, but rather than moving the hand in a back and forth motion, the hand is moved from one point on the skin of the infant or child to another, lifted off the skin, and returned to the initial point of contact.

Nurses need to use and teach parents to use firm, slow strokes when touching their infants, especially when stroking the face, palms of hands, soles of feet, and backbone. Slow, firm strokes should be utilized in a rhythmic fashion, at 12 to 16 strokes per minute. This mimics the rate of maternal respirations in utero. In addition, stroking should be done from head to toe and centrally to distally because this facilitates myelinization of nerve fibers (Coursin, 1972). Stroking the neck, arms, back, chest, and legs of well premature infants not requiring oxygen or intravenous feeding has been

found to be related to a more rapid weight gain (Solkoff et al., 1969; White and Labarba, 1976; Field et al., 1986). However, White-Traut and Tubeszewski (1986) found that stroking, rocking, talking to, or singing to and simultaneous eye contact did *not* increase weight gain over a control group. Stroking interventions for the premature infant must be totally dependent on identification of potent negative and positive infant cues given by the individual infant.

Based upon their study of 81 full-term infants, Koniak-Griffin and Ludington-Hoe (1988) state that the "beneficial outcomes reported for some stimulation programs for preterm infants may not necessarily be derived from similar protocols with other populations" (p. 75). In this controlled study, no significant treatment effects on weight gain or psychomotor development were found. However, some differences were found in scores for mood and distractibility.

Oral stimulation exercises, consisting of stroking the cheeks and the roof of the infant's mouth, stretching the infant's lip, and massaging the neck prior to tube feedings, have been shown to promote weight gain and thus decrease the number of tube feedings and shorten the length of hospital stays for premature infants (Fairchilds, 1986). Rationale for these exercises was based on Hebb's (1949) postulate that provision of stimulation to muscles will strengthen the neural pathways and increase the efficiency of the involved muscle groups. These exercises were most effective when done before the infant received a tube feeding.

In children with increased intracranial pressure (ICP) or with the potential for increased ICP, chest stroking and facial stroking have been found to have no harmful effect on ICP and, in fact, have often lowered elevated ICP readings. Parental touch most often produced decreased ICP readings, whereas nursing touch unrelated to procedures often had no effect. In addition, blood pressure and heart rate remained stable in association with these episodes of touch. In general, it is safe and possibly efficacious to increase nonprocedural stroking of critically ill children by both parents and nurses (Mitchell et al., 1985; Walleck, 1982; Pollack and Goldstein, 1981).

Stroking may also be combined with holding and rubbing to provide a very effective comfort measure for the child who is in acute distress. Triplett and Arneson (1979) carried out 100 tactile and verbal interventions on a sample of 63 children. Ninety-three interventions included combinations of touch strategies, including stroking and holding. Of these, 82 alleviated distress within five minutes. An additional three interventions were successful within ten minutes.

Schumann (1981) describes a technique that uses stroking as a method for inducing neuromuscular relaxation and sleep in young children. The technique is relatively simple. Children first need to be in an environment conducive to rest, and they need to be comfortable. As each child is told to relax, a word which the child understands, such as *heavy*, *slow*, *droopy*, or *easy* needs to be discussed in relation to the body part to be relaxed prior to starting the procedure. First, the child should stretch out and hyperextend the body while arching the back. Next, the child should take two or three cleansing breaths. It is helpful to have the child imitate the nurse. Then, the nurse should use a quiet, even voice with few inflections and repeatedly state six to eight times that the body part is getting heavy, droopy, or whatever word was chosen. Simultaneously, the nurse should use two hands and firmly stroke the body part to be relaxed. The nurse should work from the lower part of the body or toes up to the head. Intermittently, the nurse must check for relaxation. Schumann (1981) states that this technique is useful even for children younger than 18 months of age.

Sucking

Sucking is a form of touch through the oral cavity and may be either nutritive or non-nutritive in nature. Finger sucking by the fetus in utero is seen on ultrasound by 28 weeks gestation. Non-nutritive sucking, such as pacifier or finger sucking, can significantly decrease crying in newborns and older infants (Neely, 1979; Kessen and Leutzendorff, 1963). In the premature infant, non-nutritive sucking during tube feeding has been well documented to increase weight gain, to decrease time needed to complete nipple feedings, and to shorten hospital stays (Measel and Anderson, 1979; Bernbaum, 1983; Field, 1982). Placing the gavage tube through an enlarged hole in the nipple may facilitate non-nutritive sucking during feeding. Premature infants will intermittently suck on pacifiers as early as 27 to 28 weeks gestation, although their sucking patterns differ from those of full-term infants.

In using a pacifier, nurses need to be cognizant of the size and shape of the pacifier. Newborns need small pacifiers to prevent gagging. Physiologically shaped nipples, which mimic the natural shape of the breast nipple, are often better accepted by newborns and infants who are breast-feeding. Use of regular bottle nipples occluded with gauze and tape is a practice in some hospital nurseries. This practice is to be discouraged because separation of the nipple and bottle retaining ring may occur. Parents should also be taught to avoid tying a pacifier around an infants neck because the tie may present a strangulation hazard.

Hand Holding

Hand holding has been defined as "purposeful, nonprocedural touch where the hand of the patient is held by the nurse" (Knable, 1981, p. 1107). It is a simple and basic yet very effective strategy. There are many instances in which hand holding may be the touch strategy of choice. Such instances include times when the child may be alone or apprehensive, on initial contact to establish rapport, when the child is uncomfortable, prior to a procedure, when waking the child, or at the end of a day's interactions. When choosing this strategy, nurses must consider whether or not parents or other significant caretakers are present. If they are, it may be best to encourage them to utilize this strategy.

Hand holding has been utilized effectively to provide emotional support, to establish rapport, to explain and teach, to orient children to their surroundings, and to build their self-esteem. Hand holding has been shown to produce changes in blood pressure and in heart and respiratory rates. Such findings have, however, been inconclusive (Knable, 1981; Lynch, 1974; Lynch et al., 1974). Hand holding has also been shown to lower elevated ICP (Mitchell et al., 1985; Pollack and Goldstein, 1981).

Gentle Pressure

Gentle pressure at the wrist, hand, shoulder, or arm may be a very effective strategy to utilize with seriously ill and dying patients. A significant number of adult patients who were seriously ill were calmed by such touching at the wrist. This strategy has been found to be especially helpful when utilized in moments of silence. Nurses must also remember that communication with an individual who has accepted terminal illness is often more nonverbal than verbal (McCorkle, 1974; Kubler-Ross, 1969). Further, touch may be utilized not only with patients but also with family members who should be taught to use these types of touch with their ill infant or child.

Anchoring

As stated earlier, anchoring, a technique used in the field of NLP, involves touch of a specific body part and may be effectively utilized by nurses caring for children with altered health states. Nurses frequently make assumptions or at best educated guesses about the types of anchors which may elicit positive outcomes in their young clients. Examples are stroking children's heads or patting and rubbing their backs. Such actions are commonly used by caretakers to soothe and comfort young children. Nurses are searching and should continue to search for and utilize such anchors. When taking a health history, nurses may elicit from parents common actions they use to soothe and calm their child. Eliciting such information reduces the trial-and-error methodology of trying to find just the right spot to pat or rub. Whenever possible, a natural or familiar pre-established anchor should be utilized in nursing interventions (Grinder, 1986b). The phenomenon of anchoring may explain in part the decrease in ICP seen in children with Reye's syndrome when a tape recording of a parent's voice was played. Parents had previously been present and had engaged in hand holding, chest stroking, and conversation with their children. The tape recordings were found to consistently decrease ICP (Pollack and Goldstein, 1981).

By applying the technique of anchoring, specific anchors may be developed so that patients may be helped to access positive, desirable feelings at a time when they are very much needed therapeutically (King et al., 1983). There are three major points to remember regarding anchoring. First, the anchor should be unique if possible. For example, a handshake is not a unique anchor. Second, timing is crucial. To effectively utilize anchoring, the anchor must be introduced at the high-point of the experience. Subtle changes, such as an alteration in breathing pattern, slight changes in body posture, and muscle tension and coloration of the skin, must be observed carefully. These are the clues which indicate when a desired feeling state has been accessed. Finally, the anchor must be reproduced exactly. When using a kinesthetic anchor, it should be done in the same location and with the same firmness in order to elicit the same feeling. One should recall the four major characteristics of touch as described by Weiss (1979), which were discussed earlier in this chapter.

Therapeutic Touch

As discussed earlier, therapeutic touch is viewed as a controversial intervention, largely as a result of the lack of empirical evidence supporting its effectiveness. It is the belief of these authors that therapeutic touch can be a viable and useful technique for nurses, especially in this high-tech society of today.

Caution needs to be taken when utilizing therapeutic touch on the head of infants and children. Brain tissue is believed to be quite sensitive to energy input, as is the developing nervous tissue and energy fields in children. In such situations, therapeutic touch must be given in smaller, more gentle doses to prevent adverse reactions to nurses unexperienced in touch (Boguslawski, 1979; Macrae, 1979; Krieger et al., 1979).

In therapeutic touch, the nurse helps another by enhancing that person's own tendency for wellness. This is done by the transmission of universal, orderly healing energies and requires the following nine attributes: (1) the intent to help; (2) the ability to concentrate; (3) the ability to center or harmonize one's energy levels in relation to each other and to that of the universal order; (4) a state of wellness and alertness; (5) a feeling of compassion or love; (6) the uninvolvement of the ego, or the idea that the nurse is serving as a transmitter and not a supplier of energies; (7) the ability to utilize therapeutic touch in an "effortless effort"; (8) the ability to mentally visualize; and (9) a sense of confidence (Boguslawski, 1979, pp. 12–13).

First, the nurse runs his or her hands through an individual's energy field, which is approximately two to three inches away from the client's body. This area above the body surface is generally preferred because it is easier to detect alterations in an individual's energy field in that area. Alterations or dysrhythmias in the energy field may be perceived as any variety of sensations by the healer: a sensation of tingling, warmth, pressure, coolness, or a magnetic pull are common descriptions. It takes time and practice to become sensitive to these changes. As mentioned earlier, centering is also a prerequisite (Boguslawski, 1979; Krieger, 1976; Macrae, 1979).

Next, the nurse creates a field between the nurse and the patient, as was done during the assessment phase, while mentally visualizing the patient as well or whole. It is also possible to visualize colors which may help a patient: royal blue for a calming, pain-relieving, and edema-reducing interaction and yellow for stimulation for the tired client. Visualization of light green provides an interaction between that of blue and yellow (Boguslawski, 1979, p. 13). While intervening, both hands are always used to provide balance and distribution of the energy. In addition, the hands should not remain still for more than a few seconds to prevent the client from receiving too much energy. A gentle brushing or sweeping motion may be used to brush the pain away (Boguslawski, 1979; Krieger et al., 1979; Macrae, 1979).

Macrae (1979) relates several examples of her use of therapeutic touch with children. When using this little-known and controversial technique, consideration must be given to explaining actions to the patient, the family, and other staff. Explanations will vary depending upon the age of the patient. Macrae (1979) asked four and five year olds if she might "brush the pain away" (Macrae, 1979, p. 665). She found nine and ten year olds fascinated by the idea of being an energy field. When the patient was an infant, Macrae explained therapeutic touch to the parents as being derived from the ancient art of laying on of hands and added that it was being taught in some nursing schools. A similar explanation was given to the staff. It must be noted, however, that the evaluation of the success of therapeutic touch in such instances is based upon case examples, not controlled research.

Factors Modifying the Use of Touch

Various factors modify how, when, and even if we utilize touch with our young clients. These include the client's age and physiological and psychological status, the setting, a variety of sociocultural factors, and previous experience with touch (for example, the client may have experienced abuse or neglect).

With the exception of research regarding time-out cues of the premature infant, little research exists to specifically guide nurses in when and how to utilize the intervention of touch. Nurses utilize touch in any given instance frequently and in whatever manner with which they feel most comfortable. But touching is a learned behavior. Nurses can learn to touch at such times and in such a manner as to actually benefit a patient (Tobiason, 1981). Before attempting to describe specifics related to touch as a therapeutic intervention, however, it is important to acknowledge that touch has different meanings to different people. Touch is interpreted according to culture, background, mood, and the nature of the role relationship between the people who touch (Johnson, 1965; Murray and Zentner, 1975; Tobiason, 1981). It is important for nurses to be aware of their own feelings about touch and of the congruency between touch, which is nonverbal, and verbal communication (Johnson, 1965).

Age is certainly a prime factor which modifies the nurse's approach in implementing touch. Triplett and Arneson (1979) found age to be an important variable in examining young children's responses to verbal and tactile comfort. The authors speculate that the developmental stage and needs of this age group have a great impact on their ability to respond to comfort measures from strangers (Triplett and Arneson, 1979, p. 22).

Age also may affect our desire to touch our clients. Tobiason (1981) found that nursing students responded with more positive descriptive terms when describing the touching of infants than they did when describing touching the elderly (Tobiason, 1981). This corresponds with the statements of Murray and Zentner (1975) that children are touched less and less frequently as they grow older. Barnett also found that health personnel utilized touch less frequently with older than with younger children. In infants, she observed personnel to touch 83 times, 27 times with toddlers, 25 times with preschoolers, and to not touch at all with children 6 years and older.

The preterm infant requires special consideration. When born prematurely, the infant loses the continuous fluid tactile stimulus experienced in utero. In addition, premature labor is often of shorter duration (or nonexistent in the case of cesarean section) than that experienced by the full-term infant. Thus, the premature infant begins life experiencing tactile deprivation. Initially, the main issue for the premature infant is the stabilization and integration of physiological functions (Als et al., 1979). Since the preterm infant's CNS is unstable, the balance of physiological systems may be upset by movement and active postural adjustment. At this stage, tactile and vestibular manipulations by well-meaning caregivers may upset this delicate balance, leading to bradycardia, apneic episodes, mottling, and cyanosis: demonstrations of autonomic disorganization which are commonly referred to as time-out cues. Gradually, the full range of states, from being asleep to being awake to being aroused, becomes clearly identifiable in the preterm behavior repertoire. As these states become increasingly differentiated, they can also affect stability of the motor subsystem and possibly even the physiological subsystem (Als et al., 1982). Finally, the preterm infant develops the capability for a flexible, well-differentiated alert state.

For a variety of reasons, the premature and ill neonate and even older children are often deprived of social touch while being inundated with medical touch (Gorski et al., 1984) in the hospital setting. In one study, the ill compromised infant was noted to have had up to 134 touch interventions within a 24 hour period of time (Gorski et al., 1984). The majority of these were medical touch. Blackburn and Barnard (1985) reported that, of four types of caregiving studied (feeding and diapering, technical, taking out of incubator, and stroking or patting), stroking was the intervention that was least utilized by nurses caring for preterm infants with a mean gestational age of 32 weeks. This study was done between 1975 and 1978 and may be beneficial to repeat. During these medical touch types of interventions, drops in transcutaneous oxygen levels were cited (Long et al., 1980). Norris et al. (1982) also noted drops in transcutaneous oxygen levels, especially when a nurse was repositioning the infant while making no attempt to contain the infant's limbs in a flexed position. However, for those infants receiving pancuronium bromide (Pavulon), it is important that touch be minimized because touch has been shown to increase pulmonary hypertension in these infants (Moynihan and Gerraughty, 1985).

For the preterm infant receiving assisted ventilation, multisensory stimulation should be avoided. Oehler (1985) found that both talking and touching at the same interaction created twice as many avoidance or time-out cues in the ill preterm infant receiving assisted ventilation (30 to 34 weeks past conceptual age) than in the well preterm infant of the same age. Parents need to be taught that talking and touching at the same time can be overwhelming for their infant. It is important for the nurse to teach parents the time-out cues which their infant may be exhibiting and for the parents to know that their infant is not rejecting them when exhibiting some of these cues (Als et al., 1979). Time-out cues are summarized in Table 9–3.

Ludington and Cole (1987) describe five steps in their Readiness for Stimulation

Table 9–3. TIME-OUT CUES OF THE PRETERM INFANT*

Apnea
Mottling
Gaze aversion
Gagging, spitting up
Sneezing, yawning
Arching head, arms, neck, or back
Finger splaying
Sagging cheeks or chin
Tongue thrusting

*From Als, H, Lester, BM, Tronick, EZ, and Brazelton, TB. Towards a research instrument for the assessment of preterm infants' behavior (APIB). In Fitzgerald, HE, Kesterm, BM, and Yogam, MW (Eds.). Theory and research in behavioral pediatrics. New York: Plenum Press, 1982, pp. 35–63.

Scale. To prevent or decrease the possibility of stressing the premature infant, these steps of gradually introducing touch are outlined. Since the premature infant is especially prone to latency of response, it is mandatory that a minimum of 1½ minutes transpire between each of the following interventions. If any signs of physiological or behavioral overload occur, the infant is not ready for any further stimuli. The steps are as follows:

1. Uncover the infant.
2. Change the infant's position. (For the delicate premature infant, merely move an arm or leg up or down. For infants of more than than 34 weeks' gestation, turn from side to back.)
3. Place a hand on the infant's abdomen, thigh, or back and leave in place without moving (low tactile stimulation).
4. With the hand still in place, present your face to the infant, whether he or she is alert or not. Do not talk to the infant.
5. Slowly and gently yet firmly stroke the infant's abdomen, thigh, or back, keeping your face in the en face position.

There are additional studies which have found touch to have very beneficial effects on the physiological status of premature infants. Kattwinkel et al. (1975) produced a significant decrease in the frequency of apnea by rubbing an infant's extremities. Schaeffer (1982) found significantly higher hematocrit levels and a lower oxygen requirement in 13 mechanically ventilated infants. The infants in the experimental group were provided with touch to their heads and abdomens. Blackburn (1983) summarized several studies involving touch of the premature infant which have shown similar trends: that is, stimulated infants tend to score higher than control infants on various behavioral, sensorimotor, and motor scales (Blackburn, 1983, pp. 76–77). In the work of Field et al. (1986, 1987), well premature infants who received only stroking but no view of a face or sound of a voice for 15 minutes three times daily gained weight faster than a control group. It must be stressed that premature infants must be individually assessed as to their ability to handle tactile stimulation. Stroking or massage for *all* premature infants should be avoided.

Just as the physiological status of the premature infant may modify touch interventions, so may the physiological and psycho-logical status of older infants and children. The setting in which we deliver care may also invite or preclude the intervention of touch. Barnett (1972) found that patients classified as acutely ill (that is, having a serious condition with a questionable prognosis but with a chance for improvement) were touched 70% less often than those classified as being in "good" or "fair" condition.

Those patients who are experiencing psychological disturbances or who have experienced neglect or abuse will have their need and desire for touch modified (Older, 1982, p. 180). In these instances, touch interventions will need to be modified based on the specific responses and needs of each individual.

The environment in which an interaction takes place may modify how and when touch is utilized. Certainly, the entire environment of the hospital very often appears strange and frightening to children and their parents. Miles and Carter (1982a, 1982b, 1983) have developed a transactional conceptual model which provides guidelines for assessing parental stress prior to or at the time of a child's admission to an intensive care unit. Based upon this model, nurses need to assess the severity of illness and amount of uncertainty of outcome, the parents' perception of environmental stimuli, and the personal and family background factors that may affect the parents' perception of stress. Intervention strategies are directed not only at reducing environmental stressors but also the stressors arising from situational conditions and personal and family background factors. Interventions must concomitantly maximize the personal and environmental resources available to parents (Miles and Carter, 1983).

A later study utilizing the Parental Stressor Scale in a pediatric intensive care unit (PICU) found that a major source of parental stress in the PICU was change in the parent-child relationship. Nursing interventions are needed to help parents to deal with their changed parental roles. Nurses need to explain and demonstrate to parents, often repeatedly, how they can help their child by visiting, touching, and soothing (Carter et al., 1985).

Anticipatory grief and fear regarding the outcome of their child's illness add to the anxiety that parents feel. Parents may feel that harm will come to their child if they touch him or her. Wires, tubes, and restraints are far from conducive to parental touch. Possible guilt feelings on the part of the parents also contribute to the reluctance to touch. Isolation presents a special barrier to touch of the hospitalized infant or child.

In the hospital setting, parents often need "permission" from the nurse to touch their young one. Some may feel they are not allowed to touch their own child. In such instances, it is the nurse's role to encourage the parents to take control and to show them, if need be, how, where, and when to touch their child.

There are many sociocultural factors which influence the practice of touch. Males, particularly as they grow older, are touched less often and more roughly than females (Pillitteri, 1981). In touching their children, sex-linked behavior is noted. Fathers are more likely to touch so as to enliven their infant. Mothers, in contrast, touch to control, to facilitate alertness, and to soothe the child (Brazleton, 1984, p. xviii).

In the United States, the tendency is to touch less than in many other cultures (Murray and Zentner, 1975; Clark, 1981; Clay, 1968; Montagu, 1978). In one study, 75% of the cultures studied showed more nurturance and warmth toward their infants than American culture. Nurturance and warmth were measured by breast-feeding, body contact, and general attention (Whiting and Childe, 1953). Within a culture, there are also class differences regarding touching. In general, across cultures, the higher the class, the less frequently touching occurs. Further, while members of a higher socioeconomic class may touch those of a lower class, the reverse is not true (Montagu, 1978, p. 272).

How then, can the use of the touch interventions presented here be summarized? The intervention of touch varies widely depending on the nursing diagnosis of the patient, the setting, the condition and age of the child, and numerous sociocultural factors. There is no one right way to utilize touch in nursing. The following case study is but one example of how touch may be utilized with children experiencing altered health states. The outcome that is likely to be used most frequently is the observable response during and following touch, as used by Triplett and Arneson (1979).

EVALUATION

The defining characteristics of nursing diagnoses identified in assessments can also provide criteria for clinical evaluation of intervention outcomes. That is, reversal of patient-specific defining characteristics suggests that the intervention may have been effective, assuming all other factors have been controlled. In addition, other outcome measures have been identified by researchers in this area, such as Krieger (1973) and Triplett and Arneson (1979). However, development of outcome criteria for the touch intervention is an area for future researchers to study.

Case Study

Rachel was born at 26 weeks' gestation in a tertiary care center in the Pacific Northwest (Fig. 9–2). From her initial debut in this world, her parents had realistic fears about her ability to survive. Earlier, a sibling had died at 11 days of age as the result of complications related to prematurity. This, coupled with the needs of Rachel's two older siblings and the fact that her family lived some distance from the hospital, all served as obstacles to optimal bonding between Rachel and her parents. As a premature infant, Rachel also demonstrated multiple and frequent time-out cues, which greatly limited interactions, tactile or otherwise, between her and her caregivers.

Medically, Rachel was unstable. She suffered from infant respiratory distress syndrome, ventricular septal defect, atrial septal defect, and other complications of prematurity. Nursing diagnoses included *Ineffective family coping, Alterations in parenting, Decreased activity tolerance, Nutritional alterations (decreased),* and *Sensory overload.*

The nursing diagnosis of sensory overload was definitely a major and challenging problem for her. Upon tactile, auditory, or even visual stimulation (movement in the room) Rachel responded with apnea and bradycardia spells, trunk arching, and gaze and head aversion. Thus, when her parents were able to visit, their attempts to touch, to hold, and to bond were thwarted by Rachel's multiple time-out cues. Their visits became less and less frequent.

In an attempt to diminish these time-out cues and promote consistency, a primary nurse was assigned to Rachel. She was moved from the main neonatal intensive care unit (NICU), a large room with many Isolettes and a hubbub of activity, to a small, two-bed room across the hall. In this room, the nurses were better able to limit stimuli, including extraneous visual and auditory stimuli. Rachel's number of apnea and bracycardia spells immediately decreased (Fig. 9–3).

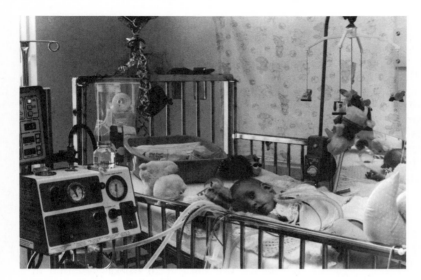

Figure 9–2. Rachel: a compromised infant. (Courtesy of Sandra Doyle.)

Given the same situation today, the nursing staff would utilize and teach the parents to use the slow, firm but gentle strokes recommended by Coursin (1972). Stroking should be done rhythmically and slowly (12 to 16 strokes per minute) because this mimics the rate of maternal respirations in utero. Stroking should also be done from head to toe and centrally to distally (Coursin, 1972). At the time of Rachel's birth, however, this information was not known nor utilized in our Center as it is today. Such a simple intervention employed early in her hospital course may have made tremendous differences in outcome. As it was, because of her strong time-out cues, touch and other stimuli were greatly limited. Rarely did caregivers hold Rachel or sit her in their lap. When this was done, she responded with her now-familiar time-out cues.

Instead of being held in someone's lap, she was propped or gently held in a sitting position on her bed. Consultations with developmental specialists from physical therapy were ongoing, helping to provide appropriate developmental stimuli as much as possible.

Rachel's aversion to different touch stimuli extended to oral touch as well. She was intubated until she was nine months old, when a tracheostomy was performed. As she progressed to solid food, textures became quite a challenge. New textures, and food in general, resulted in extreme displeasure on Rachel's part, with frequent, self-induced gagging and vomiting. In addition, she suffered from gastroesophageal reflux. One of the greatest nursing challenges was to provide Rachel with adequate calories for her growth. Again, specialists from the physical therapy department

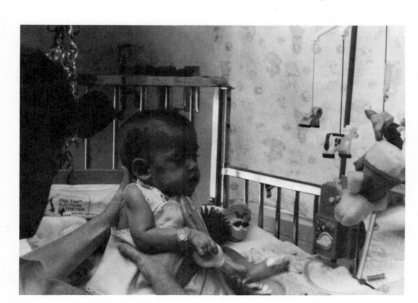

Figure 9–3. A quieter environment decreased Rachel's apnea-bradycardia spells. (Courtesy of Sandra Doyle.)

helped with oral stimulation exercises. A primary nurse helped to ensure a consistent nursing approach. Despite these attempts, a gastrostomy was performed and a tube placed to provide Rachel with the nutrition she needed.

Throughout her hospital stay, Rachel's parents, Mr. and Mrs. D., along with her siblings were encouraged to come and visit Rachel and to participate in her care. As Rachel grew, the time-out cues she so frequently gave gradually diminished. Through much encouragement, Mr. and Mrs. D. became more and more involved in her care (Fig. 9–4). Rachel remained ventilator-dependent. At the time of her most recent admission, Rachel clung to her mother and hugged her as would be expected of a child her age. She continued to be fed via her gastrostomy tube, but she did take a bottle and was gaining weight. While still developmentally delayed in her gross motor skills, she was showing significant gains, and, barring any severe medical setbacks, was expected to rapidly progress developmentally.

RESEARCH IMPLICATIONS

Most often nurses utilize touch in any given instance instinctively, in whatever

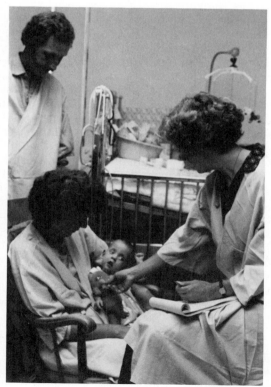

Figure 9–4. Rachel and her parents. Teaching is critical to facilitate touch by parents of compromised infants. (Courtesy of Sandra Doyle.)

manner feels comfortable. In other words, use of touch as an intervention is very often based on trial-and-error methodology. If it works, nurses assume it was needed and was utilized appropriately. Research supporting the effectiveness of touch and providing substantiation of when and more specifically how touch should be used is scant. Perhaps that is because touch, so inherent and pervasive to nursing practice, takes on so many varied forms. The challenge is to isolate and study each form or strategy of touch, then to study the variables related to strategy effectiveness.

Questions regarding touch abound. How can nurses know how others will perceive touch? As has been discussed, there are many variables or modifiers which affect touch. As of now, only educated guesses can be made in most instances about whether or not touch will produce a desirable or an undesirable effect. Weiss (1979) asks many appropriate and intriguing questions at the conclusion of her article. Does the language of touch change across the life cycle and if so, how does it change? Is the meaning of touch the same for different age groups or are there changes in the response to touch which take place? Exactly how does the meaning of touch differ between the sexes and amoung different socioeconomic groups and cultures?

Barnett (1972) lists several propositions that need further research. There is a need for substantiation of those propositions through research. Of particular application to infants and children are the following: (1) the greater the patient's dependency, the greater the nurse's responsibility regarding the appropriateness of the use of touch; (2) the greater the patient's regression, the greater his or her need for communication through touch; (3) the greater the patient's anxiety, the greater the nurse's responsibility to appropriately use touch; (4) the greater the patient's altered body image, the greater his or her need for acceptance through touch; (5) the lower the patient's self-esteem, the greater his or her need for confirmation through touch; and (6) the greater the patient's fear of death, the greater his or her need for relatedness to others through touch (Barnett, 1972, p. 109).

The four major tactile qualities of touch as described by Weiss (1978, p. 132) provide a framework and common ground upon which further touch research may be built. These qualities are as follows:

1. duration, or temporal length of touch.
2. location, or where the body is touched. This quality is best measured by the following three dimensions:
   a. threshold: referring to the degree of innervation of various parts of the body, with highly innervated areas, such as the face and hands, yielding sharply localized sense impressions.
   b. extent: the degree to which many parts of a person's body are touched rather than only a few parts.
   c. centripetality: the degree to which the trunk of the body is touched as opposed to the limbs.
3. intensity, or whether touch is weak, strong, or moderate, judged by the amount of indentation of the skin.
4. sensation, or the comfortableness or uncomfortableness of touch.

These qualities of touch provide a framework for examining the intervention more concretely. Utilizing these qualities to analytically examine the intervention of touch in the future will provide a common ground that can be used to substantiate the use of touch in nursing practice. It will enable nursing to move out of the trial-and-error period, toward the deliberate and effective utilization of touch as a nursing intervention.

The field of NLP provides promising insights into and helpful techniques for the use of touch. Most of its findings are descriptive in nature. Nursing needs to add to that descriptive data base and perhaps move to more controlled studies regarding the effectiveness of the techniques NLP promulgates. Triplett and Arneson (1979) raise many questions after discussing their data for which the field of NLP may provide some direction and answers. For example, is there a way to predict the effect of a given kinesthetic anchor? When comforted by a nurse, are children more likely to be quiet if comforted in a manner similar to that used by the mother, a manner likely to be an anchor? Does the type of tactile comfort make a difference depending on the age of the child? Longitudinal studies which examine whether the types of touch used to calm infants serve as anchors later in the life cycle to access previous feelings would also be beneficial.

In the field of therapeutic touch, research implications also abound. There is certainly a need for well-done descriptive research as well as for more controlled studies. In an extensive review of the literature, Clark and Clark (1984) cite several methodological flaws in therapeutic touch studies and state, "The current research base supporting . . . therapeutic touch is, at best, weak" (p. 40). They call for a broader, stronger research base. Connell (1984), however, argues that perhaps a holistic, humanistic treatment such as therapeutic touch cannot be examined by hard-core experimental strategies and would best be approached by descriptive research methodologies.

Yet descriptions and testimonies by people who have used and have been the recipients of therapeutic touch attest to the benefits of therapeutic touch. At this stage in its evolution, perhaps it is enough to say that we are in an initial ground-breaking phase, a trial-and-error period. If that is true, we need to focus on simple descriptive research methodologies before we can move on to more sophisticated experimental techniques to test the efficacy of therapeutic touch. Indeed, Kaiser (1988) suggests that as society becomes more high-tech, high-touch, low-tech methodologies will become more acceptable based on heuristic standards. In other words, if it works, do it!

Definitive studies also need to be done concerning how to best educate nurses to utilize touch effectively. Posthuma (1985) studied two consecutive classes of third-year occupational therapy students. Based on observations of the students in an interview situation, she found that the experimental group of students, who had practiced touching more throughout the semester, were able to "more often offer support and demonstrate concern for the patient through a caring touch" (p. 192). While some refinement of the methodology utilized in her study is warranted, the interventions utilized with the experimental group may well be found to be applicable to nursing students when future studies are concluded.

References

Als, H, Lester, BM, and Brazleton, TB. Dynamics of the behavioral organization of the premature infant: A theoretic perspective. In Field, TM (Ed.), Infants born at risk. New York: Spectrum, 1979.

Als, H, Lester, BM, Tronick, EZ. Towards a research instrument for the assessment of preterm infants' behavior (APIB). In Fitzgerald, HE, Kesterm, BM, and Yogman, MW (Eds.), Theory and research in behavioral pediatrics. New York: Plenum Press, 1982, pp. 35–63.

Anderson, GC, Marks, E, and Wahlberg, V. Kangaroo care for premature infants. American Journal of Nursing, 7:807–819, 1986.

Ballard, JL, Novak, KK, and Driver, M. A simplified score for assessment of fetal maturation of newly born infants. Journal of Pediatrics, 55:769–774, 1979.

Bandler, R. Using your brain for a change. Moab, Utah: Real People Press, 1985.

Barnard, KE, and Bee, HL. The impact of temporally patterned stimulation on the development of preterm infants. Child Development, 54:1156–1167, 1983.

Barnett, K. A theoretical construct of the concepts of touch as they relate to nursing. Nursing Research, 21:102–109, 1972.

Beaver, PK. Premature infants' responses to touch and pain: Can nurses make a difference? Neonatal Network, 6:13–17, December, 1987.

Bernbaum, JD. Nonnutritive sucking during gavage feeding enhances growth and maturation in premature infants. Pediatrics, 71:41–45, 1983.

Bibler, B. Goals and methods in a pre-school program for disadvantaged children. Children, 27:15–20, 1970.

Blackburn, S. Fostering behavioral development of high-risk infants. Journal of Obstetric, Gynecologic and Neonatal Nursing, 12:763–865, Supplement, 1983.

Blackburn, S, and Barnard, S. Analysis of caregiving: Events relating to preterm infants in the special care unit. In Gottfried, A, and Gaiter, J (Eds.), Infant stress under intensive care environmental neonatology. Baltimore, Md.: University Park Press, 1985, pp. 113–129.

Boguslawski, M. The use of therapeutic touch in nursing. Journal of Continuing Education in Nursing, 10:9–15, 1979.

Boguslawski, M. Therapeutic touch: A facilitator of pain relief. Topics in Clinical Nursing, 1:27–37, 1980.

Boortz-Marx, R. Factors affecting intracranial pressure: A descriptive study. Journal of Neurosurgical Nursing, 2:89–94, 1975.

Brazelton, TB. Introduction. In Brown, CE (Ed.), The many facets of touch. Pediatric Round Table (Vol. 10). Skillman, N.J.: Johnson & Johnson Baby Products Co., 1984, pp xv–xviii.

Brown, CE (Ed.) The many facets of touch. Pediatric Round Table (Vol. 10). Skillman, N.J.: Johnson & Johnson Baby Products Co., 1984.

Campbell, C. Nursing diagnosis and intervention in nursing practice (2nd ed.). New York: John Wiley & Sons, Inc., 1984.

Carpenito, LJ. Nursing diagnosis: Application to clinical practice. Philadelphia: JB Lippincott Co., 1983.

Carter, MC, Miles, MS, Buford, TH, and Hassanein, RS. Parental environmental stress in pediatric intensive care units. Dimensions in Critical Care Nursing, 4:180–189, 1985.

Clark, AL. Culture and childrearing. Philadelphia: FA Davis Co., 1981.

Clark, PE, and Clark, MJ. Therapeutic touch: Is there a scientific basis for the practice? Nursing Research, 1:31–41, 1984.

Clay, VS. Effect of culture on mother-child tactile communication. Family coordinator, 37:204–210, 1968.

Connell, MT. Therapeutic touch: The state of the art. In Brown, CE (Ed.), The many facets of touch. Pediatric Round Table (Vol. 10). Skillman, N.J.: Johnson & Johnson Baby Products Co., 1984, pp. 149–155.

Coursin, DB. Nutrition and brain development in infants. Merrill Palmer Quarterly, 18:180–192, 1972.

Daundivier, D. Personal communication, September 20, 1986.

DeForest, J, and Porter, A. Cuddlers: A volunteer infant stimulation program. Canadian Nurse, 7:38–40, 1981.

Dick-Read, G. Childbirth without fear: The principles and practices of natural childbirth (2nd ed.). New York: Harper and Row, 1959.

Dilts, R. Applications of neurolinguistic programming. Cupertino, Calif.: Meta Publications.

Dorland's Illustrated Medical Dictionary (24th ed.) Philadelphia: WB Saunders Co., 1967.

Dossey, L. The skin: What is it? Topics in Clinical Nursing, 2:1–4, 1983.

Fairchilds, C. Nonnutritive sucking and intraoral stimulation in prematures. Paper presented at the Developmental Enrichment Meeting: Theory and application, Costa Mesa, Calif.: March 15, 1986.

Fanslow, C. Therapeutic touch: A healing modality throughout life. Topics in Clinical Nursing, 5:72–79, 1983.

Field, T. Nonnutritive sucking during tube feedings: Effects on preterm neonates in an intensive care unit. Pediatrics, 70: 381–384, 1982.

Field, T, Schanberg, S, Scafidi, MS, Bauer, C, Vega-Lahr, N, Gorcia, R, Nystrom, J, and Kuhn, C. Tactile-kinesthetic stimulation effects on preterm neonates. Pediatrics, 77:654–658, 1980.

Field, T, Schanberg, S, Scafidi, MS, Bauer, C, Vega-Lahr, N, Gorcia, R, Nystrom, J, and Kuhn, C. Tactile/kinesthetic stimulation effects on preterm neonates. Pediatrics, 77:654–658, 1986.

Field, T, Scafidi, F, and Schanberg, S. Massage of preterm newborns to improve growth and development. Pediatric Nursing 70:385–387, 1987.

Frank, LK. Tactile communication. Genetic Psychological Monograph, 56:209–225, 1957.

Geden, EA, and Gegeman, A. Personal space preferences of hospitalized adults. Research in Nursing and Health, 4:237–241, 1981.

Gordon, M. Nursing diagnosis: Process and application. New York: McGraw-Hill Book Co., 1982.

Gordon, M. Manual of nursing diagnosis: 1984–1985. New York: McGraw-Hill Book Co., 1985.

Gorski, P, Hole, W, Leonard, C, and Martin, J. Direct computer recording of premature infants and nursing care: Distress following two interventions. Pediatrics, 72:198–202, 1983.

Gorski, P, Leonard, C, Sweet, D, Martin, J, Sehring, S, O'Harra, L, High, P, Lang, M, Diecuch, R, and Green, J. Caring for immature infants: A touchy subject. In Brown, CE (Ed.), The many facets of touch. Pediatric Round Table (Vol. 10). Skillman, N.J.: Johnson & Johnson Baby Products Co., 1984, pp. 84–91.

Gottfried, AW, and Rose, SA. Tactile recognition memory in infants. Child Development, 51:69–74, 1980.

Gottfried, AW. Touch as an organizer for learning and development. In Brown, CE (Ed.), The many facets of touch. Pediatric Round Table (Vol. 10). Skillman, N.J.: Johnson & Johnson Baby Products Co., 1984, pp. 114–120.

Grinder, J, and Bandler, R. Frogs into princes. Moab, Utah: Real People Press, 1979.

Grinder, M. The educational conveyer belt. Battle Ground, Wash.: Michael Grinder, Inc., 1986a.

Grinder, M. Personal communication, July 17, 1986b.

Guyton, AC. Textbook of medical physiology (7th ed.). Philadelphia: WB Saunders Co., 1986, pp. 580–591.

Harlow, HF. Development of the second and third affectional systems in macaque monkeys. In Tourlentes, TT, Pollack, SL, and Himwich, HE (Eds.), Research approaches to psychiatric problems. New York: Grune & Stratton, Inc., 1962.

Hasselmeyer, EG. Four premature neonates' responses to handling. American Nurses' Association, 11:15–24, 1964.

Hazinski, MF. Nursing care of the critically ill child. St. Louis: CV Mosby Co., 1984.

Hebb, DO. The organization of behavior. New York: John Wiley and Sons, Inc., 1949.

Heidt, P. Effect of therapeutic touch on the anxiety levels of hospitalized patients. Nursing Research, 1:32–37, 1981.

Hollender, M. The need or wish to be held. Archives of General Psychiatry, 22:445–453, 1970.

Hooker, D. The prenatal origins of behavior. Lawrence, Kan.: University of Kansas Press, 1952.

Huss, AJ. Touch with care or a caring touch? American Journal of Occupational Therapy, 31:11–18, 1977.

Hynd, CW, and Willis, WG. Pediatric neuropsychology. Orlando, Fla.: Grune & Stratton, Inc., 1988.

Jasmin, A, and Trygstad, LN. Behavioral concepts and the nursing process. St. Louis: CV Mosby Co., 1979.

Jay, SS. The effects of gentle human touch on mechanically ventilated very-short-gestation infants. Maternal-Child Nursing Journal, 4:199–256, 1982.

Johnson, BS. The meaning of touch in nursing. Nursing Outlook, 13:59–60, 1965.

Jourard, SM. The transparent self. New York: D. Van Nostrand Co., 1971.

Kaiser, LR. Anticipating your high-tech tomorrow. Health Care Forum, 29:12–20, 1986.

Kaiser, LR. Personal communication, June 6, 1988.

Kattwinkel, J, Nearman, HS, Fanaroff, AA, Katona, PG, and Klaus, MH. Apnea of prematurity: Comparative therapeutic effects of cutaneous stimulation and nasal continuous positive airway pressure. Journal of Pediatrics 86:588–592, 1975.

Kessen, W, and Leutzendorff, AM. The effect of nonnutritive sucking on movement in the human newborn. Journal of Comparative and Physiological Psychology, 56:69–72, 1963.

King, M, Novik, L, and Citrenbaum, J. Irresistible communication: Creative skills for the health professional. Philadelphia: WB Saunders Co., 1983.

Klaus, MH, Kennell, JH, Plumb, N, and Zuehlke, S. Human maternal behavior at first contact with her young. Pediatrics, 46:187–192, 1970.

Knable, J. Handholding: One means of transcending barriers of communication. Heart and Lung, 10:1106–1110, 1981.

Knowles, R. A guide to self-management strategies for nurses. New York: Springer Publishing Co., Inc., 1984.

Kolb, L. Disturbances of the body image. In Arieti, S. (Ed), American handbook of psychiatry (Vol. 1). New York: Basic Books, Inc., 1959, pp. 749–767.

Koniak-Griffin, D, and Ludington-Hoe, SM. Developmental and temperament outcomes of sensory stimulation in healthy infants. Nursing Research, 37:70–76, 1988.

Korner, AF. The many facets of touch. In Brown, CE (Ed.), The many facets of touch. Pediatric Round Table (Vol. 10). Skillman, N.J.: Johnson & Johnson Baby Products Co., 1984, pp. 107–112.

Kramer, M, Chamorro, I, Green, D, and Knudtson, F. Extra tactile stimulation of the premature infant. Nursing research, 5:324–334, 1975.

Krieger, D. The relationship of touch with intent to help or to heal to subjects' in-vivo hemoglobin values: A study in personalized interactions. Proceedings of the Ninth American Nurses' Association Nursing Research Conference. New York: American Nurses' Association, 1973.

Krieger, D. Therapeutic touch: The imprimatur of nursing. American Journal of Nursing, 75:786–791, 1975.

Krieger, D. Healing by the laying on of hands as a facilitator of bioenergetic exchange: The response of in-vivo human hemoglobin. International Journal for Psychoenergetic Systems, 1:121–129, 1976.

Krieger, D, Peper, E, and Ancoli, S. Therapeutic touch: Searching for evidence of physiological change. American Journal of Nursing, 79:660–662, 1979.

Kubler-Ross, E. On death and dying. New York: Macmillan Publishing Co., 1969.

Long, JG, Philipa, AGS, and Lucey, JF. Excessive handling as a cause of hypoxemia. Pediatrics, 65:203–210, 1980.

Lynch, JJ. The effects of human contact on cardiac arrhythmia in coronary care patients. Journal of Nervous and Mental Diseases, 158:88–99, 1974.

Lynch, JJ, Flaherty, L, Emrich, C, Mills, M, and Katcher, A. Effects of human contact on heart activity of curarized patients in a shock-trauma unit. American Heart Journal, 88:160–169, 1974.

Ludington, S. Effects of extratactile stimulation on growth and development of vaginally born and cesarean born infants. Communicating Nursing Research, 10:34–40, 1981.

Ludington, S, and Cole, J. Infant stimulation: 1987. A comprehensive course of study in infant growth, development and enhancement. Course Syllabus, Las Vegas, March 13–16, 1987, p. 281.

Macmillan, P. Spacing and touching and hugging. Nursing Times, 77:788–789, 1981.

Macrae, J. Therapeutic touch in practice. American Journal of Nursing, 79:664–665, 1979.

McAnarney, ER. Touching and adolescent sexuality. In Brown, CE (Ed.), The many facets of touch. Pediatric Round Table (Vol. 10). Skillman, N.J.: Johnson & Johnson Baby Products Co., 1984, pp. 138–143.

McCaffery, M. Nursing management of the patient with pain (2nd ed.). Philadelphia: JB Lippincott Co., 1979.

McCorkle, R. The effects of touch on seriously ill patients. Nursing Research, 23:125-132, 1974.

Measel, CP, and Anderson, GC. Nonnutritive sucking during tube feedings: Effect on clinical course in premature infants. Journal of Obstetric, Gynecologic and Neonatal Nursing, 8:265–272, 1979.

Mercer, LS. Touch: Comfort or threat? Perspectives in Psychiatric care, 4:20–25, 1966.

Miles, MS, and Carter, MC. Assessing parental stress in intensive care units. MCN: American Journal of Maternal Child Nursing, 8:354–359, 1983.

Miles, MS, and Carter, MC. Parental stressor scale: Pediatric intensive care unit (abstr). Nursing Research, 31:121–126, 1982a.

Miles, MS, and Carter, MC. Sources of parental stress in pediatric intensive care units. Child Health Care, 11:65–69, 1982b.

Mitchell, PH. Concepts basic to nursing. New York: McGraw-Hill Book Co., 1973.

Mitchell, PH, Habermann-Little, B, Johnson, F, Van Ingewen-Scott, D, and Tyler, D. Critically ill children:

The importance of touch in a high-technology environment. Nursing Administration Quarterly, Summer: 38–46, 1985.

Montagu, A. Touching: The human significance of the skin (2nd ed.). New York: Harper and Row, Publishers, Inc., 1978.

Moss, J, and Solomons, HC. Swaddling then, there and now: Historical, anthropological and current practices. Maternal-Child Nursing Journal, 8:137–151, 1979.

Moynihan, P, and Gerraughty, A. Low stress = higher survival. American Journal of Nursing, 85:662–665, 1985.

Murray, R, and Zentner, J. Nursing concepts for health promotion. Englewood Cliffs, N.J.: Prentice-Hall, Inc., 1975.

Muwaswes, M. Increased intracranial pressure and its systemic effects. Journal of Neurosurgical Nursing, 17:238–243, 1985.

Neely, C. Effects of nonnutritive sucking upon the behavioral arousal of the newborn. In Anderson, GC, and Raff, B (Eds.), Newborn behavioral organization: Nursing research and implications. New York: March of Dimes Birth Defects Foundation, 1979, pp. 173–200.

Nerem, RM, Levesque, MJ, and Cornhill, JF. Social environment as a factor in diet-induced atherosclerosis. Science, 208:1475–1476, 1980.

Norris, S, Campbell, L, and Brenkert, S. Nursing procedures and alterations in transcutaneous oxygenation in premature infants. Nursing Research, 31:330–336, 1982.

Oehler, J. Examining the issue of tactile stimulation for preterm infants. Neonatal Network, 4:25–33, 1985.

Older, J. Touching is healing. New York: Stein and Day Publishers, 1982.

Oremland, EK, and Oremland, JD. The effects of hospitalization on children. Springfield, Ill: Charles C Thomas, 1973.

Patton, RG, and Gardner, LI. Growth failure in maternal deprivation. Springfield, Ill: Charles C Thomas, 1963.

Pillitteri, A. Child health nursing: Care of the growing family (2nd ed.). Boston: Little, Brown and Co., Inc., 1981.

Pollack, LD, and Goldstein, GW. Lowering of intracranial pressure in Reye's Syndrome by sensory stimulation. New England Journal of Medicine, 304:732–736, 1981.

Posthuma, BW. Learning to touch. Canadian Journal of Occupational Therapy, 52:185–193, 1985.

Province, L, and Lipton, RC. Infants in institutions. New York: International Universities Press, Inc., 1962.

Quinn, JT. One nurse's evolution as a healer. American Journal of Nursing, 79:662–664, 1979.

Randolph, G. Therapeutic and physical touch: Physiological response to stressful stimuli. Nursing Research, 33:33–36, 1984.

Rausch, PB. Effects of tactile and kinesthetic stimulation on premature infants. Journal of Obstetric, Gynecologic and Neonatal Nursing, 10:34–37, 1981.

Reilly, AP (Ed.). The communication game: Perspectives on the development of speech, language and non-verbal communication skills. Pediatric Round Table (Vol. 4). Skillman, N.J.: Johnson & Johnson Baby Products Co., 1980.

Ribble, MA. The rights of infants: Early psychological needs and their satisfaction (2nd ed.). New York: Columbia University Press, 1965.

Rice, R. The effects of the Rice Infant Sensorimotor Stimulation Treatment on the development of high-risk infants. In Birth defects: Original article series.White Plains, N.Y.: The National Foundation, 15:7–26, 1979.

Robertson, J. Some responses of young children to the loss of maternal care. Nursing Times, 49:382–386, 1953.

Rubin, R. Maternal touch. Nursing Outlook, 11:828–831, 1963.

Salamaha, C, Yocke, J, Eidal, K, and Oakes, AR. Growth and development. In Oakes, AR (Ed.), Critical care nursing of children and adolescents. Philadelphia: WB Saunders Co., 1981.

Sameroff, AJ, Seifer, R, Barocas, R, Zox, M, and Greenspan, S. Intelligence quotient scores of 4-year-old children: Social environmental risk factors. Pediatrics 79:343–350, 1987.

Schaeffer, JS. The effects of gentle human touch on mechanically ventilated, very-short gestation infants. Maternal-Child Nursing Journal, 11:199–259, 1982.

Schloper, E. The development of body image and symbol formation through body contact with an autistic child. Journal of Child Psychology, 3:181–202, 1962.

Schmake, JA. Ritualism in nursing practice. Nursing Forum, 11:74–78, 1964.

Schumann, MJ. Neuromuscular relaxation: A method for inducing sleep in young children. Pediatric Nursing, 7:9–13, 1981.

Scipien, GM, Martha, MU, Chard, MA, Howe, J, and Phillips, PJ, Comprehensive pediatric nursing. New York: McGraw-Hill Book Co., 1975.

Scott, S, and Richards, M. Nursing low–birth-weight babies on lambswool. Lancet, 1:1028–1033, 1979.

Smith, JA. A critical appraisal of therapeutic touch. In Brown, CE (Ed.), The many facets of touch. Pediatric Round Table (Vol. 10). Skillman, N.J.: Johnson & Johnson Baby Products Co., 1984, pp. 156–165.

Solkoff, N, Yaffe, S, Weintraub, D, and Blase, B. Effects of handling on the subsequent development of premature infants. Developmental Psychology, 1:765–768, 1969.

Taber's Cyclopedic Medical Dictionary (14th ed.). Thomas, CL (Ed.). Philadelphia: FA Davis Co., 1981.

Tempesta, LD. The importance of touch in the care of newborns. Journal of Obstetric, Gynecologic and Neonatal Nursing, 1:27–28, 1972.

Temple, PC. Let's talk about . . . : Communicating with sick children. Indianapolis: Health and Wholeness Publications, 1979.

Tobiason, SB. Touching is for everyone. American Journal of Nursing, 81:728–730, 1981.

Triplett, JL, and Arneson, SW. The use of verbal and tactile comfort to alleviate distress in young hospitalized children. Research in Nursing and Health, 2:17, 1979.

Turkewitz, G. A sensory basis for the lateral differences in the newborn infant's response to somesthetic stimulation. Journal of Experimental Child Psychology, 18:304–312, 1974.

Turton, P. The laying on of hands. Nursing Times. 80:47–48, 1984.

Van deCarr, FR. Infant development enrichment. Paper presented at the Developmental Enrichment Meeting: Theory and applications, Costa Mesa, Calif.: March 15, 1986.

Vaughn, VC (Ed.). Nelson's textbook of pediatrics. Philadelphia: WB Saunders Co., 1979.

Walleck, CA. The effect of purposeful touch on intracranial pressure. Unpublished master's thesis, University of Maryland, College Park, 1982.

Webster's Ninth New Collegiate Dictionary. Springfield, Mass: Merriam-Webster, Inc., 1987.

Weiss, SJ. The language of touch: A resource to body image. Health Nursing, 1:17–29, 1978.

Weiss, S. The language of touch. Nursing Research, 28:76–80, 1979.

Whaley, LF, and Wong, D. Nursing care of infants and children (2nd ed.). St. Louis: CV Mosby Co., 1983.

White, J, and Labarba, R. The effects of tactile and kinesthetic stimulation on neonatal development in the premature infant. Development Psychobiology, 19:569–577, 1976.

White-Traut, R, and Tubeszewski, K. Multimodel stimulation of the premature infant. Journal of Pediatric Nursing, 1:90–95, 1986.

Whiting, JWM, and Childe, IL. Child training and personality. New Haven: Yale University Press, 1953.

Wolff, L, Weitzel, MH, and Fuerst, EV. Fundamentals of nursing (6th ed.). Philadelphia: JB Lippincott Co., 1979.

Yarrow, LJ. Maternal deprivation: Toward an empirical and conceptual re-evaluation. Psychological Bulletin, 58:459–490, 1961.

Yarrow, LJ. Research in dimensions of early maternal care. Merrill-Palmer Quarterly, 9:101–122, 1963.

CHAPTER 10

BEHAVIOR MANAGEMENT

JUDITH A. COUCOUVANIS, M.A., C.S., R.N.

Managing disruptive behavior creates unique challenges for nurses in the pediatric practice setting. Traditional approaches to behavior change are often not practical in today's busy pediatric unit where lengths of stay have decreased while patient acuity has increased. Specific, practical, and behaviorally oriented management methods are a necessity (Schroeder et al., 1983). Consequently, pediatric nurses require specialized knowledge and skill to intervene effectively when disruptive behavior occurs. The purpose of this chapter is to present the intervention of behavior management.

The hospitalized child is expected to accept separation from the familiar environment of family, school, and friends; invasions of the body; painful, uncomfortable treatments; new rules and regulations; inter-actions with strangers; unfamiliar foods; an altered time schedule; sensory underload or overload; and confinement to limited physical space. Children respond to such loss of control and unprecedented expectations in individualized fashions. One potential response is disruptive, inappropriate behavior. For purposes of this discussion, *disruptive* is defined as "to upset the order of" and "to interrupt or impede the progress, movement, or procedure of"; *behavior* is defined as "the manner in which one behaves" and "the actions or reactions of persons under specified circumstances" (Morris, 1976).

The expectations for the hospitalized child are discretionary and are generally set by authoritative adults in the hospital environment. Rationale for such norms, whether spoken or written, are usually to promote

151

rest and healing, to facilitate hospital functioning, and to expedite the giving of nursing care and treatments. When the frequency or intensity of a child's response to these expectations is judged by these adults as too high or too low, the behavior is labeled inappropriate or disruptive and management is required (Brink, 1982). Managing is defined as controlling the course of (de Mello Vianna, 1980). For example, a child's crying or screaming may be judged to occur too often, or eating may occur too seldom, and staff may determine that management is necessary.

Approaches to managing disruptive behavior must be communicated easily and implemented by all levels and classifications of personnel. The framework for such management strategies is provided by the behavioral model and social learning theory.

THEORETICAL FOUNDATION

Currently, there is no one conceptual model which explains behavior so well that it is accepted by nearly everyone. No hierarchy of importance can be established in which any single variable is selected as the decisive factor in all instances of deviant behavior. The totality of influencing mechanisms is complex, diverse, and multifaceted and varies from individual to individual (Chess and Thomas, 1984). One might consider the child's personal characteristics of temperament, motivation, and abilities; parental attitudes and child care practices; early life experiences; and stresses imposed by the school and community to initiate a discussion of relevant causative factors. Recognizing, then, that disruptive behavior evolves from a host of complex factors, this discussion will focus on the behavioral model and social learning theory as the framework from which to intervene when disruptive behavior occurs.

The Behavioral Model

The behavioral model assumes that behavior is acquired and regulated by certain principles of learning. These principles describe the relationships between behavior or operants; stimuli; and consequences such as reinforcement, punishment, and extinction.

The importance of reinforcement schedules is also emphasized in this model (Cullinan et al., 1983).

The stimuli that immediately precede the behavior are the cues to perform a certain action. These antecedents might include a person, command, setting, tone of voice, or event. Stimuli are viewed as having some control over what behaviors occur and when they occur. The stimulus can be altered to effect a change in behavior.

Consequences of behavior may strengthen, weaken, or have no effect upon behavior. Reinforcing consequences are thought to increase a behavior, while those that are punishing are believed to decrease a behavior. To provide this effect, consequences must be contingent upon the behavior's occurrence. Reinforcement can be both positive (such as praise or candy) or negative (such as withdrawing a command, disapproval, or aggression). Negative reinforcement occurs when an event is removed following a behavior that increases that behavior. For example, the child is told to put away the toys by the nurse (event). The child swears at the nurse (behavior). The nurse walks away (event removed). The child's swearing was negatively reinforced. In subsequent situations, the probability that the child will use aversive behavior is increased. Punishment can be the introduction of an aversive event, such as a reprimand, or the removal of a positive one, such as losing a privilege (Barkley, 1981).

When existing consequences are discontinued and a behavior is no longer reinforced by the environment, extinction occurs (Ayllon and Simon, 1982). There are two problems with extinction. These are (1) behavior change is gradual and too slow for the hospital setting and (2) the behavior will likely increase when the reinforcement is first withdrawn.

The schedule of reinforcements and punishments can be either continuous or intermittent. Continuous schedules are those in which every occurrence of a behavior is reinforced. In such cases behaviors increase rapidly but do not persevere once the environment suspends reinforcement. Intermittent schedules are those in which periodic reinforcement occurs. These schedules take longer to change behavior; however, the behavior is more likely to persist (Ayllon and Simon, 1982).

The related concept of secondary reinforcement or punishment occurs when a normally neutral stimuli or event is paired with a reinforcing or aversive event (Barkley, 1981). For example, pairing stickers, stars, or tokens, which by themselves are not reinforcing, with praise, and allowing them to be exchanged for food, toys, or special activities converts them to reinforcers. Pairing check marks on a piece of paper for misbehaving in public with ten minutes of lost television time makes the check marks punishing. In real life, all operant principles are likely to be acting simultaneously. The same stimulus can be a consequence for one behavior and an antecedent for another. For example, a mother's smile may be a consequence to the child's touch and an antecedent to the child's kiss. A behavior may also produce both reinforcing and punishing consequences. For example, a child's tantrum may elicit a parent's talking and soothing efforts, which positively reinforce the tantrum behavior; however, the parent's eventual resort to spanking is a punishing consequence.

Social Learning Theory

Social learning theory is a perspective on behavior that is associated with the work of Bandura (1977) and others. Bandura believes that operant conditioning principles explain much behavior-environment interaction. However, he deviates from the traditional behavioral model in his views that personal-cognitive factors such as beliefs, memories, expectations, problem-solving skills, social status, and roles have a reciprocal relationship with the individual's behavior and the environmental events. Bandura describes the phenomenon of observational learning, or the acquisition of new behavior through observing the behavior of other people. Through modeling or imitation, children learn both adaptive and maladaptive behaviors. This is particularly apparent in the learning of speech and language, self-help skills, and aggressive behavior (McGee and Saidel, 1979).

Application of the behavioral model and social learning theory to the pediatric setting is described in current literature. Jay et al. (1985) utilized a psychological intervention program which included breathing exercises, positive reinforcement, imagery, behavioral rehearsal, and modeling to effectively decrease the distress of five pediatric patients undergoing bone marrow aspirations and lumbar punctures. No patients required physical restraint after the intervention began, although several had had a history of restraint. Elliot and Olson (1983) employed a similar behaviorally oriented stress management program to decrease the distress of pediatric patients during burn treatment procedures. Substantial reductions in groans, screams, fear, resistance, and flailing occurred in the four patients. Kumchy and Kores (1981) effectively treated the disruptive behavior of a neurologically impaired pediatric patient through the use of verbal reinforcement of the patient's appropriate behavior. Abusive language, pinching, and hitting were reduced while appropriate language and attendance to a task increased.

Significance of Disruptive Behavior

All children have the potential to demonstrate disruptive behavior when reacting to a difficult situation. Such behavior may reflect a long-standing disorder or a transitory situational problem. Children with long-standing behavior disorders may have problems related to inconsistent and erratic parental attention and punishment; negative parental role models; or a chaotic, disruptive home atmosphere (Moore, 1982; Webster-Stratton, 1983b). These children generally do not have the social skills to elicit positive socializing experiences in a new environment such as the hospital. Because of disturbed family processes, their behavior repertoire is limited, and they are not oriented towards prosocial reinforcers and goals. They may continue with their disruptive behavior even when given negative feedback from others. The net result is that the child is identified as behaving in a disruptive or inappropriate manner and is excluded from normalizing social interaction (Moore, 1982). In these instances, it is unrealistic to expect such a child to automatically relate positively to peers and authority figures. However, the nurse who understands the child's limited behavioral repertoire can plan and facilitate positive interactions with others and subsequently reduce disruptive behavior.

Children with transitory problems display disruptive behavior directly related to the situation. For example, a child without a past history of eating problems may refuse to eat. A child who swallowed medicine at home might refuse to swallow pills or may spit them out in the hospital. A child who never ran from the pediatrician's office may run from the treatment room. These are attempts to gain mastery over the situation and alleviate a sense of powerlessness.

In the hospital, attempts by children to control are often labeled as resistive behavior. However, initial attempts to control are a healthy response and a successful coping strategy. If children make suggestions on how something should be done or act autonomously, their independent behavior often frustrates nurses, particularly when the behavior interferes with nursing care or schedules (Tesler and Savedra, 1981; Vulcan, 1984). However, disruptive, inappropriate behavior *is* functional in producing desired outcomes for the child. It requires managing only when it persistently interferes with prescribed treatments and nursing care, impedes the promotion of health, and consistently interrupts hospital routines and procedures or infringes upon the rights of others. Examples of such behavior include excessive motor activity (running, climbing, or fidgeting), poor impulse control (abruptly leaving, interrupting, destroying property, verbally and physically assaulting), noncompliance (acts of defiance, verbal refusals), short attention span, and teasing. Such behavior affects other patients directly. Other patients might be the targets of disruptive behavior or may receive less attention because of the extraordinary amount of staff time and energy which is spent undoing, mending, and repairing damage when the disruptive patient's behavior is mismanaged. In these instances, it is to the benefit of the child, other patients, family members, and staff to manage the disruptive behavior in a logical, consistent manner.

ASSESSMENT

The challenging task for nurses is to determine when disruptive behavior requires intervention. It is often difficult to distinguish between transient, normal, expected responses to hospitalization and long-standing behavior disorders. There are no specific rules to help with this interpretation. However, disruptive behavior represents patterns of functioning that often violate ideal or typical standards for normality. Such deviations might involve behavior that is uncharacteristic of the child's age or sex. The frequency, intensity, and persistence of a behavior are also important considerations. A child who portrays a problem, often to an extreme degree, in multiple situations or more-or-less continually over a substantial period of time is more likely to be identified as behaviorally disordered (Brink, 1982; Bumbalo and Siemon, 1983; Robinson and Siemon, 1982; Van Leeuwen, 1977; Webster-Stratton, 1983b). There may be mitigating factors in such judgments, particularly such factors as the occurrence of a highly stressful procedure, a recent change in family structure, or a change in hospitals. Validating one's perceptions of disruptive behavior is accomplished by observing the child in a variety of settings and activities, questioning parents and other staff members, reviewing pertinent patient documentation, and sharing these observations with the child and family.

Armstrong et al. (1982) used the Personality Inventory for Children (PIC) to assess the psychological impact of childhood cancer. They discovered that children with cancer exhibited cognitive development-related problems and internalized forms of psychopathology (anxiety and depression) more often than their age-matched and sex-matched cohorts. This instrument might be a useful screening tool to identify other hospitalized children in need of intervention.

Disruptive behavior can also be recognized through the use of nursing diagnoses. The defining characteristics provide data indicating disruptive behavior (Kim et al., 1984). One nursing diagnosis might be *Ineffective individual coping.* Likely defining characteristics may involve destructive behavior toward self or others, an inability to ask for help, an inability to solve problems, alterations in societal participation (such as a change in peer relationship resulting from an extended hospitalization), verbal manipulation, an inappropriate use of defense mechanisms, or a high rate of accidents.

A second nursing diagnosis is *Sensory-perceptual alteration: visual, auditory, kinesthetic, gustatory, tactile, or olfactory.* The defining characteristics are usually evident as a change in a child's behavior pattern, such as increased whining, crying, or aggressiveness. Apathy, restlessness, irritability, noncompliance, rapid mood swings, anger, or exaggerated emotional responses are other possible defining characteristics.

Alteration in thought processes is an additional prospective nursing diagnosis. Relevant defining characteristics might include distractibility, inaccurate interpretation of the environment, memory deficit or problems, decreased ability to grasp ideas, inability to follow, inappropriate social behavior, altered sleep patterns, and an impaired ability to problem solve, make decisions, or reason.

The final nursing diagnosis indicative of disruptive behavior is *Potential for violence* which is self-directed or directed at others. Usual defining characteristics encompass hostile, threatening verbalizations, including boasting or threats of violence; increased motor activity, including pacing or agitation; overt and aggressive acts, such as assault or property destruction; and threatening body language, such as rigid posture, clenched fists, or facial grimaces.

The presence of these defining characteristics indicates disruptive behavior. For example, the nursing diagnosis of potential for violence directed at others is evident in a child who throws objects or spits at staff members when they enter the child's room. When the child greets staff members with "hello" and does not throw objects or spit, one can suggest the intervention has been successful in decreasing disruptive behavior. The absence or reversal of the defining characteristics following implementation of the intervention is one method of measuring outcomes. Nevertheless, this approach to the measurement of outcomes lacks specificity and objectivity.

THE INTERVENTION

The intervention strategies for managing disruptive behavior do not focus on how to resolve or cure the disturbing behavior but instead center on how to intervene realistically to enable a child to use strengths and new ways of problem solving to restore or attain positive aspects of daily living. The primary strategies are behavior management

and cognitive intervention. Implementation of these strategies is effected by the variables of family relationship structure, setting, and the nature of the illness.

Behavior Management

Children learn in interaction with their environment. Such social learning is mediated by stimuli and consequences. In the hospital, disruptive behavior can be managed through alteration of stimuli and consequences.

Positive Reinforcement

Positive reinforcement, a powerful method of behavior change, is used to develop new behaviors or to strengthen the frequency of desirable behaviors already present in the child's behavioral repertoire (Barkley, 1981). The use of positive reinforcement is often difficult for nurses. Many adults believe children should act appropriately without praise (Webster-Stratton, 1983a). Remembering that the hospital is a new, often frightening place for a child, it is not surprising that expectations are forgotten or unknown to the child. Illness and hospitalization interfere with a child's mastery of developmental tasks. On such occasions, the child is vulnerable to regression in development with potential long-lasting effects upon personality (Belmont, 1970; Gohsman, 1981). Regressive responses such as baby talk, enuresis, or temper outbursts are common reactions but are often viewed by nurses as disruptive. However, nurses must recognize and praise any indication of a child's progress towards the set goal while remembering that perfection should not be required or expected. Behavior changes are gradual and are most likely to occur if reinforcement is consistent and goals are achievable (Patterson, 1975).

One method of changing disruptive behavior is development of a contract. A contract simply states the relationship between desired future behaviors of the child and the consequences that the child will receive when those behaviors occur. Contracts can utilize points, stars, stickers, checklists, or simple statements. Figure 10–1 shows such a contract. The older the child, the more extensively the child should be involved in

NAME: David

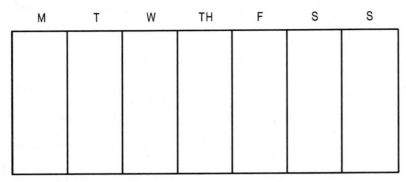

A gold star means playing nicely in the play room for 15 minutes.
   No teasing
   No hitting
   Sharing toys
6 stars = a trip to the cafeteria

Figure 10–1. Contract one.

negotiating the contract (Patterson, 1975). The contract is a positive list of desired behaviors rather than a list of don'ts. The steps are small and specific so that the child can earn the first backup reinforcer within three days. Creative, colorful charts can use pictures to identify desired behavior, or the chart itself can be made in the shape of an animal, airplane, train, or other age-appropriate item.

When implementing a contract, nurses must remain objective when a behavior does not occur and should not lecture or scold the child. Neither should nurses debate or argue with the child over points. The nurse's word is final.

Ignoring

A child will work for attention from others regardless of whether that attention is positive or negative. If a child does not receive positive attention, the child will act inappropriately in order to receive negative attention, which is considered better than no attention at all (Patterson, 1975; Webster-Stratton, 1983a). When nurses pay attention to misbehavior, they are teaching the child that misbehavior will be rewarded. By decreasing the supply of attention for disruptive behavior through ignoring (extinction), the chance the misbehavior will occur again decreases. Tantrums, whining, sulking, and swearing are best ignored. These behaviors,

although disruptive, rarely hurt anyone and usually disappear if systematically ignored. However, staff should be forewarned that ignored behaviors often get worse before they get better and that behavior change will be gradual. Ignoring requires a conscientious effort from all individuals who interact with the child. Consistency and cooperation are essential if a behavior is to be ignored immediately and every time it occurs. Effective ignoring requires that one not look at, speak to, or touch the child.

Punishment

The use of punishment methods with children usually involves one of two procedures: (1) removal of positive reinforcers or (2) the presentation of unpleasant events following a behavior. One form of punishment is termed response cost. This involves the removal or loss of previously earned tokens or points (Fig. 10–2). Response cost increases the effectiveness of secondary reinforcement systems because a reinforcer is withdrawn (Barkley, 1981).

Another form of punishment that involves the removal of positive events is called Time Out or time out from reinforcement (Patterson, 1975). The child is moved from a situation that is reinforcing problem behavior to one that is not at all reinforcing. Time Out is most appropriate for behavior that cannot be ignored, such as hitting, property destruc-

NAME: Jane

BEHAVIOR (EARNS POSSIBLE POINTS)		M	T	W	TH	F	S	S
Brush teeth	(+1)							
Takes Medicine	(3+) 8:00							
	(3+) 12:00							
	(3+) 4:00							
	(3+) 8:00							
Eats all breakfast	(+2)							
Eats 1/2 lunch	(+2)							
Eats all lunch	(+4)							
Eats 1/2 dinner	(+2)							
Eats all dinner	(+4)							
Eats all snacks	(+2) 10:00							
	3:00							
Participates with physical therapy	(+3)							
Takes bath	(+1)							
BEHAVIOR (LOSES POSSIBLE POINTS)								
SPITS OUT MEDICINE	(−4)							
TOTAL								

14 points = 1/2 hour later bedtime

18 points = 1/2 hour computer game

22 points = 1/2 hour off unit with

primary nurse

Figure 10–2. Contract two.

tion, stealing, or noncompliance. It is effective for children ages two to 12 years and for one or two behaviors at a time (Webster-Stratton, 1983a). Patterson (1975) recommends the bathroom as the ideal place for Time Out because it is dull, boring, and symbolizes all that is nonreinforcing. The Time Out place must be free of books, television, toys, and especially people. In the hospital, the bathroom can also serve as Time Out. If the child is on bed rest, the child's bed can become Time Out by removing all play articles, drawing the privacy curtain, and removing people from the room. Time Out is used for three to five minutes only. To be effective, it must be used every time the identified behavior occurs. Setting a kitchen timer at the beginning of Time Out clearly signals the end of Time Out for both staff and child.

Before a Time Out program is begun, a reinforcement contract should be in place strengthening the prosocial behavior that is replacing the disruptive, inappropriate behavior. The arrangement for Time Out is explained to the child before it is used, as suggested in the following example:

I know you have trouble playing nicely with other people. You have problems hitting and kicking other children. I also know you are tired of having the staff scold you. We have a program that will help you practice not hitting or kicking people.

First, every time you are in the playroom, you will earn one star if you play without hitting or kicking anyone. Each star is worth five points. Each time you hit or kick, you will lose one point. We will keep track on this chart in the playroom. When you have earned 20 points, you can leave the unit with your nurse, or have a comic book, or a special treat. To help with the practice, we are also going to use Time Out. Each time you hit or kick someone, we will tell you and then you go to Time Out. We will set the timer so that it rings at the end of five minutes. You go into your bathroom and wait for it to go off, then you come out.

Once Time Out has been implemented, a child may try to argue or insist upon debating the situation. This behavior is ignored and the nurse can state, "For every 15 seconds it takes you to get to Time Out, you have one more minute in Time Out." The nurse ignores the child's arguments except to state, "One minute more, two minutes more." If the child does not go into Time Out after receiving 20 minutes of Time Out, the child is informed that if he or she does not go into Time Out within one minute, playroom privileges will be lost for the rest of the day (or there will be some other consequence). The nurse waits for one more minute and then walks away. The child is not dragged into Time Out. Many children will kick the door, run the water in the bathroom, yell, or cry. This time is added on to the total time and the child is informed that Time Out will not be over until there is quiet. If a mess is made in the bathroom, the child is told that the bathroom must be cleaned before he or she can return to the playroom. The child is told where the nurse will be so that the child's return to the playroom can be approved. The child should not be reprimanded when Time Out is over. When appropriate behavior (sharing, sitting quietly) is displayed, this behavior should be praised.

One method of punishment that involves the presentation of an aversive event to a child upon the occurrence of disruptive, inappropriate behavior is the verbal reprimand. A verbal reprimand involves the use of a loud tone of voice; a verbal statement conveying disapproval; and a clear, direct, and specific command. It is most effective if used with a single child rather than a group of children and if the adult establishes eye contact with the child (Barkley, 1981). Examples of verbal reprimands are "No spitting!" and "No hitting!" A progression to a statement of consequences may or may not be necessary depending upon the child's response.

The use of punishment with hospitalized children is effective when the punishment occurs immediately following the misbehavior. It should be used consistently every time the behavior occurs. Simultaneous use of reinforcement for the alternative appropriate behavior is always recommended when a punishment approach is used.

Cognitive-Behavioral Intervention

Cognitive-behavioral intervention focuses on the training of thinking processes in order to modify a child's behavior. Typical interventions include self-instruction, problem-solving training, and social perspective–taking training (Kendall, 1984). Usual techniques include modeling by the trainer, to demonstrate strategies for dealing with situations, and role play procedures, which provide the child with opportunities to practice the newly acquired skills. The trainer provides feedback and encouragement while the child thinks out loud and evaluates the performance. Rewards are earned for accurate self-evaluation. Errors result in the loss of rewards. For example, an impulsive child can be taught on task behavior and learn to "think before acting" through the use of modeling, self-instruction, and reinforcement.

Cognitive-behavioral approaches can be adopted to teach hospitalized children frustration management skills. Such skills might lead to behavioral control and reduction in disruptive behavior. Achieving tolerance for frustrating events involves the personal acceptance that frustration is a normal part of life and an understanding of one's own threshold for emotional upset. This requires a realization that frustration is not a function of personal failure, does not reflect on one's self-worth, and cannot be avoided when facing life. Common methods that children use to deal with frustration are avoidance or violence. Teaching children alternatives to these methods can effectively reduce disruptive behavior.

Forsyth et al. (1984) in their study of chronically ill adults discovered that these adults redefined "normal" for themselves through cognitive efforts. They were realistic about limitations and frankly confronted the facts of the illness. In addition, these adults knew what was necessary to function in important areas of their lives. They adopted attitudes which conveyed that they were not helpless victims of a progressive illness but were "vying for a winning position." Such self-defined normality reordered their life values and views on accomplishments and thereby decreased frustration. For children, frustration tolerance can be modified by using role play and discussion techniques to meet specific objectives. One such objective might be to refocus the child's thinking from what the child did not accomplish to what the child did accomplish. For example, refocusing the child's thinking from what the child did not eat at mealtime to what the child did eat or from how the child pulled out the intravenous feeding line to how long the feeding line was intact would meet this objective. A second objective could be to assist the child to determine alternative methods to achieve a goal. For example, a child's goal might be to increase food intake. Strategies to achieve this goal might be to eat several small meals a day, select favorite foods from the menu, or ask the child's mother to prepare foods from home or bring in food from the child's favorite restaurant. A final objective in frustration tolerance is to revise a goal when the child is excluded, expelled, or refused participation in any activity. For example, the child's goal may be to go to the playroom for the child's birthday party. However, the child is still on bed rest. A revised goal might be to have the party in the child's room. Frustration tolerance can modify disruptive behavior because the child establishes realistic expectations for himself or herself and learns to focus on strengths rather than weaknesses.

Problem-solving approaches also help the child to reason and to verbalize about aspects of this behavior and encourages the child to discover alternative actions (Chazan et al., 1983). A problem-solving approach can lead to flexible thinking, and it demonstrates to children that there are multifaceted ways to solve a particular problem satisfactorily. Such strategies involve having the child determine the problem, list methods to solve the problem, determine consequences for each solution, and choose the best alternative to solve the problem. This approach effectively decreases inappropriate behavior because the child learns alternative

methods of interaction. The child also learns to articulate and analyze problems.

Variables Related to Behavior Management

There are numerous psychological variables which affect implementation of management strategies for disruptive, inappropriate behavior. Many of these are related to the stress of hospitalization for children, which is well documented in the pediatric literature. Consequently, rooming in, therapeutic play, communication strategies, and individualized preparation for procedures have been established as methods of intervention to minimize the stresses of hospitalization. Three other variables affecting behavioral control in pediatric patients and thereby reducing disruptive behavior are the family relationship structure, the setting, and the nature of illness.

Family Relationship Structure

Parental involvement in hospitalization minimizes emotional trauma to the child (Petrillo and Sanger, 1980). In addition, parents can be effective behavior change agents. Their knowledge of the child is of considerable value in assessing and managing disruptive behavior. However, in this age of separation, single-parent families, divorce, and reconstituted families, such support may be inconsistent at best. Parental involvement in the child's hospitalization may be compromised by a number of factors, including visiting and custody arrangements, finances, work responsibilities, interpersonal relationships, and relocation to another city or state.

Children confronted with separation, divorce, or reconstituted families often display significant behavior changes (Wallerstein and Kelly, 1980). When compounded by illness and hospitalization, it is expected that the child's reactions will multiply. Hostility, anger, and fear are not uncommon emotions in such situations, and disruptive, inappropriate behavior may intensify, particularly following parental visits.

Seegel (1978) relates that hospitalization of one's child causes concern, apprehension, and guilt for parents. These emotions are mangnified for the single parent, who may already be stressed by financial worries, care of siblings, and conflicts of responsibility. Such parents may interpret the child's hostility and negativity as rejection. They need help in understanding the nature of the child's behavior and should be given support for their efforts to manage a complex situation. They may also require assistance in learning how to manage the child's behavior.

Nurses can effectively link the child and an absent parent by using strategies that involve the parent in the child's care. White et al. (1983) found that hospitalized children who heard a bedtime story recorded by a parent fell asleep more quickly and slept longer than children who did not hear the story. This strategy appeared to help children cope with the immediate separation experience.

Stepparents may not have the same emotional attachment to a child and consequently may not provide the needed support for behavior change. Their relationship with the child may be compounded by relationships with half-siblings or stepsiblings, and they may question their role in the support of the hospitalized child. Nurses can involve stepparents with the child's care, reinforce efforts to support the child, and discuss effective strategies of behavior management.

Some families are not able to provide support for positive behavior change because the family is dysfunctional. Such families are characterized by chaos and unpredictability, poor communication patterns, unyielding responses to change, and power struggles (Steinhauer, 1977). Barron and Earls (1984), in their epidemiological survey of three year old children, related high family stress, negative parent-child interactions, and inflexibility of the child to poor behavior adjustment in the children. Knowledge of parent-child communications assists nurses in offering specific guidance to parents on ways of communication which maximize a child's development. In addition, fostering parent-child communication which conveys responsiveness to the child's concerns may help the child to accept new experiences in the hospital more easily (O'Brien, 1980).

Family structure and relationships influence assessment and evaluation methods. Collecting accurate data about prehospitalization behaviors or validating perceptions with a family member is often limited by complex visiting arrangements. Similarly, nurses may unknowingly approach a stepparent when the natural parent has the baseline information. Family members may unconsciously sabotage a behavior change plan because of their own needs or pathology. While competing for the child's affection, parents may bring in "goodies" for the child and thereby decrease the effectiveness of reinforcers. Similarly, punishment consequences may be used inconsistently.

For these reasons, nurses must be knowledgeable about family relationship structure. Establishing visitation guidelines for complex family situations may help to minimize disruptive behavior. Such guidelines should take into consideration the custody status of the child, visitor history, and the child's preferences and reactions. Examples of guidelines include establishing separate visiting times for all parties involved, monitoring visitors, establishing a visitor record, and setting limits on disruptive visitors (Coucouvanis and Solomons, 1983).

Parental support for behavior change is essential. Involving parents in determining and implementing consequences facilitates the management of disruptive behavior. Parents can be reminded that it is in the best interests of the child for family members to unite in support of the behavior change plan.

Setting

The hospital setting directly affects the application of managing disruptive, inappropriate behavior. Although multiple factors in the setting influence intervention strategies, four will be discussed here: (1) nurses' attitudes, (2) time structure, (3) play activities, and (4) rules.

NURSES' ATTITUDES

Determining how to give help to an individual disruptive child while having to care for the needs of many others taxes the skills of even the most empathic nurse. Disruptive behavior evokes strong emotions from nurses. Feelings of anger and frustration can be exacerbated by tight schedules, minimal staff, and acutely ill patients. Frustration and intolerance are common reactions to children who are uncooperative, hostile, demanding, and rejecting of the nurse's offer to help. Nurses may feel little compassion for these children and convey their skepticism and dissatisfaction through their lack of attention and concern. In addition, physical attractiveness of the pediatric patient influences how nurses assign responsibility for disturbances. The attractive patient is perceived by nurses to be less personally responsible for the negative behavior and situational causes are instead blamed, whereas an unattractive patient is reported by nurses to have a higher probability of emotional problems (Bordieri et al., 1985).

Nurses may become angry with the disruptive child and strongly critical of the child's functioning. Too often nurses engage in misguided and counterproductive psychological "prosecutions" of parents and the disruptive child during hospitalization. Many parents are already guilt-ridden and depressed over their child's illness and their inability to manage the child. Nurses' attitudes of faultfinding only reinforce these guilt feelings. Parents as well as nurses need reminders that they are not directly to blame for the disruptive behavior, but that the ways in which they choose to manage the behavior can make the problem better or worse. Nurses must adopt an attitude that is empathic, supportive, and constructive. The nurse's own emotional maturity and stability are essential. A tremendous amount of energy is also an asset. When parents are drained physically and emotionally, nurses also experience stress, which affects energy levels. Because of this demand, care for the caregivers is a necessity (Golub and Loizzo, 1985). Nurses must respond to the needs of their colleagues promptly and appropriately with evidence of support and encouragement. Peer support groups, which foster sharing of ideas and feelings; assigning a "relief" primary nurse; volunteering to help with tasks on an especially busy day; and words of praise are methods of giving such support.

TIME STRUCTURE

Hospitalization for children represents a complete disruption of their normal activities. The familiar time structure with which children have organized their day vanishes. Although nursing staff may be aware of the daily hospital routine, frequently the child is not (Volz, 1981). The loss of this familiar time structure has grave consequences for the child with hyperactive, impulsive behavior. Such children can disrupt an entire unit overnight unless strategies are implemented to increase structure. In addition, increasing a child's feeling of control over his or her environment may decrease situational disruptive behavior. Volz (1981) recommends creating a daily plan and a weekly or monthly calendar to assist the child to manage time. Suggested activities to include are (1) routine hospital activities (vital signs, meals, physician visits, medications, tests); (2) favorite television programs; (3) visitors; (4) playroom time; (5) schoolwork; and (6) phone calls. Identifying the activities through pictures in the correct time sequence is recommended for the child who cannot tell time or read.

When preparing the time schedule for the impulsive child with a short attention span, one often discovers long periods of free time. If large blocks of unscheduled time are allowed, disruptive behavior is likely to occur (White, 1983). Instead, this child can be assigned the role of helper, depending upon the child's level of wellness. Appropriate tasks might include watering plants, giving unit tours, distributing books and magazines, stapling memos, or going on office "rounds." Activities are limited only by the nurse's creativity and the child's attention span. Although staff may believe that preparing schedules is time-consuming, it is important to emphasize that schedules conserve time and energy in the long run because less time is spent managing disruptive behavior.

PLAY ACTIVITIES

Every pediatric nurse recognizes that socialization and play activities are essential for children's development. The challenge to pediatric nurses is the child who disrupts such activities either because of aggressive, impulsive behavior or short attention span and low frustration tolerance. Instead of banning such children from the playroom and restricting their use of all games, the nurse can restructure the play environment.

First of all, the disruptive child can be brought to the play area when only one or two select peers are present. This decreases the amount and kind of environmental stimulation. Because of the child's immaturity, slightly younger peers may be a better match of skills and abilities (White, 1983). While in the play area, positive reinforcement methods can be utilized for appropriate behavior. Appropriate games for the impulsive child have large pieces, simple rules, and do not require extensive counting. Two popular examples are the games Goldilocks and the Three Bears and Candyland. Other suggestions for structured activities include playing with puppets; putting together puzzles with large pieces; drawing with large crayons; modeling with clay; building with large blocks; building models that snap, not glue; and cutting and pasting collages.

Physical activity for the hyperactive child should be well planned. Encouraging this child to "run off steam" is not recommended because the overstimulation can be overwhelming and the child may return more excited and out of control than before. In addition, some physical activities can be a source of failure because of the child's poor fine and gross motor coordination. A structured physical activity program might include dancing, waterplay, supervised weight lifting, or riding on an exercise bicycle. For a more complete discussion of peer relations and therapeutic play, see Chapters 7 and 13.

RULES

Identifying which hospital rules are most important and giving the child clear, direct, and specific directions about those rules are imperative in managing disruptive behavior. When directions are unclear, nurses find they have to give the directions several times before a child complies. Some nurses may give too many commands and may be too authoritarian. They must be helped to decrease the number of directions to those that are most important. Rules that change from shift to shift and from nurse to nurse encourage confusion, manipulation, and testing by the child. Rules, or directions, should be stated positively; the nurse could say, for example, "Hands should stay by your side." When a confrontation occurs, the child's safety and self-esteem must be considered (Lamb and Rodgers, 1983). Removing the audience decreases the child's feelings of guilt and shame when the child acts in an inappropriate manner. The nurse should not try to reason the child out of any emotions, including anger, but can encourage talking about the child's feelings.

To prevent the child from harm, the nurse can utilize positive statements and physical intervention or restraint: "I understand you are angry, but I am not going to let you hurt yourself. I am going to hold your hands until you can hold them yourself." The nurse may also intervene to protect possessions valuable to the child: "I know this is important to you so I'm not going to let you break it." Demanding total obedience or forcing apologies or admissions of guilt from the child are inappropriate. These responses merely reflect the nurse's need to control.

Nurses' attitudes, time structure, play activities, and rules are four variables within the pediatric setting that can be modified to manage disruptive behavior. Making such arrangements is prudent yet creative nursing practice.

Nature of Illness

While the nature of illness affects each child differently, those children with a chronic or progressive disease require flexible, unique strategies for managing disruptive behavior. By its very nature, chronic illness represents constant stress. Using this knowledge in managing disruptive behavior is judicious nursing practice. The child with chronic or progressive illness is frequently removed from the mainstream of normal childhood activities without warning. Because of repeated and lengthy hospitalizations, the child may have limited insight into what it is like to be a member of a family (Steele, 1977) or to interact with peers in school. When the child begins to understand the ramifications of the disease, the child often becomes depressed and experiences difficulty in accepting the illness. Such depression may be visible through a change in behavior, agitation, hostility, or aggressive behavior (Rodgers et al., 1981). The child may experience intense anger because of an inability to cope with an altered self-image, and such intractable anger is never resolved entirely (Duer-Hefele et al., 1985). In addition, chronic illness affects the lifestyle of the child and the family. Established schedules and plans are often disrupted or canceled because of an exacerbation of the disease. Role expectations and assignments may shift. For example, siblings instead of parents may prepare meals. Money for leisure activities is often spent for medication and treatments while socialization patterns are restricted by treatment regimens and disease symptoms (Forsyth et al., 1984). Subsequent management strategies will capitalize on the child's strengths and mobilize the child's resources.

Behavior management plans require frequent modifications as typical reinforcers lose their effectiveness. Creative thinking will be necessary to determine alternate strategies. In addition, goals for nursing care will reflect management rather than resolution of disruptive behavior. Because of repeated hospitalizations, the child will be well aware of his or her rights, the rules, and hospital routines. Consequently, interactions with staff can be expected to be authoritarian, directive, and manipulative. This child will respond best to regular, predictable events over which he or she has specifically defined control. Such programs of care should foster the development and expression of autonomy, which is important in developing a sense of self, self-esteem, and the ability to learn and manage one's social and technical worth.

EVALUATION

Using change-in-behavior measurements is a preferable method of measuring outcomes that offers greater specificity and objectivity. This evaluation method incorporates preintervention and postintervention data sets. A baseline of behavior for a specific child is established by comparing the child's present behavior with past behavior patterns, with common patterns observed in other patients, or with response patterns described in the literature. The optimal method for determining a baseline measurement is through monitoring or counting the frequency of an identified behavior's occurrence. This target behavior, as well as the alternative behavior, is defined in observable terms and counted for a specified time period. Ideally, the monitoring record should also reflect the time the behavior occurred, the precipitating events, and the consequences. This baseline information is recorded for 48 to 72 hours prior to implementing any behavior management program. This evaluation strategy is particularly recommended for the child with a long-standing history of behavior problems. The effec-

tiveness of the intervention is then measured by comparing baseline data with postintervention data.

Case Study

After years of chronic pyelonephritis, Vicki, 12 years of age, was hospitalized for a kidney transplant. In addition, she had moderate learning disabilities. Because of frequent hospitalization, she was familiar with hospital routines.

Following her transplant, Vicki was up and about in record time, running up and down the halls, disappearing into other patients' rooms, and scurrying behind the nurses' station. She had frequent short-lived tantrums during which she screamed and threw her stuffed elephant. Although these behaviors were disruptive, the fact that Vicki clamped her mouth shut at the sight of medications or spit them out was of the most concern. Vicki would do anything to refuse her medicine. In addition, she was compulsive about her schedule and the order in which tasks were completed. She rarely napped during the day and was always up and about when the midnight shift reported for work. Her parents were divorced, and Vicki lived with her mother. Although initially supportive, both parents had reduced their visits to weekends only.

The primary nursing diagnoses for Vicki's numerous disruptive behaviors were (1) *Noncompliance with treatment regimen* and (2) *Sensory perceptual alteration resulting from a restricted environment.* A comprehensive care plan targeted compliance with medications and appropriate use of free time for structured intervention. Vicki's primary nurse discussed with Vicki the times Vicki was most willing to take her medicine. Together, they developed the medication routine, and Vicki began on a reinforcement contract. Figure 10–3 shows that contract. For the first three days of the contract, Vicki earned points only, and after three days, response cost was initiated. Staff did not plead with, bargain with, force, or argue with Vicki to take her medication. She was matter-of-factly reminded of her contract and given 60 seconds to comply. If Vicki chose not to take her pills, staff immediately left her room and ignored Vicki for ten minutes. When Vicki swallowed her medicine, she was praised, given a hug, and the nurse stayed for 15 minutes to play games and read stories. It was understood that the nurse planned her daily routine so that she had 15 free minutes at Vicki's medication times. Because of the perceived benefit to everyone on the unit, the rest of the staff supported this approach. This consensus was reached at a patient care conference and reinforced at daily shift report.

In addition, a daily schedule was planned every morning by the primary nurse and Vicki. They planned the entire day's activities, including free

Name: Vicki   (Week 1)
Behavior (Points)

Behavior (Points)		M	T	W	TH	F	S	S
Takes pills	(3) 9:00	0	3	3	3	3		
	(3) 1:00	0	0	3	-1	-1		
	(3) 5:00	3	3	0	3	-1		
	(3) 9:00	0	3	3	3	3		

Vicki loses one point when she does not take
her pills (starts Thursday).

Figure 10–3. Contract three.

Points earned and spent: 卌 卌 卌 卌 卌 卌 卌 III II III IIII

9 points = 1/2 hour walk with Karen
12 points = phone call home
15 points = $.25 trip to gift shop

time. The schedule was written in 15 minute segments because of Vicki's limited attention span. Vicki had a paper copy of the schedule with her at all times. She crossed off activities as they were completed. Staff asked to see the schedule when she appeared to be "off track" and matter-of-factly reminded her where she was supposed to be according to her schedule. The final point in Vicki's care plan was that tantrums were ignored and verbal expression of every type of feeling was rewarded.

Vicki responded very quickly to the increased structure in her day and the positive reinforcement. She thrived on the attention of staff and other patients. Ensuring that she received attention for only positive, appropriate behavior was a challenge for the staff. Some staff needed reminders not to give Vicki attention for her disruptive behavior. By the end of five days, Vicki showed 63% compliance with her medications, compared with 25% prior to initiation of the contract. She was enthusiastic about her progress, and the nurses were clearly satisfied with the decrease in disruptive behavior.

RESEARCH IMPLICATIONS

The most crucial need for research is the description of "normal" behavior of children who are experiencing health-related problems. Further analysis of disruptive behavior might refine this definition and establish norms of disruptive behavior for identified age groups, settings, health status, and developmental levels. Additional information is needed about the reliability and validity of behavior rating scales and other assessment tools.

Although management of children's disruptive behavior has been researched in home, classroom, and community settings, limited data-based reports are available regarding the effectiveness of these strategies in the hospital setting. Consequently, additional research in this area is needed. First, study might identify variables in the hospital setting which affect specific management strategies. Second, exploration of nurse perceptions and attitudes towards disruptive behavior, as well as the effect of those perceptions upon nursing care, is indicated. Longitudinal studies of chronic and progressive illness are needed to describe their relationship to disruptive behavior. Last, a comparative analysis of alternative management strategies would determine the effectiveness of specific interventions.

References

Armstrong, GD, Wirt, RD, Nesbit, ME, and Martinson, IM. Multidimensional assessment of psychological problems in children with cancer. Research in Nursing and Health, 5:205–211, 1982.

Ayllon, T, and Simon, SJ. Behavior therapy with children. In Lachenmeyer, JR, and Gibbs, MS (Eds.), Psychopathology in childhood. New York: Gardner Press, Inc., 1982, pp. 272–279.

Bandura, A. Social learning theory. Englewood Cliffs, N.J.: Prentice-Hall, Inc., 1977.

Barkley, RA. Hyperactive children: A handbook for diagnosis and treatment. New York: The Guilford Press, 1981.

Barron, AP, and Earls, F. The relation of temperament and social factors to behavior problems in three-year-old children. Journal of Child Psychology and Psychiatry, 25:23–33, 1984.

Belmont, HS. Hospitalization and its effects upon the total child. Clinical Pediatrics, 9:472–483, 1970.

Bordieri, JE, Solodky, ML, and Mikos, KA. Physical attractiveness and nurses' perceptions of pediatric patients. Nursing Research, 34:24–26, 1985.

Brink, RE. How serious is the child's behavior problem? MCN: American Journal of Maternal Child Nursing, 1:33–36, 1982.

Bumbalo, JA, and Siemon, MK. Nursing assessment and diagnosis: Mental health problems of children. Topics in Clinical Nursing, 5:41–51, 1983.

Chazan, M, Laing, AF, Jones, J, Harper, GC, and Bolton, J. The management of behavior problems in young children. Early Child Development and Care, 11:227–244, 1983.

Chess, S, and Thomas, A. Origins and evolutions of behavior disorders: From infancy to early adult life. New York: Brunner/Mazel, Inc., 1984.

Coucouvanis, JA, and Solomons, HC. Handling complicated visitation problems of hospitalized children. MCN: American Journal of Maternal Child Nursing, 83:132–134, 1983.

Cullinan, D, Epstein, MH, and Lloyd, JW. Behavior disorders of children and adolescents. Englewood Cliffs, N.J.: Prentice-Hall, Inc., 1983.

de Mello Vianna, F. (Ed.). Roget's II: The New Thesaurus. Boston: Houghton Mifflin Co., 1980.

Duer-Hefele, JT, Ekstrom, DN, Fisher, M, and Hertenstein, CJ. Managing intractable anger. MCN: American Journal of Maternal Child Nursing, 10:328–332, 1985.

Elliot, CH, and Olson, RA. The management of children's distress in response to painful medical treatment for burn injuries. Behavior Research and Therapy, 21:675–683, 1983.

Forsyth, GL, Delaney, KD, and Gresham, ML. Vying for a winning position: Management style of the chronically ill. Research in Nursing and Health, 7:181–188, 1984.

Gohsman, B. The hospitalized child and the need for mastery. Issues in Comprehensive Pediatric Nursing, 5:67–76, 1981.

Golub, L, and Loizzo, K. The ripple effect of anger. MCN: American Journal of Maternal Child Nursing, 6:333–336, 1985.

Jay, SM, Elliot, CH, Ozolins, M, Olson, RA, and Pruitt, SD. Behavioral management of children's distress during painful medical procedures. Behavior Research and Therapy, 23:513–520, 1985.

Kendall, PC. Annotation cognitive-behavioral self-control therapy for children. Journal of Child Psychology and Psychiatry, 25:173–179, 1984.

Kim, MJ, McFarland, GK, and McLane, AM. Pocket guide to nursing diagnosis. St. Louis: CV Mosby Co., 1984.

Kumchy, CIG, and Kores, PJ. Behavioral management of a neurologically impaired pediatric inpatient. Archives of Physical Medicine and Rehabilitation, 62:289–291, 1981.

Lamb, JM, and Rodgers, DR. Assisting the hostile hospitalized child. MCN: American Journal of Maternal Child Nursing, 8:336–339, 1983.

McGee, JP, and Saidel, DH. Individual behavior therapy. In Harrison, SI (Ed.), Basic handbook of child psychiatry (Vol. 3). New York: Basic Books, Inc., 1979, pp. 72–105.

Moore, DR. Childhood behavior problems: A social learning perspective. In Lackenmeyer, JR, and Gibbs, MS (Eds.), Psychopathology in childhood. New York: Gardner Press, Inc., 1982, pp. 211–243.

Morris, W. (Ed.). The American heritage dictionary of the English language. Boston: Houghton Mifflin Co., 1976.

O'Brien, RA. Relationship of parent-child communication to child's exploratory behavior and self-differentiation. Nursing Research, 29:150–156, 1980.

Patterson, GR. Families. Champaign, Ill.: Research Press, 1975.

Petrillo, M, and Sanger, S. Emotional care of hospitalized children (2nd ed.). Philadelphia: JB Lippincott Co., 1980.

Ritchie, JA, Vaty, S, and Ellerton, ML. Concerns of acutely ill, chronically ill, and healthy preschool children. Research in Nursing and Health, 7:265–274, 1984.

Robinson, MA, and Siemon, M. A nursing assessment of children. In Babich, KS (Ed.), A workbook: Assessing the mental health of children. Boulder, Colo.: Western Interstate Commission for Higher Education, 1982, pp. 23–30.

Rodgers, BM, Hillemeier, MM, O'Neill, E, and Slonim, MB. Depression in the chronically ill or handicapped school-aged child. MCN: American Journal of Maternal Child Nursing, 6:266–273, 1981.

Schroeder, CS, Gordon, BN, Kanoy, K, and Routh, DK. Managing children's behavior problems in pediatric practice. Advances in Development and Behavioral Pediatrics, 4:25–86, 1983.

Seegel, VF. The divorced parent and the hospitalized child: Implications for the hospital staff. Journal of the Association for Care of Children in the Hospital, 1:16–18, 1978.

Steele, S. General ideas in relation to long-term illness in childhood. In Steele, S (Ed.), Nursing care of the child with long-term illness (2nd ed.). New York: Appleton-Century-Crofts, 1977, pp. 107–152.

Steinhauer, PD. The child and his family. In Steinhauer, PD, and Rae-Grant, Q (Eds.), Psychological problems of the child and his family. Toronto: Macmillan of Canada, 1977, pp. 49–70.

Tesler, M, and Savedra, M. Coping with hospitalization: A study of school-age children. Pediatric Nursing, 7:35–38, 1981.

Van Leeuwen, J. Hospitalization and its meaning to the child and his family. In Steinhauer, PD, and Rae-Grant, Q (Eds.), Psychological problems of the child and his family. Toronto: Macmillan of Canada, 1977.

Volz, DD. Time structuring for hospitalized school-aged children. Issues in Comprehensive Pediatric Nursing, 5:205–210, 1981.

Vulcan, B. Major coping behaviors of a hospitalized 3-year old boy. Maternal-Child Nursing Journal, 13:113–123, 1984.

Wallerstein, JS, and Kelly, JB. Surviving the breakup: How children and parents cope with divorce. New York: Basic Books, Inc., 1980.

Webster-Stratton, C. Intervention approaches to conduct disorders in young children. Nurse Practitioner, 8:23–34, 1983a.

Webster-Stratton, C. Recognizing and assessing conduct disorders in children. MCN: American Journal of Maternal Child Nursing, 8:330–335, 1983b.

White, JE. Special nursing needs of hospitalized children with learning disabilities. American Journal of Maternal Child Nursing, 8:209–212, 1983.

White, MA, Wear, E, and Stephenson, G. A computer-compatible method of observing falling asleep behavior of hospitalized children. Research in Nursing and Health, 6:191–198, 1983.

CHAPTER 11

INTERCULTURAL COMMUNICATION

ANN R. SLOAT, M.S., M.A., R.N., and
WYNETTA MATSUURA, M.S., M.P.H., C.P.N.P.,
R.N.

Children present a unique and complex set of circumstances when they are sick. More so than for adults, children's social attachments to their primary caretakers require that they be viewed not only as individuals but also as inseparable from the family. This family holds a set of belief systems, values, and notions about health and illness that may be very different from those of the nurse or of the dominant culture. Because effective communication sets the tone for and is the foundation of nursing care, exploration of the influence a different culture has on the communication process is both timely and relevant.

Nurses consider a multitude of variables in their initial and ongoing assessment of the family to effectively implement a therapeutic plan of care. For example, the nurse considers the child's developmental level and both the child's and family's knowledge, readiness, and ability to follow through with a treatment regimen. Nurses identify the family structure and relationships, especially as they relate to the child's attachments and dependency; the immediate biological or physical needs of the child; and the effects of illness on the child's behavior. This assessment requires or is predicated on the assumption that the patient, family, and professional nurse understand each other and are able to effectively exchange information. Awareness of cultural differences and a mechanism to bridge those differences through communication becomes essential. The purpose of this chapter is to present intervention strategies to reduce the negative consequences of impaired communication related to cultural factors. A model linking the concepts of culture and communication is presented as a theoretical framework from which to derive assessment categories, nursing diagnoses, and nursing interventions.

THEORETICAL FOUNDATION

Definition of Culture

Culture is a concept frequently used in nursing as if it were a discrete and well-defined phenomenon. In actuality, definitions of culture abound and may have mixed or competing orientations (see Aamodt, 1978; Leininger, 1978; Goodenough, 1981; and Langness, 1974 for an orientation to the concept of culture). One of the more comprehensive definitions incorporating both the adaptive-ecological orientation and the ideological orientation of what is meant by culture was offered by Porter in 1972:

> When I use the word "culture," I am referring to the cumulative deposit of knowledge, experience, meanings, beliefs, values, attitudes, religions, concepts of self, the universe and self-universe relationship, hierarchies of status, expectations, spatial relations, and time concepts acquired by a large group of people in the course of generations through individual and group striving. Culture manifests itself both in patterns of language and thought and in forms of activity and behavior (p. 3).

A careful reading of this definition makes it clear that culture mediates the whole of an individual's experience. It is also important to realize that culture is a dynamic phenomenon that is lived out through and continually being shaped by its members. Culture is persistent and enduring by virtue of its continual reinforcement. It is omnipresent, encompassing and specifying the social environment permeating our lives (Samovar and Porter, 1985, pp. 19–20).

Culture has also been described as a socially "inherited lens" (Helman, 1984, p. 2) or screen through which individuals perceive, understand, and filter information. In this context, the lens or screen represents the perceptual frame of reference, which is of critical importance in communication.

The function of this lens is to select what is paid attention to and what is ignored. The child learns these very basic foundations of his or her world view through the continuous exposure to his or her culture. Culture, for instance, defines for the child what is asthetically pleasing or attractive, what is valuable, what tastes good, and what is good behavior. At a deeper level, the culture encompasses the structure of the language and through this, what is symbolized and communicated and how information is classified (Goodenough, 1981). Culture, therefore, has profound influence on the communication process; learning about different cultures has tremendous potential for expanding the nurse's understanding of people's responses to illness.

Relationship of Culture to Development

The research of Piaget has shown that children think or mentally process information differently than adults (Cowan, 1978; Piaget and Inhelder, 1969). Children are both egocentric and ethnocentric by virtue of their developmental level. Depending on their age and experience, they have a more difficult time than adults in taking another point of view or realizing that another way of interpreting things exists. Very young children often seem to expect those around them to understand what they are thinking or feeling without the prerequisite exchange of information; it is as if others' experiences must be the same as theirs and therefore their understanding, pain, or unhappiness is also the same and automatically comprehended. Similarly, it is difficult for young children to comprehend that their language, gestures, and symbols, taught to them through their culture, are not universal.

Very young children are just beginning to incorporate language and other communication tools into the task of expressing their wants and needs and of getting those wants and needs responded to effectively. They rely on the close adults in their lives to interpret their signals and respond appropriately. Those who care for them learn what each little gesture means—whether a cry, facial expression, or made-up word. However, even parents, who know their children well, sometimes experience difficulty figuring out what a child is attempting to convey. Frustration, bewilderment and even anger are often the results of this miscommunication. Young children are particularly vulnerable to confusion, stress, and separation anxiety related to miscommunication. While their parents have learned to interpret their signals, the young children have learned what behaviors work to get them attention from their caretakers. Some of these behaviors may be very subtle, such as positioning themselves beside their mother when they want to be picked up or making a particular facial expression or cry to signal distress. Separation anxiety is compounded when a young child is hospitalized and these learned behaviors no longer have the effect intended.

School-aged children are more aware of the limitations of others in understanding what is going on inside their thoughts. They have a broader base of experience which has taught them the necessity of actively communicating their ideas. They have also learned how to incorporate the subtleties inherent in the setting or context of an interaction to make communication effective and appropriate in their culture, and they may be quite skilled at it. These contextual cues, however, may be both subtle and complex (O'Keefe and Delia, 1985) and include not only proper choice of vocabulary but also such things as how to frame a message. Rules governing the framing of a message may not be obvious and therefore may occur on a much less conscious level. For instance, although language differences are initially apparent, differences in how individuals view and assign meaning to events, context, and nonverbal cues are more difficult to identify. Children, for example, are likely to speak and behave differently when they interact with their parents or other elders, an asymmetrical interaction, than when they interact with peers. The social role of each participant is an important part of the context of interaction and has a powerful influence on children's communicative competence (Gleason and Perlmann, 1985).

Politeness and respect, critical elements of the communication process in any culture, are expressed differently depending on the circumstances. For instance, the Western child is told, "Look at me when I am talking to you," encouraging eye contact and directness as a sign of paying attention. In many non-Western cultures, however, directness is considered rude, as is looking someone in the eye. In some cultures, children are taught to avert their gaze and to look down when being addressed by an adult, especially one with authority. The Western nurse who is unaware of cultural differences might interpret this behavior as disinterest or disrespect or simply an inability or unwillingness to communicate. Culturally different school-aged children may be unaware that their behavior is being misinterpreted and unaware that they are missing the important messages that are being conveyed to them by gesture, setting, or circumstance. Likewise, because differences of this sort are relatively hidden, the health provider may not be sensitive to the separateness of the child's perspective. Intercultural communication with school-aged children depends to a large extent on establishing a common frame of reference as well as on being cognizant of the influence of the asymmetrical nature of the interaction on children's ability to express themselves.

Most likely, the child from a different culture will not have benefited from adequate preparation for care in a Western medical setting. Because of this lack of familiarity, the hospital or clinic may represent a strange and sometimes hostile environment. Hospitalized children are likely to experience intrusive procedures, be examined by people they do not know, and see and hear things which make no sense to them, all of which may occur without regard to any expression of protest. This inability to exercise control over what is happening is a threat to a child's sense of mastery. Culturally different children are even more disadvantaged in this situation because of their inability to fully benefit from explanations and other sources of help. They may lack the ability to effectively grasp and interpret their experience of illness and hospitalization because it does not fit within their pre-existing cultural frame of reference. Further, their coping skills, usually effective in helping them to learn from new experiences, reduce their stress, and develop new behaviors, are also compromised by illness and hospitalization. Family patterns become disrupted, and parents themselves feel powerless within the health care setting. This situation is confusing and disturbing to children who depend on family to buffer and protect them while they are learning to explore and negotiate directly with the strangeness and dangers of the larger society.

Relationship of Culture to Communication

Culture and communication are interlocking concepts that are difficult to separate conceptually. Every step of the communication process as well as the environment or context within which an interaction takes place is culturally determined. The relationship is circular; culture is perpetuated from one generation to the next through the act of communication, and communication— the code, the context, and the meaning of a message—is in turn culturally determined or defined.

The degree of similarity in the perceptions or frame of reference among communicators relates to the degree of accuracy with which decoding messages occurs. When people share a common frame of reference, communication flows relatively effortlessly. Contextual and nonverbal cues are often transmitted and received unconsciously. Singer (1985) points out that there is a high degree of comfort within one's own group because of the predictability of the patterns of communication behavior. He states that "it is precisely such shared, often inarticulated and sometimes unarticulatable patterns of perception, communication and behavior which are referred to as a 'culture'" (p. 65). For those sharing the same "lens and filter," effective interaction takes place without the awareness of cultural influence. This is not to imply that communication between members of the same group is a simple or uncomplicated process. Active listening and the process of clarification that is characteristic of good communication takes attentiveness, energy, and skill. When the nurse is interacting with a client of a different cultural background, however, culture and communication become inseparable components of the nursing care plan. A recognized goal of the nurse is to minimize the possible negative outcomes related to the circumstances surrounding the child's treatment regimen. This goal can be more difficult to realize, however, when the child or family speaks a different language or is from a different culture. If the nurse is unaware

of the influence of culture, there is potential for serious misunderstanding between the family and nurse; therefore, the nurse may be unable to use one of the most potent therapeutic tools—communication.

Model of Culture and Communication

The goal in intercultural communication is to achieve the highest degree possible of mutual understanding between culturally different communicators—in this instance, between the nurse and child patient. A model linking culture with the communication process is presented here to facilitate this mutual understanding. The model is based on the premises that (1) culture mediates all phases of the communication process; (2) contact between communicators is dynamic and interactive, with both the initiator and receiver sending and receiving information simultaneously; and (3) the communicators can create a zone of shared experience and perceptions from which to base effective exchanges of information.

As mentioned previously, culture mediates every step of the communication process. In the model presented in Figure 11–1, culture permeates all aspects of communication and is represented or depicted as the environment or context within which an interaction between the nurse and the culturally different child and family occurs. For the purpose of facilitating a systematic cultural assessment, cultural variables are categorized into antecedent conditions; interaction processes, including both the use of language and the importance of context for the attachment of meaning to an encounter; and the resultant consequence or outcome relating to the goal of mutual understanding. The child and family are depicted separately from the nurse, with the overlapping area representing identified areas of commonality and shared experience. Both participants are equally involved in establishing this zone of learning about each other and in being able to predict the other's responses, which form the basis of effective intercultural communication. This overlapping area may become wider as the nurse works with the child and the family in establishing creative and innovative ways to communicate.

The antecedent condition represents what is currently in place. The child's develop-

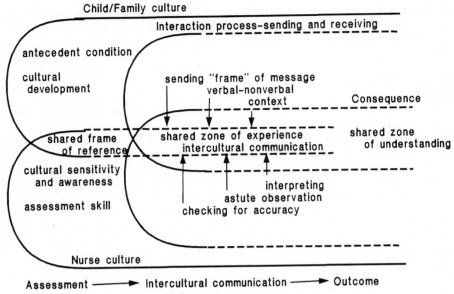

Figure 11–1. Intercultural communication.

mental level and other variables, such as the family's socioeconomic status, educational level, and amount of exposure to Western culture, are part of the antecedent conditions which could effect the quality of communication. The family's frame of reference or cultural lens is just as important as the usual variables assessed by nurses when the patient is from a different culture. The meaning of illness to the child and family, the health care model ascribed to by the family, and the caretakers' awareness of the biomedical model as a separate belief system are all part of the discrete environment that becomes the context for an interaction between the nurse, the child, and family.

The interaction process includes verbal and nonverbal language or cues as well as the context of the interaction. The importance of nonverbal communication and the critical importance of recognizing the child's ability to gain information from the context of an interaction, or how a message is framed, is stressed in this model. This framing of the message is accomplished by stressing the need to pay particular attention to environmental conditions and nonverbal cues which are present when interaction takes place. For instance, the tone of voice, the position (for example, sitting or standing) of the speaker, and the gender of the health provider may be important parts of the message. Further, the child may be pay-

ing close attention to what is happening to other children in the clinic or hospital—watching what is done to them and how they respond. Verbal interactions may be much less informative to the child than such observations as who speaks to whom, the sequence of the nurse's or doctor's activities, or what occurs in response to another child's crying.

The layout of the hospital unit or clinic, whether everything happens behind closed doors or whether most activities are visible or observable, may also be an important factor in the framing of a message and presence of cues. In addition, such things as the availability of chairs near the bedside often have more impact on visiting patterns than any encouragement the nurse might offer when there is obviously no room for parents to stay. If the unit looks like visitors are expected and welcomed, the verbal message will be consistent with the environmental cues.

In intercultural communication, the feedback mechanisms by which both parties can check the accuracy of their interpretations are confounded and require a more conscious effort. There is continuous sending and receiving of messages by both participants in the interaction process and a continuous attempt at decoding the intended meaning. The model in Figure 11–1 allows the nurse to focus on specific elements of the encounter in order to correct miscommunication.

The total intercultural communication process is shown in Figure 11–1. The outcome or consequence of successfully contrasting the frame of reference of the nurse and child or child's family and identifying or establishing an area of shared experience upon which to base efforts at communication is, it is hoped, effective intercultural communication leading to mutual understanding. The degree to which this goal is met will be reflected in the achievement of proposed outcomes. At the same time, efforts to be successful in communicating with the culturally different hospitalized child are compounded by the child's age (an antecedent condition) and the hospital setting (part of the context of the message), which is likely to be strange and unpredictable to the child.

Disease-Illness Distinction

The use of this model is predicated on the nurse differentiating between disease as it is defined in the biomedical sense and illness as experienced by the patient and family. Further, sensitivity to how children from other cultural backgrounds may differ in methods of communication is imperative. The following brief discussion elaborates these points.

The distinction between illness and disease fits well into a nursing paradigm. Dougherty and Tripp-Reimer (1985) point out that nurses mediate the biomedical and client orientations. Illness represents the client's point of view and is a subjective response to being unwell. This includes the response of the family and community, the interpretation of the origin and significance of the illness event, and how the event affects behavior and relationships (Helman, 1984; LaRargue, 1985). Disease is defined within the framework of modern medicine in terms of "abnormalities in the structure and function of body organs and systems" (Eisenberg, 1977, p. 11) and is based on such premises as scientific rationality, objectivity, and mind-body dualism (Helman, 1984). In this distinction, illnesses are posited as *experiences* and diseases are *entities*.

Cultural patterns influence every facet of the child's and family's response and experience of the illness episode. Cultural factors

determine if a symptom or symptoms will be interpreted as representing illness, how and what kind of help-seeking will take place, the manner in which symptoms are presented, and the expectations the child and family have of the health care providers. In this application of the culture and communication model, it is consideration of the illness rather than disease that most often takes precedence for the nurse. The manifestation of illness is determined by the family's beliefs and customs relating to health, causation of illness, and appropriate treatment: a folk model as opposed to a biomedical model. These variables are part of the antecedent condition about which the nurse must become knowledgeable in order to effectively communicate.

Language—Verbal

The most obvious barrier to communication between the nurse and the child and family of a different cultural background is the inability to understand and speak each other's verbal language. Young children of immigrant or refugee families may have little experience with English if they are cared for exclusively in the home where parents or caretakers converse in their native tongue. School-aged children may have reasonably competent English skills, depending upon their experience in the American educational system, but their parents may not be at all fluent or confident. The use of interpreters is sometimes imperative to convey and elicit complex information. The interpreter should be competent in both languages and ideally should be someone known and trusted by the child and family. Not all individuals are eager to share information with people they do not know simply because they speak the same language. Some cultures in particular may not be initially comfortable with strangers. For instance, distrust of strangers is part of Vietnamese cultural training and results from decades of war and wariness of spies and government informants (Hoskins, 1971). Additionally, class differences between the interpreter and client may add an element of intimidation and may influence how the message is translated. For these reasons, care should be given to choosing someone to translate and time taken to establish rapport between the client and interpreter when the interpreter is a stranger.

Language—Nonverbal and Contextual

Young children in most cultures rely heavily on nonverbal communication. Children are keen observers of body language and base their behavior as much on how and in what context something might have been said as on the verbal message itself. Even in western culture in which children are socialized into paying more attention to verbal language, the context and behavior of the communicators plus how the child views the meaning of the event play critical roles in developing meaning and interpreting the message.

It is essential for the nurse to realize the importance of nonverbal cues in intercultural communication. Within any group or society, nonverbal cues are often so subtle that they are unconscious, yet they account for the largest portion of communication that occurs (Singer, 1985). In many non-Western cultures, nonverbal or body language is emphasized for all age groups along with ritual and form as the dominant mode of expression for much of the day to day communication. This type of language is especially true for such things as addressing, greeting, and approaching others. The way a message is delivered may "speak louder" than what is actually said. Social etiquette, for example, is a major cultural variable influencing Vietnamese communication (Orque et al., 1983). For the Southeast Asian refugee, propriety and social harmony would take precedence over values a Western caretaker may hold, such as punctuality or forthrightness, in an interaction.

In some cultures, the way of showing agreement or dissent is different than in Western cultures. Western Americans expect a verbal yes or no in response to questions, especially when asking about a personal preference such as what is preferred to eat or whether a young patient would like to go to the playroom. The Vietnamese or other Asian child might respond with a nod of agreement so as not to offend or contradict the caretaker no matter what the question. A Samoan child might rely exclusively on nonverbal behavior to say yes (Metge and Kinloch, 1978) and be baffled at getting no

dessert or at being left behind when others are escorted out of the room to play. For many non-Western people, verbal behavior is not the dominant mode of expressing such things as comfort, instruction or caring, nor is it always the most effective method for the nurse to use to elicit critical information about such things as pain, distress, or a willingness to comply with a medical regimen. The nurse's attention to nonverbal behavior can help to bridge the language barrier and foster intercultural communication.

ASSESSMENT

The need for intercultural communication occurs when clients or nurses are attempting to function in a different culture. One could argue that this situation arises every time an infant, child, or parent has his or her first encounter with a hospital. Currently, there is no designated nursing diagnosis which describes communication impairment that is due to cultural differences. Therefore, the defining characteristics for impaired communication are only a beginning in the development of appropriate defining characteristics for the situation. These characteristics include the inability to speak the dominant language and an inability to name objects (Kim et al., 1984). Unfortunately, these characteristics deal strictly with language, which is only one component of culture.

Presently, then, the only available approach is the use of cultural sensitivity and awareness (Fig. 11–1) in assessment skills as the nurse determines the appropriate nursing diagnosis.

THE INTERVENTION

Orque et al. (1983) define intercultural communication as "the communication process occurring between a nurse and a patient, each with different cultural backgrounds, wherein each attempts to understand the other person's point of view from his or her own cultural frame of reference" (p. 18). Essential in this position is being aware of the cultural characteristics of both persons, contrasting these, and discovering areas of commonality. In order for this discovery to happen, the nurse must reduce his or her own ethnocentrism.

Ethnocentrism Reduction

Nurses can begin some essential intervention strategies before encountering a culturally different patient. These strategies relate to actively reducing ethnocentricity through examination of their own belief systems about health and how clients should behave. This process can be accomplished by identifying elements of their own cultures and how socialization has influenced their beliefs, health practices, and assumptions concerning what constitutes proper behavior for patients to exhibit. Members of a dominant culture, who have not had the opportunity or have not been required to question the origins or logic of their own position, may find this process particularly difficult.

Everyone, through cultural learning and through experiences, has acquired notions about people and places that are unfamiliar or different. Ideas and beliefs are necessary components of the general knowledge nurses have, but like all information, these ideas and beliefs require testing for accuracy and usefulness. Sometimes they are based on stereotypes or generalizations which have not been tested but have subtle roots in the socialization process of the nurse both as an individual and as a professional.

Ideas and beliefs direct behavior by organizing information and forming the justification for a particular approach. Self-questioning will help nurses to make explicit their own preconceived ideas which fit into the antecedent condition portion of the model. This kind of self-awareness and cultural awareness can begin with such questions as "What are my preconceived notions about a particular group of people?" and "What image comes to mind when I hear a label like *immigrant, boat person, black, poor, welfare recipient, unemployed, illiterate,* and *migrant worker?"* Henderson and Primeaux (1981) offer a self-examination in transcultural issues which may be a useful starting point. Even more useful and enlightening than individually questioning beliefs and assumptions would be forming small groups of nurses to explore attitudes and trace the genesis of ideas. Nurses initiating these groups need to be aware of what Thiederman (1988) calls ethnographic dynamite. Sensitive material such as negative stereotypes of particular ethnic groups or lumping peoples together who perceive themselves as distinct without acknowledging their differences may be offensive. An environment of psychological safety, with the freedom to fully explore, needs to be established (Thiederman, 1988). This kind of forum can assist nurses to overcome a sense of hesitancy in approaching a culturally different client, to minimize the fear stemming from a sense of strangeness, and to begin to identify the possible areas of commonality that can form a basis of mutual understanding and communication.

Awareness and respect of cultural differences are basic to effective intercultural communication. Because of this relationship, two areas of potential ethnocentrism which may be deeply ingrained in Western health care providers are highlighted. First is the assumption that Western professional health practices and beliefs are superior to the health norms and behaviors of other cultural groups (Morely, 1978; Fong, 1985). Avoidance of the posture that assumes Western medical practice are the standard from which other health care systems are to be judged is essential in intercultural communication. For example, viewing traditional treatments such as the use of herbal teas or massage as beneficial only if they can be validated "scientifically" and fit within the framework of the biomedical model may require the nurse to reject important cultural values of the child and family. This view limits the range of communication and understanding possible between nurses and clients. Martin (1987) points out that "science" can be viewed as a cultural system and that Western medicine reflects its historical roots just as do other health belief systems. For example, Martin describes the concept of "body as machine" as a mechanical metaphor which began in the 19th century as industrialization was taking hold in Europe and America. The view of the body as machine or factory separates and compartmentalizes the body and its functions from the mind or soul and permeates Western medical thought. If the nurse realizes that competing views of health and illness are similarly grounded in the experience of the cultural group, the perspective gained should make easier the ability to understand the client's point of view and mediate between the different therapeutic regimens. For instance, the family may explain the child's symptoms as resulting from a loss of soul or *Susto* (Foreman, 1985). This descriptor is a relatively common category of illness etiology and reflects the more holistic view of mind and body held by some cultures. The competing views and etiologies can coexist in any given therapeutic situation; the nurse acts to recognize both and strives to make treatment strategies compatible.

Second, it is not uncommon for health professionals to see the world revolving around health and illness (Johnson, 1977; Pfifferling, 1981). Matters associated with health and illness assume such a central position and become so important to health care providers that it is difficult to understand why others do not place an equal value on or give equal attention to health concerns. This particular form of ethnocentrism may translate into the expectation that families of child patients should place their child's illness over all of their other concerns and adjust the rest of their lives to accommodate the hospital, clinic, or health professional's schedule and perhaps even place the family in economic crisis. In some instances, the optimal health of the child or any individual member may not take precedence over the welfare of the family or group as a whole. This choice does not mean that the child lacks caring or love from his or her parents. Similarly, failure to conform to the time orientation of the hospital or clinic does not necessarily mean disinterest in the child's health or welfare. In order to be effective, nurses must appreciate the priorities and values of the child's family and be sensitive to their own cultural biases.

Cultural Brokerage

It is the nurses responsibility to function as a "cultural broker" for culturally different clients and create a bridge between the dominant health care system and the people the health system serves. Intercultural communication is the primary mechanism available to the nurse to accomplish this task.

If the initial encounter with the culturally different child and family is in the hospital or clinic, the nurse should realize that from the family's point of view, the nurse is the host and they are the visitors. The hospital is the nurse's territory and with that comes a certain responsibility to make visitors comfortable and welcome. In some cultures, for instance, small talk or what is known in Hawaii as talk story is appropriate before getting down to business or serious talk. These few minutes of greeting and what may seem like avoidance of the main issue may represent an important ritual in the process of establishing a therapeutic relationship. Participation without conveying a sense of impatience in this initial phase of the interaction may be what is necessary to set the stage for effective intercultural communication.

In some cultures, it is important to acknowledge the visitor through seating arrangements or show respect by not standing over the family members. Similarly, the order in which people are addressed may be important. When bringing a culturally different family into an examining room in a clinic situation, for instance, it may be most beneficial if the nurse focuses attention on the parents or adults first, showing through gesture where they should sit or stand, making sure that the message is not to have them "out of the way" and, in general, dealing with their need to be oriented and comfortable. This order of events may serve not only to reduce the ambiguity for the parents but also to put the child at ease. Creating an environment in which the family experiences a sense of comfort and welcome may take some creativity of the part of the nurse. The nurse will have to judge what is appropriate and possible. For instance, sometimes food should be offered—perhaps even a glass of water as a token of hospitality. In the usual hospital rules, no one except the patient should eat off the patient's tray. In family rules, maybe the parents should eat first, or at least take something as a sign of their position in the family.

The nurse's initial assessment will identify the level of English language knowledge of the child and family. If the child or family have a beginning competency or mastery of the English language, the nurse should carefully choose his or her words to be precise and unambiguous. For example, the intravenous fluid should be described as dripping rather than running, which the child or parent may only understand in the context of running a marathon.

Avoidance of symbolic language such as analogies, slang, acronyms, shortened or abbreviated words, and initials or hospital jargon will increase the possibility of a shared understanding. The nurse should use concrete terms and simple sentences but be cautious not to talk down to the child or family.

Strategies Related to the Interaction Process

The nurse as a cultural broker becomes an astute decoder of cues from the client, watching especially for signs of bewilderment and uncertainty. In this process, it is important to attempt to discover to whom or to what the child and family are responding. Nurses must pay attention to what the family is paying attention to; they must see from their eyes and hear with their ears. In this way, nurses will become sensitive to how their framing of a message influences the understanding of the child and family.

To illustrate, some members of the hospital staff, such as maintenance people, cleaning people, clerks, or candy stripers or other volunteers, may inadvertently send a message to the child and family through their behavioral cues. What information is conveyed, for instance, when the physician's arrival is accompanied by the quieting and perhaps departure of one of these people? The family may interpret this behavior as meaning silence is expected and some deference to authority is required. They may be very hesitant to ask questions or even offer a response when queried in fear of doing something inappropriate. The nurse must have astute observational skills in order to become aware of this message. This process is made difficult because in the cultural context of the nurse, the message senders the family is responding to are not central to the situation and therefore may be unnoticed or even essentially invisible. The nurse's cultural lens would not perceive the behavior of the maintenance person or candy striper as an important determinant of the family's behavior.

Once the nurse has interpreted the behavior of the family or patient as a response to an unintended message, the interpretation must be checked for accuracy. This can be done directly if both the nurse and family have sufficient understanding of the same language or if an interpreter can be made available. More often, however, the nurse must rely on systematic and purposeful observation for validation.

Using this situation as an example, the nursing strategy is to counter the environmental cues which send unintended messages. Changing the environment, in this case by encouraging hospital personnel to be sensitive to interpretation of their behavior by others, may be effective. Each intervention strategy should be aimed at increasing the quality of the interactions between the child and family and the caregivers and ensuring that both groups are able to interpret accurately the messages sent and received.

Another important strategy is to structure the environment in order to provide cues and learning opportunities for the child in a purposeful manner. One way this might be accomplished is by placing the child in a room with a cooperative child of similar age. Use of demonstration as a method will provide the culturally different child with the opportunity to observe hospital routines and what behaviors are appropriate and desirable in a situation. For example, the nurse can take the roommate's temperature, pulse, respiration, and blood pressure while explaining each step of the process and directing the child in expected and helpful behaviors by saying such things as, "Put this under your tongue," "Please be quiet while I listen for your pulse," and "Stretch out your arm while I take your blood pressure." The nurse should make an attempt to be very clear and even exaggerated with movements and other nonverbal behaviors so that the meaning and associated verbal cues are easy for the culturally different child to understand. For example, the nurse can hold up the blood pressure cuff so that it is clearly visible before showing how it goes on the arm and be conspicuous about taking the pulse. These steps allow the observing child the chance to imitate the child who is acting as a role model.

Children learn through imitation how to affect the environment and other people's actions. Seemingly simple connections are not always easy for the child to learn. The child may not immediately think, "When the nurse puts down the siderail and stretches out a hand, that is an invitation to get up; when this button is pressed, the nurse will come; and if I point to the bathroom, the nurse will know to let me go there." However, these are important connections or relationships for the child to learn. Through this method, the child can begin to experience some measure of control and can purposefully cooperate with care-giving activities.

If no other child is available to become a role model, the nurse can create other op-portunities to communicate with the child through demonstration. The use of puppets and other play can serve the same goal. If such communication is done in the parents' presence, even though directed toward the child, the parents will benefit as well.

Facial expression is a potent communica-tion tool. Delight, surprise, puzzlement, and a myriad of other messages that invite re-sponse can be effectively conveyed by expression alone. For children who do not understand the language being spoken, ap-propriate laughter and playfulness represent the kind of interactions that offer the most opportunity to develop a zone of shared experience and, thus, mutual understanding. The capacity of children to play can be enhanced by presenting recognizable mark-ers or cues that are universal. Toys or a setting such as a playroom with child-sized furniture will be recognized as a place where play and laughter are supposed to take place. It is critical, however, that smiling and laughter not be mixed with actions which the child may experience as painful or threatening. An intrusive procedure per-formed with a smile leaves the child baffled and unable to clearly sort out the messages being received. Consistent cues that match the action that is taking place are necessary for optimal communication.

EVALUATION

The desired outcome, as noted previously, is the establishment of an area of shared experience upon which to base communi-cation that will lead to mutual understand-ing. Outcome measurement can be achieved through clinical validation, but it is elusive empirically at this point in our knowledge growth. Research must operationally define areas of shared experience and develop methodologies for measurement of out-comes.

Case Study

Toan was a three year old Vietnamese child who had recently immigrated to America by way of a Thai refugee camp. As a second child in a family of three children, he had had little contact with his new world until he became too ill to be treated without help. Toan's family, in addition to his siblings, included his parents, both in their thirties, and his 60 year old grandmother. Toan's family presented complex communication prob-lems for the health care providers involved in his care. Fortunately, there was one other relative in the city where they lived: an aunt who had settled in the area years earlier. There were, however, already cultural differences between these two families because the aunt had made many adap-tations to Western culture.

Toan was ill for several weeks before his family sought help from the hospital clinic. In her initial interaction with Toan's family, the nurse recog-nized that the family's delay in bringing Toan for medical treatment was very likely based on a number of factors which were primarily cultur-ally based. The nurse identified these factors as very limited English language skills with hesita-tion in attempting to speak English, indicating a low confidence level in the use of the language and limited previous experience with the West-ern medical care system.

A cultural assessment was completed on Toan and his family. The nurse's identification of an-tecedent conditions influencing Toan's care in-cluded the family's strong religious beliefs, which affected their conceptions about illness; the choice of Toan's initial care, which had included the use of ritual and healers and indicated a belief in a different health care model; and their strong belief that the family should be responsible for the care of its own members. The structure of Toan's family, their authority patterns, and their methods of decision making were also assessed as important antecedent conditions. The socioe-conomic status of Toan's family, which was the result of the relatively short length of time since their immigration and their lack of relevant job skills, gave them access to only minimal re-sources. Compounding these characteristics was their limited command of the English language. Therefore, a nursing diagnosis of *Impaired com-munication* was made.

The nurse also recognized an overlying com-munication problem which was related to Toan's stage of development. With children, as with others, it is important that one area of concern not be overlooked while another is being consid-ered. For this reason a care plan was devised recognizing all potential sources of nursing prob-lems relating to impaired communication. The strategy to be used was cultural brokerage.

Assessment related to the cultural implications of the interaction process allowed the nurse to focus on the contextual elements of Toan's clinic and hospital visit. When Toan's family finally sought medical care for him, they entered an environment that for them was disorienting and impersonal. Their child needed a number of procedures done which they had trouble understanding and which caused them considerable anxiety. Toan's aunt, who had accompanied them, did not have the knowledge of medical terms nor the proficiency in English necessary to interpret adequately in the unfamiliar hospital setting. There were instructions on medication, temperature taking, and diet, which were confusing and frightening and which did not fit within their usual mode of behaving when caring for an ill child. What was necessary was an identification of nursing problems, a nursing diagnosis, and a plan of intervention.

The social and developmental factors that needed to be considered in order to provide an optimal level of nursing care for Toan and his family were numerous. In addition, Toan's medical diagnosis (which was pneumonia) required monitoring of his physical status and nutritional requirements. From these many areas of concern, the nurse identified the need to verbally communicate as a first priority. Once established, adequate verbal communication would become a tool for further intervention. The following plan was outlined to meet treatment goals:

Diagnoses:	1. Impaired verbal communication (cultural)
	2. Impaired verbal communication (developmental)
Defining Characteristics:	1. Speaks Vietnamese
	2. Developmentally unable to express needs well; fearful
Etiology:	1. Recent immigration
	2. Age related; three years old
Intervening Strategies:	1. Provide adequate translation through acceptable translator
	2. Simple explanations from the nurse to child; demonstration

The first strategy was to find someone who could communicate to the family about Toan's disease process and what his treatment regimen would be in order to help him recover. It was equally important for the family to be able to communicate what their concerns, desires, and needs were related to Toan's hospital and follow-up care. The clinical nurse specialist located a Vietnamese-speaking public health nurse who could communicate well with this family and who greatly facilitated the care of this child. It should be noted, however, that it is not always easy to provide adequate translators. It is often necessary to look outside the family or immediate hospital setting for a person who is familiar with both languages.

Through her assessment of family structure and authority patterns in Toan's family, the nurse had determined that the role of decision maker was held by the father, although he was influenced considerably by his own mother, Toan's grandmother. Every effort was made, therefore, to provide instructions and information about Toan's condition and treatment regimen to both parents, but the father was primarily addressed. Since Toan's grandmother was unavailable for instruc-

tion by the hospital staff, her important role in the family and in Toan's care was acknowledged by remembering to ask the parents about concerns the grandmother might have about Toan's home care. Home visits by the Vietnamese-speaking public health nurse were scheduled to ensure that both the grandmother and Toan's parents had a knowledgeable person available as a resource to clarify instructions, monitor Toan's progress, and provide encouragement.

Both of Toan's parents were working at unskilled jobs while trying to learn English. The primary caretaker for Toan and his siblings was the grandmother who, therefore, needed to be considered an integral part of his treatment regimen and follow-up care. Toan's grandmother did not speak any English and was very wary of Western health care, believing that Toan's illness was a natural part of the life cycle, and felt that she should be able to provide him with any care that he needed. She was reluctant to visit him while he was in the hospital, even though his parents came regularly. The nurse determined that both Toan and his family, especially the grandmother, were experiencing *Social isolation from impaired communication*. The strategy plan follows:

Diagnosis:	Social isolation (cultural)
Defining Characteristics:	Little extended family; sociocultural differences for grandmother; age and family duty create a barrier to entering mainstream American culture
Etiology:	Recent immigration
Intervening Strategies:	Help connect family to cultural support groups and health professionals in the community who are aware of the culture

In summary, the goal of the nurse's care plan was for a positive outcome to Toan's illness episode not only in terms of resolution of Toan's infection and improvement of his nutritional status but also in terms of the family being successfully understood and culturally respected throughout their encounter with a culturally unfamiliar health care system. In addition, long-term goals required Toan and his siblings to be followed up for well-child care through the health department and his family to be shown how to benefit from other resources in the community. In order for this positive outcome to be realized, however, Toan, his family, and the nurse needed to engage in intercultural communication. The model of culture and communication offered in this chapter provides the framework for this interaction and the foundation for intervention strategies identified.

RESEARCH IMPLICATIONS

Nurses are often innovators by developing creative solutions to problems such as the inability to effectively communicate because of cultural and language differences. However, lacking in most instances of nursing innovation is documentation and sharing of information so that strategies can be tested, fine tuned, and disseminated to other practitioners. Examination of published case reports (Sohier, 1981) of nursing in culturally different situations could give insight into the process of establishing a shared zone of experience between the nurse and client. Interviews with nurses who have experience in cross-cultural nursing and a collection and documentation of strategies they have used might also reveal patterns of intervention that could then be tested systematically for effectiveness with specific cultural

groups and age groups, or in specific nursing situations. Questions relating to the matching of strategies, child-rearing patterns, and developmental stages are also of interest. For example, an important question is, how do age and cultural expectations of children influence the response to structuring opportunities for imitation of a role model?

Toan's case study points to the need for more information about specific cultural groups. Knowledge about belief systems relating to health, illness, and preferred care needs to be available for incorporation into the assessment and planning of interventions of culturally different clients. Comparative, descriptive, and carefully documented case studies by nurses add to this important body of knowledge. In recent years, a discussion of qualitative methods appropriate for systematically gathering and interpreting information about cultural variables has become more prominent in nursing research literature (Leininger, 1985; Munhall and Oiler, 1986; Munet-Vilaro, 1988; Cohen and Tripp-Reimer, 1988). Tripp-Reimer and Dougherty (1985) point out, however, that the literature in cross-cultural nursing research frequently uses terms inaccurately and often lacks methodological and conceptual clarity. Continued efforts by nurse scientists will be required to reach consensus on definitions, and the careful analysis of concepts will be necessary for meaningful comparisons. Collaborative and interdisciplinary studies could be initiated by nurse scientists for the dual purposes of improving methodologies for cross-cultural nursing research and improving the clarity with which nurses explore culture conceptually. Nurses have an enviable opportunity because of the access their practice gives them to populations and individuals with diverse cultural backgrounds. There is an exciting potential, made possible by the availability and development of these methodologies, for nurses to make significant contributions toward the understanding and effectiveness of nursing care in practice settings.

Finally, nurses themselves represent a needed focal area for research. The process nurses use to develop cultural awareness needs to be explored. A beginning step would be to survey basic nursing curricula for content relating to culture. This would yield data on the kind and amount of relevant information available to nurses in their professional socialization process. Attempts to include anthropological approaches and content in nursing curricula could also be analyzed for successful integration strategies (Chrisman, 1982). From this baseline, questions about how best to develop respect and awareness for cultural differences through nursing education could be formulated and answered.

In this chapter, the differences relating to culture have been highlighted and intervention strategies aimed at improving communication between the nurse and culturally different clients have been explored. The need to establish effective intercultural communication is used as a pivotal point from which to draw implications for research. This need to have effective intercultural communication also serves as the focal point of the model of culture and communication. This model conceptualizes the process of establishing a shared zone of experience to lead to mutual understanding between the nurse and culturally different clients.

References

Aamodt, A. Culture. In Clark, A (Ed.), Culture/childbearing/health professionals. Philadelphia: FA Davis Co., 1978, pp. 2–19.

Chrisman, N. Anthropology in nursing: An exploration of adaptation. In Chrisman, N, and Maretzki, T (Eds.), Clinically applied anthropology: Anthropologists in health science settings. Dordrecht, Netherlands: D Reidel Publishing Co., 1982, pp. 117–140.

Cohen, MZ, and Tripp-Reimer, T. Research in cultural diversity: Qualitative methods in cultural research. Western Journal of Nursing Research, 10:226–228, 1988.

Cowan, P. Piaget with feeling. New York: Holt, Rinehart and Winston, Inc., 1978.

Dodd, C. Perspectives on cross-cultural communication. Dubuque, Iowa: Kendall/Hunt Publishing Co., 1977.

Dodd, C. Dynamics of intercultural communications. Dubuque, Iowa: Wm C Brown Group, 1982.

Dougherty, M, and Tripp-Reimer, T. The interface of nursing and anthropology. Annual Review of Anthropology, 14:219–241, 1985.

Eisenberg, L. Disease and illness: Distinctions between professional and popular ideas of sickness. Culture Medicine Psychiatry, 1:9–23, 1977.

Fong, C. Ethnicity and nursing practice. Topics in Clinical Nursing, 7:1–10, 1985.

Foreman, J. Susto and the health needs of the Cuban refugee population. Topics in Clinical Nursing, 7:40–47, 1985.

Gleason, J, and Perlmann, R. Acquiring social variation in speech. In Giles, H, and St Clair, R (Eds.), Recent advances in language, communication, and social psychology. London: Lawrence Erlbaum Associates, Inc., 1985.

Goodenough, W. Culture, language, and society (2nd ed.). Menlo Park, Calif.: The Benjamin-Cummings Publishing Co., 1981.

Gordon, M. Manual of nursing diagnosis 1984–1985. New York: McGraw-Hill, Inc., 1985.

Harwood, A. Ethnicity and medical care. Cambridge, Mass.: Harvard University Press, 1981.

Helman, C. Culture, health and illness: An introduction for health professionals. Bristol: John Wright and Sons, 1984.

Henderson, G, and Primeaux, M. Transcultural Health Care. Menlo Park, Calif.: Addison-Wesley Publishing Co., 1981.

Hoskins, M. Building rapport with the Vietnamese. San Francisco: International Institute of San Francisco, 1971.

Johnson, M. Folk beliefs and ethnocultural behavior in pediatrics: Medicine or magic? Nursing Clinics of North America, 12:77–84, 1977.

Kim, M, McFarland, G, and McLane, A. Nursing diagnosis. St. Louis: CV Mosby Co., 1984.

Korbin, J, and Johnson, M. Steps toward resolving cultural conflict in a pediatric hospital. Clinical Pediatrics, 21:259–263, 1982.

Langness, L. The study of culture. San Francisco: Chandler and Sharp Publishers, Inc., 1974.

LaRargue, J. Mediating between two views of illness. Topics in Clinical Nursing, 7:70–77, 1985.

Leininger, M. The culture concept and its relevance to nursing. In Leininger, M. Transcultural nursing: Concepts, theories, and practices. New York: John Wiley & Sons, Inc., 1978, pp. 109–120.

Leininger, M (Ed.). Qualitative research methods in nursing. Orlando, Fla.: Grune & Stratton, Inc., 1985.

Martin, E. The woman in the body: A cultural analysis of reproduction. Boston: Beacon Press, 1987.

McKenna, M. Anthropology and nursing: The interaction between two fields of inquiry. Western Journal of Nursing Research, 6:423–431, 1984.

Metge, J, and Kinloch, P. Talking past each other: Problems of cross-cultural communication. Wellington, New Zealand: Victoria University Press, 1978.

Morley, P. Culture and caring: Anthropological perspectives on traditional medical beliefs and practices. Pittsburgh: University of Pittsburgh Press, 1978.

Muecke, M. In search of healers: Southeast Asian refugees in the American health care system. Western Journal of Medicine, 139:31–36.

Munet-Vilaro, F. The challenge of cross-cultural nursing research. Western Journal of Nursing Research, 10:112–116, 1988.

Munhall, P, and Oiler, C. Nursing research: A qualitative perspective. Norwalk, Conn.: Appleton-Century-Crofts, 1986.

O'Keefe, B, and Delia, J. Psychological and interactional dimensions of communicative development. In Giles, H, and St. Clair, R (Eds.), Recent advances in language, communication, and social psychology. London: Lawrence Erlbaum Associates, Inc., 1985.

Orque, M, Bloch, B, and Monrrog, L. Ethnic nursing care: A multicultural approach. St. Louis: CV Mosby Co., 1983.

Pfifferling, JH. A cultural prescription for medicocentrism. In Eisenberg, L, and Kleinman, A (Eds.), The relevance of social science for medicine. Dordrecht, Netherlands: D Reidel Publishing Co., 1981, pp. 197–222.

Piaget, J, and Inhelder, B. The psychology of the child. New York: Basic Books, Inc., 1969.

Porter, R. An overview of intercultural communication. In Samovar, L, and Porter, R (Eds.), Intercultural communication: A reader (4th ed.). Belmont, Calif.: Wadsworth, Inc., 1985, pp. 3–18.

Samovar, L, and Porter, R. Intercultural communication: A reader (4th ed.). Belmont, Calif.: Wadsworth, Inc., 1985.

Singer, M. Culture: A perceptual approach. In Samovar, L, and Porter, R (Eds.), Intercultural communication: A reader (4th ed.). Belmont, Calif.: Wadsworth, Inc., 1985, pp. 62–74.

Sohier, R. Gaining awareness of cultural differences: A case example. In Henderson, G, and Primeaux, M (Eds.), Transcultural health care. Menlo Park, Calif.: Addison-Wesley Publishing Co., Inc., 1981, pp. 18–31.

Stern, P. A comparison of culturally approved behaviors. Health Care of Women International, 15:123–133, 1985.

Thiederman, S. Workshops in cross-cultural health care: The challenge of ethnographic dynamite. Journal of Continuing Education in Nursing, 19:25–27, 1988.

Tripp-Reimer, T, Brink, P, and Saunders, J. Cultural assessment: Content and process. Nursing Outlook, 32:78–82, 1984.

Tripp-Reimer, T, and Dougherty, M. Cross-cultural nursing research. Annual Review of Nursing Research, 3:77–104, 1985.

CHAPTER 12

PROVIDING SUPPORT

A Process Model

ALICE M. TSE, M.S.N., R.N., and
ROSANNE C. PEREZ-WOODS, Ed.D., R.N.,
C.P.N.A.

Social support of the family with an ill child is an important dimension in the realm of nursing practice and theory development. Early discharge programs have increased the demand for home nursing services and enlarged the family's role in providing health care for the child. The family has also assumed more responsibility for care of the child admitted to the hospital.

Support has been described as both an intervention and an outcome of interventions. Schoenhofer (1984) states that support is a nursing measure frequently advocated in textbooks and written care plans; how-ever, particular supportive acts are generally not specified and are presumably left to intuition. Because the family is the social network of the child, the focus of this chapter will be on the family.

In this chapter, theory, research, and practice concepts relevant to the development of social networks and associated with health status are discussed. A modification of Kane's (1988) Model of Family Social Support is provided as the framework for organizing antecedents and consequences of the support process. Interventions that are internally consistent with the Model, tools used to measure social support, and variables associated with outcomes are also discussed. A case example and indications for research to assist with the development of middle range theory characterizing and accounting for the resources needed by the family to carry out the process of social support are also included.

THEORETICAL FOUNDATION

A Process-Oriented Definition of Support

Support is defined as a process of interaction through which the family develops versatility and resourcefulness and consequently achieves health (Kane, 1988). This definition was evolved from Kahn's (1979) definition of social support as social transactions. The process of social support is dependent on the presence of the following types of resources: (1) expression of positive affect from one person to another (emotional reciprocity); (2) affirmation or endorsement of another's behaviors, perceptions, or expressed views (feedback or advice); and (3) the giving of symbolic or material aid to another (Kahn, 1979). All of these types of resources are obtained through the social network.

The Model

Antecedents of family social support identified in the literature include family characteristics, child characteristics, environmental-situational factors, and interactional factors (Kane, 1988; Cohen and Syme, 1985; Thoits, 1985; Berrera and Ainlay, 1983; Israel, 1983; Leavy, 1983; Turner et al., 1983; Greenblatt et al., 1982; Kaplan, 1977). The relationship to each other of these characteristics and factors are described in the following Model, which is based on Kane's (1988) conceptual Model of Family Support and has been adapted to include child-specific dimensions in accordance with Israel's (1983) definition of social support networks (Table 12–1).

Assumptions underlying the Model include (1) the family is a system, (2) social support is a process, and (3) social support is positive and helpful. In the family, social support is a process of social relationships through which resources may or may not be accessed.

There are a number of testable propositions associated with this Model. The propositions are listed below (Kane, 1988):

The larger a family's social network, the greater the opportunity for reciprocity, advice and feedback, and emotional involvement.

The more flexible the family structure, the more reciprocity advice, feedback, and emotional involvement.

The more esteem the family has within its social network, the more reciprocity, advice, feedback, and emotional involvement.

The more stable the family, the more substantial the reciprocity, advice, feedback, and emotional involvement.

The more reciprocity occurring, the greater the family social support.

The more advice and feedback occurring, the greater the family social support.

The more emotional involvement, the greater the family social support.

Antecedents and Consequences of the Family Social Support Process

The consequences of the family social support process are health and resources (information, goods and services, and assistance during a crisis situation). The antecedents are described in Table 12–2.

This Model identifies the construct of family social support as a process of relationships between the child, family, and social environment. Social support is not an outcome or a resource, but a process of interaction through which the family develops versatility and resourcefulness and consequently achieves health.

In the Model, a family's ability to cope is depicted as dependent on multiple interacting forces. The family is described as in continuous interaction with the child and environment. The family has an impact on the child's health outcome because the child's primary social support network is the family. The nurse should assess the family in terms of reciprocity, advice, feedback, and emotional involvement. If the family is lacking in one or more of these areas, strategies for strengthening the family process can be instituted. During the period the family is developing additional resources, the nurse may have to provide appropriate

Table 12–1. MODEL OF FAMILY SUPPORT

Family Characteristics	Child Characteristics	Interactional Factors	Environmental-Situational Factors
Social network dimension (Descriptive/structural) Family structure (Flexibility/ commonalities) Esteem (Commonalities/ positive perceptions) Stability History/developmental epoch	Personality Temperament Perception Coping	Reciprocity (Reciprocal relationships/frequency) Advice/feedback (Quantity/ quality communication) Emotional involvement (Intimacy/trust)	Physiological effects Social ecology (Informal parent social networks/social networks and the child)

resources to the family. Consideration must also be given to the possibility that although a family's social support process may be adequate, the social environment may be incapable of providing resources. If the process of family social support results in insufficient resources for successful coping, appropriate services must be provided.

The characteristics and consequences of children's behavior has been the subject of a number of investigations. Less attention has been devoted to studying the process of social support in the family with an ill child.

An analysis of the theory and research related to the social support process and its influence on the child's health outcome can be organized into the four components suggested by the Model: characteristics of the child as an individual, family characteristics, interactional factors, and environmental-situational factors.

The Child's Characteristics

The child is born with a genetic core of potentials into a social group. This group, usually the family, cares for the child's physical needs and protects the child from danger and disease. The family system also provides the child's matrix of identity. The child develops a sense of belonging and a sense of individuality within this system and becomes a member of a social group, which is recognized first by feel, and then by concept and feelings (Kegan, 1982).

Personality

When the child is born, a genetically determined group of potentials for physical, psychological (intellectual and emotional), and social competence are present. The actualization of these potentials depends on the environment. Personality evolves dependent on the interplay between genetic endowment and the environment.

Personality grows slowly, building on interactions within the family that define for children who they are and how they fit into the social structure. Children's experiences of these interactions change as they grow, as they are changing organisms with shifting needs, interests, and capacities. These interactional capacities are simple at first and become increasingly complex as children are required to organize experiences and make sense out of the patterns in which they are involved (Kegan, 1982).

Table 12–2. ANTECEDENTS OF THE FAMILY SOCIAL SUPPORT PROCESS

Child Characteristics	Environmental/Situational Characteristics
Personality	Physiological effects
Temperament	Social ecology
Perception	Parents' social network
Coping	Social networks and the child
	Family Social Support
Family Characteristics	Reciprocity
Social network	Advice/feedback
Family structure	Emotional involvement
Esteem	**Family Function**
Stability	Versatility
	Resourcefulness

Temperament

Temperament is the characteristic of the child that appears to be most associated with parental response and the resulting social interaction. In this section, the work of investigators supporting this premise will be discussed. In addition, variables associated with the outcome of the interaction between parent and child will be presented.

According to Bates (1980), temperament is the characteristic of the child that makes parenting more or less difficult. These findings imply that the social support process in this relationship is dependent on the child's temperament. Ventura (1982, 1986) states that the relationship between parent coping behaviors and infant temperament characteristics must be examined. In these studies, parents who were depressed and families that were anxious perceived their infants as less soothable and more distressed with limitations. These families focused more on resolving issues related to self rather than to the child or family. Parents who perceived their infants as smiling, laughing, and less distressed with limitations used coping patterns to maintain family integration. These studies suggest that the parents' support process is influenced both by their own mood state and by the temperament of the infant.

Infant temperament as measured by parent report has been associated with parent-infant interaction (Chess and Thomas, 1986; Bates, 1980). Campbell (1979) stated that mothers who rated their infants as having difficult temperaments at three months of age interacted with them less and were less responsive to their cries when the infants are three and eight months than matched controls. Milliones (1978) and Kelley (1976) also reported a negative association between mothers' perceptions of infant difficultness and maternal responsiveness.

These studies support the assumptions that temperament has a profound influence on the quantity and quality of the social interactions with the parent and that parental mood states are associated with perceptions of the child. The quantity and quality of social interaction is dependent on the "goodness-of-fit" between the child and parent and the environment (Lerner and Lerner, 1985). Very little work testing this position currently appears in the literature.

Perception

The work of Kiritz and Moos (1974) revealed that social stimuli do not act directly on the child. It is the child's perception of the social environment which affects him or her. Personality and behavior are mediated by the child's perceptions. In general, the child's individual temperament and personality characteristics influence the kind of social relationships established within the social network.

The social environment, composed of individuals and groups within the environment, provides a system of interpersonal stimulation for the growing child. The child forms internal representational models of self and others based on past perceptions and experiences within the social environment. Included as part of such models are aspects of one's self-image; expectations about the behavior of others; and a variety of highly valued developmental outcomes, e.g., emotional security, behavioral independence, social competence, and intellectual achievement (Bowlby, 1969, 1973, 1982; Crittendon, 1985).

Models of self are based on perceptions of experiences in the early parent-child interaction and continue to be modified by both the changing developmental perspective of the growing child and additional experiences with significant others. Ideas about the relationship between the process of social support and attachment, interaction, and cognitive competence can also be found in the literature (Colletta, 1979; Pascoe et al., 1981; Baumrind, 1967, 1971). Belsky (1984) and Belsky et al. (1984) document that social support process is related to aspects of parenting such as warmth, responsiveness, and role satisfaction.

Coping

The child's ability to cope with an illness or a disability is thought to be dependent on the social support process. During illness, stress evolves from many sources: uncertainty about the cause of the illness, expectations about the progression of the disease or change in symptoms, and cure or the perceived possibility of death. Treatment procedures often interfere with the child's ability to interact with the environment. Social interactions with the parent are often intensified, and privacy may be diminished. Repeated visits to the health care provider promote fear of relapse and isolation and alter the child's social environment and sense of accomplishment (Wolfer and Visintainer, 1975).

Many health care professionals believe children cope effectively with the stress imposed by illness. This belief is not supported in the literature (Katz et al., 1980; Patenaude et al., 1979; Powazek et al., 1978). In situations in which sufficient physical, emotional, and informational resources were absent, children become passive and ceased to engage in healthy attempts to cope with their environments (McCollum, 1981; Reddihough et al., 1977; Wolfer and Visintainer, 1975).

Coping is dependent on perceptions the child has of the social network (Caplan, 1974; Mattsson, 1972; Whitt et al., 1982), and illness can alter family interactions. These alterations put stress on the process of social support within the family. Fear, guilt, and anger may result, demanding additional alterations in coping within the family system (Moos and Tsu, 1977). The child's ability to cope is dependent on the family's ability to function adequately. Pless et al. (1972) found that families who scored low in relation to functioning were twice as likely to have poorly adjusted ill children as families that functioned well. The effectiveness of family coping strategies and support mechanisms which encouraged children with cancer to maintain a normal life while participating in family, community, and school activities was also affirmed (Spinetta, 1981).

The Family's Characteristics

Family characteristics of significance to the social support process have been identified from a review of the literature (Kane, 1988; Cohen and Syme, 1985; Greenblatt et al., 1982; Thoits, 1985; Berrera and Ainlay, 1983; Israel, 1983; Leavy, 1983; Turner et al., 1983). Significant aspects of family characteristics include (1) ties in the social network, (2) relationships in the social network, (3) economic status of the family and social network, (4) flexibility of the family structure, (5) commonalities between the family and social network, (6) positive perceptions of the family by its social network, (7) availability of the social network, and (8) history of relationships. Family ties in the social network, relationships in the social network, and the economic status of the family were found to have the greatest empirical support in the literature.

Interactional Factors

An analysis of the social support literature identified the following interactional factors of families as significant to the social support process (Kane, 1988; Cohen and Syme, 1985; Greenblatt et al., 1982; Thoits, 1985; Berrera and Ainlay, 1983; Israel, 1983; Leavy, 1983; Turner et al., 1983). The factors are (1) presence of reciprocal helping relationships, (2) frequency of interaction between family and social network, (3) quantity and quality of communication, (4) intimacy of relationships, and (5) trust within relationships.

The Social Environment

Physiological Effects

Physiological effects of the social environment have been studied (Reinhart and Drash, 1969; Powell et al., 1967). Kiritz and Moos (1974) have reviewed the influence of the social environment on the child. These authors suggest different dimensions exist within the social environment which have an influence on psychological and physiological processes. Lack of social support may make the child more vulnerable to disease. Studies suggest that at both the animal and human level the presence of another animal of the same species may under certain circumstances protect the individual from a variety of stressful stimuli. Biological evidence from animal studies (Bovard, 1962) suggests that stressful stimuli are mediated through the posterior and medial hypothalamus leading, via the release of a chemotransmitter to the anterior pituitary, to a general protein catabolic effect. Bovard further suggests that a secondary center, located in the hypothalamus, when stimulated by an appropriate social stimuli (a supportive relationship), calls forth in the organism a "competing response" which inhibits, masks, or screens the stress stimulus to such a degree that the latter has a minimal effect. These mechanisms have been well documented in animal research and provide a plausible explanation for many of the findings reported in human studies. There is no agreement about how such processes function in humans.

In an investigation of 130 infants, Spitz (1945, 1947) reported that maternal and social deprivation were associated with increased infant mortality, increased susceptibility to disease, retardation in growth, and failure to achieve developmental milestones. These observations by Spitz emphasize the importance of the social environment on the social support process and health outcomes.

Social Ecology

The social ecology within the parent and child relationship is related to the social support process (Cochran and Brassard, 1979). Transactions within this context involve child-rearing functions: nurturance, guidance, and control. Many aspects of the child's development are affected by interactions and experiences within this system. The child establishes patterns of relationship and interaction in situations of unequal power. Children learn to communicate wants and expectations to people who have greater resources and strengths (parents and social networks). They learn whether their needs will be met and how conflicts will be resolved. A generalized concept of authority is formulated as rational or arbitrary, functional or punitive, and so forth.

Influence of Parental Social Networks

Parental social networks have been described as influencing the performance of the parental role in many ways. The environment is transmitted to the child through the mediating social influence of the parent. The goal of the social support process between parents and children is augmentation of a child's strength to master the environment (Ellison, 1987; Kegan, 1982; Minuchen and Minuchen, 1974).

The social expectations, attitudes, and practices in the world beyond the immediate family are initially transmitted to the child through the family. Resources obtained by parents from social networks influence the

developing child (Cochran and Brassard, 1979). The child is exposed to a variety of other persons. The parent's social network provides a number of types of social stimulation for the child:

1. Each parent presents a unique style of interacting with the child, broadening the range of patterns available to the child.

2. The content of activities engaged with various network members may vary.

3. The network may introduce the child to new environmental settings and stimuli and new modes of interaction.

4. The characteristics of the environment have been related to the experiences of the child taking place within a given milieu (Cochran, 1977).

5. Parental networks provide people who may serve as sources of support or stress to the child as well as observational models for the child.

6. Active participation in the parent's network provides a basis for the child to develop his or her own social network.

Social networks also affect the child through the influence that network members have upon parents themselves as individuals (Cochran and Brassard, 1979). Such influence comes to the child through other competing roles maintained by the parent (e.g., worker, spouse); parental experiences linked with the outside world (e.g., parental job improvement realizing new life possibilities for the child); and the parental role itself. Network members engage in activities and exchanges which limit the child-rearing behaviors of the parent.

Network members not only provide sanction for parental behaviors but also models for parental behaviors that are acceptable within the given network (Cochran and Brassard, 1979). Access to emotional and material assistance with respect to the parental social situation is associated with the provision of a relatively consistent social environment. The parental social network may enable parents to be highly sensitive to the needs of their child.

Social Networks and the Child

Personal social networks have complex social and environmental dimensions. Adequate social environments may be distinguished on the basis of how close the members feel towards each other. For example, cohesion and involvement imply a strong affective relationship between the members of the family (Kiritz and Moos, 1974).

The child's social network is composed of persons outside the household who engage in activities with the child and engage in an exchange of an affective or material nature with the child and members of the immediate family. Included within this network are kin, neighbors, school peers, and work mates (Cochran, 1977, Cochran and Brassard, 1979). An in-depth discussion of this topic is presented in Chapter 13.

Summary

The contributions of the child and of environmental resources to the child's health have been addressed. The relationship between the family's characteristics and interactions and the child requires further investigation. Family characteristics most associated with childhood adjustment are not well defined. Interactions are determinants of the child's attitude, self-concept, and adjustment strategies. Family strategies for coping with the child's illness may indicate an attempt to adapt within the constraints of the child's impairment.

ASSESSMENT

The need for support for an individual child can be determined from an analysis of antecedents of the social support process. The quality and validity of the instruments used to measure the social support process must be taken into consideration when interpreting the findings. Instruments that can be used to measure the social support process are presented in Table 12–3.

The problem of measuring the social support process is not due to a lack of available instruments, for a great number of tools exist. The problem is that the psychometric properties for these instruments have not been consistently documented. In addition, the operational definitions of the social support process used by the investigator are not always provided. Data establishing the validity and reliability of scales need to be reported in the literature, as does the contribution the scales make in understanding the construct of social support. The applicability of the scales to families with ill children is not well documented. In addition, specific criteria against which to compare the scales is needed.

The similarities and differences in the scales must be addressed, and practitioners must choose a scale that is based on a definition of the social support process that agrees with their practice orientation. There is a significant difference between the type of assessment strategies used in a research environment and those employed in a practice environment. In a practice situation, the nurse relies primarily on information from the health and environmental history as well as on objective assessment data. No single component of the assessment, even a reliable and valid scale, should ever provide the basis for interventions.

Regularly scheduled assessments of family and child characteristics and interaction patterns may target children and families which require alteration of normal care practices. Clinical protocols for assessing parent-child conflict (Boll et al., 1978), parenting stress (Burke and Abidin, 1980), family functioning (Moos, 1974; Pless and Satterwhite, 1973; Spinetta, 1981; Stein and Riessman, 1980), or flexibility of family routines (Whitt et al., 1982) may assist with the selection of interventions.

These two nursing diagnoses suggest alterations in the social support process (Kim et al., 1986): (1) *Coping, ineffective family: compromised;* and (2) *Coping, ineffective family: disabling.*

Antecedents of the social support process are described in the Model of Family Social Support, and deficits in these resources result in alterations in coping. Thus, resources must be provided for the family in order to maintain the social support process. The Model specifies the potential intervention domains for family networks, suggests intervening variables operant in the situation, and identifies potential consequences.

Defining characteristics for each of the concepts in the Model were confirmed through the review of the literature. The tools suggested in Table 12–3 to measure the social support process as well as qualitative assessments and professional judgments must be used to evaluate the social support process in the family. A comparison of before and after measures or a design including serial measurements is needed to determine if interventions provided achieved the desired outcomes.

Text continued on page 192

Table 12–3. SUMMARY OF INSTRUMENTS USED TO MEASURE SOCIAL SUPPORT

Measure	Description	Normative Group	Reliability/Validity
Arizona Social Support Interview Schedule (ASSIS) (Barrera, 1981)	6 categories of social support: material aid, physical assistance, intimate interaction, guidance, feedback, and positive social interaction Examines characteristics of available and actual networks	45 undergraduate students	Test-retest reliability (2-day interval): .88 for total network, .54 for conflicted network (members a source both of support and stress), and .69 for support satisfaction Internal consistency: .33 for support satisfaction and .52 for need satisfaction Concurrent validity: .42 with ISSB for available network size and .32 with ISSB for conflicted network size
Diabetes Family Behavior Checklist (DFBC) (Schafer et al., 1984)	16-item scale to assess frequency of supportive and nonsupportive behaviors that influence adherence of diabetic family member to the treatment regimen; positive and negative behaviors scored separately	54 adults and 18 adolescents with diabetes	Internal consistency: .73 adult positive score, .43 adult negative score, .63 adolescent positive score, and .60 adolescent negative score Test-retest reliability (6-month interval): .58 to .72 positive scores and .22 to .27 negative scores Validity: .27 to .68 correlation between positive and negative scores for adults and .10 to .26 correlation for adolescents Significant negative correlation between scores and adherence to diabetic regimen
Family Relationship Index (FRI) (Billings and Moos, 1982)	3-component scale: cohesion, expressiveness, and conflict	185 men and 94 employed and 154 unemployed women in community sample	Internal consistency: .89 Test-retest reliability: (12- to 15-month interval): .62 (men), .64 (employed women), and .69 (unemployed women) Validity: correlation with personal functioning range: −.07 to −.27 (men), −.16 to −.44 (working women), and −.31 to −.38 (unemployed women)
Gore Social Support Index (GSSI) (Gore, 1978)	13 items focused on individual's perception of others as supportive, frequency of outside activity, and perceived opportunity to engage in satisfying outside social activity	54 rural and 46 urban unemployed blue-collar workers (mean age = 49 years)	Reliability and validity data not available

Table 12–3. SUMMARY OF INSTRUMENTS USED TO MEASURE SOCIAL SUPPORT *(Continued)*

Measure	Description	Normative Group	Reliability/Validity
Interpersonal Support Evaluation List (ISEL) (Cohen et al., 1985)	40-item scale (48-item student version) 4 subscales: tangible, self-esteem, belonging, and appraisal Measure perceptions of available support	7 undergraduate samples and 5 general population samples	Test-retest reliability (6 week interval): .71 to .87 student version and .63 to .70 general population version Internal consistency: .77 to .86 student version and .88 to .90 general population version Construct validity: (student version) .46 with ISSB Discriminate validity on student version: −.52 to −.64 with measures of social anxiety; on general population version: −.52 to −.60 with measures of psychiatric symptoms and −.19 to −.39 with measures of physical symptoms
Interview Schedule for Social Interaction (ISSI) (Henderson et al., 1980)	45-minute interview to determine availability and perceived adequacy of attachment and social integration	756 registered voters (age 18 to 65 years)	Test-retest reliability (18-day interval, 231 individuals): .75 to .79 Internal consistency: .67 to .81 Construct validity: modest correlations with Eysenck Personality Inventory
Inventory of Socially Supportive Behaviors (ISSB) (Barrera, 1981)	40 items, respondents rate the frequency with which each item occurred in the preceding month using a 5-point scale	30 male and 41 female undergraduate students	Test-retest reliability (2-day interval): .88 with range of individual items from .44 to .91 Internal consistency: .93 first administration and .94 second administration Validity: .36 correlation with the cohesion subscale of the FES and .42 with the ASSIS
Norbeck Social Support Questionnaire (NSSQ) (Norbeck et al., 1981)	Seld-administered; respondent lists 20 network members and answers 9 questions about each: 6 questions on functional properties of social support 1 question on duration of relationships 1 question on frequency of relationships 1 question on recent losses	75 first-year nursing graduate students (mean age = 30.3 years) and 60 senior nursing students (mean age = 27.3 years)	Test-retest reliability (graduate nursing students): .85 to .92 Internal consistency: .69 to .98 Poor to modest concurrent validity with other measures of social support (Schaefer's SSQ): .03 to .56 Discriminate validity evidenced by lack of correlation with measure of mood states
Perceived Social Support from Friends and Perceived Social Support from Family (PSS-Fa) (Procidano and Heller, 1983)	2 scales of 20 items each measuring perceived support information and feedback	222 undergraduate students	Test-retest reliability .83 Internal consistency: .88 friends and .90 family Correlations with psychiatric symptom scales demonstrated

Table continued on following page

Table 12–3. SUMMARY OF INSTRUMENTS USED TO MEASURE SOCIAL SUPPORT *(Continued)*

Measure	Description	Normative Group	Reliability/Validity
Personal Resource Questionnaire (PRQ) (Brandt and Weinert, 1981)	2 parts: 1. Descriptive information about resources, satisfaction, and presence of a confidant 2. 25 item Likert Scale and 5 item Self-Help Ideology Scale	149 white middle-class spouses of individuals with multiple sclerosis	Test-retest reliability not available Internal consistency: .89 (part 2) Concurrent validity (part 1): .21 to .23; (part 2): .30 to .44 with a measure of family integration Construct validity: −.25 to −.14 with the self-help inventory (those who rely more on themselves have lower scores)
Quantitative Social Support Index (QSSI) (Holahan and Moos, 1982)	Quantitative measure of numbers of supports, including visits with friends and relatives, number of club memberships, and availabilty of significant others Score derived by summing the number of contacts	267 familes, 2 adults from each, in San Francisco area (median age about 43 years)	Data not available
Satisfaction with Social Network Scale (SSNS) (Stokes, 1983)	8-item scale in which respondents rate network structure on 4 dimensions: general satisfaction, amount of change desired, satisfaction with assistance in daily activities, and satisfaction with emotional support	Data not available	Internal consistency: .92 Reliability and validity data not available
Social Network List (SNL) (Stokes, 1983)	Respondents list up to 20 individuals who provide support and describe characteristics of the network (size, density)	82 respondents identified by undergraduate students	Reliability and validity data not available
Social Relationship Scale (SRS) (McFarlane et al., 1981)	6 categories of potential life stress Individuals indicate individuals with whom they have discussed each area and rate helpfulness of each person on 7-point scale and indicate reciprocal nature of relationship	73 community college students	Test-retest reliability: .91 for number of individuals in the network and .78 for average degree of helpfulness of these potential supports Validity measure: clinical judgment
Social Stress and Support Interview (SSSI) (Jenkins et al., 1981)	Brief, semistructured interview which assesses stress and support in major life domains of occupation, finance, housing, social life, marriage, and family	100 individuals with minor psychiatric morbidity	Interrater reliability: .75 to .95; Internal consistency: Kendall's tau: .65 to .72
Social Support Index (SSI) (Wilcox, 1981)	18 items with 6 items from each of the following catagories of support: emotional, tangible, and informational	320 community residents	Test-retest reliability (4-week interval): .89 Internal consistency: .92 Validity data not available except that items were reported to buffer respondents from stress

Table 12–3. SUMMARY OF INSTRUMENTS USED TO MEASURE SOCIAL SUPPORT *(Continued)*

Measure	Description	Normative Group	Reliability/Validity
Social Support Questionnaire (SSQ1) (Sarason et al., 1983)	2 parts: 1. List of individuals in network 2. Level of satisfaction with support received	602 undergraduate students	Test-retest reliability (4-week interval): .90 (part 1) and .83 (part 2) Internal consistency: .97 (part 1) and .94 (part 2) Validity demonstrated with a number of other measures
Social Support Questionnaire (SSQ2) (Schaefer et al., 1981)	2 parts: 1. 9 situations measuring tangible support 2. List of network members and ratings for informational support and emotional support	100 adults, ages 48 to 64 years (48 men and 52 women)	Test-retest reliability (100 adults): .56 tangible support and .66 emotional support over 9 months Internal consistency: .81 informational support, .95 emotional support, and .31 tangible support Validity data not available
Social Support Questionnaire (SSQ3) (Wilcox, 1981)	Questions regarding number of supporters, relationship to respondents, and proximity and number of organizations to which respondents belong	Not available	Reliability and validity data not available
Social Support Satisfaction Scale (SSSS) (Blaik and Genser, 1980)	Both long and short form available, each consisting of a series of questions Respondent draws a line from feel worst possible to feel best possible for each question	Description of normative population not available	Test-retest reliability: .96 long form and .91 short form Internal consistency: .93 long form and .69 short form Interform substitutability: .85 Data on construct or concurrent validity not available
Social Support Scale (SSS1) (Dean et al., 1981)	4 parts: 1. Confidant characteristics 2. Family problems 3. Community and neighborhood support 4. Instrumental or expressive support	99 adults from New York State, based on census data	Factor analysis resulting in 5 items, .54 to .83 on instrumental or expressive support Interitem correlations among confidant characteristics: .28 to .82; family problems: .59 to .76; community and neighborhood support: .67 Validity data not available
Social Support Scale (SSS2) (Lin et al., 1979)	9-item scale measuring interaction and involvement with friends, neighbors, people nearby, and the subcultural community	121 male and 49 female Chinese-Americans (76% foreign born)	Internal consistency: .52 Interitem correlations: .36 to .74 Validity: correlation with number of psychiatric symptoms: .364
Social Support Vignettes (SSV) (Kaplan, 1977)	16 vignettes: Respondents pick which of the 3 fictitious people they resemble the most	293 family volunteers, 65 maladaptive parents, 420 hearing-impaired adults, and 100 mentally ill adults	Internal consistency: .79 for family volunteers, .82 for maladaptive parents, .83 for hearing-impaired adults, and .83 for mentally ill adults
Work Relationship Index (WRI) (Billings and Moos, 1982)	3 components: (1) involvement, concern and job commitment, (2) peer cohesion and support for co-workers, and (3) support to and from supervisors	185 employed men and 94 employed women community members	Test-retest reliability (12- to 15-month interval): .59 (men) and .53 (women) Internal consistency: .88 Validity: correlation with personal functioning range: −.20 to −.33 men and −.10 to −.15 women

THE INTERVENTION

Social network characteristics are related to health status and have implications for clinical assessment, community level needs assessment, and program planning. Assessment data related to the concepts in the Model are the basis for the intervention program. The steps in the process (Israel, 1983) include (1) determining social networks; (2) identifying need to strengthen existing networks and develop new networks; (3) providing services in a manner which is conducive to the development of interactions that provide feelings of caring, closeness, and moral support (interdependent and mutual, e.g., peer counseling and home visitors); (4) providing services that encourage the development of interactional skills (such as self-help groups); and (5) developing community-based promotion, prevention, treatment, and rehabilitation programs.

In addition, the kind of task or crisis facing the child and family, the stage of crisis, the needs of the individual child or family member, and the individual's orientation toward using network resources must be taken into consideration (Israel, 1983). The nurse should also keep in mind that (1) lay persons and professionals have expertise that can be shared, and (2) professionals need to acknowledge, respect, and respond appropriately to different value systems, norms, and customs. Intervention programs must focus on the child's and family's strengths and resources as well as their problems and needs. Lay persons should be involved in and should control to every extent possible programs for everything from defining the problem to evaluating the effectiveness of solutions. Social conditions that limit the effectiveness of health-promoting social networks must be identified and altered.

Determining Social Networks

Determination of social support should be part of every initial patient evaluation. The nurse should find out who the family counts on for comfort during times of trouble and ask who provides moral and emotional support. Future research may show instrumental aid, information or appraisal to be more important than the emotional aspect of the social support process; however, at the present time there is reason to believe that the emotional sustenance is what matters the most, so questions must be phrased with this belief in mind (Israel, 1983).

The nurse can do the following to intervene: Make a list of people who are close to the family using Norbeck's tool (Norbeck, 1981). Ask the family members to list all individuals who provide support or who are important to them. Ask who helps the family with problems or who they would call to provide help with a problem. Also, ask about social activities. When you are done with the list, give it to the family and ask them if there is anyone else they would like to add. Ask the family to select people on the list who they feel closest to. Inquire about the nature of these social relationships (type, strength, reciprocity). Now comes the hard part: You must make a judgment about the adequacy of the network. Try to reach your conclusion from the family's perspective. If the network is adequate, intervention is directed toward pointing out the strengths and effectiveness of the network to the family, as cognitive affirmation is important.

If you judge that there are deficits, you must consider the following possibility: Is the family doing well even though there is social isolation? If the answer is yes, monitor the situation. Do not intervene unless the family wants assistance. You might ask the family for ideas about who might help with a problem and reinforce opportunities within the social network for interaction. Make suggestions about how the relationship might be strengthened and ascertain the potential for change in existing resources. Help the family to understand the importance of reciprocity, and encourage them to interact with other members of their network. It is not necessary for a deficit to be present for intervention to occur.

Norbeck (1981) suggests minimal disruption or alteration in the natural support system unless it is a pathological system. If the family's needs cannot be met through the informal network, supplementation may be necessary, i.e., self-help groups. Additional resources may be provided through referral to community agencies or through the use of the family's network. Strategies that communicate factual information in terms that children can understand may help them anticipate their needs for resources and help them use the right amount and type.

Prioritizing Strategies

Different environments and situations require different supportive intervention strategies to optimally promote the family social support process (Unger and Powell, 1980; Croog et al., 1972). Qualitative differences in the types of support have been identified as emotional and supportive, instrumental and material, and informational and referential (Kaplan et al., 1977). The choice of intervention mode or strategy is dependent on the nurse's assessment of deficits based on antecedent variables in the Model.

It is important to prioritize and determine the cost of the intended intervention strategies. Children and their families have the right to collaborate in the development of the intervention plan and choose the plan which is most appropriate and affordable for them. Failing to determine the potential cost of the intervention plan denies the family the right to make an informed decision. This right is especially important in relationship to the family support process. A broad range of alternatives should be provided to the child and family. The social, psychological, physical, and financial implications of each alternative must be considered for truly informed decision making to occur.

Certain aspects of social networks are related to health status. The quality of interactions (emotional intensity, mutual sharing) rather than their frequency is most significantly related to well-being. Strategies for integrating network concepts into the nursing management of families have been suggested. Such approaches will recognize and build upon the potential influence of social networks on health-related behavior changes.

Consideration must be given to where the child and family assign responsibility for the child's needs, solutions, and the role of others. These decisions are made by the family social system based on their value system. Several types of value systems and their consequences are described in Table 12–4.

It also important for the nurse to identify his or her own value system regarding responsibility for needs and the provision of resources. Once an awareness of the value systems of both the nurse and family has developed, strategies appropriate for the family can be selected.

Social programs aimed at assisting the child to cope with one or more of the aspects of his or her medical management may also be considered. Such programs many include peer modeling and group or play therapy (Melamed and Seigel, 1975). These programs serve to provide feedback to the child and parents. Providing information serves the function of supplying reassurance through fostering a trusting relationship between the child and parents and the health care worker. The anxiety of the child and parents can also be reduced by decreasing uncertainty about what is going to happen (Clough, 1979; Becker, 1972).

Involving the Family in Care

Family-oriented programs for the family of an ill child can be conceptualized to include a continuum from general strategies appropriate to most families to more intensive specific approaches appropriate only to a specific problematic child or family. There is little empirical data to validate the effectiveness of family-oriented programs. However, parents report they value these types of groups (Tonkin, 1979; Vermilion et al., 1979). Parent care units are an example of a family-oriented program.

Chronically ill children are often hospitalized for diagnosis and initial treatment. Parental support during these times is recognized to be so important that most hospitals offer liberal visiting privileges. In a study by Hardgrove and Kermoian (1978), two thirds of the hospitals provided sleeping arrangements for parents and one half allowed well siblings to visit. One third of the hospitals provided parents with an educational program either prior to or following the child's hospitalization. Only a small percentage of the hospitals provided parental support groups; parents were often barred from medical tests and procedures administered to their child. Since the time of the Hardgrove and Kermoian study, several hospitals have developed parent care units.

In these units, parents are encouraged to take a major role in providing care for their hospitalized child. This type of social program is ideal for parents who need to develop expertise in managing their child's care or treatment once the child returns home. These programs appear to cost less

Table 12-4. VALUE ORIENTATION TO THE FAMILY SUPPORT PROCESS*

Types of Models

Dimensions of Model	Moral Model	Compensatory Model	Medical Model	Enlightenment Model
Responsibility for child's needs	All children's and parent's problems are of their own making	Children and parents are not blamed for problems but are seen as suffering from a lack of resources and services to which they are entitled	The child and parents are not responsible for their problems and are expected to adopt sick-role behavior	Children and parents are not blamed for causing their problems
Responsibility for solutions	Each child and parents must find their own solution	Children and parents are responsible to solve their own problems by seeking and using help from significant others or professionals	The child and parents are not responsible for finding a solution and are expected to seek and use expert help	The child and parents are not responsible for solving their problems
Role of other persons	Help may be given by significant others who provide strong emotional support or who exhort the child and parents to change and improve	Provides resources or opportunities that the child and parents need. The child and parents are responsible for deciding what will be helpful and if it will be used	Help is given by experts who know what the problem is, prescribe appropriate solutions, and determine if the solutions were successful	To enlighten persons about the true nature of their problems and the course of action that is needed to deal with their problems
Value of model	Compels the child and parents to take action on their own behalf and assume full responsibility for change	Increased competence of the child and parents	Allows the child and parents to claim and accept help without being blamed for their problem	This model is helpful when people are unable to control what they believe is undesirable behavior on their part
Problems of model	The belief that the child and parents always get what they deserve or deserve what they get. Conducive to loneliness	The child and parents are continually held responsible for solving their own problems even when the problems are not created by them. Poses a bitter view of the world	Fosters dependency rather than competency and compliance with agency procedures	May introduce guilt in those children and parents for whom the solution does not work

*From Cronenwett, L., and Brickman, P. Models of helping and coping in childbirth. Nursing Research, 32:84–88, 1983.

than routine hospital care (Tonkin, 1979; Vermilion et al., 1979). Another type of program is described in a study by Pless and Satterwhite (1972), in which lay persons were trained to serve as family counselors for other families of chronically ill children. All counselors had a child with a chronic disease in their family. The counselors served to listen, educate, and advise, as well as to help provide and coordinate services. Mothers who received this assistance were pleased and saw their children as better adjusted psychologically than control families who were not assigned a family counselor. This program appeared less effective with families who had multiple problems.

EVALUATION

Outcomes of interventions to promote the social support process are described in the community mental health literature (Caplan, 1974; Mitchell and Trickett, 1980). Three outcomes have been identified: (1) the child uses psychological resources and masters emotional burdens following emotional support from significant others; (2) the child shares tasks when provided with instrumental assistance; and (3) the child's ability to handle situations is improved with additional skills, materials, and cognitive guidance.

These outcomes reflect emotional, educational, and instrumental resource provision for the child. They can be modified to serve as outcome criteria for nursing intervention programs to promote the process of social support in the family.

Case Study

Mr. and Mrs. LeHare, ages 35 and 34, respectively, and their son Jacquo, age 5, resided in a lower-income section of a large metropolitan area. The LeHare family came to the attention of the public health nurse working in a pediatric outpatient clinic when appointments arranged for Jacquo at the asthma and immunology clinics were repeatedly missed. Jacquo had been diagnosed as having bronchial asthma when he was hospitalized at age three. Upon his discharge, the family was instructed about the treatment regimen by their local pediatrician. Since the initial admission, 12 hospitalizations had occurred because of acute exacerbation of the asthma. Three to four acute asthmatic attacks had been documented daily for the past several months.

During the nurse's visit, Mrs. LeHare contin- ually stated how she worried day and night about Jacquo's asthma and felt that he was too fragile to play with other children. She stated that she always anticipated "bad news" about Jacquo. In response to inquiries about the missed clinic visits, Mrs. LeHare seemed indifferent, stating that they had been too busy. Several covert statements were noted by the nurse throughout the conversation with Jacquo's mother: "He can spend all day playing; I know he can't really be that sick." Mrs. LeHare was unwilling to discuss Jacquo's asthmatic exacerbations except to say that they were Jacquo's way of getting attention.

During the home visit, Jacquo was observed to respect his mother's authority. Sitting quietly on the floor near his mother, he did not make any comments until he was directly asked a question. He answered quickly while looking at his mother for approval. Mrs. LeHare told the nurse that she believed that she must remain alongside of Jacquo all the time because of the frequent asthma attacks.

Mrs. LeHare related that the family had moved to their present location a year ago from a small town because Mr. LeHare had been transferred. Two months earlier, Mr. LeHare had lost his job and had been unable to find another. This had resulted in the family receiving welfare, which made both of Jacquo's parents feel ashamed.

The Model of Family Social Support provides the foundation for intervention strategies for the LeHare family. The strategies should be focused on the four categories of antecedent variables identified in the Model: characteristics of the child and family, the environment and situation, and interactions. Supplemental resources, new resources, or reinforcement of existing resources should be provided to promote the process of social support within the family.

Evaluation of the assessment data regarding the LeHare family supported the nursing diagnosis of *Compromised coping within the family*. This problem was thought to be associated with the inability of Jacquo's parents to generate adequate and appropriate resources through the social support process for Jacquo's comfort, assistance, and encouragement. Jacquo needed specific types of resources because of his individual characteristics to adapt to bronchial asthma and achieve his developmental potential.

Following review of the data from the home visit, it became evident that Jacquo's mother lacked a clear understanding of his needs. In fact, she was preoccupied with personal and emotional conflicts of her own that consumed her own resources to participate in the family social support process. Mrs. LeHare's lack of personal resources made it difficult for her to perceive Jacquo's needs (interactional factors). The temporary family disorganization and resultant role changes because of the relocation, job loss, and request for public assistance, (environmental and situational factors) were identified as intervention priorities. The ability of the LeHare family to cope with Jacquo's needs was dependent on the provision of additional supportive resources for the family as a whole. At that time, the family's resources were exhausted. Provision of resources from the community was deemed essential.

The data supporting the conclusions mentioned earlier included many of the antecedent variables associated with the process of family social support: missed clinic appointments (environmental and situational factors), Jacquo's repeated hospitalizations (child characteristic), and the disproportionate amount of maternal protective behavior demonstrated (interactional factor). Mrs. LeHare's lack of adequate knowledge about asthma, Mr. LeHare's loss of his job, and the application submitted by the family for public assistance also compromised the family's ability to engage in reciprocity, advice giving and feedback, and appropriate emotional involvement. Mrs. LeHare's attempt to deny the severity of Jacquo's condition while she worried constantly about him and about the family's relocation to an unfamiliar community further compromised the family social support process.

The plan for Jacquo's care should focus on continued assessment; the strengthening of existing social networks and the development of new networks; and the provision of services in a manner which is conducive to the development of interactions and feelings of closeness, caring, and moral support. Specific assessments should include a complete nursing history (including an assessment of the LeHare family's knowledge about asthma), a complete physical assessment of Jacquo, and administration of one of the instruments used to measure social support (see Table 12–3). Therapeutic and educational interventions needed are referral of the family to the appropriate social service and provision of transportation to the appointment; a possible home visit by the parent of another asthmatic child; and arrangements for Jacquo's transportation to clinic appointments, which should reduce the existing drain on the family's resources. These interventions should provide additional resources (emotional, instrumental, and educational) for the family and strengthen the internal family social network as well as the family's relationships with external social networks.

Information about Jacquo's condition supported with the use of visual aids, demonstrations, and reinforcement should be provided for both of Jacquo's parents (educational resources). Opportunities for privacy and questions should also be provided because it is essential that the LeHares perceive that they are competent and receiving the information correctly, not merely being told what to do (emotional resources). The family should be encouraged to learn at their own pace and allowed to make mistakes, but not to feel that they have failed. Plans for care of the LeHare family should be revised dependent on the assessment data and the response of the family to the intervention plan.

Outcomes identified for the LeHare family include the following: a list of the LeHare family's problems and resources; a family understanding of Jacquo's illness that includes physiological, developmental, and psychosocial implications; a relationship with social services; and enrollment in appropriate available community resources. In addition, the provision of support (e.g., listening, sharing information, affirming, and clarifying) by a home visitor and the offering of membership in a parent support group are also essential outcomes. Provision of transportation so that Jacquo can attend his next clinic appointment and revision of Jacquo's plan for care within one month based on the assessment data are also important outcomes for the LeHare family. Achievement of these family-specific outcomes will result in the following: (1) Jacquo will be better able to use his psychological resources and successfully cope with the emotional burdens associated with his illness because of the resources generated through his interaction with his family, (2) Jacquo should share in responsibility for tasks associated with his care as well as in maintenance of the family unit; and (3) Jacquo's ability to deal with responsibilities within the family system should improve because of additional skills, materials, cognitive guidance, and emotional reassurance.

RESEARCH IMPLICATIONS

In this section, implications for research related to the process of social support are considered from two points of view: conceptual clarity and theoretical alternatives.

Variables associated with support are inconsistently conceptualized and operationalized and are often not derived from a theoretical framework. It is difficult to detect relationships between social support and health outcomes with measures having less than optimal reliability. At the present time there is no consensus on the operational or conceptual definition of social support (Gottlieb, 1981). This makes it difficult, if not impossible, to compare studies that link social support to stress, health outcomes, and general and psychological well-being. This results in problems in generalizing findings related to the support process from one study to another. A definition of what is meant by family, beliefs about health and illness, and children's health concepts is also urgently needed.

A review of the results of investigations related to the support process revealed that investigators failed to differentiate between support as a process that buffers the impact of stress and as a main effect (Cohen and Wills 1985). The interplay between social health, of which the process of social support is a part, and physical health (Renne, 1974) has also not been well developed. In addition, the interaction between resources, stress, and the support process is not documented (Thoits, 1985).

Problems associated with construct independence are also prevalent in the existing literature. The embryonic nature of procedures established within the discipline of nursing to study holistic constructs poses an additional methodological problem. A comprehensive discussion of these problems extends beyond the boundaries of this chapter. However, researchers must address these concerns in any investigation of the family support process.

Although it is reasonable to assume, as the Model does, that parental characteristics are related to the health outcome for the child, the mechanisms by which this occurs are often undefined. Family characteristics are often associated with child outcome variables without considering intervening variables associated with the child's characteristics (e.g., the child's knowledge of the disease or perceptions of the treatment plan). Consideration must also be given to family members other than the mother. To date, most studies focus on the mother-child relationship. All contextual environmental variables must also be defined and measured. Thus, methods need to be developed to measure the intervening variables specified in the Model as well as new variables as they emerge from future studies.

The well-accepted assumption that all families benefit from intervention needs to be re-examined from the evolving data base. Studies conducted to date do not answer questions of primary importance, such as the following: Who needs resources? How should resources be provided and by whom and at what time? Current policies that allow parents to participate in administering care in health care settings provide unique opportunities for naturalistic studies in which the interactions of children and their parents involved in the process of social support can be studied. Intervention measures related to

theoretical postulates need to be developed and examined empirically, with reference to specific outcome criteria. Collaboration between different disciplines incorporating direction from both the research literature and practice appropriate to the discipline should advance our understanding of the social support process within families of ill children.

Future studies must consider the difference between the availability of resources versus satisfaction with resources. McNett's (1987) work indicates that perceived availability of social support, but not the use of social support, was significantly related to coping effectiveness. In contrast with the relationship usually reported between marital status and coping, unmarried subjects in this study coped more effectively and perceived less threat. Personal constraints related to the use of resources must also be considered.

Criterion validity of measures of the social support process continues to be a problem because validity is dependent on demonstration of association between a score and some well-defined criterion. At the present time no criterion measurement of the social support process is available. Demonstration of construct validity while simultaneously defining a construct and developing an instrument to measure is a problem of significant magnitude.

A need also exists to develop and refine the Model as presented here so that relationships between the child's characteristics, the family's characteristics, and interactional factors can be explicated. The existing lack of data, combined with lack of both conceptual clarity and articulated theory, suggests a theoretical breakthrough may be somewhat distant.

At this point in time, most of the research available in this area is correlational in nature. A need for longitudinal studies also exists. Children grow and change, altering the nature of appropriate interventions. Thus, the social support process must be studied within a developmental context using a longitudinal design.

In summary, research problems related to the process of social support are based on the fact that little strong evidence to confirm the role the social support process plays in health and illness exists. This situation is not surprising because attempts at conceptualization and measurement have been inadequate and discipline bound and usually based on retrospective interpretations of unexpected findings. Future investigations must focus on (1) the place of social support in understanding health, (2) the question of what social support alters in the person, (3) clarification of the concept of social support, (4) definition of the relevance of the concept for the individual, (5) testing the propositions associated with the Model, and (6) nursing care implications based on what is known.

We have attempted to link the theory, research, and practice concepts relevant to social support process and their association with child health status. Applied action-oriented research is needed involving the collaboration of researchers, practitioners, and community members to generate new knowledge and understanding of behavioral science principles. This interaction will also facilitate the development of effective counseling and educational programs that build on the individual and collective expertise found in social networks.

The strength, courage, and determination of children who are able both with adequate support and with minimal resources to live fully should challenge us to address these challenging research issues. It is hoped that enlarging our knowledge base will offer increasingly effective support for children, who grow and develop and must struggle to live, adapt well, and experience a positive quality of life.

References

Barrera, M. Preliminary development of a scale of social support. American Journal of Community Psychology, 9:435–447, 1981.

Bates, J. The concept of difficult temperament. Merrill-Palmer Quarterly, 26:299–319, 1980.

Baumrind, D. Child care practices anteceding three patterns of preschool behavior. Genetic Psychology Monographs, 75:43–88, 1967.

Baumrind, D. Current patterns of parental authority. Developmental Psychology Monographs, 4, 1971.

Becker, RD. Therapeutic approaches to psychopathological reactions to hospitalization. International Journal of Child Psychotherapy, 2:64–97, 1972.

Belsky, J. The determinants of parenting: A process model. Child Development, 55:83–96, 1984.

Belsky, J, Robins, E, and Gamble, W. The determinants of parental competence: Toward a contextual theory. In Lewis, M (Ed.), Beyond the dyad. New York: Plenum Publishing Corp., 1984.

Berrera, B, and Ainlay, SL. The structure of social support: A conceptual and empirical analysis. American Journal of Community Psychology, 11:113–143, 1983.

Billings, AF, and Moos, RH. Social support and functioning among community and clinical groups: A panel model. Journal of Behavioral Medicine, 5:295–311, 1982.

Blaik, R, and Genser, SG. Perception of social support satisfaction: Scale development. Personality and Social Psychology Bulletin, 6:172–178, 1980.

Boll, TJ, Dimino, E, and Mattsson, AE. Parenting attitudes: The role of personality style and childhood in long-term illness. Journal of Psychosocial Research, 22:209–213, 1978.

Bovard, EW. The balance between negative and positive brain system activity. Perspectives in Biological Medicine, 6:116, 1962.

Bowlby, J. Attachment and loss (Vol. 1). Attachment. New York: Basic Books, Inc., 1969.

Bowlby, J. Attachment and loss (Vol. 2). Separation. New York: Basic Books, Inc., 1973.

Bowlby, J. Attachment and loss. American Journal of Orthopsychiatry, 52:664–678, 1982.

Brandt, PA, and Weinert, C. The PRQ: A social support measure. Nursing Research, 30:277–280, 1981.

Burke, WT, and Abidin, RR. Parenting stress index: A family system assessment approach. In Abidin, RR (Ed.), Parent education and intervention handbook. Springfield, Ill.: Charles C Thomas, 1980.

Campbell, S. Mother-infant interaction as a function of maternal ratings of temperament. Child Psychiatry and Human Development, 10:67–76, 1979.

Caplan, G. Support systems and community mental health. New York: Human Sciences Press, Inc., 1974.

Chess, S, and Thomas, A. Temperament in clinical practice. New York: The Guilford Press, 1986.

Clough, F. The validation of meaning in illness-treatment situations. In Hall, D, and Stacey, M (Eds.), Beyond separation. London: Routledge and Kegan Paul, Inc., 1979.

Cochran, MA. A comparison of group day and family child-rearing patterns in Sweden. Child Development, 48:702–707, 1977.

Cochran, MA, and Brassard, JA. Child development and personal social networks. Child Development, 50:601–616, 1979.

Cohen, S, and Wills, TA. Stress, social support and the buffering hypothesis. Psychological Bulletin, 98:310–357, 1985.

Cohen, S, and Syme, SL. Issues in the study and application of social support. In Cohen, S, and Syme, SL (Eds.), Social support and health. New York: Academic Press, Inc., 1985.

Cohen, S, Mermelstein, R, Kamarck, T, and Hoberman, HN. Measuring the functional components of social support. In Sarason, I, and Sarason, B (Eds.), Social support: Theory, research, and applications. Dordrecht, Netherlands: Martinus Nijhoff, 1985.

Colletta, N. Support systems after divorce: Incidence and impact. Journal of Marriage and the Family, 41:837–846, 1979.

Crittendon, PM. Social networks, quality of child rearing, and child development. Child Development, 56:1299–1313, 1985.

Cronenwett, L, and Brickman, P. Models of helping and coping in childbirth. Nursing Research, 32:84–88, 1983.

Croog, SH, Lipson, A, and Levine, S. Helping patterns in severe illness: The roles of kin and non-family resources, and institutions. Journal of Marriage and the Family, 2:32–41, 1972.

Dean, A, Lin, N, and Ensel, WM. The epidemiological significance of social support systems in depression. Research in Community Mental Health, 2:77–109, 1981.

Ellison, ES. Social support and the Constructive-Developmental Model. Western Journal of Nursing Research, 9:19–28, 1987.

Gore, S. The effect of social support in moderating the health consequences of unemployment. Journal of Health and Social Behavior, 19:151–165, 1978.

Gottlieb, BH. Social networks and social support. Beverly Hills, Calif.: Sage Publications, 1981.

Greenblatt, M, Becerra, RM, and Serfetinides, EA. Social networks in mental health: An overview. American Journal of Psychiatry, 139:977–984, 1982.

Hardgrove, C, and Kermoian, R. Parent-inclusive pediatric units: A survey of policies and practices. American Journal of Public Health. 68:847–850, 1978.

Heitzmann, CA, and Kaplan, RM. Assessment of methods for measuring social support. Health Psychology, 7:75–109, 1988.

Henderson, S, Duncan-Jones, P, Byrne, DG, and Scott, R. Measuring social relationships: The interview schedule for social interaction. Psychological Medicine, 10:723–734, 1980.

Holahan, CJ, and Moos, RH. Social support and adjustment: Predictive benefits of social climate indices. American Journal of Community Psychology, 10:403–415, 1982.

Israel, BA. Social networks and health status: Linking theory, research, and practice. Patient Counseling and Health Education, 4:65–79, 1983.

Jenkins, R, Mann, AH, and Belsey, E. The background, description, and use of a short interview to assess stress and social support. Social Science and Medicine, 15:195–203, 1981.

Kahn, RL. Aging and social support. In Riley, MD (Ed.), Aging from birth to death: Interdisciplinary perspectives. American Association for the Advancement of Science: Selected Symposium No. 30. Boulder, Colo.: Westfield Press, 1979, pp. 77–91.

Kane, CF. Family social support: Toward a conceptual model. Advances in Nursing Science, 10:18–25, 1988.

Kaplan, A. Social support: The construct and its measurement. Unpublished bachelor of arts thesis, Brown University, Providence, R.I., 1977.

Kaplan, BH, Cassel, JC, and Gore, S. Social support and health. Medical Care, 15:47–57, 1977.

Katz, ER, Kellerman, J, and Siegel, SE. Behavioral distress in children with cancer undergoing medical procedures: Developmental considerations. Journal of Consulting and Clinical Psychology, 48:356–365, 1980.

Kegan, R. The evolving self: Problem and process in human development. Cambridge, Mass.: Harvard University Press, 1982.

Kelley, P. The relation of infant's temperament and mother's psychopathology to interactions in early infancy. In Riegel, KF, and Meacham, JA (Eds.), The developing individual in a changing world (Vol 11). Chicago: Aldine, 1976.

Kim, MJ, McFarland, GK, and McLane, AM. Pocket guide to nursing diagnosis. St. Louis: CV Mosby Co., 1986.

Kiritz, S, and Moos, RH. Physiological effects of social environments. Psychosomatic Medicine, 36:96–114, 1974.

Leavy, RL. Social support and psychological disorder: A review. Journal of Community Psychology, 11:3–21, 1983.

Lerner, R, and Lerner, J. Temperament-intelligence reciprocities in early childhood: A contextual model. In Lewis, M (Ed.), Origins of intelligence (2nd ed.). New York: Plenum Publishing Corp., 1985.

Lin, N, Simeone, R, Ensel, W, and Kuo, W. Social support, stressful life events and illness: A model and an empirical test. Journal of Health and Social Behavior, 20:108–119, 1979.

Mattsson, A. Long-term physical illness in childhood: A challenge to psychosocial adaptation. Pediatrics, 50:801–811, 1972.

McCollum, AT. The chronically ill child. New Haven: Yale University Press, 1981.

McFarlane, AH, Neale, KA, Norman, GR, Roy, RG, and Streiner, DL. Methodological issues in developing a scale to measure social support. Schizophrenia Bulletin, 7:90–100, 1981.

McNett, SC. Social support, threat, and coping responses and effectiveness in the functionally disabled. Nursing Research, 36:98–103, 1987.

Melamed, BG, and Siegel, LJ. Reduction of anxiety in children facing hospitalization and surgery by use of filmed modeling. Journal of Consulting and Clinical Psychology, 43:511–521, 1975.

Milliones, J. Relationship between perceived child temperament and maternal behavior. Child Development, 49:1255–1257, 1978.

Minuchin, S, and Minuchin, P. Families and family therapy. Cambridge, Mass.: Harvard University Press, 1974.

Mitchell, R, and Trickett, E. Task force report: Social networks as mediators of social support. Community Mental Health Journal, 16:27–44, 1980.

Moos, RH. The family environment scale preliminary manual. Palo Alto, Calif.: Consulting Psychologist Press, 1974.

Moos, RH, and Tsu, VD. The crisis of physical illness: An overview. In Moos, RH (Ed.), Coping with physical illness. New York: Plenum Publishing Corp., 1977.

Moos, RH, and Moos, BS. Family environment scale manual. Palo Alto, Calif.: Consulting Psychologists Press, 1981.

Norbeck, JS. Social support: A model for clinical research and application. Advances in Nursing Science, 3:43–59, 1981.

Norbeck, JS, Lindsey, AM, and Carrieri, VL. The development of an instrument to measure social support. Nursing Research, 30:264–269, 1981.

Pascoe, JM, Loda, FA, Jeffries, V, and Easp, JA. The association between mothers' social support and provision of stimulation to their children. Developmental and Behavioral Pediatrics, 2:15–19, 1981.

Patenaude, AF, Szymanski, L, and Rappeport, J. Psychological costs of bone marrow transplantation in children. American Journal of Orthopsychiatry, 49:409–422, 1979.

Pless, IB, and Satterwhite, BB. Chronic illness in childhood: Selection, activities, and evaluation of nonprofessional family counselors. Clinical Pediatrics, 11:403–410, 1972.

Pless IB, and Satterwhite, BB. A measure of family functioning and its application. Social Science and Medicine, 7:613–621, 1973.

Pless, IB, Roughmann, K, and Haggerty, RF. Chronic illness, family functioning, and psychological adjustment: A model for the allocation of preventive mental health services. International Journal of Epidemiology, 1:271–277, 1972.

Powazek, M, Goff, JR, and Paulson, MA. Emotional reactions of children to isolation in a cancer hospital. Journal of Pediatrics, 92:834–837, 1978.

Powell, GF, Brasel, JA, and Blizzard, RM. Emotional deprivation and growth retardation simulating idiopathic hypopituitarism: Clinical evaluation of the syndrome. New England Journal of Medicine, 276:1271–1278, 1967.

Procidano, ME, and Heller, K. Measures of perceived social support from friends and from the family: Three validation studies. American Journal of Community Psychology, 11:1–24, 1983.

Reddihough, DS, Landau, L, Jones, HJ, and Rickards, WS. Family anxieties in childhood asthma. Australian Paediatric Journal, 13:295–298, 1977.

Reinhart, F. Drash A. Psychosocial dwarfism: Environmental induced recovery. Psychosomatic Medicine, 31:165–172, 1969.

Renne, KS. Measurement of social health in a general population survey. Social Science Research, 5:25–44, 1974.

Sarason, IG, Levine, HM, Basham RB, and Sarason, BR. Assessing social support: The social support questionnaire. Journal of Personality and Social Psychology, 44:127–139, 1983.

Schaefer, C, Coyne, JC, and Lazarus, RS. Health-related functions of social support. Journal of Behavioral Medicine, 4:381–406, 1981.

Schafer, LC, McCaul, KD, and Glasgow, RE. Supportive and nonsupportive family behaviors: Relationships to adherence and metabolic control in persons with Type I diabetes. Unpublished manuscript, North Dakota State University, Fargo, N.D., 1984.

Schoenhofer, SO. Support as legitimate action. Nursing Outlook, 32:218–219, 1984.

Spinetta, JJ. Adjustment and adaptation in children with cancer: A 3-year study. In Spinetta, JJ, and Deasy-Spinetta, P (Eds.), Living with childhood cancer. St. Louis: CV Mosby Co., 1981.

Spitz, RA. Hospitalism: Psychoanalytic study of the child (Vol 1). New York: International University Press, 1945.

Spitz, RA. Hospitalism: A follow-up report. Psychoanalytic study of the child (Vol 2). New York: International University Press, 1947.

Stein, RK, and Riessman, CK. The development of an impact-on-family scale: Preliminary findings. Medical Care, 18:465–472, 1980.

Stokes, JP. Predicting satisfaction with social support from social network structure. American Journal of Community Psychology, 11:141–152, 1983.

Thoits, PA. Social support and psychological well-being: Theoretical possibilities. In Sarason, IG, and Sarason, BR (Eds.), Social support: Theory, research, and applications. Dordrecht, Netherlands: Martinus Nijhoff, 1985.

Tonkin, P. Parent care for the low risk and terminally ill child. Dimensions in Health Service, 56: 42–43, 1979.

Turner, RJ, Frankel, BG, and Levine, DM. Social support: Conceptualization, measurement and implications for mental health. Research in Community Mental Health, 3:67–111, 1983.

Unger, DG, and Powell, DR. Supporting families under stress: The role of social networks. Family Relations, 29:566–574, 1980.

Ventura, J. Parent coping behaviors, parent functioning, and infant temperament characteristics. Nursing Research, 31:268–273, 1982.

Ventura, J. Parent coping: A replication. Nursing Research, 35:77–80, 1986.

Vermilion, B, Ballantine, T, and Grosfeld, J. The effective use of the parent care unit for infants on the surgical service. Journal of Pediatric Surgery, 14:321–324, 1979.

Whitt, JK, Brantley, HT, and Wise, E. Family, child, and school factors in academic "re-entry" of children with chronic illness. Unpublished research report to the Spencer Foundation, University of North Carolina at Chapel Hill, N.C., 1982.

Wilcox, BL. Social support, life stress and psychological adjustment. American Journal of Community Psychology, 9:371–386, 1981.

Wolfer, J, and Visintainer, M. Pediatric surgical patients' and parents' stress responses and adjustment. Nursing Research, 24:244–255, 1975.

CHAPTER **13**

USING FRIENDS AS A SOCIAL SUPPORT SYSTEM FOR CHILDREN

DIANE PFLEDERER, M.A., R.N.

The relationships that children share with their friends serve as one of the central ingredients of childhood. These relationships account for a large portion of the lives of children through the outer world of shared experiences between friends and the inner world of thoughts and fantasies that children have about their friends (Rubin, 1980). Although most children interact with many other children in a variety of social situations, only a small number of these interactions will evolve into friendships. Friendships can be defined as relationships between children that are based upon affec-

tive preferences and are emotionally rewarding to each child (Suelzel, 1981).

Because of the supportive nature of friendships, it is vital that these relationships be maintained when children are experiencing altered health status. The purpose of this chapter is to discuss the concept of friendship as a support system for children. In the theoretical framework, friendship formation will be traced from its early foundations in infancy to its full development during childhood and adolescence. The function of friendship will be discussed as well as the supportive role that it can play in helping children cope with illness. Support will be defined as "promot[ing] the interests or cause of [and] defend[ing] as valid or right" (Webster, 1987).

THEORETICAL FOUNDATION

The Function of Friendship

Throughout childhood, friendships provide children with opportunities for the development of social skills and psychological growth. Friendships play a vital role in helping children understand themselves. In the safe environment of a close friendship, sense of self is nourished through mutual validation of ideas, thoughts, and feelings. Along with strengthening self-awareness, friendships provide the opportunity for children to appreciate the value of interdependent relationships with others and to develop the social skills that are necessary for harmonious interactions with others in various social situations. The research literature reveals an association between childhood peer relationships and later mental health (Crockett, 1984). Significant relationships have been found between childhood peer relationships, high school activity, and young adult mental health. In a longitudinal study that followed over 2000 grade school children into young adulthood, Roff and Wirt (1984) reported that children with low peer status had a two to three times greater risk for mental health treatment during young adulthood.

The development of intimacy between friends is one of the most valuable functions of friendship. Sullivan (1953) hypothesized that intimacy begins during preadolescence as children learn to adjust their own behavior to the expressed needs of a friend of the same sex, resulting in a relationship that involves validation of all components of self-worth. Intimate friendships include providing satisfaction to one another and sharing experiences as the two friends move toward common goals.

Child development theories vary in their view of the role that friends play in the socialization of children. Traditional socialization theories emphasize the important role that adults have in helping children understand society. The child is viewed as a passive individual who is influenced by praise, instruction, and other forms of communication from adults. Cognitive theories view the child as a more active participant in social development. These theories emphasize the cognitive capacities that are needed to form relationships. As cognitive skills are developed, children move away from an egocentric world and learn to understand and take on the perspectives of others. Piaget (1969) placed more emphasis on the role that peers have in transmitting societal norms to children. According to Piaget, adult interactions with children communicate the belief that all situations are governed by rules. This belief is transformed through interactions with other children because children learn that they are equal to their peers, and, therefore, new rules can be constructed through cooperation and negotiations with peers. Sullivan (1953) valued the contribution that friends make in social development. He believed that friends provide new opportunities for social exchange and consequently enable children to discover meaningful insights about themselves. Sullivan viewed close friendships as opportunities for children to develop a capacity for intimacy (Skolnick, 1986; Youniss, 1980).

The Supportive Role of Friendship During Illness

Several social support researchers have postulated that the need for supportive relationships is increased when individuals encounter unwanted and unpredicted changes in their lives. The presence of a supportive network of family and friends often facilitates the ability of the individual to cope with these changes. Additionally, this network may protect people as they pass through the transitions and crises of the life cycle (Cobb, 1976; Kahn and Antonucci, 1981). Support from friends can also decrease the potential for development of a state of learned helplessness, which may occur when individuals feel they cannot overcome uncontrollable negative events in their lives. Supportive actions that help an individual gain a sense of control and predictability will diminish the undesirable effects of unwanted and unpredictable circumstances (Wallston et al, 1983).

The way in which an individual responds

to a crisis is not only related to the support received from family and friends but also to the coping behavior of that particular person. Broadhead and colleagues (1983) define this interaction between individuals and their social environments in terms of goodness of fit. A good fit depends on the following factors: (1) a match between the *demands* of the environment and the ability of the individual to handle those demands and (2) a match between the *needs* of the individual and the resources from the environment that are available to satisfy those needs.

The ability of the child to handle demands and seek resources from the environment is dependent upon age and experience. The initial mother-infant relationship serves as a pattern for later supportive interactions. Therefore, in early infancy, patterns of altering and controlling the social environment are established that are later expanded and reinforced through the numerous stressful experiences of childhood and adolescence (Broadhead et al., 1983). Because the needs of the child change with age and experience, the form and amount of support that is needed change with time. In early childhood, parents provide the majority of support to the young child experiencing illness. As the child grows older, other people, such as siblings, grandparents, and friends, are incorporated into the expanding social world of the child. If initial interpersonal experiences are warm, responsive, and encouraging, the behavioral patterns and beliefs of the child about supportive relationships will be reinforced. Eventually, the social environment of the child will include a network of supportive people who are available to provide support for the child who is coping with the developmental challenges of growing up, handling unexpected illness, or facing an aversive event (Kahn and Antonucci, 1981).

Development of Friendship Patterns Throughout Childhood

Numerous psychoanalytic, child development, and social learning theories emphasize the significance of the early dyadic relationship between an infant and mother. As mentioned earlier, this dynamic relationship may serve as a pattern for later supportive interactions because it provides the infant with opportunities to receive support and actively acquire gratification from the mother. Both the infant and mother are actively involved in this relationship and bring unique backgrounds to it, such as the temperament and genetic endowment of the infant, the temperament and experiences of the mother, parental expectations, and parenting style (Kahn and Antonucci, 1981). The nature and quality of early social interactions within the family influence the development of social behaviors between infants.

Infants begin to demonstrate the beginnings of social interaction with other infants by the end of the first year. Early in the first year, it is common for infants to engage in similar activities in close proximity to one another without any interaction. Interaction between prelinguistic infants generally involves accidental exploration of each other because of a mutual interest in a toy or object. As language formation begins near the end of the first year, interactions between infants gradually result in an appreciation of the socially responsive nature of communication. During the second year, toddlers begin to direct social behaviors, such as smiling and vocalizing, toward one another and eventually coordinate these behaviors so that social interchanges occur (Rubin, 1980).

Toddler friendship has been studied by videotaping eight toddlers in an adult-supervised peer group over a one year period. These videotapes demonstrated that two of the toddlers developed a relationship through a sequence of identifiable stages. Although this relationship did not include many of the elements of friendships between older children, the tapes revealed the presence of proximity seeking, positive affect, shared activities, and empathetic behavior (Press and Greenspan, 1985). Thus, by the end of the second year, the toddler has a beginning awareness of friendship as a relationship that offers the opportunity for sharing enjoyable activities with familiar peers who respond in particular ways.

During the span from three to five years, social relationships between children involve momentary interactions with playmates who are physically available to each other at any particular point in time. In order for these relationships to develop, there must be opportunities for children with similar interests to interact over repeated occasions. Because of the need for adult supervision of this age group, such opportunities may be either common or unusual, depending on the schedule of the supervising adult. One setting where these opportunities occur regularly is the day care center. Over a three year period of time, Suelzel (1981) studied friendship formation by observing two to five year old children enrolled in full-time day care. In her study, she identified the following types of social exchanges, which occurred in the following hierarchical order: (1) situational relationships that occurred because children were aggregated as classmates, (2) interactions that occurred when children engaged in ongoing verbal dialogues and shared activities, (3) alliances that occurred when children were attracted to one another through mutual interests, and (4) friendships that were selectively initiated by children who were emotionally involved with other children of similar interests or skills. Her study revealed examples of all levels of interaction between various ages of children in the day care setting with some interactions eventually advancing to the friendship stage. Some friendships occurred between children of differing ages from two to five years when there were frequent opportunities for children with similar interests to interact. Some children were more apt to form friendships because they had basically altruistic personalities or were consistently positively responsive to the interactions of others. Older or more experienced children often had an advantage in establishing friendships because their seniority enabled them to easily initiate interactions and respond to interactions from others (Suelzel, 1981).

The Suelzel study relates to earlier research by Duck (1973) on personal constructs in adult friendship formation. Duck concluded that individuals pass through several stages from initial attraction to one another to actual friendship formation. He demonstrated that individuals in new groups relied on physical constructs in evaluating new acquaintances. In subsequent encounters with the same individuals, psychological traits and interaction styles became important determinants in friendship formation (Duck, 1973).

During the elementary school years, relationships between children progress from momentary encounters with many peers to frequent interactions with several favorite peers. According to Sullivan (1953), friendships become more important during this time, because children become more sensitive to the needs of others. These changes occur because of growth in several areas of social development. The first area is the growing ability of the child to understand the point of view of another person. Very young children are egocentric, whereas older children are beginning to be able to understand the viewpoints of their peers, which definitely contributes to growth in social relationships. Second, children learn to recognize and value psychological qualities of their peers rather than only physical traits. When describing their friends, older children are more likely to use abstract concepts that relate to behavioral dispositions, such as, "She's a real showoff" (Rubin, 1980). Over time, psychological qualities have an increasing significance in friendship formation. Third, the child's perception of friendship changes from momentary encounters to emotionally rewarding relationships that endure over time (Rubin, 1980).

There are a variety of developmental research studies that illustrate the change in friendship behavior over the school years. Childhood friendship has been studied by comparing the stated intentions and actual behaviors of two age groups toward their friends. Berndt (1981) found that fourth graders were more likely to share with their friends than first graders. Newcomb and Brady (1982) studied mutuality in second grade and sixth grade boys by comparing differences in socially responsive behaviors of friends and acquaintances in each age group. Study outcomes led them to the conclusion that social responsiveness to friends developed in early childhood and remained stable throughout childhood.

As early adolescence approaches, there is a growing tendency for children to form close relationships with a few friends along with a continuing emphasis on peer group membership. Crockett and colleagues (1984) studied early adolescent peer relations by observing students over a two year period of time from sixth grade to eighth grade. Their study revealed that most boys and girls had well-developed friendship networks that included a group of good friends and one best friend of the same sex who they interacted with on a frequent basis at school. With each grade level, there was an increase in the number of students reporting that they were able to confide in their friends. At the same time, most students also reported feeling close to their parents. The authors concluded that early adolescents began to expand their close relationships with their parents to include their friends.

During adolescence, close relationships with friends of the same sex assume an even greater importance than in earlier years. These friendships endure over time, are based on affective preferences, and are highly valued. Adolescents spend most of their time with their friends, away from the presence of their parents. In a study that contrasted the daily experiences of adolescents with family and friends, Larson (1983) found that adolescents felt open and free with their friends, their talk was joking, and they received positive feedback from friends, whereas adolescent interactions with their families were more closed and restrained. However, Larson also found poorer school performance and mood variability in adolescents who spent more time with their friends than with their families.

Over a four year period of time, Youniss and Smollar (1985) carried out eight studies on various aspects of interpersonal relationships between adolescents and their parents and adolescents and their friends. In one study, they surveyed 180 subjects with 60 subjects in each age level of 12 to 13 years, 14 to 16 years, and 18 to 20 years. Their questionnaire was designed to assess the range of topics and quality of communication in adolescent relations with their mothers, fathers, and friends. Study results revealed that 66% of the females appeared to have close friendships based on shared activities; mutual understanding; a respect for differing opinions; and a perception of self as open, relaxed, accepted, and accepting. Fewer than 50% of the males reported this form of shared friendships, while 33% of the males had close friendships characterized by nonunderstanding, absence of intimacy, and a sense of guardedness or defensiveness.

ASSESSMENT

The challenge for nurses in the health care and school setting is to identify those chil-

dren who are undergoing excessive or continuing physical or psychological stressors that could be mitigated by support from friends. Examples of such stressors include sudden hospitalization, chronic illness, the return of a child with an altered physical appearance to school, and teenage pregnancy. Such experiences place unique demands on the child or adolescent and increase the need for support from friends. However, the unusual nature of these events may result in a strain on relationships between friends and ultimately hinder the potential for support, especially if the child becomes physically separated from friends. Therefore, it is important for nurses to recognize the support needs of the child in crisis as well as the needs of the friends who may be able to help.

When sudden hospitalization occurs, the child is unexpectedly separated from the familiarity of home and friends and placed in a strange new environment. During the initial crisis period in the hospital, the majority of support will probably be provided by family members. However, as the child improves, there will be opportunities for friends from home to provide support through letters and calls, especially if hospitalization is prolonged. The hospital nurse must recognize that friends can help and then establish an environment that allows for supportive interactions to occur between friends. Friends at home may be very curious and even frightened because of the sudden departure of the ill child. The school nurse can help by identifying the children who are close to the ill child and then providing ongoing explanations about the child in the hospital and encouraging correspondence with the ill child.

Chronic illness usually places a strain on friendships between school-aged children because of repeated hospitalizations and absences from school. Consequently, there are limited opportunities for establishing and strengthening friendships. The recurring nature of chronic illness places continuous demands on the child and may cause feelings of loss of control and helplessness. Supportive friends can help the child maintain a sense of control through frequent visits and conversations about school happenings, whether the child is hospitalized or recuperating at home. Hospital and school nurses must recognize the importance of ongoing support from friends when a child has a chronic illness. The teacher can also play a key role by identifying school friends who can help and then encouraging these friends to remain involved with the ill child.

For children who experience physical changes, such as an amputation or alopecia, the potential for re-establishing previous friendships or establishing new friendships after hospitalization may be jeopardized if peers perceive the physical change as a stigma. During initial interactions with peers, the physical change in the child may serve as a salient cue that interferes with the process of friendship formation. Here again, the school nurse can help by recognizing the potential for altered relationships between friends, and then steps can be taken to minimize this potential.

When adolescent pregnancy occurs, the presence of supportive friends may influence the adjustment of the adolescent. Barrera (1981) conducted a study that illustrated this relationship. To assess social support systems of pregnant adolescents, Barrera utilized the Inventory of Socially Supportive Behaviors (ISSB), which measures the frequency and type of helpful behaviors, and the Arizona Social Support Interview Schedule (ASSIS), which determines support satisfaction, need, and social network indexes. Negative life events and symptomatology of participants were also assessed. Assessment procedures included self-administered scales and structured interviews of the participants. Study outcomes revealed that the ISSB and ASSIS were effective measures of the frequency with which various forms of support were given. However, the consequences of receiving various supportive interventions were not demonstrated. The women who reported the most stress during pregnancy received the most support, but the particular benefit of each intervention could not be demonstrated.

In addition to determining situations that create a need for friendship to be utilized as an intervention, two nursing diagnoses will assist the nurse to recognize this need: (1) *Coping, ineffective individual*; and (2) *Self-concept, disturbance in: body image* (Kim et al., 1984). The defining characteristics of these diagnoses provide the nurse with data which indicate that friendships of the child may be jeopardized or that the child will benefit from support from friends.

For the diagnosis of *Ineffective individual coping*, key defining characteristics are non-verbal behaviors or verbal statements by the child which demonstrate an inability to cope with an illness or unexpected event. Expressions of ineffective coping will vary greatly with the age of the child. Examples of this wide variance range from subtle behavior changes in problem solving ability in a school-aged child to overt statements from an adolescent which indicate an inability to handle the unexpected event.

The diagnosis of *Disturbance in self concept* is justified when the child demonstrates a negative response to an actual or perceived change in body structure or function. Since changes in the physical appearances of children influence the feelings that they have about themselves, it is not unusual for children to respond negatively to such experiences. Examples of cues of a disturbed self-concept include single or frequent negative comments about self during play sessions or nursing care activities, withdrawal of the child from social situations with peers, and refusal of the child to look at self in the mirror (Arneson and Triplett, 1978).

THE INTERVENTION

Using Existing Friends

An essential first step in implementing support from friends is assessing the quantity, quality, strengths, and limitations of significant relationships. The awareness by the nurse that the child has significant friends who are potential supporters will be heightened by asking questions during the admission process about relationships with friends. This measure is especially important for children of junior high-school and high-school age since by this age most children have well-developed peer networks (Crockett et al., 1984; Larson, 1983). The nurse can learn the names of friends during the admission process and include those names in the care plan, so all nurses caring for the child will ask about friends in daily conversations. By asking the child a question such as, "Shall I invite Mary to visit you today?" the nurse provides a valuable opportunity for a visit from a significant friend. Another method of promoting visits from friends is to call the parents of friends and ask them to bring their child to the hospital to visit.

The barrier of physical distance can be overcome partially by encouraging phone conversations and written correspondence between hospitalized children and their friends. Although friends may be unable to personally visit the ill child, other forms of communication can be helpful forms of support. Drawings and letters from friends can be displayed in the room of the ill child, where they will serve as visual reminders of happy experiences the child has shared with friends.

The interpersonal skills of both the child and friends influence supportive interventions from friends. To provide support, friends must initiate and maintain social contact with the child or teenager who has a health problem. At the same time, communication skills are necessary for the child to express needs and accept support. Inadequacies by either child will pose a serious obstacle to effective support. The nurse can help by modeling effective communication techniques through demonstrations of appropriate body posture, gestures, eye contact, and verbal expressions of support.

The barrier of psychological distance can be minimized through discussion with both the parents and friends of the child who has experienced a physical change in appearance. Parental attitudes of the child with the disfigurement will influence how the child copes with the new appearance. Helping parents understand how their attitudes are transmitted to the child may ultimately enhance the adaptation of the child to the change (Arneson and Triplett, 1978). Discussions with friends about the reasons for changes in appearance will help to reduce fears of the friends and, it is hoped, decrease the teasing and irritating questions that often occur when children do not understand why there has been a change in the appearance of their friend. By working with the friends of the affected child, the nurse can help preserve the friendships and, ultimately, help the friends become advocates for the child (Goodell, 1984). As friends learn to support the child, the nurse may want to change classroom seating arrangements and play group assignments so that several friends are physically close to help thwart teasing attempts from uninformed or insensitive children.

In addition to an inquiry about the names and availability of friends, the quality of these relationships must be determined, particularly with adolescent populations. Questions such as "What do you and your friend talk about?" and "How does your friend make you feel liked?" will help the nurse determine quality. The nurse will also want to assess the potential of each child for forming friendships, especially during lengthy hospitalizations.

Encouraging New Friendships

Several health professionals in hospital settings have reported favorable outcomes from the offer of support groups for adolescents hospitalized with chronic illness, physical trauma, or terminal illness. Such groups provide a safe atmosphere in which adolescents can share common needs and feelings, gain emotional support from peers, and learn new coping skills (Pazola and Gerberg, 1985; Bryne et al., 1984). Support groups are also valuable in school settings for children with similar problems such as support groups for those experiencing chronic illness, handicaps, or pregnancy. If group meetings are not possible, the school nurse can encourage the development of relationships between children and adolescents with similar problems even though they may be in different classes. For example, the newly diagnosed seven year old diabetic child who has just returned to school after hospitalization can gain valuable support and reassurance by talking with an older diabetic child who has successfully managed diabetes for several years. In the hospital setting, new relationships can be encouraged by placing children with similar diagnoses together as roommates and by encouraging ambulatory patients to play together in the playroom.

The child with a chronic or terminal illness may experience difficulty in maintaining existing friendships because of recurring hospitalizations or extended periods of recuperation at home. Encouraging these children to become involved in community activities and clubs such as scouts and 4H will provide regular opportunities for new friendships to develop and flourish.

Although many children possess the skills needed for making friends, some children are socially isolated from their peers, and others experience intense feelings of loneliness. School nurses may be consulted for suggestions about helping socially isolated children gain necessary social skills for developing peer acceptance. With specific individualized interventions from adults, these children may be able to learn to make friends. For example, the Oden and Asher study (1977) of socially isolated third graders and fourth graders revealed that specific coaching helped these children gain acceptance from peers. Coaching by an adult included giving instructions about the social skills needed for friendship formation, encouraging the children to play games to practice social skills, and holding a postplay review session with the children. Control groups who did not receive the coaching were unable to gain peer acceptance.

Showing Friends How to Help

Once friends are identified, the next intervention is to incorporate them into the plan of care by helping them learn how to provide support. This intervention is especially relevant for nurses who are working with children who have chronic illnesses. The hospital nurse usually becomes very familiar with the physical and psychological needs of these children because of their repeated hospitalizations. The nurse can begin building a communication link between the hospitalized child and school friends early in hospitalization. In some hospitals, a phone hookup can be established between the hospital and school so the child will be able to listen in on classroom discussions. The teacher can help by including the child in classroom conversations and by keeping classmates informed about progress on the hospitalized child. Letters from friends at school will also help to maintain relationships between the ill child and school friends.

Because of the strong support network that develops among adolescent friends, the intervention of showing friends how to help is especially useful for nurses who work with adolescent populations in clinics and physicians' offices. Illness or pregnancy during the adolescent years creates complex physical and psychosocial demands for the teenager who is already coping with the major developmental tasks of this time period. An unexpected event, such as pregnancy, may result in a forced dependency on parents and other adults at a time when support from friends is essential for reality testing. Therefore, it is vital that the nurse incorporate close friends into the plan of care of the adolescent client. Once friends are identified, the nurse can determine the unique emotional, social, and informational needs of the adolescent. This information can then be used as a framework for determining appropriate helping behaviors that can be carried out by close friends of the adolescent.

Gottlieb's classification scheme of informal helping behaviors (1978) identifies useful examples which the nurse can utilize when designing interventions for close friends who are available to offer support to the adolescent. First, needs for emotional support can be met by talking, listening, and reflecting understanding to the teenager. These behaviors will create a supportive environment for the teenager that will encourage ventilation of concerns. When tangible support is needed, offering services, such as help with studies, may be useful. Further, informational needs can be met by providing information that helps the adolescent solve problems. Similarly, offering to discuss the problems could provide a new self-understanding in the adolescent and result in a greater potential for problem resolution. The key to instructing friends about how to offer support is to determine unique ways to help the teenager mobilize resources and effectively cope with emotional burdens and physical demands (Gottlieb, 1978).

Helping a Child When a Friend Dies

The death of a friend can be a serious trauma, especially if the child or adolescent experiences intense feelings of loss of a special relationship. During the weeks and months after the death, strong emotions such as denial, guilt, anger, and sadness are very common as the child yearns for the closeness and companionship that were once part of the friendship. The experience of grief is influenced by the developmental level of the child, family expectations, and the unique way in which the child relates to the world (Arnold and Gemma, 1983).

In the hospital or school environment, the death of a child usually creates unanswered questions and confusion for surviving children who knew the child. Therefore, a key nursing intervention is to provide careful explanations about the circumstances and causes of the death. Friends of the dead child need an opportunity to discuss their observations and questions about the death with a trusted adult. Because young children are unable to verbalize thoughts and feelings, the nurse can help the child express concerns and fears by asking the child to draw a picture or act out past experiences with the friend through puppets or toys. There are also many stories about death that can help the young child share feelings through identification with the experiences of the characters in the story.

Variables Influencing Support from Friends

The success or failure of support from friends is influenced by a variety of factors including availability of friends, size and quality of the peer network, level of demands on friends, and sociocultural factors. Sociocultural factors include family perceptions of the value of support from friends and family coping styles.

The availability of friends is a major concern during hospitalization because of the physical distance between friends at home and the hospitalized child. This is especially true if hospitalization occurs in a distant medical center. Even when hospitalization occurs near the homes of friends, the visiting regulations may not allow for visits from young friends. Adequate provisions for privacy during visits from friends and explanations to prepare friends for changes in the appearance of the ill child will positively influence the quality of peer interaction in the hospital environment.

The size and quality of the peer network will vary with the age of the child. However, having a large number of friends does not always mean that the child or adolescent will receive adequate support during a crisis. Porritt (1979) has shown that the quality of support is more helpful to the person in a crisis than the number of supporters. He studied social support during crisis by interviewing 70 males three to four months after they had been injured in a road accident. He asked each subject to identify sources of support and describe the quality of support provided by each source. The quality of support for the subjects was identified as more important than the quantity of support. He also found that dimensions of empathetic understanding, respect, and genuineness were key components of support.

The potential for support from friends is also influenced by the level of demands on friends of the child. Some friends might be undergoing their own unique crises, which will seriously limit the support they can provide. Family as well as school and work responsibilities could seriously restrict the time and energy that is available from supporting friends.

How a family perceives the value of support from others and the family's coping style affect implementation of support from friends. Some families may not recognize that friends can make a valuable contribution to the recovery of their child. Discussing the value of support from friends during the admission process will help parents recognize the importance of friends. It is not unusual for families to withdraw from contact with friends when a life-threatening illness, such as a malignancy, occurs. Parents may be reluctant to allow the child to return to school, even when the cancer is in remission. These children often miss out on valuable opportunities for support from friends if they are tutored at home. Office nurses can encourage parents to invite friends to the home. Also, explanations for parents to give to friends when they ask questions about physical body changes are helpful.

EVALUATION

The criterion for measurement of the value of support from friends is a positive change in the data which led the nurse to make the nursing diagnosis of *Ineffective individual coping* or *Disturbance in self-concept*. During unexpected events such as sudden illness, appropriate supportive interventions from friends create a strong potential for the mitigation of feelings of unpredictability and loss of control in the child. Consequently, these interventions will result in improved coping behaviors (Wallston et al., 1983). For the child with a disturbed self-concept resulting from an altered appearance, support from friends will positively influence the feelings the child has about self. If withdrawal from friends was occurring prior to the intervention, this withdrawal will diminish as the child begins to demonstrate improved self-confidence during interactions with friends. Negative statements and behaviors directed toward self will diminish and will be replaced by more positive comments from the child.

In health care settings such as clinics and physicians' offices in which nurses interact with the same children or teenagers periodically, the effectiveness and outcome of support from friends can be evaluated through the use of research tools such as the ASSIS and the Norbeck Social Support Questionnaire (NSSQ). These tools are especially helpful for nurses who are working with pregnant adolescents and children with chronic illnesses. The ASSIS (Barrera, 1981) is an interview tool that was developed to identify key individuals in the support network, their support functions, and the degree of satisfaction or dissatisfaction that the client has toward each support person. The NSSQ (Norbeck et al., 1981) measures multiple dimensions of social support, i.e., affect, affirmation, and aid. These tools can be used individually or in combination by the nurse to determine the effectiveness of support from friends when the child or adolescent comes to the clinic for periodic visits.

Case Study

Ms. Smith, a school nurse in a large Midwestern high school, met Mandy, a 16 year old sophomore, for the first time when Mandy walked into her office and exclaimed, "What should I do? I think I'm pregnant." Although Mandy and her boyfriend, Brad, had been having sexual intercourse for several months, they had not been using birth control. In their first meeting, Ms. Smith helped Mandy talk about her fears about being pregnant and arranged an appointment for medical care in a nearby community clinic. The pregnancy was confirmed the next week.

In her second meeting with Mandy, Ms. Smith began to assess the family and peer support network. Mandy often stayed at home after school and on weekends with her ten year old sister because her divorced mother managed a floral shop. Her father had remarried and lived in another state, so Mandy had only infrequent opportunities to visit him. Mandy had two close friends, and she mentioned that she wanted to

maintain a close relationship with Brad, the father of the baby.

During subsequent weekly meetings with Ms. Smith, Mandy made several statements indicating that she was very angry about the pregnancy. She expressed a desire to end the pregnancy so she could resume a normal teenage lifestyle. These statements, coupled with her refusal to seek medical care, demonstrated an initial inability to cope with the unexpected pregnancy. Therefore, Ms. Smith identified a priority nursing diagnosis of *Ineffective individual coping* in the plan of care for Mandy.

Over the next two weeks, Ms. Smith developed several nursing interventions which centered on friendship as a way of helping Mandy cope with the pregnancy. The nurse encouraged the development of a new friendship with Karen, a teenage mother in the same school. Karen had recently returned to school after the birth of a baby girl. Mandy was reluctant to meet Karen at first but eventually agreed to talk with her in the school nurse's office. The meeting was helpful because Karen encouraged Mandy to ventilate her strong negative feelings about the pregnancy. As the friendship between the girls grew during the early months of the pregnancy, Mandy began to talk more positively about becoming a mother. Ms. Smith also urged Mandy to talk with her two close friends about the pregnancy and rely on them for support. Ms. Smith met individually with Brad and discovered that he was very concerned about Mandy and the welfare of the baby. He volunteered to help Mandy with her homework and to occasionally take her to the clinic for prenatal visits.

The intervention of utilizing friends to assist Mandy in coping more effectively with the pregnancy was successful because there were noticeable behavior changes in Mandy by the end of the first trimester. Comments from Mandy revealed a more realistic acceptance of the pregnancy. She selected a physician and began going to the office for regular prenatal checkups. She seemed more interested in the baby, and she asked Ms. Smith appropriate questions about the birth process.

At 33 weeks of gestation, Mandy developed signs of toxemia, which resulted in hospitalization in the antepartum unit of a nearby tertiary medical center. The medical condition of Mandy required that she remain hospitalized throughout the remainder of the pregnancy with some restrictions on her activities. Ms. Smith visited Mandy several days after her admission to the hospital and found Mandy to be quite bored and discouraged. Ms. Smith talked with the primary nurse assigned to Mandy about regular visits and phone calls from her friends. Arrangements were made for Brad and her two close friends to visit frequently and bring in her school work.

Mandy also met Michelle, another pregnant

teenager, who was hospitalized with gestational diabetes. A friendship developed between the two teenagers, and the nursing staff arranged for the nurse educator to teach the birthing and child care classes to the two teenagers together. Their friendship continued to grow during their hospitalization as they shared common concerns and feelings about labor, childbirth, and the future responsibilities of child rearing. Mandy's mother was also a valuable support person, but because of her floral business, she was unable to visit every day. Since her mother was not sure that she could be present during the birth process, the childbirth educator suggested that Mandy select another significant person to be available as an alternate coach. Mandy chose one of her close friends from school who was able to attend most of the evening childbirth classes at the hospital with Mandy.

Her ability to cope with pregnancy and prolonged hospitalization was strengthened because Mandy expressed her need for support to her friends, and her friends, in turn, provided appropriate forms of support. The school nurse initiated and encouraged supportive interactions from friends by promoting the development of a friendship between two teenagers undergoing similar life experiences and by preserving Mandy's close relationships with several established friends.

RESEARCH IMPLICATIONS

Much research is available on the protective value of social support for individuals who are experiencing crises in their lives. However, the majority of these studies have used adult populations, and therefore the study conclusions can only be generalized to adults. The use of friendship as an intervention for children and adolescents facing unexpected changes in their lives has not been studied extensively. Because intimate friendships begin to develop during early adolescence, social support studies that identify adolescent concerns and clarify helpful interventions for this age group are needed. Tools such as the NSSQ which assess the quality of support networks can be adapted for study of adolescents. Development of reliable and valid instruments to measure the unique dimensions of support required by adolescents facing various crises would be helpful for professionals in community as well as hospital settings.

There is also a need to more clearly delineate which helping behaviors are most appropriately performed by professionals and which behaviors can be effectively utilized

by friends. Some situations undoubtedly require that interventions be developed and performed by a partnership of professionals and lay persons. Experimental research is indicated to test and refine these behaviors and then determine how friends can appropriately use the interventions.

Further study is also needed in elementary school and high school settings to identify ways that children can be shown how to give and receive support from friends. Providing this information to young children will help to lay the groundwork for helping children to cope with the developmental changes and unexpected crises that are part of childhood, adolescence, and adulthood.

References

Arneson, S, and Triplett, J. How children cope with disfiguring changes in their appearance. MCN: American Journal of Maternal Child Nursing, 3:366–370, 1978.

Arnold, JH, and Gemma, PB. A child dies: A portrait of family grief. Rockville, Md: Aspen Systems Corp., 1983.

Barrera, M. Social support in the adjustment of pregnant adolescents: Assessment issues. In Gottlieb, BH (Ed.), Social networks and social support. Beverly Hills, Calif.: Sage Publications, 1981, pp. 69–97.

Berndt, TJ. Age changes and changes over time in prosocial intentions and behavior between friends. Developmental Psychology, 17:408–416, 1981.

Broadhead, WE, Kaplan, BH, James, SA, Wagner, EH, Schoenback, VJ, Grimson, R, Heyden, S, Tibblin, G, and Gehlback, SH. The epidemiologic evidence for a relationship between social support and health. American Journal of Epidemiology, 117:521–535, 1983.

Bryne, CM, Stockwell, M, and Gudelis, S. Adolescent support groups in oncology. Oncology Nursing Forum, 11:36–40, 1984.

Cobb, S. Social support as a moderator of life stress. Psychosomatic Medicine, 38:300–314, 1976.

Crockett, L, Losoff, M, and Petersen, AC. Perceptions of the peer group and friendship in early adolescence. Journal of Early Adolescence, 4:155–181, 1984.

Crockett, MS. Exploring peer relationships. Journal of Psychosocial Nursing, 22:18–25, 1984.

Duck, SW. Personal relationships and personal constructs: A study of friendship formation. London: John Wiley & Sons Inc., 1973.

Eckenrode, J, and Gore, S. Stressful events and social supports: The significance of context. In Gottlieb, BH (Ed.), Social networks and social support. Beverly Hills, Calif.: Sage Publications, 1981, pp. 43–68.

Goodell, A. Peer education in school for children with cancer. Issues in Comprehensive Pediatric Nursing, 7:101–106, 1984.

Gottlieb, BH. The development and application of a classification scheme of informal helping behaviors. Canadian Journal of Behavioral Science, 10:105–115, 1978.

Kahn, RL, and Antonucci, TC. Convoys over the life course: Attachment, roles, and social support. In Baltes, PB, and Bream, O (Eds.), Life span development and behavior. New York: Academic Press, Inc., 1981.

Kim, MJ, McFarland, G, and McLane, AM. Pocket guide to nursing diagnosis. St. Louis: CV Mosby Co., 1984.

Klinzing, DR, and Klinzing, DG. The hospitalized child: Communication techniques for health personnel. Englewood Cliffs, N.J.: Prentice-Hall, Inc., 1977.

Larson, RW. Adolescents' daily experience with family and friends: Contrasting opportunity systems. Journal of Marriage and the Family, 45:739–750, 1983.

Mercer, RT. Assessing and counseling teenage mothers during the perinatal period. Nursing Clinics of North America, 18:293–301, 1983.

Newcomb, AF, and Brady, JE. Mutuality in boys' friendship relations. Child Development, 53:392–395, 1982.

Norbeck, JS, Lindsey, AM, and Carrieri, VL. The development of an instrument to measure social support. Nursing Research, 30:264–269, 1981.

Oden, S, and Asher, SR. Coaching children in social skills for friendship making. Child Development, 48:495–506, 1977.

Pazola, KJ, and Gerberg, AK. Teen group: A forum for the hospitalized adolescent. MCN: American Journal of Maternal Child Nursing, 10:265–269, 1985.

Piaget, J, and Inhelder, B. The psychology of the child. New York: Basic Books, 1969.

Porritt, D. Social support in crisis: Quantity or quality? Social Science and Medicine, 13A:715–721, 1979.

Press, BK, and Greenspan, SI. Ned and Dan: The development of a toddler friendship. Videotape. Washington, D.C.: National Center for Clinical Infant Programs, National Institute of Mental Health, 1985.

Richardson, SA. Children's values and friendships: A study of physical disability. Journal of Health and Social Behavior, 12:253–258, 1971.

Roff, JD, and Wirt, RD. Childhood social adjustment, adolescent status, and young adult mental health. American Journal of Orthopsychiatry, 54:595–602, 1984.

Rubin, Z. Children's friendships. Cambridge, Mass.: Harvard University Press, 1980.

Schaefer, C, Coyne, JC, and Lazarus, RS. The health-related functions of social support. Journal of Behavioral Medicine, 4:381–405, 1981.

Skolnick, AS. The psychology of human development. San Diego: Harcourt Brace Jovanovich, Inc., 1986.

Smith, DL. Meeting the psychosocial needs of teen-age mothers and fathers. Nursing Clinics of North America, 19:369–379, 1984.

Suelzel, M. The structuring of friendship formation among two- to five-year-old children enrolled in full day care: Research in the interweave of social rules. Friendship, 2:51–73, 1981.

Sullivan, HS. The interpersonal theory of psychiatry. New York: WW Norton & Co., Inc., 1953.

Wallston, BS, Alagna, SW, DeVellis, BM, and DeVellis, RF. Social support and physical health. Health Psychology, 2:367–391, 1983.

Webster's Ninth New Collegiate Dictionary. Springfield, Mass: Merriam-Webster, Inc., 1987.

Youniss, J. Parents and peers in social development: A Sullivan-Piaget perspective. Chicago: University of Chicago Press, 1980.

Youniss, J, and Smollar, J. Adolescent relations with mothers, fathers, and friends. Chicago: University of Chicago Press, 1985.

CHAPTER 14

COPING WITH FAMILY LOSS

The Death of a Sibling

KATHLEEN ROSS-ALAOLMOLKI, Ph.D., R.N.

Coping with the death of a child can be one of the most stressful and poignant experiences that a family can encounter. Research indicates that the impact of the death of a child on each family member can have short-term and long-term disruptive effects on the family (Brown, 1986; Davies, 1983; Miles and Demi, 1983–84; Pearlin and Aneshensel, 1986; Rando, 1984, 1986; Sanders, 1982–83; Schumacher, 1984; Spinetta et al., 1981). The child's death can lead to divorce, separation, depression in one or more of the members, and an increased incidence of alcoholism in the parents (Heller and Schneider, 1978; Kaplan et al., 1976). In the literature on bereavement in adults, it

has been demonstrated that unresolved grief in childhood tends to inhibit the ability to grieve in later adulthood (Bowlby, 1981; Parkes, 1972). The death of a child may contribute to the development of behavioral problems, psychosomatic symptoms, and depression in the siblings (Cain et al., 1964).

Upon the death of a child, all family members face challenges such as despair, isolation, vulnerability, withdrawal from others, helplessness, guilt (Miles and Demi, 1983–84; Rando, 1984; Worden, 1982), anxiety, and depression (Bowlby, 1961, 1963, 1970, 1979; McClowry et al., 1989). Adolescent siblings are also faced with the challenges of coping with parental reactions. Ambiva-

213

lent feelings may range from anger and fear to guilt, sadness, and a lack of understanding (Balk, 1983; Rosen, 1986; Schumacher, 1984).

Family relationships and the coping mechanisms of individual family members are believed to be related to such variables as the age of the child who died (Barnes, 1978; Schumacher, 1984), the age of the siblings (Barnes, 1978; Schumacher, 1984; Woosley et al., 1978), the ordinal position of the child who died and the siblings in the family structure, and the function that these children played within the family (Bowen, 1978). Bowen (1978) states that "few human events provide as much emotional impact as serious illness and death in resolving unresolved emotional attachments" (p. 331). He suggests that the death of either parent when a child is young or the death of an important child can alter the family equilibrium for several years as the family adapts to the loss. The loss of a child can also affect extended family members as well as other persons who have close connections to the family.

There are additional variables that are important considerations when intervening with these families, such as the financial strain incurred by the child's illness and death as well as the availability of a supportive network that can be drawn upon as a resource for the family during the weeks and months following a child's death (Rando, 1984, 1986; Rosen, 1986; Ross-Alaolmolki, 1985).

THEORETICAL FOUNDATION

Loss and Children

Grief is a normal response to loss (Bowlby, 1979, 1981; Rando, 1984; Rosen, 1986). The terms grief, grieving, and bereavement are all expressions found in nursing literature. In the literature regarding nursing diagnosis, the term dysfunctional grieving is used to denote that grieving has not taken place. This author would prefer to use the term unresolved grief, because it focuses on the potential for resolution and change. Viewing grief as an expression or signal that loss has taken place serves the function of signaling to the attachment figures that protection is needed. Viewing loss from a family systems perspective rather than as a process within the individual alone provides a broader perspective from which to intervene.

The family perspective is stressed because children's capacity to grieve is affected by their parents' reactions and ability to grieve. It is the family, both parents and children in interaction, that, in the final analysis, gives permission to its members to grieve. The family members must recognize and validate the feelings of grief that each member is experiencing so that grief can be resolved. It is the open, explicit acknowledgment of each person's feelings of grief that will facilitate grief work.

Grief has been beautifully articulated by Rando (1984):

Grief: The process of psychological, social, and somatic reactions to the perceptions of loss. This implies that grief is (a) manifested in each of the psychological, social, and somatic realms; (b) a continuing development involving many changes; (c) a natural, expectable reaction (in fact, the absence of it is abnormal in most cases); (d) the reaction to the experience of many kinds of loss, not necessarily death alone; and (e) based upon the unique, individualistic perception of loss by the griever, that is, it is not necessary to have the loss recognized or validated by others for the person to experience grief. It is also hypothesized that grief is a product of biological evolution that has adaptive value (Averill, 1968). By making separation from the group or from its members an extremely stressful event, it helps assure the group's cohesiveness. This is important for those species in which the maintenance of social bonds is necessary for survival and those bonds are based upon individual recognition and attachment (p. 15).

There is a large body of literature that addresses loss and its effects on adults (Bowlby, 1973, 1981; Parkes, 1972). However, there is a lack of literature that examines the effects of stress and loss on the behavior and subsequent development of children (Bowlby, 1979, 1981; Garmezy, 1983, 1986). Unfortunately, children are not strangers to either stress or loss.

Several losses that can be experienced by children include separation and the threatened loss of one or both parents (Bowlby, 1979; Rutter, 1977); divorce, with the threatened loss of a close relationship with one parent (Wallerstein, 1983); death of a parent (Bowlby, 1981; Gardner, 1983); death of a sibling; and chronic illness in the child, parent, or sibling (Bowlby, 1979; Armstrong and Martinson, 1980; Rando, 1984; Rosen, 1986). Less often a reality in North America, but nonetheless a reality for many of the world's children, are the effects of war on children and the consequences of forced separation. Many children experience loss, family disruption, and psychological and physical suffering in the face of dramatic social and economic chaos and change (Garmezy, 1983; Rosenblatt, 1983). Thus culture and sociopolitical conditions are important factors to consider when working with families who have experienced a loss, regardless of whether the family has recently immigrated or has been in the country for several generations (Landau, 1982; McGoldrick, 1982; Speigel, 1982).

The purpose of this chapter is to present loss as it relates to the sibling within the family system when a child has died. Loss for a child when a sister or brother dies an untimely death belongs within a particular category of stress that is initially acute and probably unexpected, even though it may have been anticipated. The intensity of the impact of such a death irrevocably changes the child's world. The child is required both to recognize that a major life change has taken place and to adapt rapidly to the changed conditions within the family (see Chapter 3).

Loss and Attachment Theory

Loss must be considered within the context of attachment theory, since the feelings resulting from the perception of loss flow from connections that one human being has for another. Worden (1982) underscores the linkage between Bowlby's attachment theory and the concept of loss, pointing out that one must first understand attachment theory in order to understand loss. The importance of attachment theory cannot be overlooked by clinicians and researchers working with children and their families who have experienced loss or a series of losses. Attachment theory has already been discussed in depth in Chapter 1.

Loss, as defined by Webster's dictionary (1987), is "the harm or privation resulting from loss or separation." Loss can be physical (tangible) or psychosocial (symbolic) (Rando, 1984). Physical losses can include the loss of possessions or a friend or family member. A psychosocial or symbolic loss as explained by Rando is that resulting from

divorce or from a change in status, such as the loss of a job. The loss of a relationship that results from person-to-person interaction in which an emotional bond is formed is the type of loss that is discussed in this chapter.

The response to loss, or the different forms in which emotional distress can be manifested, is expressed in many ways. Commonly, there are feelings of anxiety, anger, depression, and emotional detachment, which are signals of distress resulting from unwilling separation and loss (Bowlby, 1973).

Bowlby's attachment theory provides a way to conceptualize the tendency in human beings to make strong affectional bonds with others and a way to understand the strong emotional reaction that occurs when these bonds are broken (Bowlby, 1979; Worden, 1982). Bowlby (1979) posited that "attachment behavior is any form of behavior that results in a person attaining or retaining proximity to some other differentiated and preferred individual, who is usually conceived of as stronger and wiser" (p. 129). His thesis proposes that these attachments come from a need for security and safety, developing early in life, and are usually directed toward a few specific individuals. He believes that these attachments endure throughout the life cycle of the individual. Forming attachments is normal behavior for children and adults according to Bowlby, who argues that it serves a protective function, having as its goal survival of the species.

If it is the goal of attachment behavior to maintain an affectional bond, situations that endanger this bond give rise to certain very specific reactions. The greater the potential for loss, the more intense and varied these reactions will be. The most powerful indicators of attachment behavior may become activated, such as clinging, crying, and anger. If these signals are successful, the bond may be restored, the signaling attempts will end, and the feelings of distress will be alleviated. If the threat of loss or actual loss is not reversed, then sadness, withdrawal, apathy, and despair will emerge.

Loss of a Sibling

The behavioral responses of siblings whose brother or sister has died are influenced by their ability to understand and integrate the meaning of the death as well as by the relationship that they had with that child (Weiner, 1970). Another factor related to childhood grieving is the way in which the parents cope with the loss (Rosen, 1986; Schumacher, 1984; Vernon, 1970). Others, in particular the parents, must acknowledge that the child has experienced a significant loss. In addition to coping with the loss of a sibling, the child may be attempting to cope with the functional loss of grieving parents (Rosen, 1986). Cobb (1958) suggested that children suffered detrimental effects after the death of a sibling and that younger children suffered more ill effects than older children. Parents described ill effects as "apathy, loss of time, loss of appetite, and wandering around in a daze" (p. 749).

Other authors have reported that after the death of a child, the previously well-adjusted siblings demonstrated altered behavior patterns such as severe enuresis, headaches, poor school performance, school phobia, depression, severe separation anxiety, and persistent abdominal pains. During the terminal illness and after the death of a child, siblings have reported feelings of resentment and anger. Resentment was expressed toward the parents because of the time they spent with the dying child and anger at the parents for allowing the child to die. These children also expressed fears that they themselves would incur a fatal illness and die (Binger et al., 1969).

One member of a family such as a parent or sibling may take the blame for the child's death (Cain et al., 1964); this person will carry the grief for the family (Landau-Stanton and Stanton, 1985). If the child who died was perceived as a favored child or particularly outstanding at some activity, there may be normal sibling rivalry, which can result in guilt and remorse after the child's death (Raphael, 1983; Schumacher, 1984). Cain et al. (1964) documented several responses in children to their sibling's death, in particular "depressive withdrawal, accident-prone behavior, punishment seeking, constant provocative testing, exhibitionistic use of guilt and grief, massive projection of superego accusations, and many forms of acting out" (p. 743).

Three hypotheses were suggested by Krell and Rabkin (1979) about the three types of children that result from families in which there has been a conspiracy of silence surrounding the death of a child: (1) the haunted child, (2) the bound child, and (3) the resurrected child. Haunted children are terrified of what may happen to them, often becoming the caretakers of their parents. These children frequently develop somatic symptoms, misbehave in school, or develop phobias. The bound child is overprotected by the parents because they are afraid of losing another child. Krell and Rabkin believe that these children become angry and may reject their parents. The resurrected child becomes a substitute for the dead child and is often treated as if he or she were the child who died. This approach will interfere with the sibling's developing an identity of his or her own and also may impede the important task of grieving for both the siblings and the parents.

In a study of the surviving siblings of 15 families in which a child had died from cancer, suicide, or an accident (Schumacher, 1984), several major concerns were identified. The first was about taking a direct, open, and honest communication approach with the parents. This approach was seen as important to assist the siblings to incorporate the realities of the death, thereby enabling them to participate actively in shared emotions. Siblings also identified the need to share their own feelings, which were very changeable. They feared revealing anger and resentment for fear of being hurt or rejected by the parents. Their anger was usually counterbalanced by feelings of sadness, and these conflicting feelings led to confusion. Schumacher reported that feelings of guilt were very difficult for the siblings to identify and understand. In the course of normal development and sibling relationships, conflicts arise in which children wish their sibling dead or away. This process, frequently reported in the literature, may lead to a child thinking that he or she caused the sibling's death.

According to the siblings, what to tell their friends was a critical concern for them. Friends often did not understand their feelings of loss, and the siblings reported feeling avoided, rejected, or isolated. School, then, became a place of painful experiences. Other concerns which resulted in feelings of anxiety included trying to appear happy out of fear that displays of sadness would lead to rejection. Concerns were also expressed about being sad on holidays when they wanted to feel happy. Thus holidays, potentially happy occasions, created more ambivalent feelings.

Martinson and colleagues (1987) examined the long-term effects of sibling bereavement on self-concept in siblings eight to 18 years of age seven to nine years following the death of the sibling. They reported that bereaved siblings had statistically significant higher self-concept scores than a normative group of siblings. Generally these siblings reported that they had gained maturity and psychological growth from the experience. Siblings who had lower self-concept scores reported a feeling of "I'm not being good enough." This feeling was characteristic of children who perceived that they did not compare favorably with the deceased sibling.

There are conflicting reports in the literature on the short-term and long-term effect of sibling loss on the surviving siblings. Two important factors, however, stand out as important to sibling growth after a death: open communication in the family system and fostering feelings among the surviving siblings of being valued.

Grieving in Children

Several reviews and studies on the development of children's concept of death exist in the literature (Anthony, 1971; Gartley and Bernasconi, 1967; Koocher, 1981; Nagy, 1948; Piaget, 1929; Safier, 1964; Schilder and Weschler, 1934). It is important that the child's age and cognitive development be considered when intervening during the grief process. Concepts of death in children are age related and differ according to intellectual ability, environment, and culture. It is believed that healthy children up to two years of age have no understanding of death. However, children of this age fear separation from protective figures who give comfort and protection. Further, they may be influenced by the grief of other members of the family.

Children between the ages of three and five years of age have a vague concept of death, generally believing that it is something that happens to someone or something else. These children are beginning to learn about and tolerate brief periods of separation from protective figures.

Children from six to ten years gradually begin to accommodate their thinking about death. They begin to understand death as inevitable, final, personal, and universal; however, their thoughts about death are future oriented. By ten to 11 years of age, death is understood as universal and permanent. Thus, by adolescence, children have the intellectual capacity to understand life and death in a logical way.

The developing concept of illness and death is continuously evolving and varies with each child. Some studies have revealed that children who are faced with their own fatal illness and death may come to understand or be aware of the meaning of death at a much earlier age than their healthy peers (Bluebond-Langner, 1974, 1978; Spinetta et al., 1973, 1974; Waechter, 1971).

Bowlby (1961) articulated a framework for grief that included three distinct phases: (1) the drive to recover the lost object; (2) disorganization and despair; and (3) later reorganization. In 1981, Bowlby added a phase called numbing that he and Parkes had recognized earlier (Bowlby, 1970, 1979; Parkes, 1972). Bowlby suggested that there are more similarities than differences between childhood grieving and adult grieving and that children may grieve for much longer periods than was previously supposed. Children who do experience loss and unresolved grief may be at increased risk for the development of adverse psychological and social outcomes (Rutter, 1977, 1980).

The Phases of Grieving

The four phases of grieving as described by Bowlby (1981) are numbing, yearning, disorganization, and reorganization. These phases are consistent with the views of several other authors on grief and grieving (Parks, 1972; Rando, 1984; Worden, 1982).

The phase of numbing is characterized by feelings of disbelief, of being stunned, and of being unreal. This phase can have intervals of anxiety and feelings of panic. This phase is usually brief, but sometimes may last for weeks or months.

The phase of yearning and searching for the lost person may continue for months or even years. During this phase, the bereaved person exhibits behaviors that signal a desire to search, find, and recover the lost person. Insomnia, restlessness, and preoccupation with thoughts of the lost person may occur in addition to spasms of distress and sobbing. Anger, a common feeling exhibited in this stage, may be directed at persons who are seen as responsible for the loss or may be a sign of frustration at not being able to find the lost person. Beneath these more obvious feelings is a feeling of deep, pervasive sadness.

The phase of disorganization and despair is characterized by conflicting emotions of despair; aching loss; and, as in the previous phase, anger at those perceived by the bereaved person as responsible for the loss. In order to achieve a new level of synthesis, the dialectic of the emotional extremes must be bridged. The person may give up the search; however, feelings of despair and frustration may continue until old patterns of thinking and responding to familiar situations are gradually given up for new patterns.

The last phase, reorganization, is characterized by an attempt by the individual to redefine oneself. The redefinition of self without the person to whom one was attached can be a painful process. However, redefinition must take place so that plans for the future can be made.

It is often believed that time heals; however, time heals only if the grieving person deals with the loss. The intensity and duration of grief vary with each individual and fluctuate over time. Grief responses may be intensified at particular times, such as birthdays, holidays, or with experiences that trigger memories of the deceased person. Each person must be considered individually according to his or her own specific grief responses as the response to loss is an expression of his or her own way of coping and making meaning out of the loss (Arnold and Gemma, 1983).

Tasks of Grieving

Lindemann (1944), in his classic work on grieving, conceptualized the grief process as including three tasks: (1) emancipation from the bondage of the deceased; (2) readjustment to the environment in which the deceased is missing; and (3) formation of new relationships. The first task can be reformulated as an untying of the invisible threads of loyalty that connect one person to another in families. Parents owe loyalty to their own family of origin in addition to each other and their own children; children owe loyalty to their parents and to each other as siblings. These invisible loyalties span past, present, and future generations (Boszormenyi-Nagy and Spark, 1984).

Rando (1984) suggests that the most critical task in grief work is "untying the ties that bind" (p. 19) the griever to the child who has died. In order to resolve grief and establish new emotional ties and relationships, the relationship to the deceased child must be altered. This does not mean that one forgets or thinks any less of the person who died. The relationship with the child who has died can be thought of in special ways through memories shared with other family members, with friends, or with other parents and children who have experienced a similar loss.

Readjustment to an environment without the deceased child is different for both siblings and parents. For parents, it means a readjustment of roles and a shift in responsibilities. The deceased child may have played a particular role in the family, such as that of the bright child or the child who always was the one to joke; the loss of such a child would be painful for all family members. Both the siblings and the parents will have to adjust to the loss in some way. The siblings who were the closest in age to the deceased child may have the most difficult time adjusting, for they will have to form new identities as siblings.

Family members regulate the expression of their emotions by modifying their behavior according to their experience with the life situation confronting them. Siblings and parents monitor and modify feelings as they struggle to maintain a comfortable homeostatic state. In order to do this, they often, although not very successfully, try to conceal their anguish and pain. Parents and siblings try to protect themselves and one another in order to maintain normal family functions and relationships.

The formation of new relationships requires that all family members take that part of their emotional energy that was invested in the deceased child and reinvest it in other relationships. The siblings may invest energy in new or special friendships and, in some instances, in new activities. If they have had to curtail some of their activities because of the prolonged illness and death of their sibling, this is a good opportunity to resume their familiar routines. Parents have to redefine their relationship with their children and with each other, for they are now parents of a child who has died and the parents of a child or children whose sibling has died.

Grief Work

Lindemann (1944) used the term grief work to describe the physical and emotional energy that resolving grief requires. Grief, the "emotional response to the loss of a close relationship" (Raphael, 1983, p. 33), includes a complex series of painful feelings, including sadness, anger, helplessness, guilt, and despair. Grieving is a crucial aspect of grief work and refers to the psychological processes that occur during bereavement. Grieving enables the bereaved to loosen the emotional bonds that linked the person to the deceased. The very same bonds that formed the relationship to the deceased person must be undone. All the various aspects of that relationship include memories associated with the lost person, such as happy, difficult, and sad moments. Memories also include intense feelings about the past development of the relationship. If grieving proceeds naturally and is not inhibited, negative as well as positive aspects of the relationship are remembered. Gradually, the ambivalence that is felt about the good and the bad aspects of the relationship are worked through. Support of ambivalent feelings by family members and peers in the social network enables grief work to proceed. Acceptance of these feelings means that the family members have the support as well as the freedom to express their grief and to review both their positive and negative memories.

Grieving the death of a child is in the truest sense a transition for the family. Transition refers to a period of change, disequilibrium, and growth that serves as a bridge between one relatively stable period in life and another relatively stable but different period. Normative transitions are those that are expected to occur, such as the continuous process of life span development (Kim-

mel and Weiner, 1985). Non-normative transitions or idiosyncratic transitions occur at unpredictable times, such as the transition that occurs with the death of a child (Neugarten, 1976).

ASSESSMENT

Evaluation of the family system must include an assessment of intergenerational losses. This evaluation should be initiated at the first or second session. In taking the family history, the nurse should cover at least three generations to assess losses and conflicts that may have occurred during transitions (Bowen, 1978). This assessment, using a genogram to map the nuclear family and extended family network, becomes a tool for designing therapeutic interventions (McGoldrick and Gerson, 1985). The genogram, a schematic diagram of the family structure and intergenerational relationships, can be used with the family members as an assessment, planning, and intervention tool. It is a visual map of the family members' connections and relationships (Wright and Leahey, 1984).

It is important to assess what functions or roles the deceased child and the surviving siblings played in the family (Worden, 1982). Children may play many roles in families, including that of caretaker, nurturer, scapegoat, the intelligent one, the quiet one, and the good child, to name a few. The nurse can ask each family member in turn, including the siblings, for their perspective of the deceased child's role.

An assessment of the ways in which each of the family members is grieving (Rando, 1984) and what factors are influencing the grieving process is essential before the family can be given tasks or directives to be completed outside of the counseling sessions. Questions eliciting the relationship that each of the family members had with the child who died can be asked to assess the quality of the relationship and the feelings surrounding the loss.

For the case study presented later in this chapter, two nursing diagnoses are appropriate and will be considered as interrelated. The first is *Alteration in family process* (Kim and Moritz, 1982; Kim et al., 1984), which involves a situational transition or crisis; in this case, the crisis is the family's responsibility and need to deal with the suicide gesture of their 12 year old daughter. Included in this transition or crisis is the family's need to deal with the death of their younger son several months prior to their daughter's suicide gesture. Several of the defining characteristics of the diagnosis focus on the emotional, developmental, communication, and security needs of the family system.

A second nursing diagnosis that is included in this case study is *Dysfunctional grieving* (Kim and Moritz, 1982; Kim et al., 1984), for this family system is still experiencing grief without being able to communicate their grief and emotional pain to each other. The consequence of this unresolved grief or inhibition of the grief process is itself the signal, in the form of a suicide gesture from the surviving sibling, that things in this family are not healthy. The defining characteristics focus on affect, the ability to express loss, activity levels, and interference with life functioning. The defining characteristics help to guide the assessment process and the development of strategies to intervene and also provide criteria to evaluate efficacy of the intervention outcome.

THE INTERVENTION

Even though a child seems to have the problem with grieving, the intervention must focus on the family system. Because most childhood losses take place within the context of the family, one must consider the impact of the death on the family system (Bowen, 1978; Minuchin, 1974; Worden, 1982). Interventions based on a family systems perspective assume that the family is an interacting unit, with each member influencing every other member in the system (Bowen, 1978; Haley, 1976; Minuchin, 1974). The reactions of the parents themselves to their child's death will affect the siblings' abilities to resolve the loss (Bowlby, 1981; Rosen, 1986; Schumacher, 1984; Worden, 1982). Parents who are anxious or depressed cannot hide their feelings from each other or the surviving siblings and will be less available emotionally.

Several authors have observed that little is known about time and the grief processes (Bowlby, 1973; Lindemann, 1944; Pine and Bauer, 1986; Rando, 1983, 1986). Rando (1983) suggests that general models of grieving are inadequate to describe the grieving processes of parents. She states that the criteria used for identification and classification of pathological grieving are to be found in bereaved parents. She further suggests that the patterns characteristic of parent-child relationships are the reasons that parents are more vulnerable to experiencing unresolved grief. Moreover, parents who have sustained several losses in the past are also more susceptible to experiencing unresolved grief.

Therefore, it is not unusual for self-destructive behaviors by children to be associated with deaths or losses in the family (Paul and Grosser, 1965; Rando, 1984; Landau-Stanton and Stanton, 1985; Rutter, 1977). Suicide rates among adolescents ten to 14 years old were 0.8 per 100,000 in 1978 and have shown a small increase (1.1 per 100,000 in 1982) over the years. However, these statistics are much lower than those among adolescents 15 to 19 years old (National Center for Health Statistics, 1978; 1982). It should be noted, however, that there are serious problems when examining suicide statistics because many suicide attempts and deaths are not reported. Loss, unsupportive family relationships, and an accumulation of stress, such as the overwhelming stress associated with the death of a family member (Hawton, 1986), have been linked with suicide in the young adolescent. Intervention strategies are approached throughout this discussion in terms of facilitating the expression of grief that families experience after the death of a child, when grief is unresolved or too painful for parents to express openly. These strategies to facilitate the expression of grief and open communication in families can be used by nurses in a variety of practice settings.

It is essential that the nurse work with the family over an extended period of time. This long-term interaction enables the nurse to explore any unresolved issues with the family, open communication among family members and give the family and child tasks to facilitate their grieving. Weekly sessions are necessary during the first few weeks, during which time strategies can focus on grief work and the absolution of acute or chronic family grief. The nurse must be sensitive to the family and advance at their pace.

Providing Safety During Intense Grief

If a sibling is suffering intense grief, it is essential during the first session with the family to address the issue of the possibility of an attempted suicide and focus on the safety of the child. One of the most important strategies to prevent a suicide attempt by any surviving sibling is to implement a safety watch with the parents in charge to ensure the safety of the surviving sibling. When implementing a safety watch, the nurse must focus on the parental dyad. The nurse can point out to the parents that the distressed sibling may be carrying grief for the family. This measure enables the parents to become more aware of the sibling's sadness and grief. The safety watch pushes the family members closer together, thus re-establishing boundaries, opening up communication, and reconnecting linkages between the nuclear and extended family and the supportive network (Landau-Stanton and Stanton, 1985).

During this first session when the safety watch is being planned with the parents, it is necessary to coach the parents in implementing the procedures that they must follow. By discussing their plans, the nurse can suggest options. For instance, when informing the parents that someone must be physically present with their child at all times, the nurse can assist the parents to establish a shift schedule and discuss anticipated problems and their solutions. The nurse can have the parents plan how they will supervise the child's daily schedule in terms of school, recreation, homework, sleeping arrangements, bathroom privileges, eating, and time with peers.

Fostering Resource Mobilization

It is crucial to mobilize the resources of the family immediately after a suicide attempt. The parents can be encouraged to bring as many family members to the counseling sessions as possible. If there are older siblings in the family or an extended family nearby, the nurse should encourage the parents to include them in the safety watch.

The parents should be asked to bring grandparents, aunts, uncles, and even close friends involved with the family to the sessions.

The nurse must work to mobilize the family and empower the parents so that they will feel a sense of mastery. It is important to assist the family to (1) identify family resources and support systems, (2) decide how support systems can be mobilized and used, and (3) make a detailed schedule for the safety watch (Landau-Stanton and Stanton, 1985, p. 322). This plan may need to be very explicitly detailed for some families. The nurse can help the parents construct a daily schedule, enlisting the support of family members and friends.

In a review of the research literature examining the nature of protective factors in children under stress, Garmezy (1986) identified three recurring factors contributing to resilience in children. These factors grouped into three broad categories include (1) the personality disposition of the child; (2) a supportive family milieu; and (3) an external support system that encourages and enhances a child's coping efforts by reinforcing the child's positive values. These protective factors are congruent with a family systems perspective of interventions with families. A nurse can foster a supportive family environment and assist the family to expand their support network. This approach will have a positive effect on the family members and the distressed child.

Encouraging Communication

Because parents are anxious and sometimes angry with the behavior of the surviving sibling, the nurse can initiate parent-to-sibling communication immediately in the first session. The nurse can ask the parents to tell their child what it would have been like for them if the suicide attempt had been successful and the child had died. This strategy emphasizes the seriousness of the suicide attempt to the parents and lets the child know how much they care. It is important at this time that the parents be given permission by the nurse to express their love and caring openly. The nurse can direct the parents to tell their child in session how much the child is valued and loved. This move helps to change a behavior pattern in the family and facilitates more open communication. When initiating this strategy, the nurse should have each of the parents speak directly to the child. This communication can be difficult for parents, and they may need the nurse to coach them in speaking to and looking directly at the child. During this process the emotional integration of the family should be noted (Worden, 1982). Does the family seem connected to one another? Are the family members able to help each other cope with their loss, or do they need external sources to assist them? A family that is not emotionally integrated may have one or more members develop physical, emotional, or behavioral symptoms.

An effective strategy is to ask family members to track down information missing from the genogram as a task to be completed between family sessions. This includes asking extended family members, such as grandparents, aunts, and uncles, about relationships, losses, illnesses, deaths, or other crises that have occurred in the family. This task can be therapeutic, for it facilitates family communication and reinforces the family's extended network. Another strategy in the form of a task is to have the parents and the children bring in a written list of strengths that they see existing in their family. The nurse can ask the parents to list the strengths that they brought with them from their families of origin. This process lets the family, and in particular the parents, see that they do have strengths and that they received positive strengths from their family that have enabled them to survive as a family. Maintaining a family systems perspective for the counseling sessions enables the nurse to use the resources of each of the family members, including their strengths, which will be valuable in supporting one another (Rando, 1984; Rosen, 1986).

Sharing Grief

The next several sessions can be planned with the family to address grieving, the circumstances surrounding the death of the child, the funeral, and the relationship between siblings. Questions surrounding the death itself and where each person was that day inform the nurse of the circumstances surrounding the illness and the subsequent

death and whether it was expected or unexpected. It is also helpful to ask about the funeral, including who participated in the planning as well as who participated in the funeral service.

It may be appropriate to plan one session around the funeral service itself. This strategy can be potent because it gives permission to the family members to grieve openly and to share special memories of the service. The family can be directed to plan the session at home. In this way, they can bring selected readings or music to share with one another. The family may want to plan a memorial service and invite friends and relatives who were unable to attend the funeral.

Questions about what has been happening since the death of the child in terms of relationships outside the family and the reestablishment of family patterns, such as family activities, especially activities for the siblings, will give the nurse a look at the family and its support systems (Rando, 1984). What other stresses have they been experiencing since the child died? Are the siblings playing with their friends? Are they going to school? Are they having any difficulties with homework or grades? What is happening at school with friends and other students? Do they fear questions about the sibling who died? Do their friends understand why and how the death occurred? If one of the children is experiencing difficulties in school or with friends, the school counselor or teacher should be included in one or more of the family sessions. Friends who are important to the siblings can be included in selected sessions to enhance their supportive network.

Sharing Memories

Family discussion of which tasks have been accomplished in the grieving process will give the nurse the information necessary to assist the grieving family to complete the unfinished tasks (Rando, 1984; Worden, 1982). When appropriate, the rest of the family members along with the siblings can be asked to share special memories about the child who died. This discussion can include memories of fun times together, with secrets that only the siblings knew about and perhaps laughed about together.

Another strategy to assist parents and children to come to terms with their loss is to review and share very special family transitions, such as the months prior to the deceased child's birth, the birth itself, and the period after the birth. The nurse can ask how the name for the child was chosen and what traditions surrounded the naming or the christening of the child. Using the genogram as a family map can help the interventions to be implemented in a nonthreatening way. Were there communions or bar mitzvahs in this family? What were birthdays like in the past? What school and extracurricular activities did the child enjoy or not enjoy? Certificates and prizes that were won by the child can be brought in to share with the nurse as well as any other possession that has special meaning to the parents and to the siblings. This strategy facilitates synchrony of grieving in all the family members and leads to greater understanding and acceptance among them.

Absolving Grief

A strategy to help absolve any guilt over disagreements and fights that siblings had experienced is for the nurse to ask the siblings to share memories with the parents about some mischief that they had shared together and perhaps been reprimanded for by the parents. This strategy can normalize the disagreements that siblings experienced, and they can then be reframed by the nurse to be positive memories.

Letting Go

During an active interchange as just described, the nurse can take the opportunity to encourage each family member to facilitate the expression of emotions and can identify those members who seem to have difficulty (Worden, 1982). To resolve grief adequately, the family members need to be able to experience and freely express feelings, intense emotions, and memories. Open discussion in the family can facilitate the identification and exploration of these feelings with each other. The nurse must assist the grieving children and family to release their emotional ties to the deceased child, even though this process will involve hurt and discomfort. The children and the par-

ents, for their own growth, must be encouraged to actively participate in the grief work (Rando, 1984; Worden, 1982).

Nurses must be certain to give the family members permission to grieve. In addition, the parents must give permission to the surviving siblings to grieve. If the parents develop coping skills to deal with the death of their child, they will then be better able to assist their children in grieving (Rosen, 1986; Spinetta et al., 1981). These interventions will help the family members to redefine their relationships without the deceased child. In this way they are assisted in readjusting to their new environment and in reinvesting their emotional energy in each other and in new relationships or in redefining old relationships. The nurse must be aware that parents who never resolve their grief over the death of a child are out of sync with the natural phases of the life process. Appropriate interventions can only ease the pain of the family's loss. They cannot completely eradicate the memories and the sadness that will drift intermittently through their thoughts (Arnold and Gemma, 1983; Rando, 1986; Schoeneck, 1986; Viorst, 1986).

The following case study illustrates the tendency of adults to be unaware of or to overlook the sadness and pain that a preadolescent or young adolescent may be experiencing as a result of the death of a sibling. Oftentimes the pain of loss is difficult for adults, in particular parents, to express or to acknowledge to one another, and the difficulty is compounded when that loss must be shared with other young members of the family. A protective barrier or a conspiracy of silence may be the only way in which the family can cope with the overwhelming feelings of sadness that are experienced when a child in the family dies. A therapeutic intervention that includes all family members can serve to identify and enhance the already existing strengths inherent in that family and each of its individual members.

Case Study

Twelve year old Debbie and her mother and father were encouraged by Debbie's teacher to seek counseling because of an unsuccessful suicide attempt by Debbie that was discovered by the teacher. Debbie's younger seven year old brother, Sean, had died a few months previously. Sean had been diagnosed as being in an advanced stage of leukemia and had died four weeks later.

Sean's death had been unexpected and traumatic for Debbie and her parents.

Debbie, unbeknownst to her parents, had attempted to hang herself with a rope in her closet during the weekend; she had jumped off a ledge, but changed her mind at the last minute and managed to pull herself back to a shelf. She went to school as usual for a few days. The physical education teacher noticed marks around her neck and talked to Debbie, who then told her what she had done. The teacher contacted the parents and discussed the seriousness of the distress that Debbie felt and the suicide attempt. The parents had no idea that Debbie had made a suicide attempt, nor had they noticed any difference in her behavior.

On first meeting this family, it was evident to the nurse that the parents were very close and that Debbie was peripheral to them. The mother and father were both involved in their professions and in community service groups. They saw Debbie as the problem. At this session, Debbie's safety was the main concern, and ways of ensuring her safety were discussed. The parents were asked how they would implement ways to keep her safe. By doing this, the nurses involved them in Debbie's care; they were also able to demonstrate their love and care for her while doing so.

It was decided to counsel the family together to facilitate grieving. This direction was taken after the family had been assessed from a systems perspective. That is, a family history of losses was taken that included losses incurred by members in past generations. In that way, the nurse was able to assess how grief might be handled in this generation.

The parents and Debbie were asked to list family strengths. This engendered some anger from the mother, for she viewed the family as being very strong, caring, and warm; she reminded the nurse that Debbie's suicide gesture was the problem. From that point on, it was decided to focus on actual expressions of grief. Another nurse, who herself had lost a child, was brought in to assist with the counseling sessions. The parents were able to relate well to her experience and how it had affected the siblings in the family.

Between counseling sessions, Debbie and her parents were given tasks to accomplish at home and were asked to share the outcome or bring in evidence of the task being worked on to show at the following sessions. They were asked to share what was special about Sean and their relationships with him. They were directed to share their memories with each other so that communication between them could be opened up. These memories included activities shared by Debbie and Sean as well, secrets shared between them, and their fights and the resolution or nonresolution of those fights; this type of task was important to help alleviate any guilt. At the following session,

the family members laughed and cried as they shared their memories. The parents were then encouraged to join a bereavement group for parents who have had a child who died. Debbie herself said that she wanted to join a sibling group where there were other teenagers her age with whom she could talk about what it was like to have a brother die. The nurses were able to facilitate the family's entry into the appropriate groups. At this session, it was discovered that Debbie had been hospitalized for an infection since her brother had died, and she was terrified that the medicine would not be effective for her, as it had not been for her brother.

One session focused on Sean's illness and his funeral; the participation of Debbie, her friends, and Sean's friends was acknowledged. The parents shared their role in the funeral and what the service had meant to them. They acknowledged that they had been unable to talk about the funeral or Sean's death. During this session, it was discovered that they had not entered Sean's room since his death; the mother said that she was unable to go into the room.

The task for the next session flowed from this information. The parents and Debbie were directed to talk about Sean's possessions and activities that had special meaning either to Sean, to them as parents, or to Debbie as his sister. When they arrived for the following session, the mother was carrying a large bag. She, the father, and Debbie had been able to enter Sean's room to reorganize his belongings—to put them away or to give them to others. Each of them kept a memento that was special to him or her. The session was spent talking about Sean's baptism, his communion suit, and the prizes and certificates he had won for essays and activities at school. It was evident toward the end of the session that Debbie had become reunited with her parents. Her mother was able to talk to her more freely and with genuine caring as well as to touch her affectionately. The mother no longer interrupted when the father talked to Debbie.

Because the holiday season was approaching, the nurses asked the family about their plans and how they planned to deal with Sean's absence. The nurse told them that some families set a place for the child who has died and that they should do what they felt comfortable doing as a family. Debbie, because she was an accomplished violin student, decided to practice music that was special to Sean and herself and to perform for her parents. During one session the nurse asked Debbie to bring her violin and play the music that she herself had played at Sean's funeral. This let Debbie know that she was special too; she loved sharing her talents.

Toward the end of the sessions, the family relationship structure had been changed and the parents were again involved with Debbie. Debbie, through her parents, had been given permission to grieve with them openly. Up to this time, neither the parents nor Debbie had been able to express their grief at the loss of Sean. The parents and Debbie became involved in bereavement groups, in which they were able to continue to redefine their lives and their identities with others at the same developmental phase. The parents were now able to spend special times with Debbie providing the love and nurturance that is so critical for healthy development.

RESEARCH IMPLICATIONS

There is a paucity of research on the concepts of loss and grief and what effect loss and grief in children may have on future psychological, physical, and social development. There is an extensive body of literature that has been reviewed by Bowlby (1973, 1981), Rutter (1977, 1980), and Garmezy (1983) suggesting that loss has long-term adverse effects on developmental outcomes in adolescence and later adulthood. Several examples of actual or potential loss were mentioned earlier in this chapter. In addition to exploring the effects of loss on children, it is essential to examine the association between loss and the developmental issues within the family system that are a part of the transition phase of adolescence. There have been no systematic longitudinal investigations, however, examining the effects of loss over time.

There are a variety of situations in society today that can expose children of all ages to the experience of loss. Because there has been little systematic development of knowledge in nursing science on the responses of children to loss and how the coping behaviors of children and parents may facilitate their adjustment, childhood and family response to loss is a fruitful area for nursing research.

Situations that expose children to loss are varied and numerous and can be examined situationally as well as developmentally. A few examples are (1) an unplanned teenage pregnancy and parents who may be angry or depressed at this situation; (2) parents who are unable to interact with their children in a healthy way because of their own depression and loneliness; (3) living with parents who are threatening to separate or divorce; (4) the death of a parent, sibling, grandparent, or close friend (whether a peer or older friend); (5) children who live in foster care

or institutions; (6) runaway children; (7) children involved with addictive substances or who live with parents using addictive substances; and (8) children who have to cope with the experience and consequences of incest and sexual abuse. Further, there are children who must learn to cope with losses resulting from their own chronic illness or chronic illness in their parents and children who have lost the use of a body part because of unexpected trauma or planned surgical intervention. Loss related to critical care environments is only beginning to be addressed in nursing textbooks (Jones and Peacock, 1988).

Programs of research could be built around these various situations, using both qualitative and quantitative approaches to research, as appropriate. There are also areas of research that still would best be done by careful observation and categorization of behaviors or responses (Hinde, 1979); this is particularly true of research on children and on family interactions and relationships. For such research projects to be effective, they must focus on narrowly defined experiences.

Bowlby (1979) suggests two strategies for research on loss: (1) to examine a sample of older children and adults who have had the experience of loss in their early years and compare them with a sample of those who have not had a comparable experience and (2) to study children's responses at the time of the experience and during the period immediately following the experience. Problems with the first strategy are sample location and selection and the selection and examination of controls. Also, there are problems in both strategies with the selection and development of appropriate instruments to measure the phenomenon of loss.

To measure the response to loss in children and their families, certain variables must be included for investigation such as (1) past experiences of loss for children and their family and their responses, including coping behaviors; (2) family relationships, because it is the relationship that will determine the response to loss and the ensuing behaviors; and (3) coping behaviors used by the children and the family members to cope with the grief engendered by the loss. In the future, theoretical approaches to coping with loss in narrowly defined situations may be built into experimental designs so that interventions to facilitate the grieving process can be tested empirically.

References

Anthony, S. The discovery of death in childhood and after. London: Penguin Books, 1971.

Armstrong, GD, and Martinson, IM. Death, dying, and terminal care: Dying at home. In Kellerman, J (Ed.), Psychological aspects of childhood cancer. Springfield, Ill.: Charles C Thomas, 1980, pp. 292–311.

Arnold, JH, and Gemma, PB. A child dies: A portrait of family grief. Rockville, Md.: Aspen Systems Corp. 1983.

Averill, JR. Grief: Its nature and significance. Psychological Bulletin, 70:712–748, 1968.

Balk, D. Adolescents' grief reactions and self-concept perceptions following sibling death: A study of 33 teenagers. Journal of Youth and Adolescence, 12:137–161, 1983.

Barnes, MJ. The reactions of children and adolescents to the death of a parent or sibling. In Sahler, OJ (Ed.), The child and death. St. Louis: CV Mosby Co., 1978, pp. 185–201.

Binger, CM, Ablin, AR, Feuerstein, RC, Kusher, SH, Zoger, S, and Mikkelsen, C. Childhood leukemia: Emotional impact on patient and family. New England Journal of Medicine, 280:414–418, 1969.

Bluebond-Langner, M. I know, do you? Awareness and communication in terminally ill children. In Schoenberg, B, Carr, A, Peretz, D, and Kutscher, A (Eds.), Anticipatory grief. New York: Columbia University Press, 1974, pp. 171–181.

Bluebond-Langner, M. The private worlds of dying children. Princeton, N.J.: Princeton University Press, 1978.

Boszormenyi-Nagy, I, and Sparks, GM. Invisible loyalties. New York: Brunner/Mazel, Inc., 1984.

Bowen, M. Family therapy in clinical practice. New York: Jason Aronson, Inc., 1978.

Bowlby, J. Childhood mourning and the implications for psychiatry. American Journal of Psychiatry, 118:481–498, 1961.

Bowlby, J. Pathological mourning and childhood mourning. Journal of American Psychoanalysis, 11:500–541, 1963.

Bowlby, J. Separation and loss within the family. In Anthony, EJ, and Koupernik, C (Eds.), The child in his family (Vol. 1). New York: John Wiley & Sons, Inc., 1970, pp 197–216.

Bowlby, J. Separation: Anger and anxiety (Vol. 11). New York: Basic Books, Inc., 1973.

Bowlby, J. The making and breaking of affectional bonds. London: Tavistock Publications Limited, 1979.

Bowlby, J. Loss: Sadness and depression (Vol. 3). New York: Penguin Books, 1981.

Brown, GW. Mental illness. In Aiken, LH, and Mechanic, D (Eds.), Applications of social science to clinical medicine and health policy. New Brunswick, N.J.: Rutgers University Press, 1986, pp. 175–203.

Cain, AC, Fast, I, and Erickson, ME. Children's disturbed reactions to the death of a sibling. American Journal of Orthopsychiatry, 34:741–752, 1964.

Cobb, B. Psychological impact of long illness and death of a child on the family circle. Journal of Pediatrics, 49:746–751, 1958.

Davies, EB. Behavioral responses of children to death of a sibling. Unpublished doctoral dissertation, University of Washington, Seattle, 1983.

Gardner, RA. Children's reactions to parental death. In Schowalter, JE, Patterson, PR, Tallmer, M, Kutscher, AH, Gullo, SV, and Peretz, D (Eds.), The child and death. New York: Columbia University Press, 1983, pp. 104–124.

Garmezy, N. Stressors of childhood. In Garmezy, N, and Rutter, M (Eds.), Stress, coping, and development in children. New York: McGraw-Hill Book Co., 1983, pp. 43–84.

Garmezy, N. Developmental aspects of children's responses to the stress of separation and loss. In Rutter, M, and Izard, CE (Eds.), Depression in young people: Developmental and clinical perspectives. New York: The Guilford Press, 1986, pp. 297–323.

Gartley, W, and Bernasconi, M. The concept of death in children. Journal of General Psychology, 110:71–85, 1967.

Haley, J. Problem-solving therapy. San Francisco: Jossey-Bass Inc., 1976.

Hawton, K. Suicide and attempted suicide among children and adolescents. Beverly Hills, Calif.: Sage Publications, 1986.

Heller, DB, and Schneider, CD. Interpersonal methods for coping with stress: Helping families of dying children. Omega, 8:319–330, 1978.

Hinde, RA. Family influences. In Rutter, M (Ed.), Scientific foundations of development. London: Heinemann Medical, 1979, pp. 47–66.

Jones, MB, and Peacock, MK. Loss. In Howell, E, Widra, L, and Hill, MG (Eds.), Comprehensive trauma nursing: Theory and practice. Glenview, Ill.: Scott, Foresman Co., 1988, pp. 223–246.

Kaplan, DM, Grobstein, R, and Smith, A. Predicting the impact of severe illness in families. Health and Social Work, 1:71–81, 1976.

Kim, MJ, McFarland, GK, and McLane, AM. Pocket guide to nursing diagnoses. St. Louis: CV Mosby Co., 1984.

Kim, MJ, and Moritz, DA (Eds.). Classification of nursing diagnoses. New York: McGraw-Hill Book Co., 1982.

Kimmel, DC, and Weiner, IB. Adolescence: A developmental transition. Hillsdale, N.J.: Lawrence Erlbaum Associates, Inc., 1985.

Koocher, GP. Children's conceptions of death. In Bibace, R, and Walsh, ME (Eds.), Children's conceptions of health, illness, and bodily functions. San Francisco: Jossey-Bass, Inc., 1981, pp. 85–99.

Krell, R, and Rabkin, L. The effects of sibling death on the surviving child. Family Process, 10:471–477, 1979.

Landau, J. Therapy with families in cultural transition. In McGoldrick, M, Pearce, JK, and Giordano, JD (Eds.), Ethnicity and family therapy. New York: The Guilford Press, 1982, pp. 552–572.

Landau-Stanton, J, and Stanton, MD. Treating suicidal adolescents and their families. In Mirken, P, and Koman, SL (Eds.), Handbook of adolescents and family therapy. New York: Gardner Press, Inc., 1985, pp. 309–328.

Lindemann, E. Symptomatology and management of acute grief. American Journal of Psychology, 101:141–148, 1944.

Martinson, IM, Davies, EB, and McClowry, SG. The long-term effects of sibling death on self-concept. Journal of Pediatric Nursing, 2:227–235, 1987.

McClowry, S, Gilliss, CL, and Martinson, IM. The process of grief in the bereaved family. In Gilliss, CL, Highley, BL, Roberts, BM, and Martinson, IM (Eds.), Toward a science of family nursing. Menlo Park,

Calif.: Addison-Wesley Publishing Co., Inc., Health Sciences Division, 1989, pp. 216–225.

McGoldrick, M. Ethnicity and family therapy: An overview. In McGoldrick, M, Pearce, JK, and Giordano, JP (Eds.), Ethnicity and family therapy. New York: The Guilford Press, 1982, pp. 3–30.

McGoldrick, M, and Gerson, R. Genograms in family assessment. New York: WW Norton & Co., Inc., 1985.

Miles, MS, and Demi, AS. Toward the development of a theory of guilt: Sources of guilt in bereaved parents. Omega, 14:299–314, 1983–84.

Minuchin, S. Families and family therapy. Cambridge, Mass.: Harvard University Press, 1974.

Nagy, M. The child's theories concerning death. Journal of General Psychology, 73:3–27, 1948.

National Center for Health Statistics: Vital Statistics of the United States (Vol. II). Mortality, Part A. DHHS Publication PHS 83–1101. Public Health Service, Washington, D.C.: U.S. Government Printing Office, 1978.

National Center for Health Statistics: Vital Statistics of the United States (Vol. II). Mortality, Part A. DHHS Publication PHS 86–1122. Public Health Service, Washington, D.C.: U.S. Government Printing Office, 1982.

Neugarten, BL. Adaptation and the life cycle. The Counseling Psychologist, 6:16–20, 1976.

Parkes, CM. Bereavement: Studies of grief in adult life. New York: International Universities Press, Inc., 1972.

Patterson, PR, Tallmer, M, Kutscher, AH, Gullo, SV, and Peretz, D (Eds.). The child and death. New York: Columbia University Press, 1983, pp. 125–133.

Paul, NL, and Grosser, GH. Operational mourning and its role in conjoint marital therapy. Community Mental Health Journal, 1:339–345, 1965.

Pearlin, L, and Aneshensel, CS. Coping and social supports: Their functions and applications. In Aiken, LH, and Mechanic, D (Eds.), Applications of social science to clinical medicine and health policy. New Brunswick, N.J.: Rutgers University Press, 1986, pp. 417–437.

Piaget, J. The child's conception of the world. London: Routledge & Kegan-Paul, Inc., 1929.

Pine, VR, and Bauer, C. Parental grief: A synthesis of theory, research, and intervention. In Rando, TA (Ed.), Parental loss of a child. Champaign, Ill.: Research Press, 1986, pp. 59–96.

Rando, TA. An investigation of grief and adaptation in parents whose children have died from cancer. Journal of Pediatric Psychology, 8:3–20, 1983.

Rando, TA. Grief, dying, and death: Clinical interventions for caregivers. Champaign, Ill.: Research Press, 1984.

Rando, TA (Ed.). Parental loss of a child. Champaign, Ill.: Research Press, 1986.

Raphael, B. The anatomy of bereavement. New York: Basic Books, Inc., 1983.

Rosen, H. Unspoken grief: Coping with childhood sibling loss. Lexington, Mass.: Lexington Books, 1986.

Rosenblatt, R. Children of war. New York: Anchor Press, 1983.

Ross-Alaolmolki, K. Supportive care for families of dying children. Nursing Clinics of North America, 20:457–466, 1985

Rutter, M. Separation, loss and family relationships. In Rutter, M, and Hersow, L (Eds.), Child psychiatry: Modern approaches. Philadelphia: JB Lippincott Co., 1977, pp. 47–73.

Rutter, M. The long-term effects of early experience. Development, Medicine and Child Neurology, 22:800–815, 1980.

Safier, G. A study in relationships between the life and death concepts in children. Journal of General Psychology, 105:283–294, 1964.

Sanders, CM. Effects of sudden vs. chronic illness death on bereavement outcome. Omega, 13:227–241, 1982–83.

Schilder, P, and Weschler, D. The attitudes of children toward death. Journal General Psychology, 45:406–451, 1934.

Schoeneck, TS. Hope for bereaved: A handbook for understanding, coping and growing through grief. Syracuse, N.Y.: Hope for Bereaved, 1986.

Schumacher, JD. Helping children cope with a sibling's death. In Hansen, JC, and Frantz, JT (Eds.), Death and grief in the family. Rockville, Md.: Aspen Systems Corp., 1984, pp. 82–94.

Speigel, J. An ecological model of ethnic families. In McGoldrick, M, Pearce, JK, and Giordano, J (Eds.), Ethnicity and family therapy. New York: The Guilford Press, 1982, pp. 31–54.

Spinetta, JJ, Rigler, D, and Karon, M. Anxiety in the dying child. Pediatrics, 52:841–845, 1973.

Spinetta, JJ, Rigler, D, and Karon, M. Personal space as a measure of the dying child's sense of isolation. Journal of Clinical and Consulting Psychology, 42:751–756, 1974.

Spinetta, JJ, Swarner, JA, and Sheposh, JP. Effective parental coping following the death of a child from cancer. Journal of Pediatric Psychology, 6:251–263, 1981.

Vernon, GM. Sociology of death. New York: Ronald Press, 1970.

Viorst, J. Necessary losses. New York: Ballantine Books, 1986.

Waechter, EH. Children's awareness of fatal illness. American Journal of Nursing, 71:1168–1172, 1971.

Wallerstein, JS. Children of divorce: Stress and developmental tasks. In Garmezy, N, and Rutter, M (Eds.), Stress, coping, and development in children. New York: McGraw-Hill Book Co., 1983, pp. 265–302.

Webster's Ninth New Collegiate Dictionary. Springfield, Mass.: Merriam-Webster Company, Inc., 1987.

Weiner, JM. Reaction of the family to the fatal illness of the child. In Schoenberg, B, Carr, A, Peretz, D, and Kutscher, A (Eds.), Loss and grief: Psychological management in medical practice. New York: Columbia University Press, 1970, pp. 87–101.

Woosley, SF, Thornton, DS, and Freidman, SB. Sudden death. In Sahler, OJ (Ed.), The child and death. St. Louis: CV Mosby Co., 1978, pp. 100–111.

Worden, JW. Grief counseling and grief therapy: A handbook for the mental health practitioner. New York: Springer Publishing Co., Inc., 1982.

Wright, LM, and Leahey, M. Nurses and families: A guide to family assessment and intervention. Philadelphia: FA Davis Co., 1984.

CHAPTER 15

PROMOTION OF SELF-CARE

MARY KAY KOSTER, M.A., R.N.

In 1959, Dorothea Orem introduced the concept of self-care into nursing practice (Fawcett, 1984). Orem's model is based on clients assuming a more active role in their own health care and on nurses assisting clients with their self-care activities. Although the promotion of self-care as an intervention is receiving increased attention in the literature, little is known about the uniqueness of this intervention for either the well child or the ill child. The purpose of this chapter is to present the intervention of promotion of self-care for the child who has an alteration in health state that results in hospitalization. Using Orem's model, self-care will be discussed in relation with growth and development, thereby providing a conceptual framework for understanding

the need to promote self-care as an intervention during illness and hospitalization.

THEORETICAL FOUNDATION

Orem (1985) defines self-care as "the practice of activities that individuals initiate and perform on their own behalf in maintaining life, health and well-being" (p. 84). This definition is based on the belief that a person has an innate ability to care for self and that each person is a rational being capable of choosing behavior designed to promote or maintain health. Using this framework, an outcome of nursing intervention is to maximize each client's potential for self-care (Anna et al., 1978; Bililtski, 1981; Dickson and Lee-Villasenor, 1982; Joseph, 1980; Porter and Shamian, 1983; Walton, 1985).

Self-care is undertaken by individuals to meet three types of self-care requisites (Orem, 1985). Universal self-care requisites are common to all human beings and include the maintenance of air, water, food, elimination, activity and rest, and solitude and social interaction; the prevention of hazards; and the promotion of human functioning. Developmental self-care requisites promote the processes of development and prevent conditions deleterious to maturation. Health deviation self-care requisites exist for persons who are ill or injured or who have defects and disabilities. All three types of self-care requisites result in a therapeutic self-care demand. When the individual is unable to meet this demand, a self-care deficit is said to exist.

The nurse assists individuals to meet their own therapeutic self-care demands through one of three types of nursing systems. In the wholly compensatory system, the nurse acts for the client who does not have the resources to engage in self-care activities. When the client is able to meet some, but not all, therapeutic self-care demands, the client and nurse work together, sharing the responsibility in a partly compensatory system. Within the educative-supportive system, the client has resources to meet self-care demands but needs nursing assistance to do so.

The ability to care for self is referred to as self-care agency (Orem, 1985). Agency is used in the sense of taking action. Orem believes there is a difference in self-care agency throughout the life span. Children are in a stage of dependent care. "Infants and children require care from others because they are in the early stages of development physically, psychologically, and psychosocially" (Orem, 1985, p. 84). The adult becomes a dependent care agency, and "care of others becomes an adult's contribution to the health and well-being of dependent members of the adult's social group" (Orem, 1985, p. 84). Based on this perspective, the parent or parent surrogate becomes a dependent self-care agency for the child.

Self-Care Agency in Children

As a human response, self-care becomes a "phenomenon of concern to nurses" (Bar-

nard, 1984, p. 5). Understanding of a phenomenon includes determining its antecedents or the "factors that precede or influence a particular event" (Walker and Avant, 1983, p. 150) and the consequences of a phenomenon or the "effects which occur after some event" (Walker and Avant, 1983, p. 150). The individual's practice as a self-care agent changes throughout the life span. When do individuals begin to demonstrate the human response of self-care agency?

One of the propositions that underlies Orem's conceptual model of self-care is that "the ability to engage in self-care is conditioned by age, developmental state, life experience, sociocultural orientation, health and available resources" (Orem, 1985, p. 35). Using empirical data, the factors listed in this proposition will be interpreted as antecedents to support the phenomenon of self-care agency in children. As a result of performing self-care activities, a person experiences one or more of three types of self-care requisites: universal, developmental, and health deviation (Orem, 1985). These self-care requisites, whether achieved or not, are interpreted as consequences of the phenomenon of self-care agency (Chang, 1980).

Age and Developmental Stage

Although the number of research studies on self-care in children using Orem's model is limited, the available data suggest that the phenomenon of self-care agency in children becomes measurable during the school-age years (six to 12 years). Therefore, both age and developmental stage can be viewed as antecedents to children being capable of acting on their own behalf in performing self-care activities.

Stullenbarger (1984) developed a pictorial Q-sort instrument to describe health-related self-care abilities of seven to nine year old children. Sixty items, bipolar representations of 30 self-care actions, were derived in part from Orem's universal self-care requisites. Line drawings of these actions were placed on cards for children to sort as "most like me" to "least like me" in graduated steps to describe what they did to stay healthy. This study demonstrated that children were capable of deciding self-care actions using Q-sort methodology.

In a descriptive correlational study, Saucier (1984) determined the relationship between the self-concept of ten to 12 year old diabetic children and their participation in self-care activities of diabetes management. Self-concept was measured by the Piers-Harris Children's Self-Concept Scale, and self-care was measured by a Self-Care Questionnaire (SCQ) developed by Saucier. Sixty-four children were able to respond to the 15 item SCQ by checking the frequency of performance of self-care activities related to diabetes management, ranging from never to always. The scores on the SCQ indicated that these children participated in self-care activities of diabetes management most of the time; the scores on the Self-Concept Scale were higher than the norm.

Experiences and Sociocultural Orientation

In a clarification of the self-care model, Orem (1983) recognized that it is the health situation, not the dependencies resulting from age and developmental state, that initiates the requirements for nursing care. As an antecedent, an individual's health state could result in a limitation in the ability to act as a self-care agent, thereby increasing the need for nursing intervention, or it could act as a stimulus for the practice of self-care. Therefore, health-related experiences affect the individual's orientation to wellness and illness.

The societal expectation that individuals should have responsibility regarding their health state is congruent with Orem's model (Fawcett, 1984). An individual is more likely to engage in self-care behavior if the outcome is perceived as dependent on the antecedent behavior of self-directed action or internal locus of control. The Children's Health Locus of Control Scale (CHLCS) measures the extent to which children view health event outcomes as being the result of their own actions rather than the result of others' whims and manipulations or simply fate or chance (Parcel and Meyer, 1978).

Blazek and McClellan (1983) investigated the effects of self- care instruction on locus of control, using the CHLCS, in two groups of fifth grade children. The children in the experimental group actively participated in a health care program whereas the children in the control group attended a health discussion. The results suggest that active participation in self-care instruction can in-crease the extent to which children view health event outcomes as being the result of their actions.

In a study also using a pretest–post-test control group design, Kubly and McClellan (1984) investigated the effects of an instructional program designed to promote self-care in second grade, third grade, and fourth grade asthmatic children. The experimental group received self-care instruction in breathing exercises, medication, and basic knowledge of asthma. The experimental group showed a significant change in scores on the CHLCS. Again, the results suggest that participation in a program oriented toward self-care may increase a child's perception of control over health-related experiences.

Availability of Resources

Resources which serve as antecedents to the child's practice of self-care activities can be divided into three areas: personal, environmental, and health promotional information. Although not based on Orem's model, descriptive studies by Lewis et al. (1977) and Stephenson (1983) indicate that elementary school children can make self-care choices in their decision to utilize the environmental resource of the school nurse for care, which includes health promotion information. This suggests that children know how to use the system to meet personal self-care needs.

Self-Care Requisites

Universal self-care requisites focus on life processes and the maintenance of human structure and function, whereas developmental self-care requisites specifically focus on life cycle events as part of developmental processes (Fawcett, 1984). Health deviation self-care requisites arise from disabilities or from deviations or defects in human structure or function (Fawcett, 1984). In studies previously cited by Saucier (1984) and Kubly and McClellan (1984), children with diabetes or asthma have a positive perspective of their ability to manage their health state. These studies support the consequence of meeting both universal and developmental self-care requisites through adaptation of the child in accord with human potential as well as the limitations of health deviation on self-care requisites.

ASSESSMENT

Based on the available empirical data, the phenomenon of the self-care agency in children is a plausible reality. Consideration of the antecedents and the consequences of this phenomenon provides a rationale for promotion of self-care as an appropriate intervention for children. The cited antecedents and consequences become critical factors to be noted in assessment and in outcome criteria when developing a nursing process that includes the intervention of promotion of self-care.

The concept of self-care is most often viewed in the context of wellness. Although a person may be ill, elements of wellness remain as part of the human response. It is generally agreed that the nurse's goal with the ill hospitalized child is to return that child to the highest level of wellness possible. It is for this reason that the author has provided data to support the promotion of self-care agency as opposed to focusing on self-care deficit. This approach builds upon the developmental strengths of the child and supports the holistic nature of nursing care (Eichelberger et al., 1980).

Data obtained through assessment of the child's response as a self-care agent to an actual or potential health need establish the basis for making a nursing diagnosis. Pertinent diagnoses include (1) *Alteration in health maintenance* and (2) *Self-care deficit* (Kim et al., 1984).

Defining characteristics for both of these diagnoses are incorporated in the following three categories as prerequisites for self-care: (1) knowledge for decision making about self-care, (2) motivation for self-care, and (3) ability (including psychomotor skill) to initiate and perform self-care practices (Joseph, 1980). These three categories also serve as a source for outcome criteria to determine the effect of nursing intervention on altering, maintaining, or increasing the child's response as a self-care agent (Clinton et al., 1977).

Competence for Self-Care

Although knowledge level and skill level may be factors of the child's growth and development, it is motivation that "moves a person to action or inaction" (Steiger and Lipson, 1985, p. 115). The interaction between cognitive processes, behavior, and motivation is described by social learning theory. Bandura's (1977) sociobehavioristic approach to development emphasizes personal efficacy or a "sense of personal mastery" (p. 194) or "personal competence" (p. 198).

"Perceived self-efficacy is concerned with judgments of how well one can execute courses of action required to deal with prospective situations" (Bandura, 1982, p. 122). Although efficacy expectations are measured independently of the performance of the behavior, the stronger the perceived self-efficacy, the more active the efforts to execute the behavior (Bandura, 1977). Social learning theory provides a framework for understanding how children develop skills and confidence in their ability to make health care choices for self-care. Indicators of cognitive processing and self-efficacy provide predictions on the child's ability to perform self-care activities. Taking action is dependent on perceived efficacy of self-regulatory capabilities for self-care.

Assuming responsibility for self-care occurs as a result of perceived competence which, in turn, produces a feeling of efficacy. Competence is the ability to assume responsibility for one's individual health, which includes self-directing health behavior and the ability to make appropriate use of available health resources (Parcel, 1976). "Competence is the ability to master self as well as one's life style; it is self-direction for self-care" (Koster, 1983, p. 40). The development of competence occurs throughout life. At around eight years of age, there is an emergence of a type of self-theory in which children make discrete judgments about their competence in different domains (Harter, 1982).

A health care environment that is conducive to the development of competence is one in which the child's attempts at mastery are encouraged and realistic feedback is given. Even though external factors of family and the health care environment have an impact on competence and efficacy, intrinsic motivation supports continuation and persistence of behavior (Bandura, 1977). The child is more likely to engage in a self-care behavior if the outcome is perceived as dependent on self-action. Locus of control describes the nature of the expectation held by the individual that a particular event will occur as a result of a specific act of behavior (Parcel et al., 1980a). If the person perceives that this event is contingent upon luck or upon powerful others, the person is said to have an external locus of control. If this person believes the event is contingent upon his own behavior, then this person has an internal locus of control (Parcel et al., 1980a). An internal locus of control can be reinforced by making health care choices related to self-care.

Utilizing Privacy for Competence Development

Growth in competence of self-care also occurs as a result of provisions for privacy. As described in internal locus of control, the affairs of the self are best conducted when the individual senses control of events and the environment. Privacy allows for maintenance of total system integrity, because privacy protects the self from threats to loss of autonomy and intrusions on basic dignity (Oland, 1978). Arriving at a state of comfort through freedom in the performance of self-care is the goal of privacy.

Solitude is one of Orem's (1985) universal self-care requisites. Hospitalization, with its attendant technology in the form of invasive needles, tubes, and machines, violates this solitude because nurses routinely enter intimate space of the ill client for the purpose of monitoring some bodily function.

Privacy is interpreted as the exclusive access of a person to a realm of his or her own (Rawnsley, 1980). Privacy is a social privilege associated with status. Children are often viewed as lacking status and therefore the privacy of children in the hospital may be overlooked. For the child who is not expected to exert control through decision making and is dependent on others for health care choices, status is decreased even more.

Privacy provides the child with quiet time to integrate the experience of illness and bodily changes into a meaningful perspective (Bloch, 1978). It is an opportunity for freedom to discover inner resources while creatively exploring self-care choices in making decisions. Withdrawal may be ac-

tively used as a way to establish privacy for thinking that is free from interaction and intrusion (Oland, 1978).

Withdrawal may also be used as a means to ensure privacy while performing a self-care task associated with activities of daily living, which include feeding, bathing, dressing, grooming, and toileting. These activities may be taken for granted (Chinn, 1978) and may be of concern only when there is a self-care deficit. For the child, maintenance of a familiar routine in meeting basic physiological needs increases "everyday self-care competence" (Benoliel et al., 1980, p. 4).

Overcoming setting constraints of decreased privacy by restructuring the environment allows for the child's activation of self-care agency. The use of pulled curtains, closed doors, knocking when entering, and privacy during phone calls may be forgotten while caring for children. Performance of activities in the room by the nurse without an explanation or the rearrangement of the child's personal items, including toys, may be perceived as an interruption of privacy. Organizing nursing care with as few intrusions as possible supports an environment that is conducive to performance of self-care activities and reinforces competence in self-care.

THE INTERVENTION

Alteration in health state that results in hospitalization affects a person's usual self-care practices. The nurse identifies not only self-care deficits or an interruption in the ability to engage in self-care but also self-care assets or actions that contribute positively to a client's state of health (Dickson and Lee-Villasenor, 1982). The role of the nurse is to facilitate the self-care agency of the client through the intervention of the promotion of self-care. Nursing measures which promote self-care include acting or doing for the client, guiding, teaching, supporting, and providing a developmental environment (Orem, 1985). Guiding is viewed by Orem as assisting the child and family in making choices, and teaching is the providing of health information. From a developmental perspective, Barnard (1982) views support as providing the child and parent with validation that normal developmental progress is occurring. All of these nursing measures are collectively reflected in the approach of advocacy to be discussed later as an intervention for promotion of self-care.

As noted previously, the parent may take on the role of dependent care agency for the child. Based on the severity of alteration in the child's health state, the parent or another family member may serve as a substitute self-care agent to assist the child in maintaining health and well-being. The nurse and the family work together to determine the optimum level of self-care that the child can achieve. The nurse then assists the family with measures to meet this outcome.

During illness, self-care as a priority may appear to be overshadowed by other issues facing the child and family. The practice of self-care may also be perceived differently by each individual and each family. As a reciprocal interaction between behavior and the environment, self-care demands active participation in selecting from alternative options. The family, as part of the environment, becomes a major influence on the child's initiation and maintenance of self-care. The family system provides communication and a support network through its intergenerational health traditions (Forrest, 1981).

Individuals as well as families are in the process of developing throughout life, with each stage of development being a transition or a time of change (Connell and Furman, 1984). Illness and hospitalization also involve change in both the child and family. Transitional periods, whether from normal growth and development or from an altered health state, can be times of positive growth. It becomes clear that to implement an intervention for a child and family, the nurse needs to consider the potential for growth during transitional periods. The nursing intervention then includes "instituting conditions that support the individual's adaptation, mastery or growth" (Barnard, 1982, p. 363).

Self-Care As a Developmental Process

The intervention of promotion of self-care focuses on development of the self-care capabilities of the child. Children at every developmental level exhibit the potential and ability for self-care (Facteau, 1980). The infant's potential for self-care is based on a capacity to interact with others to meet both universal or basic human needs and developmental needs. Infants have signaling behaviors or actions which stimulate the parent or adult caretaker to respond (Facteau, 1983). The infant signals by crying for milk in response to hunger. The infant sustains human interaction through preference for the human face as a visual object and through alerting with eyes, head, and body to animate sounds and human holding (Brazelton, 1969). The parent or adult caretaker who wishes to foster self-care allows for infant self-regulation "by responding to signals from the infant rather than presuming the infant's need" (Facteau, 1983, p. 17). In this way, the child is initiated into a pattern of self-care behavior which includes self-regulation of the environment (Barnard and Blackburn, 1985).

During the toddler years, self-care behavior is fostered primarily through the developmental milestones of ambulation, language acquisition, and toileting behaviors. Whereas ambulation allows the child to get what he needs, the development of language enables the child to ask directly for assistance with self-care (Facteau, 1983). Both ambulation and the ability to communicate needs are included as part of the determining factors in the accomplishment of the self-care task of toileting.

The preschool child is able to learn specific psychomotor skills needed in the practice of self-care. These include self-feeding and the daily hygiene tasks of brushing teeth, washing hands and face, toileting, and dressing. Repeated positive experiences in performing these skills, reinforced through supportive adult feedback, help the child incorporate them as continual self-care behaviors (Bruhn and Cordova, 1977). It is through family experiences that children first learn self-care as a daily expectation. The self-care behaviors learned are mediated by parents within the context of the family's sociocultural beliefs.

As the child enters school, self-care practices such as eating and dressing are monitored through the social environment of the school setting. It is in the school-age years that children become cognitively capable of taking responsibility for self-care. By the end of the school years, the child should be able to make appropriate self-care decisions in the areas of nutrition, exercise, sleep, and safety (Koster, 1983). Self-care for this age group has been described frequently in the literature (Corry and Galli, 1985; Gantz, 1980; Gorman, 1980; Groninza and Ojala, 1981; Gulbrandsen et al., 1981; Igoe, 1980; Lasky et al., 1981; Lewis, 1974; Ozias and Peterson, 1984).

Adolescence is a critical period during which the synthesis of cognitive skills and social responsibilities can result in maximum self-care decision making. The adolescent's enthusiasm for independence, alternating with the need to seek refuge in a peer group, often results in confusion (Jordon and Kelfer, 1983). The questioning and doubting characteristic of adolescence may make it difficult for the adolescent to make self-care choices (Bruhn and Cordova, 1978). Because of the incomplete acquisition of formal thought, an adolescent may make a health care choice which involves a risky rather than a growth-enhancing behavior.

After administering a self-assessment questionnaire on health to 125 seventh and tenth grade students, Benedict et al. (1981) found that the most frequently identified concerns were in the area of psychological and social adjustment. One recommendation was that interventions be directed at individual and peer support. Michael and Sewall (1980) found that support in the form of an adolescent peer group for those from ages 14 to 20 years functioned as a developmental force in fostering the responsible use of alcohol, thereby serving as an effective modality in increasing or strengthening the self-care agency of adolescents.

In addition to the developmental level of the child, other variables which may affect the outcome of the intervention include family influence, health status of the child, cultural factors, and constraints of the setting or environment. These variables influence advocacy, which is a major nursing strategy appropriate to implementation of the intervention of self-care promotion.

Advocacy

Promoting self-care to the maximum extent of the child's capabilities is the goal of advocacy. Kohnke (1980) describes advocacy in nursing as providing information and support so that a person can make the best decisions possible. In a similar approach, Orem (1985) refers to the supportive-educative role of the nurse. In the advocacy role, the nurse recognizes and facilitates the developmental strengths and growth potential of the child in achieving the highest level of health possible. There is an expectation that the child can be an active participant in health care and can be responsible for self-care.

For the child who has an alteration in his or her health state resulting in hospitalization, a common expectation is that the child is in a dependent role that is due to the development and regression associated with illness. Although these variables must be assessed, the nurse needs to resist the temptation to be a "rescuer" beyond the time when it is necessary (Kohnke, 1980). Rescuers of the sick see themselves as making decisions for others because they have the knowledge and "know best"; clients come to them for help, thereby relinquishing their autonomy. This attitude of paternalism is believed to "protect" individuals, especially children, from making choices that are not in their best interests. Such a belief raises ethical questions about a client's right to act responsibly on his or her own behalf (Free, 1984; Gadow, 1983). Advocacy, however, is an attitude whereby the nurse adopts an affirmative role to intervene with professionals and health care agencies to assure that a child's rights are respected.

Advocacy assists children and parents to have freedom of individual self-determination. The nurse acting as an advocate helps clients to assess their level of self-care agency, to become aware of existing and needed resources, to prioritize health values, and to estimate potential health outcomes (Bilitski, 1981). McCorkle (1983) emphasizes that clients "need to be seen as competent, responsible and well-motivated for maintaining their health" (p. 17). Through the advocacy role, nurses can place the responsibility for health care where it belongs—with the client.

In addition to the previously cited literature, the following reports indicate that children can be included in the category of responsible client. Children on renal dialysis (Grossman, 1981), with hemophilia (Tetrick, 1978), phenylketonuria (Hurst and Stullenbarger, 1986), asthma (Blessing-Moore et al., 1985; Dyer 1977; Parcel et al., 1980b; Pituch and Bruggeman, 1982), and diabetes mellitus (Fow, 1983; Loman and Galgani, 1984; Pridham, 1971) are reported to manage their chronic illnesses with self-care. Children are also capable of intermittent self-catheterization (Altshuler et al., 1977; Clarkson, 1982). Again, the literature supports the school-age years as the age when the emergence of self-care can be expected.

If self-care is viewed as a developmental process and if each child is seen as a unique individual, children of any age can be expected to exhibit aspects of self-care. When the child does not have the developmental ability and skills necessary for meeting universal and health deviation self-care requisites (Orem, 1985), a self-care deficit may exist. The influence of the family then becomes an operating variable affecting the outcome of the promotion of self-care. Through advocacy, the family is approached as a responsible client.

Hospitalization may be the first sustained contact with a health professional for the child and family. It is an opportune time for the philosophy of self-care to emerge through an advocacy relationship between the nurse and the child and family. The focus on self-care becomes especially critical with the current trend toward short hospital stays and the increased use of home care for the ill and recovering child. The practice of self-care bridges the transition from hospital care to home health care.

Problem Solving for Self-Care As an Advocacy Strategy

Activation of self-care involves more than an awareness that a health need exists and more than exposure to information about health care practices. The practice of self-care requires active participation in making health care choices through problem solving. Support from others through reinforcement of attempts and successes is also essential. Such participation strengthens motivation for the continued practice of self-care.

Through the use of a problem-solving approach, advocacy involves the client as a responsible decision maker in his or her health care. This partnership or shared relationship between the nurse and client is referred to as the Mutual Participation Model (Erickson, 1976; Szasz and Hollander, 1956; Trandel-Korenchuk, 1982), the Mutual Interaction Model (Williamson, 1981), and Nurse/Patient Peer Practice (Bayer and Brandner, 1977). Specific approaches for helping children with decision making have been described by Kaufman (1985), Koster (1981), and Ozias (1982).

To implement the problem-solving process in self-care, the nurse guides the client through every step of the process. Collection of both subjective and objective data is the first step. As the nurse analyzes the data, an actual or potential problem may be perceived that can be managed with self-care. Problem solving with the client then is initiated. The nurse also helps the child or parent to put the data together so that the client becomes aware that a health need exists. Identification of the problem or making a diagnosis or clinical decision is the next step in problem solving. Parents make good clinical judgments every day about their children. They know when there is a change in their child. Using the problem-solving process and making decisions with a professional person's guidance gives reassurance to the parent and lets the parent know that his or her judgment is sound. This same feeling of positive self-confidence occurs if the child is the decision maker. The child or parent then reaches a conclusion about what will be done to solve the problem. In this next step, a solution is selected from possible options. The nurse helps the client recognize available alternatives, consider the probable outcomes for each alternative, and then make a choice or decision about how to approach the problem.

Up to this point, the problem-solving process as well as positive reinforcement by the nurse has helped the child or parent feel increasingly competent and self-directive in being able to manage self-care. This feeling is important because the client must carry out the next step of the problem-solving process. This step involves implementing the plan or the solution. In the hospital, nursing assistance is still available. But once clients leave the hospital, they are essentially on their own, although a nurse from a home health care agency may visit (Pierce and Giovinco, 1983). Through problem solving for self-care, clients should be able to manage care, since decisions may have been already made about problems that may arise.

The final step of the problem-solving process occurs when the child and family have the next contact with the nurse. The outcome or results of the plan are evaluated. The child or parent is asked to evaluate the plan and suggest what could be done differently the next time to enhance success. This step is often omitted, but it can serve to remind the client that the focus is on self-care. The client can expect to receive continuity of care and to be an active participant in self-care.

The problem-solving process for self-care is more than the giving of information or advice (Forti, 1981; Levin, 1978). In giving information only, the nurse becomes the decision maker. Compliance will most likely be minimal. Information-giving alone also increases the client's dependence on health care professionals. Dependent behavior by the client is not consistent with self-care, for which the client is motivated to use his or her own resources.

Problem solving with the child or parent as a method of promoting self-care requires a role change by the nurse, who may feel the need to be in power or to control the child's management. Further, this method not only encourages parents to make decisions about their child but it also gives the child a voice in self-care.

As can be seen by the description of the problem-solving process for decision making, the promotion of self-care does not absolve the nurse from continued client involvement and professional responsibility. As an advocate, the nurse guards the child's right to make health care choices and to have an appropriate level of autonomy when the child is in less control of self and the environment because of illness and hospitalization.

For the child, participation in self-care is a learning process. Using the child's own health-related experiences, self-care in both wellness and illness can be promoted by the nurse in an advocacy relationship. As a result, beliefs of children that they are the most important health care providers for themselves and that their wellness is the result of their health behavior and lifestyle practices are reinforced. Children will be more likely to grow into adulthood believing, "Being well is my responsibility. I am the best advocate for my personal wellness" (Kandzari and Howard, 1981, p. 40). Thus, advocacy by the nurse can lead to self-advocacy.

Case Study

After a bicycle accident, emergency surgery to immobilize a fractured tibia with traction was performed on eight year old Larry. He was accompanied to the hospital by both of his parents, and one parent was in attendance throughout most of the hospital stay. Larry was an energetic third grade student who participated in Little League and miniature car racing. This was his first experience with hospitalization. Prior to the accident, Larry was an active self-care agent, taking responsibility for self-nourishment, bathing and hygiene, dressing and grooming, and managing self-toileting. Minimal prompting had been needed by his parents with these activities of daily living.

Postoperatively, Larry was placed on a nursing unit that subscribed to the self-care model of nursing care. Immediately postoperatively, Larry was unable to participate in self-care activities, and therefore the nurse met his self-care needs for him through wholly compensatory nursing care. Larry alternated between no verbal responses and quietly asking about his leg, his bicycle, and when he could go home. He gradually resumed self-feeding and self-toileting activities, and partly compensatory nursing care was provided as the nurse helped Larry to provide his own self-care.

Larry displayed little interest in participating in his bath. He would lie passively while either the nurse or one of his parents bathed him. One day, as the nurse was organizing the bath supplies, Larry, almost in a whisper, said, "I can wash myself." On further discussion with the nurse, Larry revealed that he didn't know how to reach the leg that was not in traction while he was on his back. He asked, "What if I move too much? Then I couldn't go home."

Based on the antecedent variables of Larry's developmental capability, his current health state, resource availability, and his expression of self-care agency, two nursing diagnoses were established. The first was *Self-care agency deficit* (Gordon, 1982, p. 73) in bathing and hygiene related to the environmental constraint of traction and decreased opportunity for decision making. The second was *Alteration in health maintenance* related to interruption in prior ability to meet basic health practice.

While in a supportive-educative role (Orem, 1985), the nurse initiated mutual problem solving with Larry regarding his active involvement in bathing. It was agreed that Larry could do all of his bath except his back. Because of the inaccessibility of that area to Larry and the importance of skin care, the nurse would continue to perform back care. Several practice sessions in moving in the bed with traction were held. Larry proudly informed his parents of the plan.

As a result, Larry changed from asking about *if*

he would go home to how he would manage *when* he went home. Since Larry would be going home with a cast, discharge problem solving was begun with both Larry and his parents. The return of Larry to the active self-care agent he was prior to his accident enabled Larry to continue growth in developmental strengths while hospitalized.

RESEARCH IMPLICATIONS

Kearney and Fleischer (1979) note that the construct of self-care agency "is conceptually complex, since it is relative to the person's agency or power to engage in self-care actions" (p. 26), and therefore measurement of a person's exercise of self-care agency should not rely solely on behavioral observation. Kearney and Fleischer (1979) developed an instrument to measure a person's exercise of self-care agency using a sample of 84 associate degree nursing students and 153 psychology students. The instrument contains 43 items that are rated on a five-point Likert scale. Construct validity, content validity, and test-retest reliability were established. Their findings suggest that people who exercise a high degree of self-care agency describe themselves as self-controlled, dependable, assertive, intelligent, confident, responsible, helpful, and adaptable. Additional studies using this tool need to be done to validate the results· of this study with other age groups.

Denyes (1982) developed an instrument to measure self-care agency using a sample of 161 adolescents ages 14 to 18 years. The instrument is a Likert scale questionnaire of 35 items related to ego strength and health decision-making capability, valuing of health, health knowledge, physical energy levels, feelings, and attention to health. Internal consistency and stability across alternate forms and content and construct validity of the tool were demonstrated. This tool should serve as a stimulus for development of an instrument to measure self-care agency in younger age groups.

Little is known empirically about the development of self-care agency in children. Interventions performed by nurses as "treatment of human responses" (American Nurses' Association, 1980, p. 9) need validation. "Testing of nursing interventions is the challenge of the next decade" (Barnard, 1985, p. 63) using both quantitative and qualitative methods.

Several research designs are needed to test nursing interventions designed to promote self-care. Experimental studies would demonstrate causal relationships (Polit and Hungler, 1983) that may help identify antecedents and consequences of the child acting as a self-care agent. A time series design or repeated measures design (Huck et al., 1974) could help establish patterns of self-care by the child. A single subject design that is a case study which includes an intervention (Barnard, 1983) may be a realistic approach to studying the promotion of self-care in nursing practice.

Generating a sound knowledge base for the practice of nursing is the goal of research (Barnard, 1986). Further evaluation of Orem's conceptual framework is needed, especially as it applies to children. A measure of self-care agency with children of different ages needs to be developed and utilized as a predictor in determining outcomes of the intervention of promotion of self-care. This chapter has provided information to support the idea of the child as capable of acting as a self-care agent and the promotion of self-care as a nursing intervention. Research needs to continue on both the deductive testing of Orem's self-care theory with children and the inductive generation of a self-care intervention model appropriate to children.

References

Altshuler, A, Meyer, J, and Butz, A. Even children can learn to do clean self-catheterization. American Journal of Nursing, 77:97–101, 1977.

American Nurses' Association. Nursing: A social policy statement. Kansas City, Mo.: 1980.

Anna, DJ, Christensen, DG, Hohon, SA, Ord, L, and Wells, SR. Implementing Orem's conceptual framework. Journal of Nursing Administration, 8:8–11, 1978.

Bandura, A. Self-efficacy: Toward a unifying theory of behavioral change. Psychological Review, 84:191–215, 1977.

Bandura, A. Self-efficacy mechanism in human agency. American Psychologist, 37:122–147, 1982.

Barnard, K. Determining the role of nursing. American Journal of Maternal/Child Nursing, 7:363, 1982.

Barnard, K. The case study method: A research tool. MCN: American Journal of Maternal Child Nursing, 8:36, 1983.

Barnard, K. The American Nurses' Association's social policy statement on nursing implications for the conference group's work on classification of nursing diagnoses. In Kim, MJ, McFarland, GK, and McLane, AM (Eds.), Classification of nursing diagnoses: Proceedings of the Fifth National Conference. St. Louis: CV Mosby Co., 1984, pp. 2–12.

Barnard, K. Blending the art and the science of nursing. MCN: American Journal of Maternal Child Nursing, 10:63, 1985.

Barnard, K. Research utilization: The researcher's responsibilities. MCN: American Journal of Maternal Child Nursing, 11:150, 1986.

Barnard, K, and Blackburn, S. Making a case for studying the ecologic niche of the newborn. March of Dimes Birth Defects: Original Article Series, 21:71–88, 1985.

Bayer, M, and Brandner, P. Nurse/patient peer practice. American Journal of Nursing, 77:86–90, 1977.

Benedict, V, Lundeen, KW, and Morr, BD. Self-assessment by adolescents of their health status and perceived health needs. Health Values: Achieving High Level Wellness, 5:239–245, 1981.

Benoliel, JQ, McCorkle, R, and Young, K. Development of a social dependency scale. Research in Nursing and Health, 3:3–10, 1980.

Bilitski, JS. Nursing science and the laws of health: The test of substance as a step in the process of theory development. Advances in Nursing Science, 4:15–29, 1981.

Blazek, B, and McClellan, MS. The effects of self-care instruction on locus of control in children. Journal of School Health, 53:554–556, 1983.

Blessing-Moore, J, Fritz, G, and Lewiston, NJ. Self-management programs for childhood asthma. Chest, 87:1075–1105, 1985.

Bloch, DW. Privacy. In Carlson, CE, and Blackwell, B (Eds.), Behavioral concepts and nursing intervention. New York: JB Lippincott Co., 1978, pp. 226–239.

Brazelton, TB. Infants and mothers. New York: Delacorte Press, 1969.

Bruhn, JG, and Cordova, FD. A developmental approach to learning wellness behavior, part I: Infancy to early adolescence. Health Values: Achieving High Level Wellness, 1:246–254, 1977.

Bruhn, JG, and Cordova, FD. A developmental approach to learning wellness behavior, part II: Adolescence to maturity. Health Values: Achieving High Level Wellness, 2:16–21, 1978.

Chang, BL. Evaluation of health care professionals in facilitating self-care: Review of the literature and a conceptual model. Advances in Nursing Science, 3:43–58, 1980.

Chinn, PL. Activities of daily living for the hospitalized child. In Brandt, PA, Chinn, PL, Hunt, VO, and Smith, ME (Eds.), Current practice in pediatric nursing. St. Louis: CV Mosby Co., 1978, pp. 45–52.

Clarkson, JD. Self-catheterization training of a child with myelomeningocele. American Journal of Occupational Therapy, 36:95–98, 1982.

Clinton, J, Denyes, MJ, Goodwin, JO, and Koto, EM. Developing criterion measures of nursing care: Case study of a process. Journal of Nursing Administration, 7:41–45, 1977.

Connell, JP, and Furman, W. The study of transitions. In Emde, RN, and Harmon, RJ (Eds.), Continuities and discontinuities in development. New York: Plenum Press, 1984, pp. 153–173.

Corry, JM, and Galli, N. The role of the school in consumer health education. Journal of School Health, 55:145–147, 1985.

Denyes, MJ. Measurement of self-care agency in adolescents (abstr). Nursing Research, 31:63, 1982.

Dickson, GL, and Lee-Villasenor, H. Nursing theory and

practice: A self-care approach. Advances in Nursing Science, 5:29–40, 1982.

Dyer, B. Asthmatic kids: Independence, one giant step. Pediatric Nursing, 3:16–23, 1977.

Eichelberger, KM, Kaufman, DN, Randall, ME, and Schwartz, NE. Self-care nursing plan: Helping children to help themselves. Pediatric Nursing, 6:9–13, 1980.

Erickson, ML. Assessment and management of developmental changes in children. St. Louis: CV Mosby Co., 1976.

Facteau, LM. Self-care concepts and the care of the hospitalized child. Nursing Clinics of North America, 15:145–155, 1980.

Facteau, LM. The need to teach self-care skills. In Thornton, SM, and Frankenberg, EK (Eds.), Child health care communications. New Brunswick, N.J.: Johnson & Johnson Baby Products Co., 1983, pp. 14–19.

Fawcett, J. Analysis and evaluation of conceptual models of nursing. Philadelphia: FA Davis Co., 1984.

Forrest, J. The family: The focus for health behavior generation. Health values: Achieving High Level Wellness, 5:138–144, 1981.

Forti, TJ. Advice: A well-intentioned ineffectual notion. Nurse Practitioner, 7:25–27, 1981.

Fow, SM. Home blood glucose monitoring in children with insulin-dependent diabetes mellitus. Pediatric Nursing, 9:439–442, 1983.

Free, TA. Paternalism in pediatric care. MCN: American Journal of Maternal Child Nursing, 9:9–14, 1984.

Gadow, S. Basis for nursing ethics: Paternalism, consumerism, or advocacy? Hospital Progress, 64:62–78, 1983.

Gantz, SB. A fourth-grade adventure in self-directed learning. Topics in Clinical Nursing, 2:29–38, 1980.

Gordon, M. Nursing diagnosis: Process and application. New York: McGraw-Hill, Inc., 1982.

Gorman, G. The school-age child as historian. Pediatric Nursing, 5:39–40, 1980.

Groninza, S, and Ojala, E. Participatory health care for children: The pros and cons. Journal of School Health, 51:193–194, 1981.

Grossman, MB. Self-care for children and adolescents on dialysis. American Association of Nephrology Nurses and Technicians Journal, 8:36–42, 1981.

Gulbrandsen, MG, Lasky, PA, and Scoblic, M. Translating health knowledge into health behavior. Issues in Comprehensive Pediatric Nursing, 5:177–184, 1981.

Harter, S. The perceived competence scale for children. Child Development, 53:87–97, 1982.

Huck, SW, Cormier, WH, and Bounds, WG. Reading statistics and research. New York: Harper & Row, Publishers, Inc.,1974.

Hurst, JD, and Stullenbarger, B. Implication of a self-care approach in a pediatric interdisciplinary phenylketonuria (PKU) clinic. Journal of Pediatric Nursing, 1:159–163, 1986.

Igoe, JB. Project health PACT in action. American Journal of Nursing, 80:2016–2021, 1980.

Jordon, D, and Kelfer, LS. Adolescent potential for participation in health care. Issues in Comprehensive Pediatric Nursing, 6:147–156, 1983.

Joseph, LS. Self-care and the nursing process. Nursing Clinics of North America, 15:131–143, 1980.

Kandzari, JH, and Howard, JR. The well family: A developmental approach to assessment. Boston: Little, Brown and Co., Inc., 1981.

Kaufman, DH. An interview guide for helping children

make health-care decisions. Pediatric Nursing, 11:365–367, 1985.

Kearney, BY, and Fleischer, BJ. Development of an instrument to measure exercise of self-care agency. Research in Nursing and Health, 2:25–34, 1979.

Kim, MJ, McFarland, GK, and McLane, AM (Eds.). Classification of nursing diagnoses: Proceedings of the Fifth National Conference. St Louis: CV Mosby Co., 1984.

Kohnke, MF. The nurse as advocate. American Journal of Nursing, 80:2038–2040, 1980.

Koster, MK. Anticipatory guidance. In Steele, S (Ed.), Child health and the family. New York: Masson Publishing, 1981, pp. 45–57.

Koster, MK. Self-care: Health behavior for the school-age child. Topics in Clinical Nursing, 5:29–40, 1983.

Kubly, LS, and McClellan, MS. Effects of self-care instruction on asthmatic children. Issues in Comprehensive Pediatric Nursing, 7:121–130, 1984.

Lasky, PA, Gulbrandsen, M, and Scoblic, M. Health education translated into health behavior. Issues in Comprehensive Pediatric Nursing, 5:167–175, 1981.

Levin, LS. Patient education and self-care: How do they differ? Nursing Outlook, 26:170–175, 1978.

Lewis, CE, Lewis, MA, Lorimer, A, and Palmer, BB. Child-initiated care: The use of school nursing services by children in an adult-free system. Pediatrics, 69:499–507, 1977.

Lewis, MA. Child initiated care. American Journal of Nursing, 74:652–655, 1974.

Loman, D, and Galgani, C. Monitoring diabetic children's blood-glucose levels at home. MCN: American Journal of Maternal Child Nursing, 9:192–196, 1984.

McCorkle, R. Nurses as advocates for self-care. Cancer Nursing, 6:17, 1983.

Michael, MM, and Sewall, KS. Use of the adolescent peer group to increase the self-care agency of adolescent alcohol abusers. Nursing Clinics of North America, 15:157–176, 1980.

Norris, CM. Self-care. American Journal of Nursing, 79:486–489, 1979.

Oland, L. The need for territoriality. In Yura, H, and Walsh, MB (Eds.), Human needs and the nursing process. New York: Appleton-Century-Crofts, 1978, pp. 97–140.

Orem, DE. The self-care deficit theory of nursing: A general theory. In Clements, IW, and Robert, FB (Eds.), Family health: A theoretical approach to nursing care. New York: John Wiley & Sons, Inc., 1983, pp. 205–217.

Orem, DE. Nursing: Concepts of practice (3rd ed.). New York: McGraw-Hill, Inc., 1985.

Ozias, JM. Self-care: Partnership for problem solving. Journal of School Health, 52:621–622, 1982.

Ozias, JM, and Peterson, FL. Facilitating a self-care practicum experience in consumer health education. Journal of School Health, 54:392–393, 1984.

Parcel, GS. Skills approach to health education: A framework for integrating cognitive and affective learning. Journal of School Health, 46:403–406, 1976.

Parcel, GS, and Meyer, MP. Development of an instrument to measure children's health locus of control. Health Education Monographs, 6:149–159, 1978.

Parcel, GS, Nader, PR, and Roger, PH. Health locus of control and health values: Implications for school health education. Health Values: Achieving High Level Wellness, 4:32–37, 1980a.

Parcel, GS, Nader, PR, and Tiernan, K. A health education program for children with asthma. Journal of Developmental and Behavioral Psychology, 1:128–132, 1980b.

Pierce, PM, and Giovinco, G. REACH: Self-care for the chronically ill child. Pediatric Nursing, 9:37–39, 1983.

Pituch, M, and Bruggeman, J. Lungs unlimited: A self-care program for asthmatic children and their families. Children Today, 11:6–10, 1982.

Polit, DF, and Hungler, BP. Nursing research: Principles and methods. Philadelphia: JB Lippincott Co., 1983.

Porter, D, and Shamian, J. Self-care in theory and practice. Canadian Nurse, 79:21–23, 1983.

Pridham, KF. Instruction of a school-age child with chronic illness for increased responsibility in self-care, using diabetes mellitus as an example. International Journal of Nursing Studies, 8:237–246, 1971.

Rawnsley, MM. The concept of privacy. Advances in Nursing Science, 2:25–31, 1980.

Saucier, CP. Self-concept and self-care management in school-age children with diabetes. Pediatric Nursing, 10:135–138, 1984.

Stephenson, C. Visits by elementary school children to the school nurse. Journal of School Health, 53:594–599, 1983.

Steiger, NJ, and Lipson, JG. Self-care nursing: Theory and practice. Bowie, Md.: Brady Company, 1985.

Stullenbarger, B. A Q-analysis of the self-care abilities of young, school-aged children (abstr). Unpublished doctoral dissertation, University of Alabama, Birmingham, Ala., 1984.

Szasz, TS, and Hollander, MH. The basic models of the doctor-patient relationship. Archives of Internal Medicine, 97:585–592, 1956.

Tetrick, AP. Ambulatory care of the hemophiliac. Journal of the Association for the Care of Children in Hospitals, 7:19–27, 1978.

Trandel-Korenchuk, DM. Patient participation in decision making. Nurse Practitioner, 8:46–52, 1982.

Walker, LO, and Avant, KC. Strategies for theory construction in nursing. Norwalk, Conn.: Appleton-Century-Crofts, 1983.

Walton, J. Orem's self-care deficit theory of nursing. Focus on Critical Care, 12:54–58, 1985.

Williamson, JA. Mutual interaction: A model of nursing practice. Nursing Outlook, 29:104–107, 1981.

CHAPTER 16

HOME CARE

ELIZABETH L. DOWD, M.A., R.N., C.P.N.P., and
LINDA D. VLASTUIN, M.S., R.N.

Three month old Jonathan was born at 29 weeks gestation and quickly developed respiratory distress syndrome. He was ventilated for two weeks and then gradually weaned to 1/4 liter of 100% oxygen per minute. Jonathan has remained on an apnea monitor because of his history of bradycardia and apnea. Because of his severe difficulty with oral feedings and the danger of aspiration with gastroesophageal reflux, a gastrostomy tube was placed when Jonathan was ten weeks old. He now weighs 2600 grams and appears stable. His parents, grandparents, and sitter have received instruction in assessing his cardiopulmonary status, use of the apnea monitor and oxygen equipment, technique of gastrostomy tube feedings, and appropriate interventions, such as cardiopulmonary resuscitation.

Just a few years ago, Jonathan might have remained hospitalized for several more weeks or even months. However, technological advances in recent years as well as increased emphasis on and acceptance of home care now make it possible for Jonathan to be cared for safely in his home. Client or parent education takes place at an accelerated pace or even on an outpatient basis. Thus, both new equipment and philosophical changes mean Jonathan is able to go home much sooner than he would have in the past.

In order to promote quality and consistency in home care programs, a group of four national organizations, the Assembly of Outpatient and Home Care Institutions of the American Hospital Association, the National Association of Home Health Agencies, the National Home Caring Council, and the Council of Home Health Agencies and Community Health Service of the National League for Nursing, has proposed the following definition of home care:

Home health service is that component of comprehensive health care whereby services are provided to individuals and families in their places of residence for the purposes of promoting, maintaining, or restoring health or minimizing the effects of illness and disability. Services appropriate to the needs of the individual patient and family are planned, coordinated, and made available by an agency or institution, organized for the delivery of health care through the use of employed staff, contractual arrangements, or a combination of administrative patterns. These services are provided under a plan of care which includes medical care, dental care, nursing, physical therapy, social work, nutrition, homemaker, home health aide, transportation, laboratory services, medical equipment, and supplies.

Stewart (1979, pp. 1–2)

This definition encompasses all levels of care encountered when considering home care: preventive, acute, chronic, and progressive. Preventive home care includes all health teaching aimed at avoiding episodes requiring acute care. Home care in acute illness involves those activities which assist a child and family to cope with an episode of illness from which the child will recover. Home care in chronic illness refers to nursing functions which are designed to help a child and family live with a condition which has the characteristics of permanence; residual disability; nonreversible pathological alteration; and the need for long-term supervision, rehabilitation, and care (Hymovich, 1981; Lawson, 1977; Rodgers, 1981). Home care in progressive illness assists children and families in dealing with a progressive illness that will culminate in death.

THEORETICAL FOUNDATION

The idea of home care is by no means a recent development in the health care field. Caring for ill people in their homes or assisting the family to do so dates back to the earliest times of recorded history. From the medicine man to the midwife, patients have received home care for their illnesses for thousands of years. Organized nursing services had their origin in the early 17th century when St. Vincent de Paul founded the Sisters and Ladies of Charity in France. This group visited the sick in their homes, saw that adequate food was provided, and arranged for a nurse if the patient was very ill

(Bullough and Bullough, 1969). In 19th century Great Britain, William Rathbone and Florence Nightingale collaborated to develop Visiting Nurse Services (Bullough and Bullough, 1969; Heinrich, 1983).

In the United States, home care was initially sponsored by religious and private groups. It eventually gained public support through Lillian Wald's establishment of settlement houses in New York City. Miss Wald, who emphasized the reduction of mortality rates, was the first to use the phrase public health nursing. As the health of mothers and children became an important concern, milk stations were established, and communicable diseases were attacked. Federal and state governments became involved in public health between 1930 and 1940, with home care becoming identified with government health departments (Bullough and Bullough, 1969; Heinrich, 1983).

Hospitals entered the home care field between 1940 and 1950, and the Medicare and Medicaid programs were enacted by Congress in 1965. These programs were designed to assist the elderly and the poor with medical care costs. However, home care received little attention or funding; it was considered nursing care at home (Hall, 1985). In 1966, Title XVIII of the Social Security Act created the Medicare Home Benefit Entitlement Program. Medicare-certified home health agencies could receive partial payment for skilled, intermittent care to homebound elderly patients if the care was considered medically necessary and was ordered by a physician. This program is still in effect but is restrictive in its funding. Most clients are over 65 years of age, and reimbursement is only allowed for a specified number of visits (Suther and Ricciardelli, 1985). Payment for long-term home services remains a serious concern, not only for the elderly but also for children.

Several trends have developed to increase the emphasis on home care for children, particularly those who have chronic health problems. Home care for persons with chronic illness is fast becoming an alternative to institutional care for infants, children, and teenagers as well as for adults, even in cases demanding the use of expensive, highly technological equipment. Advanced medical knowledge and technology have resulted in an increasing population of children with chronic health problems (Feetham, 1986). Parents and other child advocates are making the public aware of the effects of long-term hospitalization on the development of a child.

Payment for services plays an important role in the discharge of the child from the hospital in this era of cost containment, private insurance companies, and health maintenance organizations. Third party payers are realizing the value of home care in decreasing the overall cost of care for a particular episode of illness. As prospective payment for diagnostic-related groups (DRGs) and early discharge become the standards, the need for more and different home care services will continue to rise dramatically. The 1981 case of a 3½ year old, Katie Beckett, demonstrates how home care can drastically lower the cost of medical care. Katie had been hospitalized since the age of four months for the treatment of complications of viral encephalitis. When approval was granted for Medicare payment of her home care expenses, the monthly cost of her care dropped from $6000 to $1000 (Schrader, 1982). Other cases have shown equally dramatic savings (Cabin, 1985). Home care addresses the health needs of children and families in the home and in the community. Tinkham and Voorhies (1977) define community health nursing as "the field of nursing in which the family and the community are the patients. Although it is concerned with the total health-illness spectrum, its primary focus is on the prevention of disease, and the promotion and maintenance of the highest level of health and well-being" (p. 113). They state that "the community health nurse works collaboratively with families and groups in identifying their health problems and nursing needs, in determining the nursing care plan, in mobilizing appropriate community resources, and in evaluating the nursing services given" (Tinkham and Voorhies, 1977, p. 113). The community health nurse may provide the care directly or serve as coordinator for others who provide direct service. The American Nurses' Association's *Standards of Community Health Nursing Practice* (1973) also identifies the consumer as the client or patient. The consumer may be an individual, a group, or the community as a whole. The *Standards* states, "Health promotion, health maintenance, health education, coordination, and continuity of care are utilized in a holistic approach to the family, group, and community" (American Nurses' Association, 1973, p. 3).

Home care specifically deals with clients in their places of residence. Stewart (1979) cites health promotion and disease prevention, health restoration, and health maintenance as objectives of home health care. Home care services for children can range from lay visitor programs aimed at facilitating maternal-infant bonding to hospices organized to care for children with progressive illnesses. Mothers are assisted in treating childhood illnesses at home, infants at risk for sudden infant death are monitored, and children with chronic illnesses are supplied with nursing and physical therapy sessions (Stein, 1984).

The benefits, or value, of home health care to clients are numerous. The clients are afforded more privacy and can maintain control of their environment. Activities of daily living are pursued as the clients see fit, and clients may more easily refuse unwanted or inappropriate services. Emotional support may be more readily available. The coordination and multidisciplinary aspect of home health care helps assure that referrals among health team members will mobilize the services needed by the clients. Home health care can be highly personalized since only one client can be served at a time (Stewart, 1979).

The home environment is a good setting for teaching and learning to occur. Redman (1976) states that "the environment can be used to focus the patient's attention on what he is to learn" (p. 48). Since the client is likely to be more at ease in his home and because family members are present, learning about the client's condition may take place more readily. Further, reinforcement of procedures learned in other settings can be given (Stewart, 1979). The need for adaptations of procedures to a client's specific environment will be more apparent in the home. For example, assisting a child in a long-leg cast with use of the home's bathroom will initially require inspection of the facilities available.

Children in particular can benefit from home care because the emotional and separation problems seen during hospitalization can be partially avoided (Petrillo and Sanger, 1980). People with whom children are familiar can provide their care and are likely to be more readily available in the home.

The confidence of parents in their ability to care for the child is also enhanced by a familiar environment and by adaptations the parents make to suit procedures to their own homes. The self-care requisites discussed by Orem (1980) can more readily be fulfilled in the home. In addition, exposure to infection, which is a common problem with hospitalization, is reduced (Chinn, 1979; Stamm, 1981).

Benefits to the community are also realized when home health care is utilized. Use of more expensive sources of care, such as hospital emergency rooms, can be reduced. Length of hospitalization can be decreased, as can readmission rates and uses of other forms of institutional care (Chinn, 1979; Stewart, 1979).

Home care for children with progressive illness has become increasingly acceptable over the past 15 years, largely through the efforts of Ida Martinson (1976). Her studies have shown home care to be feasible and even desirable for many families with children dying of cancer (Martinson et al., 1986). Financial costs were reduced substantially when children dying of cancer were cared for at home (Lauer and Camitta, 1980; Moldow, 1982). In addition, parents' adaptation after the death of a child appeared to be more favorable with progressive care at home. The parents of 37 deceased pediatric oncology patients were interviewed following the deaths of their children. Those parents who cared for their child at home displayed more positive adjustment patterns as measured by their perception of the effect of the death of the child on their marriage, social orientation, religious beliefs, and views on the meaning of life and death. On a guilt-rating scale administered to the parents, those who provided home care indicated significant reductions in guilt feelings. These reductions were maintained at six and 12 months following the death of the child. The parents who did not provide home care reported increased guilt feelings during the final hospitalization of their child. These feelings were still unresolved at one year after the death of the child (Lauer et al., 1983).

Smith et al. (1983) also studied parents' adaptations to their child's cancer. When parents were asked directly about themselves in subjective interview questions, interdependence or self-concept concerns

were elicited. Responses to objective questions about the child or the effect of the diagnosis tended to fall into the areas of self-concept and physiological concerns. The results suggested that questions relating to the various categories of adaptation can be used to assist parents with the identification of their own adaptive strengths as well as those of the child.

In a study of how parents choose between hospital and home care in progressive illness, Edwardson (1983) found that the influence of the physician over care and treatment choices was the dominant influence in the choice of site for progressive care. However, parents reported they were also influenced by their own desires and beliefs about their ability to provide care. Moldow and Martinson (1980) described how a pilot program providing home care to children dying of cancer helped local health care institutions develop home care programs.

Home care for chronically ill children is also being researched. The Pediatric Ambulatory Care Treatment Study (PACTS) by Stein and Jessop (1983) evaluated a Pediatric Home Care (PHC) program provided by an interdisciplinary team to chronically ill children and their families. Analysis of interviews conducted at enrollment, after six months, and after one year indicated family satisfaction with the care, improved psychological adjustment of the child, and decreased psychiatric symptoms of the mother. Functional status of the home care children was equally well maintained when compared with hospitalized children. Those children in the home care program for the longest period appeared to show the greatest psychological benefit.

In a study of a hospital discharge protocol, Kruger and Rawlins (1984) gave parents verbal or written instructions covering physician's visit, diet, activity, medication regimen, and special instructions. In phone call interviews after four days, the responses of those parents receiving written instructions were significantly more accurate in the categories of physician's visit, diet, and special instructions. Accuracy of knowledge regarding activity also approached significance. In addition, the parents who received written instructions had significantly fewer problems with follow-through in the categories of visits to the physician and diet. The findings suggest that written as opposed to verbal instructions for home care can assist parents in the areas of accuracy of knowledge and follow-through (Kruger and Rawlins, 1984).

Ahmann's book dealing with high-risk infants covers such topics as discharge planning, the nursing process, health maintenance, and nutrition. Specific chapters address home care of infants requiring tube feeding, oxygen therapy, mechanical ventilation, tracheostomy care, and seizure precautions. Assessment guides, record forms, and nursing care plans are provided (Ahmann, 1986). Other current literature is also available to assist home care nurses with chronically ill children (Jackson, 1986; McCarthy, 1986; Norris-Berkemeyer and Hutchins, 1986; Wildblood and Strezo, 1987).

For a home care program to be successful, it must fulfill several criteria. Feetham (1986) and Stein (1984) both identify these ingredients as family willingness; individualized, flexible plans; emergency back-up systems; back-up or respite care alternatives; financial resources; continuing emotional and social support; and program evaluation. In addition, the program must meet community needs. Stein (1984) also states that families need to have alternatives such as long-term placement available to them in case home care does not appear to be appropriate.

Although home care can make an important difference for many families, it also has pitfalls. Stein (1984) identifies these as rigidity and bureaucracy. Examples of these pitfalls include rigid eligibility criteria, inflexible structures, and focusing only on costs and savings. Bock (1985) states that home health care programs require flexibility and "constant vigilance for the home environment is ever-changing and does not have the predictability of the institution" (p. 26). These pitfalls can be avoided partially through careful selection of clients for home care.

ASSESSMENT

Jonathan, the infant discussed previously, is medically ready for discharge from the hospital. However, his parents and significant others may require further instruction, reinforcement of hospital instruction, support and encouragement, or referral to other agencies for assistance with specific problems in order to make the home care of Jonathan safe and realistic. The need for these further services makes Jonathan and his family candidates for referral to a home nursing care agency.

Identification of the candidate for home care is essential. The process begins in daily or weekly multidisciplinary case conferences in which each hospitalized child is evaluated as a potential home care candidate. The American Academy of Pediatrics' task force on home care (1984) has outlined several factors that should be considered when selecting candidates for home care. These include patients factors, family factors, and community factors.

Patient Factors

Patient factors include potential benefits and risks of home care for the child and family. Stein (1984) discusses the level of care needed for a child in terms of the health condition of the child. Factors to be considered include the need for medical and nursing care, fixed deficits, age-inappropriate dependency in activities of daily living, disruption in normal family routine entailed in the prescription for care, and the psychological burden of the prognosis. It is also important to look at the skills, capacities, style, and needs of the child (Sargent, 1984). Although the effect of any chronic condition, such as cerebral palsy, on the normal growth and development of a child should be carefully assessed, it is also important to identify those characteristics of a child which are not affected by the condition. These individual, as well as family, strengths will be used by the nurse to help the child and family achieve independence.

Family Factors

Family factors are perhaps the most important considerations in the assessment of a child and family for home care. Family factors include the presence of involved family members and an appropriate home setting. Stein (1984) discusses the physical, emotional, and educational resources of the primary caretakers. Social supports and available assistance are also considered, as are other demands competing for the time and energy of the caretaker. Tinkham and Voorhies (1977) outline questions that can be used to gather data on family characteristics, socioeconomic and cultural factors, environmental factors, and health history.

The family assessment is extremely important in making the decision as to the appropriateness of home care. The initial interviews should offer the family the opportunity to identify and reflect upon their own goals so that they can make a decision about future care of the child in the context of the family. Other factors to be considered in family assessment include the current and past effects of the condition of the child on the family; the style of caring for the child, including distribution of roles and level of assistance routinely received from others; the quality of family cohesiveness; the attitudes of parents, siblings, and other family members toward the child; the presence of psychosocial stressors; the relationship of the family to extended family and other support systems; the ability of the family to identify and utilize community resources; and the financial status of the family (Feinberg, 1984). The communication and self-advocacy skills of the family should also be explored. Families that function poorly may need special consideration, and the nurse may need to serve as a liaison for these families in their contacts with resources. The following example illustrates this:

Matthew, a seven year old male, has been hospitalized for six weeks following an automobile accident in which he experienced multiple fractures of both arms and his right leg. Following surgery to pin the fractures in his leg, he developed osteomyelitis. Further surgery was necessary to treat the infection. Matthew's condition is now stable. He receives physical therapy twice a day, and a teacher visits three times a week. He is medically ready for discharge if adequate care can be provided at home.

Matthew's parents are divorced; the father has custody of Matthew and his nine year old sister. The father frequently works ten hours a day to make ends meet. The family lives 15 miles from Matthew's school. No relatives live nearby. The father's insurance policy will not pay for home care. After careful evaluation of these factors, the health care team determines that the family is not a good candidate for home care at this time. Discharge is postponed until the school system can arrange transportation for Matthew and his wheelchair to

school. Matthew's father will contact neighbors and friends or will advertise for a sitter before and after school to assist with the care of Matthew. When these and other options have been explored, the case will be re-evaluated for home care.

The family assessment process affords the staff the opportunity to learn about the style, culture, and expectations of the family. The knowledge and skill needed to care for a child and the ability of the family to deliver this care should be considered carefully. Stein (1984) identifies the role of home care as an equalizer in the relationship among the burden of the condition, the care of the child, and the resources available to the family. Deficits in any of the three areas must be corrected through education or professional assistance to produce a successful outcome.

Home care is not for everyone. Therefore, families should be given information regarding options for types of home care, such as group living, residential care, and respite care. The ultimate decisions about postdischarge placement will be made by the family. The home care nurse provides support to the family during the decision-making process and after the family has made its decision.

Community Factors

Community factors to consider in assessing the appropriateness of home care include medical, social, and educational resources. Availability of emergency services is particularly important to families, especially to those who are caring for ventilator-dependent children or infants with apnea. Home care options depend on the nature and extent of the health care system supports that exist in each community. These range from well-developed, well-organized, comprehensive tertiary care programs providing skilled nursing and therapy services to small county agencies which may have no health workers with specialized training (Stein, 1984). For example, a family with a six month old oxygen-dependent child living in a small rural community with no private transportation available may not be a good candidate for home care until the child can be weaned from oxygen.

Selecting families for home care can be a relatively simple matter when preventive care is the primary intervention needed. For example, many single adolescent parents will benefit from anticipatory guidance regarding basic well-child care, such as nutrition, normal growth and development, management of minor illnesses, and recommended scheduling of checkups and immunizations. The nursing diagnoses of *Knowledge deficit* and *Potential for alteration in parenting* are appropriate diagnoses because young single mothers often know little about child care and are at risk for child abuse or neglect (see Chapter 5).

Whether a family can manage treatment of an acute condition such as pneumonia or acute diarrhea at home depends on a more detailed assessment. The health care provider needs to answer several questions. Is the child ill enough to warrant hospitalization? Is the hydration level of the child adequate? Is the child experiencing respiratory distress? Can the child receive adequate nutrition orally? What is the knowledge level of the parents concerning signs of dehydration, assessment of body temperature, and signs of respiratory distress? Are the parents reliable to give needed medication? Are the parents comfortable with their ability to care for the child at home and to recognize warning signs? The answers to these and other similar questions will determine, in part, the appropriateness of home care in a particular situation. Nursing diagnoses appropriate in such cases might be *Potential fluid volume deficit, Ineffective breathing pattern, Impaired gas exchange,* and *Knowledge deficit.*

Any child with a chronic condition may potentially be cared for in the home. Chronic conditions range from diabetes, congenital heart disease, cystic fibrosis, and asthma to bronchopulmonary dysplasia with mechanical ventilation and cerebral palsy. Careful assessment of the child, the family, and community factors discussed above will help determine the appropriateness of home care for a particular situation. Appropriate nursing diagnoses might include *Potential for infection, Alteration in nutrition, Impaired skin integrity, Ineffective breathing pattern, Self-care deficit, Knowledge deficit, Potential alteration in parenting, Social isolation,* and *Ineffective family coping.* The nursing diagnoses involved will depend on the particular chronic condition of the child, the family, and the available resources.

Assessing families of children with progressive illness requires special care. Availability of adequate professional services, such as hospice care, as well as support from friends, family, and community may be especially critical to assist with care of the child and to provide respite for parents and other family members. The willingness and desire of the child and family for home care as well as confidence of the family in their ability to provide the care are primary considerations in determining the appropriateness of home care in progressive illness. As indicated by Edwardson (1983), these factors play an important role in the decision of parents to opt for home care.

Many nursing diagnoses are appropriate in home care of the progressively ill child. These may include *Potential for infection, Potential for physical injury, Fluid volume deficit, Alteration in nutrition, Impaired skin integrity, Decreased activity tolerance, Impaired mobility, Alteration in comfort related to pain, Fear, Anticipatory grieving, Potential alteration in parenting, Social isolation, Ineffective coping,* and *Spiritual distress.*

THE INTERVENTION

The goal of any home health care program for a child is to promote the health and well-being of the child and family in the home while minimizing the effects of any illness or health problem the child may experience. Ideally, the family becomes the primary caretaker, functioning independently within the community and utilizing available resources.

Linking Hospital and Home Care

The establishment of a successful home health care program begins with discharge planning. It involves a process of correctly evaluating the ability of a family to provide adequately for the child, while it also serves the needs of other family members. To achieve a successful discharge, the health team seeks to understand the family's circumstances, ability to manage stress, strengths and vulnerabilities, relevant history, resources, and support systems.

The discharge-planning process begins at

the time of hospital admission and may be the responsibility of the primary nurse caring for the child, a social worker, or a combination of health care providers (Rasmusen and Buckwalter, 1985). Other disciplines involved with nursing may include social work, medicine, physical therapy, occupational therapy, speech therapy, respiratory therapy, and nutrition services.

With home care assuming such a prominent position in the health care system, new concerns have arisen which influence the coordination of care. Communication is often the greatest potential obstacle which blocks the continued progress of clients. Kruse (1985) states communication barriers may be interpersonal, interdisciplinary, organizational, or societal. Each professional involved must be aware of those in other disciplines working with a particular client. Further, a clear knowledge of each plan of care is imperative to avoid duplication of services and perhaps even contradictory actions. Frequent, open communication and mutual respect among professionals are essential. Information transfer forms between professionals and agencies aid in presenting an accurate picture of the total care required by a client. Referral forms with multiple copies facilitate communication, and copies should remain in the client's chart to document referrals made. The agency receiving the referral keeps a copy and sends one back to the referral source with feedback on the progress of the client. Some hospitals and home care agencies jointly hire a person to fulfill these functions. This discharge planner fills out the appropriate forms, discusses home care with the client and family whenever possible, and obtains release-of-information signatures so the flow of information necessary for home care is enhanced. The discharge planner may be responsible for delivering referral information to the home care agency by hand, thus speeding up the process of communication. Return information to the referring agency can also be delivered by the discharge planner.

Communication and mutual goal seeking are facilitated by use of a discharge plan of care. This care plan includes input from all health team members, including home care staff. Family members are present at the discharge planning case conferences whenever possible. The child should also be included in the conference when appropriate.

For example, a ten year old child with diabetes would attend such a conference since he or she will be responsible for much of his or her own care under parental supervision. It is critical that family and health team perceptions of needs and anticipated problems are congruent. Interventions are then developed that maximize the ability of the family to meet the needs of the child (Sargent, 1984).

Realistic goals are set by the entire team, which includes the family. Individual family goals take priority whenever possible and should include health maintenance for the affected child as well as prevention of normal childhood illnesses, an area often overlooked when a major illness or handicapping condition is present. When the health of the child permits, some aspects of well-child care, such as an update of immunizations, can be handled during hospitalization. Referring the child to a primary care provider prior to discharge assists in the coordination of well-child care. At well-child visits, the primary care provider assists the family to understand information presented to them by specialists. By communicating closely with the parents and with the specialists, the primary care provider acts as a liaison for the child and family.

Designing a contract with the family may be useful when planning home care. Areas covered might include mutual goal setting and problem solving, scope of visits, tentative length of involvement with the family, role with the family, and the family's responsibilities. A written contract may be essential with multiproblem families. Discharge planning also includes educating the child and family to perform care and treatments for the child, providing necessary information to the family, and emotionally preparing the family for discharge. Educating parents to provide care encompasses many areas. It may, for example, involve developing new skills, such as problem solving and decision making, regarding the condition of the child.

Adjustment of hospital schedules to incorporate the lifestyle of the family will assist them in developing a plan of care for the child at home. A schedule for procedures, medications, feeding, sleeping, and bathing should be developed and integrated into the daily routine (Levine and Rice, 1984). In addition, encouraging parents to provide complete care for their child in the hospital assists parents in adjusting to the caretaking process while increasing their skill level in a secure environment where assistance is available. Praising the parents for their efforts increases their confidence and reassures them that they are capable of caring for the child at home.

Consistency in the information presented to parents from all health team members helps the parents understand the material presented and prevents confusion. Further, health teaching should incorporate the learning styles of individual family members. If verbal information is to be reinforced with written material, the reading level of the parents must be ascertained. For parents with low reading levels, drawings are helpful. Providing an opportunity for return demonstrations of learned skills is essential, particularly if the parents are insecure regarding their ability to perform the procedure. Information given in the hospital should be transferred to home care staff so reinforcement can continue at home. It is equally important that information provided to parents after discharge be consistent.

Emotional preparation of the family for discharge is essential, because parents often experience guilt, fear, and anger and need the opportunity to discuss these feelings. They may find it helpful to share concerns with other parents who have experienced similar situations (Levine and Rice, 1984). Support groups, such as Candlelighters, an organization for parents of children with progressive illness, can provide needed support to the parents. Iscoe and Bordelon (1985) discuss the implementation of a parents' support group, highlighting the strengths and concerns of the program (see Chapter 12).

Sophisticated, high-technology equipment is now being used in home care. Making arrangements for equipment, maintenance, and supplies is a critical part of the discharge planning process. Hartsell and Ward (1985) suggest that contacting vendors prior to discharge decreases the frustration and confusion parents may experience when working with various health care providers, equipment vendors, and insurance companies. It is essential that the vendor provide instructions regarding operation and trouble-shooting of the equipment prior to discharge.

A home visit by home care staff prior to discharge facilitates the transition from hospital to home. Evaluation of the home environment includes assessment of the layout and the arrangements of the house itself to determine its compatibility with the level of surveillance necessary to ensure the well-being of the child. Availability of a telephone and the capability of the home to accommodate specialized equipment are important considerations (Staggs, 1984). The assessment also includes checking for safety hazards specific to the care of the child, such as cigarette smoking or use of a wood-burning stove when the child will need oxygen. When extra equipment, such as a suction machine or a ventilator, is involved, adequate wiring to handle the increased energy load must be ensured. A safe water source is essential. If the home uses well water, it should be tested for nitrates, bacteria, parasites, and other impurities to protect the health of the child. A telephone directory of health care providers, including emergency telephone numbers, should be posted by the telephone for easy access. The list should include the emergency number of the equipment vendor for assistance with repairs as well as the names of people who can help with care of the child on a temporary basis.

Utilizing Family Resources

The outcome of a particular home care experience will depend to a large degree on the availability of a support system and on how well the support system copes with the situation. The support system of each child is different and must be assessed carefully when determining individual needs and considering how these needs can best be met. The support system of a child includes the immediate family and those who work together to meet the family responsibilities, described as "(1) procreation, (2) provision of safe environment, (3) promotion of growth and development potential, and (4) socialization of the young" (Sahin, 1986, p. 153). However, with the broad societal changes observed over the last 20 to 30 years, family may no longer mean only natural parents and siblings. It often includes a stepparent and stepsiblings, and in some cases it involves foster parents. In some families, members of the extended family, such as a grandparent or an aunt, function as part of the immediate family.

In a broader sense, any person involved with children is part of their support system. These people could include extended family, friends, neighbors, and persons from the family's church or other organizations. A person the family meets because of the condition of the child may become part of the support system, such as another child with the same condition, a parent of such a child, or a professional who becomes a close friend.

The support system of a child can also be involved directly in the care of the child. For example, a grandmother of a child with a tracheostomy may learn and perform tracheostomy care. The total care of the child may be provided for a period of time to allow the parents respite time. Family and friends can assist with the educational and diversional needs of the child. Helping a child in a body cast with homework or reading to a young child with muscular dystrophy can be a tremendous help to the parents. These helpers can also serve as listeners for the child with a chronic or progressive illness. The child may discuss his or her feelings more freely with a friend or family member than with a parent.

Use of the support system is an important intervention. The nurse should advise the family to explore this resource thoroughly and should assist them in determining who will be the most successful sources of support. The nurse should also help the family explore methods of explaining the situation to other family members. Assisting a family in this way may be one of the most important roles the nurse can play.

Dealing with Rapid Physiological Changes

Home care for children in the acute stages of an illness includes careful instruction of the primary caregiver regarding the plan of care. Topics covered may include diet, medication, level of activity allowed, and treatments specific to the disease involved. The nurse should assist the family with implementation of treatment and instruct the caregiver about which symptoms or circumstances warrant contacting a member of the health care team. Activities which promote recovery from acute illness also need to be discussed, including the importance of rest, minimizing stress, improving nutrition, and encouraging interactions between the child and his or her siblings and peer group.

Long-Term Problems

The family with a chronically ill child presents special challenges to the home care nurse. Although most of the functions discussed in connection with acute care are applicable to the care of the chronically ill child, one striking difference is present: There is no readily predictable end in sight. Further, remissions and exacerbations may occur unexpectedly. The nurse should help the child and family adjust to these characteristics of chronic illness.

Parents may need support and assistance as they grieve the loss of the "normal" child and accept their child as he or she is. Providing anticipatory guidance in matters of well-child care may be just as important to these parents as is help with the element of chronicity. Obtaining immunizations; providing a well-balanced diet; and coping with developmental issues such as toilet training, school entry, and adolescence are important tasks for all parents. Steele (1983) provides guidelines for families in these areas and discusses communication through play and how chronically ill children perceive their condition.

The child's condition and diagnosis determine the specific treatments necessary to meet the physical needs of the child. For example, children with diabetes require instruction regarding diet, insulin injections, and signs of hyperglycemia and hypoglycemia. The asthmatic child needs to know how to use inhalation treatments and how to recognize an impending asthma episode. Numerous organizations have developed materials to assist with the education and management of children with long-term illnesses. Detailed care plans are also available to assist parents in caring for children with complex care, such as ventilator-dependent infants. Ahmann (1986) has developed care plans and suggestions for home care of high-risk infants.

It may be necessary to develop economical adaptations of hospital equipment to continue some treatments in the home. Some expensive equipment which is disposable in the hospital can be sterilized or cleansed thoroughly and reused several times at home. Syringes and extension tubes used for gastrostomy tube feedings are examples of equipment which can be safely reused after proper cleaning. However, the advisability of reusing syringes for injections, such as for insulin for the diabetic, has been questioned (Poteet and Reinert, 1986). Normal saline solution for maintaining airway moisture in the child with a tracheostomy and acetic acid for irrigation of urinary catheters can be made inexpensively with recipes using ingredients found in the home. Care of the child at home provides the nurse with many opportunities for creative improvisation.

Care of the Dying Child

The responsibilities of the nurse in home care of the dying child are largely supportive and consist of promoting the interests of the child and the family. The parents have chosen to be the primary caregivers of their child for as long as possible. The major advantage of home care for dying children is that children will remain in familiar environments with the people most important to them as death approaches, instead of in a hospital filled with strangers, treatments, tests, and procedures which disturb sleep.

Since curative treatment has been discontinued, the aim of care is to keep the child comfortable. Although the nurse may be responsible for administering pain medication, it is also possible for the family to assume this function. Teaching parents other comfort measures, such as use of a water bed, massage, and helping the child to be close to family and other loved ones, is an important function for the nurse. Martinson (1983) stated that a child who has had a good night's sleep is better able to enjoy the daytime. This can be facilitated through the use of medications; a comfortable bed; and, for the child with respiratory distress, suctioning and upright positioning. Nutrition and fluid intake are important to counteract the effects of medication and immobility; however, because appetites are often not good, Martinson urges giving children whatever they request to eat. Graner (1976) states that many parents are fearful of giving their children too much pain medication, not understanding the action and importance of such medication to the rest and comfort of their child. Medication, coupled with other techniques such as relaxation, distraction, and imagery, is helpful to many children and families in coping with pain.

Frequent communication with the physician is necessary as the status of the child deteriorates; the role of the nurse may become a liaison between the family and health team. Counseling the family and child in dealing with stress and in grieving both before and after the death of the child is also an important role of nursing. Martinson (1976) advocates support groups for parents of dying children as a source of information and comfort. Family therapy may be useful for families as they cope with the strain of caring for a dying child. She also believes that parents should receive honest information, because this is the basis for trust in the health care system and helps parents deal with fear and uncertainty realistically. Supporting parents in the decision-making process, based on realistic data and consideration of the alternatives, gives parents the confidence they need to continue caring for or adjusting to the death of their child (Martinson, 1976).

Some families may opt for home care and then realize this decision is not appropriate for them. Others may find after a period of time providing home health care that they no longer have the energy to cope physically or emotionally with the needs of the dying child. The nurse should assist the family during this decision-making period by providing information about alternative forms of care and should support the family once their decision has been made. The nurse should help the family continue the support of their child, whether in an institution or at home. Reassuring the family they have not failed their child is an important nursing function when the family decides to rehospitalize the child.

Because caring for children with progressive illness is stressful for nurses as well as for families, nurses also need a support system to discuss their feelings of anger, frustration, and grief. The nurse who is able to maintain a healthy perspective of the situation is better able to provide needed support to families during their home care experiences.

Resources in Home Care

It is essential for the home care nurse to be aware of resources available in the community and make appropriate referrals. Compiling a list of services which deal directly with children and their families is beneficial. Such a list needs to be updated periodically by contacting the services directly. Ahmann (1986) discusses community resources for the family of the high-risk infant. Included are financial resources such as insurance, Medicaid, and Social Security; therapeutic resources such as infant stimulation and physical therapy; family support resources such as back-up caregivers and parent groups; and informational resources such as newsletters and pamphlets. Addresses should be given of helpful organizations and publications. Many support groups and organizations have developed and will provide educational materials and lists of resources available to families and will personally assist families in accessing these resources (Shannon, 1985).

When a new situation arises and the nurse is not aware of specific resources for the problem, other agencies can be contacted for ideas. Solutions to the problem should then be shared with other nurses and agencies. Communication and a spirit of cooperation will help produce a successful outcome for the family.

Planning Termination

Dependence on home care staff is a problem which can negatively influence the outcome of home care. The nurse can help prevent dependence by early preparation of the family for total care. Continual feedback to the family and positive reinforcement guide the family in the provision of care and give them confidence in their ability to provide the needed care and to manage future problems. The nurse can also assist parents in resolving psychosocial problems which may interfere as the family strives to achieve independence.

Stewart (1979) states that, ideally, clients decide when home care services will be discontinued. When clients have been involved from the beginning in planning their care, they can determine jointly with staff members when their goals have been met and home care services are no longer needed. However, the realities of present funding often force reduction or termination of services sooner than clients and staff would prefer. When this point is reached, clients are often referred to other community agencies that may help continue to meet client needs. The nurse should help families understand and accept the necessity of these changes. Feetham (1986) states that while the principle of termination is emphasized in public health nursing, the home care nurse will need assistance and supervision in carrying out this process.

Rehospitalization

It is important that parents be reminded that progress is not always straightforward. Temporary setbacks or unanticipated problems may be expected, depending upon the disease or condition of the child. The nurse should encourage parents not to feel guilty or feel that they have failed when setbacks occur. Since the parents of a child with a long-term problem may view hospitalization as a welcome break, the nurse can help the family identify and address these feelings. During periods of rehospitalization, the home care staff communicates closely with the hospital staff and the family, thus ensuring continuity of care in the transition from home to hospital and back to the home.

Communication

Continuity of care is maintained by reviewing and updating the plan of care frequently. Frequent case conferences that include the physician, parents, child, and home care staff allow problems to be resolved and maintain the ongoing planning process. Whenever possible, case conferences should be held in the home of the child to assist parents in feeling that they retain control of the situation. The nurse should help the family in deciding when a conference would be appropriate to clarify misunderstandings or to update the care plan. Whenever possible, members of all disciplines involved with the child are present at such a conference to ensure continued clear communication. Each team member then gives a progress report and discusses problems identified.

At the beginning of each case conference, one team member is identified to function as secretary for the meeting. This member records all suggestions and decisions made during the meeting. At the end of the session, the secretary summarizes the discussion and reviews actions to be taken by various team members prior to the next meeting of the team. This information is then recorded and sent to each team member to facilitate communication and follow-through.

EVALUATION

Nursing care provided to a child and family in the home must be evaluated in terms of changes seen in clients as in any nursing care setting. Concurrent or retrospective reviews may be used. Concurrent review is concerned with identifying nursing care priorities and providing optimal service while a client is receiving service from an agency. Client charts are reviewed by an audit team according to standard criteria previously identified by the team. In this manner, outstanding care can be recognized and deficiencies in care can be identified and corrected. Retrospective chart review is performed in the same manner but occurs following discharge of a client from agency services. Either method can help an agency improve the care given to a client and family as well as improve the documentation of that care. Davidson (1980) discusses methods of evaluating care and provides examples of evaluation formats for specific conditions.

Evaluation of nursing care will only benefit the clients and staff members of an agency if the results of the evaluation are communicated to the staff. A review of the types of deficiencies identified is shared with all nursing staff members with the goal of improving care and documentation. Quality of nursing care can also be assessed by surveying former clients about their satisfaction with the care provided and by obtaining their suggestions on ways to improve care. An objective questionnaire can be developed to serve this purpose. This form of evaluation is best used following discharge so the family will not feel that their responses could affect the quality of care provided.

Evaluating the effect of home care involves continual assessment and reassessment of the child and family, their progress, and their adherence to the plan of care as determined mutually by the family and the health care team. If successful, the goal of the highest level of independence possible for the child and family will be attained.

The progress of the condition of a child can be strongly influenced by whether the family follows the plan of care determined by the health care team, which includes the family. The nurse should monitor the effectiveness of prescribed medication, treatments, and nursing interventions. This monitoring, of necessity, includes observing the degree of compliance of the family. In nursing, compliance, "a disposition to yield to others" (Webster, 1987), indicates a position of submission on the part of the patient and places the nurse or other health professional in authority. Literature dealing with compliance qualifies this definition to reflect a prescribed regimen of some sort, such as "the positive behaviors that patients exhibit when moving toward mutually defined therapeutic goals" (Rutkowski, 1982b, p. 461). Placing the emphasis on patient behaviors facilitates evaluation of the effectiveness of the nurse-patient relationship. Because of the coercive implications of the term compliance and its definitions, many writers prefer the terms adherence or alliance. These terms "more nearly describe the ideal process" (Rutkowski, 1982a, p. 449).

To promote adherence to therapeutic regimens, Sallis (1985) suggests that behavioral goals of treatment should be determined and the regimen made as simple as possible. The problem and treatment recommendations should be explained clearly to the parents and child. The care provider should explore for questions and problems that may arise during treatment. The schedule for treatment should be negotiated with the parents and child with the use of cues, reminders, and rewards being considered. Roles of the parents, the child, and other family members in treatment and in keeping records should be determined. New skills needed must be identified. Plans for follow-up should be specified. The care provider should ask the family for a restatement of the instructions and provide them with the directions in written form.

What, then, can health care providers do to produce the greatest degree of adherence possible? Rapoff (1982) states that although research has not shown education to be the most important element in ensuring patient adherence, it is still highly desirable and is most effective when it is brief and to the point. The most essential elements should be given first and repeated several times, if possible. A concise written handout is also helpful.

Follow-up by telephone or by actual home visits can be very helpful in promoting adherence. The patient's knowledge can be assessed, and misunderstandings can be clarified. Actual adherence to the regimen can be monitored, and positive reinforcement given for adherence. All staff members should be informed of the relationship between the health care experience and patient adherence. Every effort should be made to make the experience pleasant and to assist the patient and family in any way possible.

Case Study

Three month old Jonathan, introduced at the beginning of this chapter, was born at 29 weeks gestation. Following delivery, Jonathan quickly developed respiratory distress, was ventilated for two weeks, and was weaned to 1/4 liter of 100% oxygen per minute. Jonathan's respiratory status then stabilized, but he still required oxygen at all times and remained on an apnea monitor. Because of the difficulty Jonathan had with feedings, a gastrostomy tube was placed, and all feedings were given through the tube.

Early in Jonathan's stay, his primary nurse, who was responsible for planning his care and for his discharge, interviewed Jonathan's parents to determine resources and to assess readiness for discharge. A case conference was called with representatives present from all disciplines involved—nursing, medicine, respiratory therapy, social services, and others as appropriate. The conference was scheduled at a time the parents could attend. Areas of concern for discharge were addressed, alternatives were explored, and decisions were made with the parents' full involvement.

The nurse helped the parents plan the physical setup needed at home to safely care for Jonathan. A referral for a home visit was made to the home care agency to assess the home environment as well as to determine if any physical modifications would be necessary for Jonathan's care. Back-up and respite care were discussed. The parents were advised to contact the power and telephone companies to minimize problems caused by power outages. Emergency numbers were provided. In-struction was given regarding use of the apnea monitor and oxygen equipment, the technique of gastrostomy tube feedings, and administration of cardiopulmonary resuscitation. Precautions to be taken when using oxygen were stressed. Individual concerns expressed by the parents were addressed as they arose.

The home care nurse visited Jonathan's home prior to discharge. This nurse had attended the care conference and discharge conference. Another home visit was made to the home within one to two days after discharge. Nursing diagnoses identified as appropriate included *Potential impairment of gas exchanges, Potential for altered nutritional status, Altered developmental pattern,* and *Potential for alterations in parenting.* Care plans were designed to address the problems identified in the nursing diagnoses with outcomes to be measured in terms of oxygen saturation levels, weight gain, and assessment of development and parental ability to manage home care.

Regular visits to Jonathan's home began the day following hospital discharge. At the first visit, contacts made by the family with the power and telephone companies and the equipment vendor were reviewed to ensure safe care in the event of an emergency or an equipment failure. Parental follow-through with instructions relating to gastrostomy feeding, oxygen, care of equipment, and modifications in the physical environment were continually evaluated. In addition, weight gain and oxygen saturation levels measured by an ear oximeter were obtained twice weekly to evaluate Jonathan's physical status.

When it was demonstrated that oxygen levels remained stable and weight showed slow but continuous gains, home visits were reduced to one a week. The home care nurse continued to provide positive reinforcement and support to Jonathan's parents as well as the opportunity to express fears and concerns. Reports were made to Jonathan's physician, and referral was made for developmental follow-up and well-child care.

The home care nurse functioned as a liaison between Jonathan's family and the various agencies involved. One month following hospital discharge, a case conference organized by the home care nurse was held to evaluate Jonathan's progress and home care management. The conference was held in the home and was attended by the hospital discharge planner, home care nurse, equipment vendor, high-risk infant follow-up team member, physician, and grandparents. Because weight gains and oxygen saturation levels were satisfactory, plans were made to decrease oxygen levels and to introduce oral feedings under the supervision of the nurse during the next two weeks. Parental management of care and equipment were evaluated. The grandparents were providing regular care for Jonathan to give the parents an opportunity to care for other responsibilities and to have an occasional evening out. A schedule for developmental assessment was outlined by the high-risk infant follow-up team, including sessions for the parents to discuss and promote development. Another case conference was planned for two months later, at which time physical and developmental progress would be evaluated. In the interim, the home care nurse would manage the case and make visits as appropriate as oral feedings began and oxygen was decreased. The nurse also continued as a liaison between the team members, communicating progress and concerns about Jonathan and preparing the family for discharge from the home care program.

RESEARCH IMPLICATIONS

Home care for children with health problems is a growing trend in this decade, and indications are that it will continue to gain in popularity. Bock (1985) points out that prevalence and epidemiology statistics will be important in determining the need for in-home services and ensuring precise allocation of these services. She advocates a standardized data base to facilitate longitudinal prospective studies of children receiving home care. Needs assessment studies should be conducted to identify how many children are still routinely kept in the hospital unnecessarily. The problems or disabilities these children face will need to be determined as well as the primary diagnosis and prognosis of each child. These figures will be helpful in planning for future services. Research should also attempt to identify which children are not well suited for home care and in which cases further damage might actually be caused by home placement (Bock, 1985). The impact of home care on the family should also be studied in terms of physical drain, emotional stress, and financial difficulty. Feetham (1986) states there may often be discrepancies between the family's perception of the care needs of the child and that of the health care professional. Larger and more varied samples are needed to define objective criteria for home care and to develop a timely process which will ensure readiness of a child and family for home care or for an alternate form of care.

The true cost-effectiveness of home health care must be evaluated more closely. Most studies examine hospital costs compared with home care costs. Although hospital costs include such things as food, laundry, housekeeping services, electrical power, and administrative costs, these items are often not included in the determination of home care costs. As a result, preliminary cost studies may not accurately reflect true cost comparisons. Studies also need to be conducted to facilitate policy formulation on financial responsibility for home care; should the federal government, private insurance, or the family be responsible? When money is involved, home care becomes a difficult issue. Yet, if comparisons of true costs continue to show a significant savings when the child is cared for at home, funding must be found to support families in their efforts.

Current research has evaluated parent and patient satisfaction immediately after discharge. However, few studies have investigated satisfaction with home care and quality of life on a long-term basis. The actual interventions and care plans used to assist children and their families should be evaluated for their effectiveness as measured by client outcome in order to ensure appropriateness and quality of care. Those interventions which seem most useful should be evaluated in research studies and then shared with other professionals. This type of research is especially applicable to children facing lifelong dependency on respirators and other life support systems. Further, this research could also address ethical decisions in sustaining life as well as the effect of stress on the family unit.

Part of the process of ensuring high-quality home care involves the professional providing the care. Research is needed to determine what educational preparation and work experience best prepare a nurse to provide quality home care services. The home care nurse must be knowledgeable about providing care to patients who have complex health problems and depend on technologically advanced equipment to maintain life. At the same time, the home care nurse must be able to work with the family unit in their environment, assist the family in providing case management services, and be a referral source for community resources. The home care nurse must have the skills of a community health nurse as well as those of an intensive care nurse. Perhaps a multisetting work background would prove beneficial.

Thus, research to ensure high quality in home care must be conducted in several areas. The consumers themselves should be investigated to assess prevalence and epidemiological statistics and to assess satisfaction with care. The home care process needs to be studied to determine what works best in preparation of families for home care and in the actual provision of care. Finally, the qualifications of professional providers of home care should be scrutinized and standards developed for the educational preparation of these professionals. Since home care appears to be here to stay, it deserves the same rigorous study that is applied to other fields of nursing in order to ensure the highest quality of care possible for children and their families in the home.

References

Ahmann, E. Home care for the high risk infant. Rockville, Md.: Aspen Publishers, Inc., 1986.

American Academy of Pediatrics. Ad hoc task force on home care of chronically ill infants and children. Pediatrics, 74:434–436, 1984.

American Nurses' Association. Standards of community health nursing practice. Kansas City, Mo.: American Nurses' Association, 1973.

Bock, RH. State of the art: Pediatric home care in 1985. Caring, 4:26–28, 1985.

Bullough, VL, and Bullough, B. The emergence of modern nursing. Toronto: Macmillan Publishing Co., 1969.

Burr, BH, Guyer, B, Todres, ID, Abrahams, B, and Chiodo, T. Home care for children on respirators. New England Journal of Medicine, 309:1319–1323, 1983.

Cabin, B. Cost effectiveness of pediatric home care. Caring 4:48–51, 1985.

Chinn, PL. Child health maintenance. St. Louis: CV Mosby Co., 1979.

Davidson, SV. Evaluating home health care. In Reinhardt, AM, and Quinn, MD (Eds.), Family-centered community nursing. St. Louis: CV Mosby Co., 1980, pp. 221–240.

Edwardson, S. The choice between hospital and home care for terminally ill children. Nursing Research, 32:29–34, 1983.

Feetham, SL. Hospitals and home care: Inseparable in the '80s. Pediatric Nursing, 12:383–386, 1986.

Feinberg, EK. Criteria for admission to programs, for funding, and for discharge home. In Home care for children with serious handicapping conditions. Houston: Proceedings of the Home Care Conference of the Association for the Care of Children's Health, 1984, pp. 35–39.

Graner, A. The effects of pain on child, parent, and health professional. In Martinson, IM (Ed.), Home care for the dying child. New York: Appleton-Century-Crofts, 1976, pp. 61–69.

Hall, HD. Historical perspective: Legislative and regulatory aspects of discharge planning. In McClelland, E, Kelly, K, and Buckwalter, KC (Eds.), Continuity of care: Advancing the concept of discharge planning. Orlando, Fla.: Grune & Stratton, Inc., 1985, pp. 11–19.

Hartsell, MB, and Ward, JH. Selecting equipment vendors for children on home care. MCN: American Journal of Maternal Child Nursing, 10:26–28, 1985.

Heinrich, J. Historical perspective on public health nursing. Nursing Outlook, 31:317–320, 1983.

Hymovich, DP. Assessing the impact of chronic illness on the family and parent coping. Image, 13:71–74, 1981.

Iscoe, LK, and Bordelon, KW. Pilot parents: Peer support for parents of handicapped children. Children's Health Care, 14:103–109, 1985.

Jackson, DF. Nursing care plan: Home management of children with BPD. Pediatric Nursing, 12:342–348, 1986.

Kruger, S, and Rawlins, P. Pediatric dismissal protocol to aid the transition from hospital care to home care. Image, 16:120–125, 1984.

Kruse, KA. Analysis of roles in discharge planning. In McClelland, E, Kelly, K, and Buckwalter, KC (Eds.), Continuity of care: Advancing the concept of discharge planning. Orlando, Fla.: Grune & Stratton, Inc., 1985, pp. 67–78.

Lauer, ME, and Camitta, BM. Home care for dying children: A nursing model. Journal of Pediatrics, 97:1032–1035, 1980.

Lauer, ME, Mulhern, RK, Wallskog, JM, and Camitta, BM. A comparison study of parental adaptation following a child's death at home or in the hospital. Pediatrics, 71:107–112, 1983.

Lawson, BA. Chronic illness in the school-aged child: Effects on the total family. MCN: American Journal of Maternal Child Nursing, 2:49–56, 1977.

Levine, S, and Rice, N. Facilitating transition from hospital to home. In Home care for children with serious handicapping conditions. Houston: Proceedings of the Home Care Conference of the Association for the Care of Children's Health, 1984, pp. 54–60.

Martinson, IM (Ed.). Home care for the dying child. New York: Appleton-Century-Crofts, 1976.

Martinson, IM. Care of the dying child. Nursing Times, 80:56–57, 1983.

Martinson, IM, Moldow, DG, and Armstrong, GD. Home care for children dying of cancer. Research in Nursing and Health, 9:11–16, 1986.

McCarthy, MF. A home discharge program for ventilator-assisted children. Pediatric Nursing, 12:331–335, 1986.

Moldow, DG. The cost of home care for dying children. Medical Care, 20:1154–1160, 1982.

Moldow, DG, and Martinson, IM. From research to reality: Home care for the dying child. MCN: American Journal of Maternal Child Nursing, 5:159–160, 1980.

Norris-Berkemeyer, S, and Hutchins, KH. Home apnea monitoring. Pediatric Nursing, 12: 259–262, 1986.

Orem, DE. Nursing: Concepts of practice. New York: McGraw-Hill, Inc., 1980.

Petrillo, M, and Sanger, L. Emotional care of hospitalized children (2nd ed.). Philadelphia: JB Lippincott Co., 1980.

Poteet, GW, and Reinert, BR. Letter to the editor: Controversy over reuse of disposable syringes. Pediatric Nursing, 12:466, 1986.

Rapoff, MA, and Christophersen, ER. Improving compliance in pediatric practice. Pediatric Clinics of North America, 29:339–357, 1982.

Rasmusen, L, and Buckwalter, KC. Discharge planning in acute care settings: An administrative perspective. In McClelland, E, Kelly, K, and Buckwalter, KC (Eds.), Continuity of care: Advancing the concept of discharge planning. Orlando, Fla.: Grune & Stratton, Inc., 1985, pp. 57–66.

Redman, BK. The process of patient teaching in nursing. St. Louis: CV Mosby Co., 1976.

Rodgers, BM, Hillemeier, MM, O'Neill, E, and Slonim, MB. Depression in the chronically ill or handicapped school-aged child. MCN: American Journal of Maternal Child Nursing, 6:266–273, 1981.

Rutkowski, B. Foreword to symposium on patient compliance. Nursing Clinics of North America, 17:449–450, 1982a.

Rutkowski, B. The nurse: Also an educator, patient advocate, and counselor. Nursing Clinics of North America, 17:455–466, 1982b.

Sahin, ST. The physically disabled child. In Johnson, SL (Ed.), High-risk parenting. Philadelphia: JB Lippincott Co., 1986, pp. 152–171.

Sallis, JF. Improving adherence to pediatric therapeutic regimens. Pediatric Nursing, 11:118–148, 1985.

Sargent, J. Assessing and building family coping skills and confidence. In Home care for children with serious handicapping conditions. Houston: Proceedings of the Home Care Conference of the Association for the Care of Children's Health, 1984, pp. 44–49.

Schrader, E. Home care keeps children out of the hospital. AORN, 35:684–706, 1982.

Shannon, K. Sick kids need involved people. Caring, 4:64–65, 1985.

Smith, CE, Garvis, MS, and Martinson, IM. Content analysis of interviews using a nursing model: A look at parents adapting to the impact of childhood cancer. Cancer Nursing, 6:269–275, 1983.

Staggs, K. Pediatric discharge and home care planning. The Coordinator, 3:20–23, 1984.

Stamm, WE. Nosocomial infections: Etiologic changes, therapeutic challenges. Hospital Practice, 16:75–88, 1981.

Steele, S. Health promotion of the child with long-term illness. Norwalk, Conn.: Appleton-Century-Crofts, 1983.

Stein, R. Home care: A challenging opportunity. In Home care for children with serious handicapping conditions. Houston: Proceedings of the Home Care Conference of the Association for the Care of Children's Health, 1984, pp. 2–8.

Stein, R, and Jessop, D. Does pediatric home care make a difference for children with chronic illness? Findings from the pediatric ambulatory care treatment study. Pediatrics, 783:845–853, 1983.

Stewart, IE. Home health care. St. Louis: CV Mosby Co., 1979.

Suther, MCS, and Ricciardelli, TP. Impact of discharge planning and home care on health care delivery in the United States. In McClelland, E, Kelly K, and Buckwalter, KC (Eds.), Continuity of care: Advancing the concept of discharge planning. Orlando, Fla.: Grune & Stratton, Inc., 1985, pp. 121–133.

Tinkham, CW, and Voorhies, EF. Community health nursing. New York: Appleton-Century-Crofts, 1977.

Webster's Ninth New Collegiate Dictionary. Springfield, Mass.: Merriam-Webster, Inc., Publishers, 1987.

Wildblood, RA, and Strezo, PL. The how-to's of home IV therapy. Pediatric Nursing, 13:42–68, 1987.

PART 2

Biophysiological Interventions for Enhancing Homeostatic Mechanisms

Overview

MARTHA J. CRAFT, Ph.D., R.N.

The last section of this book includes interventions that place infants and children in the best condition for nature to act. The first five interventions in this part of Section II affect systemic homeostatic mechanisms, and the last two interventions have a specific action. They represent interventions that are crucial to survival, recovery, and maximal functional status for which nurses are responsible. The number of interventions in this last category will continue to grow and be tested into the next century.

The first intervention provides an environment which promotes healing and growth. Karen Thomas is a scholar from the University of Washington who writes that the responses of children and families to actual or potential health problems are determined by the nature of the environment as well as individual characteristics. Thus, environmental manipulation can be used as an intervention to alter responses.

The next intervention acts upon the interaction of infants with their environment. The author, Debra Leners, began her interest in vestibular stimulation during her master's program at The University of Iowa, and she is now finishing doctoral study in Colorado. She writes that the vestibular mode of stimulation will accommodate sensoridynamic needs and discusses strategies to use it.

These interventions are followed by an intervention that is essential to survival, recovery, and health maintenance, presented by Kathy Schibler, a nurse educator, and Susan Fay, a nurse clinician. They present the biophysical characteristics of sleep and discuss measures to promote sleep in children.

The chapter on pain management is written by three authors who are internationally known for their work: Marilyn Savedra, Joann Eland, and Mary Tesler. These authors have long-standing programs of research relating to pain. They present a model of what should and will be done in the future. That is, nurse scientists should and will focus on a particular intervention to test and refine throughout a career of scientific inquiry.

In contrast, the intervention of nutritional support is understudied, and the author presents a beginning of what needs to become a program of research for many nurse scientists who wish to develop and test strategies to support nutrition as an intervention for infants and children. An example of one such strategy is that of non-nutritive sucking, developed by Meier, Anderson, and Gill at the University of Florida.

The last two chapters include interventions that modify a specific type of biophysical problem. The first intervention is intended to reduce cerebral cellular damage. The second intervention is intended to promote normal elimination and to increase functional status for children with disabilities. Both interventions represent the best in nursing practice and science because they deal with interventions nurses use to make a difference directly in the course of pathology in the case of cerebral edema, and in the course of functional status in the case of bowel and bladder maintenance.

In their discussion of cerebral edema management, Rojann Alpers and Vicki Hertig incorporate the work of Nancy Woods, a nurse scientist who pioneered the development and testing of strategies to manage cerebral edema. These strategies are used by scholarly practitioners and continue to be studied for their effectiveness in infants and children.

The management of cerebral edema is just one of the thousands of biophysical nursing interventions used commonly in every type of care setting to control pathology and promote recovery. It is time for nursing to recognize, test, and publicize the use of these interventions to facilitate public awareness of the role nurses play in human survival and quality of life.

The intervention of bowel and bladder maintenance is another used commonly by nurses to improve functional status. Patricia Smigielski and Janet Maple are two very experienced and knowledgeable practitioners who describe an intervention to increase functional status and self-esteem for children with disabilities. This intervention belongs in the highest tradition of nursing interventions used to increase functional status and quality of life, and it is one for which nurses are assuming greater autonomy. For example, at a recent National Nursing Research Symposium, Diane Newman, from the University of Pennsylvania, described private practice opportunities for nurses who are experts in this intervention.

It is an honor to introduce the work of this elite group of scholars, scientists, clinicians, and educators. They are showing the way for nursing to refocus upon, respect, and reward the crucial part nurses play in biophysical assessment, diagnosis, and intervention.

CHAPTER 17

ENVIRONMENTAL MANIPULATION

KAREN A. THOMAS, Ph.D., R.N.

The environment encompasses social and psychological aspects and stimuli which are associated with the physical environment. Nursing science centers on the study of the human-environment interaction (Roy and Roberts, 1981), with health status resulting as a product of that interaction (Dubos, 1965), and is experienced by the senses through the processes of reception and perception of environmental stimuli. The impact of environmental stimuli is measured in terms of responses, and responses are the phenomena used for assessing the impact of the environment on human functioning. Nursing, defined as the diagnosis and treatment of human responses to health problems (American Nurses' Association, 1980), entails consideration of responses in relation to context.

The interventions discussed in this book deal with the responses of children and their families to actual or potential health problems. These responses are determined by the nature of the environment as well as individual characteristics. Nursing interventions are designed to alter responses through manipulation of the environment in addition to interventions which focus on other aspects of health care. In this chapter, the manipulation of environmental stimuli as a nursing intervention is presented.

THEORETICAL FOUNDATION

Contact with the health care system involves contact with physical environments which are unfamiliar and stress-provoking for infants and children as well as for adults. The health care system, whether experienced as a well-child clinic or an in-hospital acute care unit, presents an environment which is different from a child's usual surroundings. For children who have had limited experience with a variety of environments and who are developing sophistication in interacting with the environment, the physical surroundings of an acute care setting are challenging. Research in the field of environmental psychology indicates the effects of the physical environment on human functioning include both behavioral or physiological responses. The stimuli provided by the physical qualities of the health care environment are pervasive, involving every aspect of health care. The environment provides the stage on which all nursing interventions are performed. The therapeutic process must include assessment of both individual and environmental characteristics and incorporate recognition of the unique effects produced by this interaction.

Manipulation of environmental stimuli is an indirect intervention which does not require actual contact between the client and caregiver. For the purposes of this discussion, manipulation of environmental stimuli will be limited to the physical environment of the acute care setting and will center on those forms of physical stimuli which do not come into direct contact with the client or the client's physical sensory environment. Manipulation of environmental stimuli is defined as planned modification of the environment to alter the physical stimuli presented and produce changes in responses. This form of intervention has been a prominent component of nursing care. Nightingale (1969) has eloquently depicted the influence of the physical environment on recuperative processes and highlighted nursing's role as an environmental control agent. In the 20th century, however, the role of the environment in caregiving has received less attention because of the increased emphasis on technological aspects of care (Kornfeld, 1977). Rising acuity levels coupled with innovations in medical treatment result in care units which often depersonalize clients. Environmentally based interventions include disease-specific interventions, such as darkened rooms for clients with cerebral aneurysm and isolation for clients with impaired immune response or infection, as well as more general actions, such as adjusting room lighting to facilitate sleep. As the technology of health care becomes more complex, nurses must be increasingly sensitive to the context in which nursing care is performed. Manipulation of the physical environment entails interventions based on rationales supported by research findings.

Sensory Stimulation: A Basic Need

Adequate sensory stimulation is a necessity for all individuals. Reception and perception are the neural processes through which contact with the environment is maintained (Shelby, 1978). Neurological function underpins all considerations of the sensory needs of infants and children (see Chapter 18). Neurological alterations influence the reception of stimuli, the central processing of sensory information, and the ability to respond to stimuli. These alterations may be long-term or situational. Impairment of a particular modality, such as vision, restricts sensory input. Blindness alters sensory reception as does eye patching; however, the implications for these restrictions vary as do the individual adjustments. Increased intracranial pressure affects central processing of sensory information as does barbiturate sedation; again, the implications and consequences vary. The immobility imposed by degenerative muscle disease reduces the ability to respond, as does the use of restraints. Thus, in diverse ways, many factors are related to sensory needs.

Most of the research dealing with sensory needs has focused largely on quantitative differences in sensory input—too much or too little stimulation. Additionally, much of the experimental research in this area has been limited to adults. The empirical evidence supporting adequate sensory input as a basic need has been derived from laboratory settings in which adults, primarily college-aged, volunteer research subjects, have been placed in restricted sensory environments (Schultz, 1965). The experiments have included restrictions such as immobilization, use of diffuse lighting, sound reduction, lack of human contact, water submersion, and serving of bland food. Such conditions of sensory deprivation have been criticized for their contrived nature; however, similarities between research findings and the experiences reported by individuals in "natural" conditions of sensory restriction, such as those of Arctic explorers or individuals who were adrift in lifeboats, suggest that the experimental research described above has tapped the severe forms of sensory restriction.

Research has documented the following responses to limited sensory input: (1) alteration of affective state producing conditions such as depression or anxiety; (2) reception-perception changes such as heightened responsiveness, altered sensations, and hallucinations; and (3) physiological changes, including electroencephalogram and endocrine alterations. Research on overstimulation has utilized experimental laboratory settings as well as naturally occurring environments and has similarly documented affective, receptive-perceptual, and physiological responses to excess sensory input. Responses to such conditions include anxiety, frustration, fatigue, withdrawal, elevated blood pressure, and tachycardia (Kellerman et al., 1979; Mitchell, 1981; Schultz, 1965; Shelby, 1978).

The research on sensory deprivation and overload suggests a stimulation continuum in which a midrange of appropriate stimulation is bounded by excess and inadequate stimulation (Fig. 17–1A). Human responses to stimulation are depicted by a U-shaped curve. Sensoristasis is a term used by Schultz (1965) to indicate the degree of cortical arousal preferred by an individual; above or below this level of stimulation, behavior is initiated to either increase or decrease sensory input. An adequate level of stimulation is therefore a product of the interaction between the individual and the environment. Behavioral cues are one indication of an inappropriate environment. The width of the central area of the stimulation curve, indicating the range of appropriate stimulation, varies with factors pertinent to the individual and the context. Thus, a healthy, vigorous child may tolerate a wider range of stimulation than a child who is ill, anxious, and exposed to the sensory environment of the acute care setting. As discussed in a later section, a child's development and the illness experience itself modify this range.

Thus far, sensory stimulation has been discussed quantitatively with a focus on how much. It is interesting to note that the U-shaped curve depicting human responses to stimulation which is suggested by research findings (Schultz, 1965) is not consistent with practice. Nursing interventions which simply add or subtract sensory stimuli fail to distinguish the appropriate range of stimulation, given the characteristics of the infant or child; the responses of the infant or child are not used as a guide for such interventions. Although considering the appropriate range of stimulation for an infant or child is of importance in modifying the physical environment, there are two additional aspects of the environment which are significant, yet are often ignored—pattern and contingency.

Stimuli can be conceived of as relaying information about the environment. The amount or intensity of stimulation may not be as influential as the pattern variability of the stimulus (Mitchell, 1981). Pattern describes the intensity (how much), frequency (how often), and period length (how long) of sensory input. The pattern of sensory input provides information about the environment. Novelty is associated with variation in amount, timing, and duration of stimuli whereas redundancy is associated with lack of change (Ilardo, 1973). The newness of information is related to predictability. Figure 17–1B depicts the dual nature of information provided by pattern variation. Here novelty, or unfamiliar input, creates uncertainty, whereas redundancy produces predictability (Ilardo, 1973). The amount of stimulation may not be as influential as the pattern variability of the stimulus. Pattern incorporates intensity, frequency, and the period length of sensory input (Mitchell, 1981). Variation in amount, timing, and duration of stimuli produce novelty, whereas lack of change leads to redundancy (Ilardo, 1973). Novelty entails uncertainty, whereas redundancy creates predictability. As with amount of stimulation, predictability and uncertainty form a continuum. Predictability facilitates synchrony or togetherness in the interaction between the individual and the environment. When patterns of stimuli may be anticipated with accuracy, cognitive control may be exercised; however, at the extreme, redundant information is monotonous. Novelty is essential for enriching and expanding an individual's information about the environment and inducing new and more sophisticated behavioral responses;

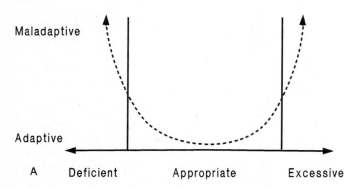

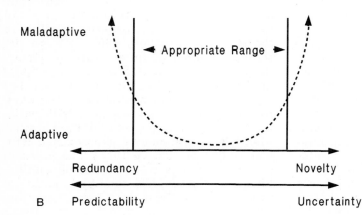

Figure 17–1. Sensory stimulation continuum. *A*, Range from deficient to excessive. *B*, Ranges from redundancy to novelty and predictability to uncertainty.

however, excessive novelty is associated with a high degree of uncertainty, which impairs the ability of the individual to competently interact with the environment. Appropriate patterns of stimuli variation therefore include a blend of novelty and redundancy. As with the amount of stimulation, the need for pattern variation is determined by both individual and environmental factors and is modified by developmental status and the illness experience.

In addition to pattern, contingency is a factor pertinent to the sensory environment. Contingency means that changes in the sensory environment are responsive to or conditional on actions taken by the individual to initiate, terminate, or in some way modify stimuli. In other words, the individual is capable of exerting control over particular forms of sensory input. Listening to the radio is an example. The radio may be turned on or off, the volume may be adjusted, or the station selected. Similarly, an infant or child uses behavioral cues to elicit sensory input. The ability to control the sensory environment improves responses to aversive stimuli; one research project found that individuals who were allowed to control noise intensity exhibited decreased evidence of distress (Lundberg and Frankennauser, 1978). The concept of sensoristasis (Schultz, 1965) presented earlier describes the sensory environment appropriate for the individual. In the contingent environment, the individual self-regulates sensory input, and behavioral cues indicate the attempt to control the amount and pattern of stimulation. Research by Thoman (1987) indicates that preterm infants who elicited contingent breathing motions from a mechanized stuffed bear experienced more quiet sleep and more regular respiration than infants who did not receive this type of stimulation.

In summary, sensory input is a basic life

requirement. The physical environment is a source of stimulation and may be described in terms of amount, pattern, and contingency of stimuli. Although these three areas provide a framework for discussing the sensory environment, in reality, amount, pattern, and contingency of stimuli are not separate entities, because the sensory environment is experienced as a whole. In the following sections, the rationale supporting manipulation of the physical environment focuses on the association between sensory experiences and development as well as the impact of illness on sensory needs.

Development Related to the Sensory Environment

Sensory stimulation is a basic need; however, the need is not static throughout the life span. Research substantiates the need for sensory stimulation during early development. Studies in which infant animals were raised in deprived environments have demonstrated neurological impairments as well as behavioral abnormalities. Specific deprivations, such as inhibiting or altering visual input through a darkened environment or use of blinders that produce selective reduction of vision, have been found to block normal maturation in corresponding areas of the visual cortex (Monshon and Van Sheyters, 1981). Conversely, animals raised in enriched environments have displayed evidence of improved neurological functioning, including intellectual abilities (Ferchmin et al., 1975; Ferchmin and Eterovic, 1980; Goldman and Rakic, 1979; Rosenweig et al., 1972). Although these studies used animal models, which do not maturationally correspond with human infants, and examined extremes in terms of sensory environment alterations, research on augmenting the sensory environment of infants has produced comparable improvements in motor and intellectual development (Barnard, 1973; Chapman, 1978; Katz et al., 1980; Levine, 1973; Schaefer et al., 1980). Additionally, the sensory component of the infant's home environment has been related to cognitive development.

Development is an ongoing process of increasing integration and complexity. Development is dependent on the central nervous system. Maturation of the central nervous system includes changes in neural structure and function (Parmelee and Sigman, 1983). These neurophysiological changes are observable as increasing behavioral competence (Smart, 1980). Als and colleagues (1979) have postulated a hierarchical model of neurobehavioral development. In their formulation, development entails increasing neurobehavioral organization and results in an expanding capacity to respond in an organized fashion. The infant uses environmental stimulation to organize behavior (Als et al., 1979). The infant may "hook into" subtle environmental patterns; preterm infants have been found to breathe in synchrony with the cycling air temperatures produced by incubators (Thomas, 1986b). Further, the infant elicits sensory input from the environment and uses this input to organize behavior. A contingent environment is therefore paramount for the developing infant and child. Research with preterm infants has found that rocking and auditory stimulation contingent on activity by the infant effectively promoted sleep and rest patterns, growth, and developmental outcomes (Barnard, 1973).

Although sensory input is essential for development, the reception and perception and processing of and the response to stimulation in the immature organism is unlike that of the adult because of differences in central nervous system maturation. The central nervous system of the infant exhibits limited branching of axons and dendrites, limited interconnectedness between neurons, changing neurotransmitters, increasing differentiation of neurons, and increasing myelinization (Cowan, 1981; Yokoulev and Lecourst, 1967). As a result, neurological function in the infant is characterized by decreased spontaneous neural activity, slower conduction velocity and transmission time, decreased ability to sustain neuronal activity, and increased ability to achieve temporal and spatial summation to facilitate neuron firing. These limitations affect the ability to receive and respond to the sensory environment and, consequently, affect interaction with the environment. Responses, therefore, are a window allowing a view of ability to receive and process sensory information (Gorski et al., 1979). In the infant, responses are frequently physiological in nature and tend to be more global. Lack of neurological maturation impairs the infant's ability to sustain attention to sensory input and makes the infant prone to being overwhelmed by stimuli. These limitations are more prominent in the very young; the trajectory of neurological maturation indicates that interaction with the sensory environment is correspondent with development. Thus, development is a primary factor influencing sensory needs and, as described in the following section, illness also affects sensory needs.

The Relationship between the Illness Experience and the Sensory Environment

In considering the responses to the physical nature of the care environment, it must be noted that illness alters the individual-environment interaction. Illness produces changes in the infant or child as well as in the environment (Rose, 1975, 1984; Tesler and Savedra, 1981). Fever, fatigue, immobility, pain, hypoxemia, and alterations in consciousness are examples of illness-related factors which affect the way in which stimuli are received and perceived, the processing of information by the central nervous system, and response capacity. Treatment of health problems may involve alterations in the sensory environment (such as protective isolation), suppression of central nervous system activity (such as sedation), or inhibition of responses (such as restraints). When illness necessitates hospitalization, not only are the usual means of interacting with the environment modified but also the infant or child is placed in a strange environment.

The Physical Environment of the Acute Care Setting

The previous sections have considered the basic need for sensory stimulation, the role of sensory input in development, and the impact of illness on the individual's interaction with the sensory environment. With these perspectives in mind, the physical aspects of the care environment are reviewed. Oftentimes, the sensory environment presented by the acute care setting is inappropriate for the infant or child. The aberrant nature of the acute care environment is not appreciated by health care personnel, who have developed psychological defense mechanisms for dealing with the peculiarities of their work environment (Kornfeld, 1977). Because of these defense mechanisms, nurses and other health care personnel suppress their own reactions to the acute care environment and, consequently, may lack appreciation of how the environment affects clients and their families (Kornfeld, 1977). It is essential that nurses sensitively evaluate the context in which they practice. The acute care setting influences not only the client but also health care providers (Fagernaugn et al., 1980). Continual light, noise, and human traffic produce tension, anxiety, and fatigue. Job stress is related to the nature of the work environment, and nurses are not immune to the stress caused by the physical environment. It is encouraging, however, to realize that many of the negative aspects of this particular environment can be modified for the benefit of the infant or child—as well as for the nurse.

The infant or child, subjected to the sensory environment of the acute care setting, is engulfed by unfamiliar visual stimuli. Much of the visual input is related to technological equipment found in the care setting, such as monitors, infusion pumps, and suction canisters. The infant or child views the multitude of persons who are involved in health care delivery or supportive services. Institutional settings are often painted drab beige or gray and offer little color variation. A prominent form of visual input is the lighting found in the care unit. Lighting varies in type (fluorescent, incandescent, or natural light or sunlight). In one study, newborn nursery lighting varied from 15 to 2500 foot-candles per square foot, depending on the location of light fixtures and the presence of windows as well as outside weather conditions (MacLeod and Stern, 1972). Oftentimes lighting is not patterned. Although the natural pattern of light is diurnal, acute care settings notoriously fail to maintain this pattern. Lights are often left on continuously for nursing convenience. The design of many units does not include windows, which can provide not only a sense of diurnal variation but also a view outside the client's room.

The auditory stimuli associated with the acute care environment are equally unfamiliar, disruptive, and unpatterned. The persistent sounds of monitor alarms, call bells, and the intercom blend with human voices to produce a pervasive acute care unit problem—noise. Noise can be an antecedent to energy-consuming arousal responses and, at high decibel levels, a possible source of cochlear damage and hearing loss. Noise in the acute care setting is characterized by lack of pattern and lack of meaning to the patient (Gottfried, 1985). In the neonatal intensive care unit, the acoustic environment has been found to be composed of a large proportion of high-frequency sounds and a high level of background noise (Linn et al., 1985; Newman, 1981). Such sounds not only muffle the human voice but also produce withdrawal behavior as the infant attempts to "turn off" auditory input. In critically ill infants, the arousal produced by noise has precipitated hypoxemia (Long et al., 1980). Sounds in the acute care setting also do not often exhibit a daily pattern of variation. As with light, sound in the normal environment of the infant or child has a diurnal pattern.

Although vision and sound are the forms of stimulation most readily apparent in the physical environment, olfactory and thermal sensory input are also present. Olfaction is a phylogenetically old sensory function which is often ignored and seldom studied in relation to the care environment. Smells may include draining wounds, stool, urine, medications, cleaning solutions, as well as freshly perked coffee, fragrant bouquets, or perfume. Olfaction is a primary determinant of human behavior; consider the increase in salivation and gastric motility which occur when visiting the bakery or the revulsion experienced when finding spoiled food in the refrigerator. Temperature is another forgotten sensation. Thermoreception is not only a component of thermoregulation but is also a sensory experience (Hensel, 1982). Manipulations of environmental temperature, such as tent administration of heated, humidified oxygen, are frequently part of health care.

Although the acute care environment may sometimes affect the intensity of a particular sensory modality, the more common problems encountered entail pattern and contingency of sensory input. Sensory modalities are often separated in the acute care setting (Newman, 1981): Alarms can be heard but the monitor is unseen. Sensory input may be monotonous, such as the continuous beeping of a cardiac monitor or hum of the incubator motor. Television often becomes a substitute sensory input for the hospitalized child. A study of hospitalized children revealed that in an eight-hour day, these children watched television an average of 3.9 hours total, more than their nonhospitalized peers, and the majority of programs observed were adult oriented (Guttentag et al., 1981). The acute care environment is largely noncontingent. Hospitalized children and their families have little if any control over the environment. For example, the human traffic in and out of a child's room provides visual and auditory stimuli. In one study of a child hospitalized in a six-bed room, there were 300 entrances by 100 different people noted in a 12-hour day (Grant, 1983). Most visits were less than one minute in duration and the majority were by nurses.

Examining the limitations of the acute care setting's sensory environment in conjunction with the need for appropriate sensory input sets the stage for nursing action. Consideration of these aspects is an essential component in nursing care of infants and children.

ASSESSMENT

The data indicating the need for manipulation of environmental modification are derived from a number of physiological systems as well as psychosocial behaviors. The responses listed in Table 17–1 were derived from both the literature and clinical observations. Data support the following nursing diagnoses according to Gordon's (1982) schema: *Fear* (self-perception, self-conception pattern); *Sensory perceptual alterations* (cognitive-perceptual pattern); *Sleep pattern disturbance* (sleep-rest pattern); *Mobility impairment* (activity-exercise pattern); and *Coping, ineffective, individual* (coping-stress-tolerance pattern)

There is no clear and precise set of responses defining the need for manipulation of the physical environment. The general areas of response in Table 17–1 suggest, and rightly so, that the sensory environment affects many processes and functions. Responses are highly individual, depending on the infant or child and the particular envi-

Table 17–1. DATA SUPPORTING INTERVENTIONS THAT MODIFY THE PHYSICAL SENSORY ENVIRONMENT*

General Areas of Alteration
Mentation-impaired reasoning and concentration
Reception-perception processes
Sympathetic-parasympathetic nervous system
    activity
Motor activity
Affect
State organization, sleep-wake patterns
Eating patterns
Social interaction
Achievement or maintenance of developmental
    milestones

Responses Indicating Withdrawal
Passivity, decreased responsivity
Closed eyes, gaze aversion
Turning from source of stimulation
Protective positioning, posture
Depression, helplessness, apathy
Parasympathetic activity—stooling, decreased heart
    rate and respiratory rate
Decreased motor activity
Decreased social activity and communication
Dependency

Responses Indicating Arousal
Vigilance
Increased sensitivity to stimuli
Irritability, tension
Increased motor activity, muscle tension
Restlessness, insomnia
Heightened perceptions
Sympathetic activity—peripheral vasoconstriction,
    sweating, increased heart and respiratory rate and
    blood pressure, high-pitched voice, dry mouth
Aggression, anger, hostility, behavioral outbursts
Sedation requirement

Responses Indicating Sensory-Seeking Activity
Self-stimulation—head banging, rocking, sucking,
    masturbation
Activity eliciting sensory input from the
    environment
Hallucinations, illusions, delusions

*Based on data compiled from Kellerman, et al., 1979; Mitchell, 1981; Sallustra and Atwell, 1978; Schultz, 1965; and Shelby, 1978.

ronment. There is not a direct, one-to-one correspondence between specific aspects of the physical sensory environment and a particular response. General areas of altered responses which are related to the physical sensory environment are listed in Table 17–1. In reviewing these responses, three clusters emerge: (1) responses indicating withdrawal, (2) responses indicating arousal, and (3) responses indicating sensory-seeking activity. These clusters are presented only as a beginning schema for identifying patterns of response and are not distinct or mutually independent and exclusive. It is feasible that an infant or child may show portions of various patterns or may exhibit different patterns at different points in time. Some alterations may exist across several patterns, such as reduced appetite or increased food intake. The specific category is not as important as what the response cluster means.

THE INTERVENTION

Intervention strategies include planned manipulation of the environment and focus on the intensity, patterns, and contingency of the physical sensory environment provided in the acute care setting. Interventions modify the physical environment as a way of indirectly altering the responses of the infant or child. Given the multitude of individual and environmental factors which ultimately affect responses to the physical environment, there are no clear-cut prescriptions for individual infants or children. Rather, interventions are based on knowledge of sensory input as a basic human need, the role of sensory input in development, and the impact of illness on sensory experiences. The environmental modifications required by a toddler undergoing cardiac surgery differ from those required by an adolescent receiving chemotherapy for leukemia. In each situation, sensory stimulation is recognized as a basic requirement; however, developmental level and health status also determine the appropriateness of the environment.

Additionally, intervening variables which moderate the effects of the physical environment must be considered. These include duration of exposure to the acute care setting; previous experiences with the acute care setting; competence in controlling and eliciting sensory input; and sensory, neurological, or motor limitations.

A short period of hospitalization may preclude the establishment of adaptive responses which assist in the adjustment to the physical sensory environment whereas a longer hospitalization and greater experience with the hospital environment may be positive factors. The life history of the infant or child, including contingency in parent-child interactions, will affect competence and mastery exhibited in dealing with the physical environment. Any limitations involving processing of sensory information, including limited cognitive development, will influence the need for sensory stimulation and the resulting responses.

Interventions are guided by responses. Following implementation of interventions which manipulate the physical environment, the responses are the basis for monitoring the effectiveness of the intervention and modulating the intervention. Although specific interventions cannot be prescribed, suggestions for manipulating the physical environment are presented. These environmental changes are discussed as variations of modality intensity, pattern, and contingency. Intervention possibilities are a challenge to creativity in nursing.

Auditory Strategies

As ecologists, nurses must monitor sound levels within the care environment. The loudness or intensity of sound is easily measured using a sound-level meter. Although this instrument is not a standard piece of clinical equipment, sound-level meters can often be borrowed from an audiology clinic or environmental-safety department. Sound intensity is measured in decibels (dB). In measuring sound levels or reading research which reports sound levels in the care environment, it is important to recognize that decibels constitute a logarithmic scale: i.e., a 10-dB increase in sound intensity indicates a tenfold increase whereas a 20-dB increase indicates a 100-fold increase in sound level (Patton, 1976, p. 250). Therefore, even a small change in decibel level indicates a large change in sound intensity.

Measurements of sound intensity or loudness reflect the total auditory environment. Sometimes radios or televisions are played in acute care settings as a means of muffling the noise of equipment or talking. Although such sounds, particularly music, may provide a form of patterned stimuli, the sound of radio and television adds to the auditory environment, increasing the decibel level. Adding an additional source of sound can never decrease the existing decibels. For the infants or children who are alert and responding to the sensory environment, radio and television may be a welcome form of stimulation; however, if their ability to receive and respond to stimulation is im-

paired, the addition of noise must be carefully considered. Imagine being confined to a hospital bed and continually hearing a radio program broadcast in a foreign language. This example of meaningless auditory stimulation provides some appreciation for the situation of the compromised infant or child exposed to the continuous noise of radio or television.

Since noise is a major problem in the acute care environment, interventions should be aimed at its reduction. A prominent source of noise is talking—physicians on rounds, nurses conversing at the front desk, people talking "over" the infant or child while in the client's room, and chatter in the hallways. Conversation is a normal part of human function, and talking is often a stress-reducing technique for health care professionals. However, nurses must be cognizant of the effect of such noise on their clients and must monitor their own contribution to the sound environment. Health care personnel need to have locations in the unit, such as staff lounges or conferences rooms, where conversations may be carried on without disturbing clients. Unit designs which enclose the work station or front desk in glass help contain noise. Other design issues include the high resonance and reverberation of sounds when floors and walls are constructed of hard surfaces; carpeting and draperies help absorb sounds (Izumi, 1976). Many forms of noise are related to caregiving activities. A study of the intensity of sounds recorded inside an incubator located in a neonatal intensive care unit revealed that the loudest sounds experienced by the infant were related to caregiving events such as closing the incubator porthole, writing on top of the incubator, setting formula bottles on top of the incubator, and elevating the head of the bed (Thomas, 1986a). Many of the sounds on care units can be reduced easily. Switching to plastic wastebaskets is a means of reducing the noise created by metal wastebaskets. Placing a pad, such as a washcloth, over the top of a room door prevents noise made by the door closing.

Technology is another source of noise. Even though the beneficial nature of equipment often competes with the negative aspect of noise, nurses should not resign themselves to noise being a necessary evil. Monitor alarms should not be allowed to sound for long periods of time. Nurses must be involved in equipment purchases by institutions, and the sound of operation of the equipment should be a priority when deciding what to purchase. Monitor alarms do not need to be loud; rather, the alarm should provide health care personnel with a novel stimulus, drawing attention to the monitor.

The sound environment may be enriched in a variety of ways. Music played on a tape recorder, radio, or phonograph not only provides auditory stimulation but may also be used to produce a therapeutic atmosphere, depending on the type of music played. Music may be soothing and relaxing or upbeat and invigorating. For example, a preschooler confined to bed because of a fractured femur may benefit from rhythmical, active music. Tape recordings of books are commercially available. Recordings of books, favorite stories, or songs can be inexpensively made by parents. Many toddlers enjoy recordings of parents reciting nursery rhymes. Relaxation tapes, which include the sounds of waves breaking on the beach or gentle rainfall, are also available. These latter forms of stimulation are suited to older children and adolescents. Headphones allow the child to enjoy such recordings privately without disrupting roommates. Battery operated tape recorders and radios are desirable for safety purposes. Heartbeat recordings are commercially available and may be an appropriate intervention for neonates.

Visual Strategies

Variations of visual stimuli involve the use of color, form, texture, and lighting. Posters and fabric wall hangings add interest to the visual environment of the acute care setting. Some hospitals offer an art library that allows clients to select paintings for their rooms. Safe, nonbreakable mirrors are particularly suited to an infant's environment, as are mobiles suspended over the crib. Windows are a desired addition to the design of the care unit, providing variation in the visual environment. Infants and children hospitalized for prolonged periods of time should be given the highest priority when assigning rooms with windows. Reducing harsh lighting, including eliminating a variety of reflective surface textures, and reducing the gloss of polished floors and painted hallways and rooms increases the

personal feeling created by the care environment (Lacy, 1981). A lamp rather than harsh overhead lighting provides indirect light and a more soothing lighting environment. Lighting controlled by a rheostat allows the level of light to be easily adjusted. Printed linens add color to the client's room; allowing personal choice of such bed linens is also desirable. Cartoon characters, bold abstract designs, or petite prints are examples of colored bed linens which might be used with various age groups. In multiple-bed rooms, colors may be used to define personal space. Colors may also be used to produce a particular atmosphere, such as bright yellow for an invigorating atmosphere or subdued pastels for a restful environment. Outdoor areas provide a pleasant change in visual stimulation for the hospitalized child.

Although the aim of the suggestions just mentioned is to make the visual environment pleasant, nonthreatening, and appropriate for the infant or child, the importance of "visual noise" must also be noted. As discussed earlier, the visual environment of the acute care unit contains visual stimuli which are frightening or lack meaning to the infant or child, particularly the sight of equipment and people. Nurses must critically examine the visual environment available to the child. Unnecessary equipment should be removed. Equipment and materials used at intervals should be stored in closets or drawers to reduce visual noise. Infants and children should not be peripheral witnesses to procedures performed on other clients, such as their roommates.

An example of visual and auditory noise is the television turned on continuously. Although television is a source of entertainment for children, constant television viewing is monotonous. Additionally, not all television programming is suitable for children. Although television viewing is not controlled in many homes, health care facilities should demonstrate health-promoting behaviors, including the use of appropriate sensory stimulation. Of particular concern are televisions operating continuously as "stimulation." Appropriate stimulation is geared to the developmental level and is patterned or contingent on the child's responses. Continuous television viewing does not meet these requirements. Nurses should carefully observe responses to television. Are the infants and children in an alert state?

Are they making direct eye contact with the television? What are the attention spans of each child? Answers to these questions will assist in evaluating television as a source of stimulation for infants and children.

Olfactory Strategies

The olfactory environment is often ignored. Sources of unpleasant odors must be removed, such as used diapers or dressings left outside the infant's or child's room. Sachets can be used to add interesting or pleasant odors. They can be inexpensively made with fabric—a sewing project for volunteers, parents, or older children—or a tea ball can be used as a recyclable sachet holder. A bag filled with spices, orange or lemon peel, or dried flowers or a cotton ball soaked with cologne are a few ideas for homemade sachets.

Thermal Strategies

Environments that are too warm or too cool not only impose physiological demands on the infant or child but also are a form of sensory input. With time, however, thermoreceptors adapt to steady temperatures, decreasing sensory input to the central nervous system. For example, neonates who become drowsy while feeding are often unwrapped to awaken the infant and promote feeding; one result of this unwrapping is the arousal produced by the change in temperature. Interior temperatures often lack pattern and are generally monotonous; a change in thermal sensory input can be produced by an outdoor excursion or a warm bath.

Pattern Variation

Pattern encompasses variation in intensity (how much), frequency (how often), and phase (how long) of stimuli. Pattern variation reduces monotony in the environment (Lacy, 1981). One natural pattern is diurnal variation. Acute care settings must maintain daily light-dark cycles as well as activity patterns that follow the usual diurnal cycle. Interventions include turning off or dimming lights in conjunction with reducing sound levels during nighttime hours. Promoting a diurnal pattern of activity in the environment requires that nurses question unit procedures such as passing out ice water or restocking room supplies during the night shift. In the acute care setting, pattern is often imposed by caregiving events (Blackburn and Barnard, 1984), shift schedules, routines, meals, and physician rounds, which all contribute to the activity pattern in a care unit. Such patterns may be advantageous in that events are predictable; however, the pattern of sensory input often is not compatible with the needs or usual routines of infants or children. Some care units are experimenting with a daily afternoon quiet time in which lighting is dimmed, traffic reduced, and talking limited. Adherence to this time-out period is difficult. However, nurses report that not only patients but also parents and staff benefit from this arrangement. Interventions may be employed to specifically provide patterned stimuli more suitable to the client. Stimuli may be patterned by linking sensory input to caregiving activities (for suggestions, see Verzemnieks, 1984), such as operating a musical mobile while vital signs are measured. Pattern may also be used to moderate arousal. A decrease in pattern variation reduces arousal; continuous auditory stimulation produces soothing, whereas increased novelty and pattern variation result in arousal and increased attention (Brackbill, 1971). To illustrate, pattern variation can be used with an infant who is fed by lavage tube every three hours. To establish the feeding pattern, the infant is aroused prior to the feeding by softly calling the infant's name, increasing the lighting, or playing a music box. The infant is then fed while alert and awake, promoting interaction with the infant during the feeding event. Following completion of the feeding and related nursing care, the infant is soothed and calmed by using dimmed lights and a repetitive stimulus, such as a simulated heartbeat.

CONTINGENCY

The environment can promote contingency at a variety of levels. For older children, the focus of environmental manipulation may be the provision of sensory experiences the child can turn on and off. Examples include the use of videocassette recordings and audio cassettes. Hand-held controls allow the child to operate televisions or videocassette players independently. The control of lighting and window coverings and the operation of television in the hospital room can be delegated to the child. Children should be allowed and encouraged to arrange their physical environments. The case history that follows includes an illustration of using an infant's responses to guide sensory input. The subtle cues employed by younger children and infants to control sensory input require a sensitive observer to recognize and respond to such behavior. Toys designed for infants and toddlers frequently use the principle of contingency—the child's action produces action from the toy. Toys can be used to provide contingent sensory input and may be as simple as a string of bells sewn securely to a strip of fabric and hung from the crib rail; the infant rings the bells by shaking or kicking the strip.

EVALUATION

Responses indicating arousal are noted when stimuli increase in intensity or there is pattern variation or novelty. The arousal response shows that the infant or child is "turned on," with increased attention to the stimulus, and the child is prepared for action. Such turning on is advantageous in interacting with the environment; however, arousal is energy consuming because of increased metabolism and oxygen needs and can lead to depletion of physiological resources. Responses indicating withdrawal signify an inability to sustain interaction with the environment—the infant or child is overwhelmed. Such turning off is a protective mechanism whereby sensory input is reduced to a manageable level. This pattern of response may be seen following repeated or prolonged arousal associated with intense stimuli or excessive pattern variation. The message conveyed by such withdrawal responses is, "I can't deal with this." Conversely, withdrawal may also occur when the sensory environment lacks intensity, has little pattern variation (redundancy), or lacks contingency. In this type of situation, the message is, "I give up." The environment does not provide adequate sensory input and

is unresponsive to the infant or child's attempts to self-regulate sensory input.

The goal of modifying the physical environment is to provide a supportive environment in which sensory input is of an intensity, pattern, and level of contingency appropriate for the infant or child. The responses listed in the assessment section are not entirely specific to the effects of the physical environment. Because of this, outcome criteria are difficult to measure since responses may also be caused by interpersonal aspects of the environment or by pathophysiology related to illness. Therefore, specification of the above goal must include recognition of factors other than the physical environment contributing to the identified responses. It must also be noted that interventions which modify the physical environment are a component of a total plan of care. When the physical environment is supportive, the infant or child maintains appropriate eating, sleeping, and motor activity patterns. Affect and social interaction are consistent with usual levels, and the infant's or child's development is promoted. Withdrawal or arousal responses are reduced as are inappropriate sensory-seeking behaviors.

Case Study

Bobby was a term gestation neonate at four days postnatal age. His birth history included a difficult low forceps delivery to a woman who became febrile during labor. At the time of delivery, Bobby was noted to have meconium aspiration, and he rapidly developed moderate respiratory distress requiring oxygen therapy. Prophylactic antibiotic therapy was instituted. Because of a problem with temperature stability, Bobby remained in an incubator.

His incubator was located adjacent to the entrance to the acute care nursery; the unit desk, including paging system and telephone, were nearby, as were a scrub sink and a supply center. Bobby's extremities were mottled and his face presented a furrowed brow and worried expression. His nurse stated that he looked "wasted." When handled, Bobby experienced a decrease in heart rate and evidenced gaze aversion when held face-to-face. When alone, Bobby lay in a limp position, with his head turned toward the wall and eyes closed. Noises, such as closing of the incubator porthole, produced a startled reaction, including Moro's reflex. He was unable to sustain periods of quiet sleep. When Bobby's mother visited, she stated, "He doesn't seem to know I'm here."

Bobby's behaviors indicated a mismatch between his capacity to handle sensory input and the environment in which he had been placed. His age indicated a level of neurological maturation that limited his ability to tolerate intense or extremely novel sensory input and that produced responses which were global in nature. Bobby had little experience in interacting with the extrauterine environment, and his physiological status was compromised. Hypoxemia, acid-base imbalance, and possible sepsis affected his central nervous system function. Although many of Bobby's behaviors indicated withdrawal, he was also easily aroused, which increased his oxygen consumption and further complicated his respiratory status. Additionally, he was unable to participate in social interactions appropriate for his age, which interfered with the development of maternal-infant attachment. Appropriate nursing diagnoses included *Sensory-perceptual alteration* and *Sleep pattern disturbance.*

The approach required by these diagnoses included manipulation of the physical environment. Bobby's incubator was moved to a quiet corner in the unit, away from the traffic and noise. The lights in Bobby's cubicle were dimmed. Sources of noise were closely monitored. A *Quiet, please* sign was placed on Bobby's incubator as a reminder to staff. Incubator portholes were gently closed. The incubator temperature was maintained in the thermal neutral zone. In addition to reducing the intensity and novelty in the environment, sensory experiences were planned. When Bobby appeared aroused, particularly following caregiving activities, continuous auditory stimulation was provided by a simulated heartbeat; when arousal decreased, the heartbeat was discontinued. Once extraneous sources of stimulation were limited, it was noted that Bobby began to open his eyes spontaneously. When Bobby's eyes were open, the nurse gently called his name. Bobby turned to focus on the nurse's face. The nurse noted that although Bobby could maintain eye contact for short durations, the combination of eye-to-eye contact and speaking precipitated gaze aversion, a furrowed brow, and increased mottling. For this reason, only a single modality (eye-to-eye contact or voice) was presented. As Bobby improved, multiple modes of stimulation were tolerated. These brief episodes of planned stimulation were linked to the feeding schedule to establish pattern. Bobby's mother received teaching about his interactional abilities and learned to observe his cues and provide appropriate sensory input.

RESEARCH IMPLICATIONS

The body of knowledge supporting interventions which modify environmental stimuli requires expansion. Much of our present knowledge is based on animal studies or studies of adults under extreme conditions. Although animal research is an important contribution to basic science, the comparability between animal and human research models is limited (Dubowitz, 1980). Study should focus on the effect of the sensory environment during the rapid development of infancy and childhood. Although the focus of research has been on extreme sensory conditions, more investigation of subtle variations in pattern, contingency, and intensity are needed. There is particular need to examine the mutual effects of illness and development on sensory needs. Research will facilitate an understanding of sensory needs and how these needs are best met. As research assists in decoding infant's and children's behavioral cues, nursing interventions can use these cues as a guide in providing adequate physical environments.

Research examining environmental manipulation must be centered on the interaction between the infant or child and the environment. The relationship between individuals and their environment is extremely complex. Theory is currently being stretched beyond simple, linear models suggesting the need for an ecological approach to the acute care setting. Intense observational studies will facilitate recognition of responses and response patterns among infants and children. Behavioral cues are the only key to understanding the infant's or child's interactions with the environment. Too often data on such interactions are gathered from the interpretations of health professionals or childhood experts rather than from the purest source of information— the infant's or child's responses.

Research on interaction calls for varied approaches to methodology. Studying response patterns entails measurement over time, such as intensive, within subject design. Such designs produce time-dependent data and require suitable statistical approaches. Instrumentation to capture environmental events and the response of infants or children is essential. Use of videotapes, polygraphic records, and computer-recorded data are examples. However, use of such instrumentation requires safety considerations, and such instrumentation must not become an obtrusive component of the environment. Qualitative research is an additional means of studying the effects of the physical environment. The rich information derived from the phenomenological approach is an essential contribution to the present state of knowledge.

Experimental studies, based on sound theoretical and empirical work, are needed to test nursing interventions. Conducting such studies in the uncontrolled setting of the acute care unit is a methodological challenge. To be successful, clinical experimentation requires extensive support within the acute care setting, including nurses who have a vested interest in promoting nursing science through research. Intervention studies designed to test the effectiveness of environmental manipulation must be valued in the larger context of health care delivery to assure funding.

References

Als, H, Lester, BM, and Brazelton, TB. Dynamics of the behavioral organization of the premature infant: A theoretical perspective. In Field, TM (Ed.), Infants born at risk: Behavior and development. New York: SP Medical and Scientific Books, 1979, pp. 173–192.

American Nurses' Association. Nursing: A social policy statement. Kansas City, Mo.: 1980.

Barnard, K. The effect of stimulation on the sleep behavior of the preterm infant. Communicating Nursing Research, 6:12–33, 1973.

Blackburn, ST, and Barnard, KE. Analysis of caregiving events relating to preterm infants in the special care unit. In Gottfried, AW, and Gaiter, JL (Eds.), Infant stress under intensive care. Environmental neonatology. Baltimore: University Park Press, 1985, pp. 113–129.

Brackbill, Y. Cumulative effects of continuous stimulation on arousal level in infants. Child Development, 42:17–26, 1971.

Chapman, JS. The relationship between auditory stimulation and gross motor activity in short-gestational infants. Research in Nursing and Health, 1:29–36, 1978.

Cowan, WM. The development of the vertebrate central nervous system: An interview. In Garrod, DR, and Feldman, JO (Eds.), Development in the nervous system. London: Cambridge University Press, 1981, pp. 3–33.

Dubos, R. Man adapting. New Haven, Conn.: Yale University Press, 1965.

Dubowitz, V. Correlation between animal and human studies. Developments in Neuroscience, 9:505–517, 1980.

Fagernaugh S, Strauss, A, Suczek, B, and Wiener, C. The impact of technology on patients, providers, and care patterns. Nursing Outlook, 28:666–672, 1980.

Ferchmin, PA, Bennett, EL, and Rosenweig, MR. Direct contact with enriched environments is required to alter cerebral weights in rats. Journal of Comparative and Physiological Psychology, 88:360–367, 1975.

Ferchmin, PA, and Eterovic, VA. Genetic learning deficiency does not hinder environment-dependent brain growth. Physiology and Behavior, 24:45–50, 1980.

Goldman, PS, and Rakic, PT. Impact of the outside world upon the developing primate brain: Perspective from neurobiology. Bulletin of the Menninger Clinic, 43:20–28, 1979.

Gordon, M. Nursing diagnosis: Process and application. New York: McGraw-Hill, Inc., 1982.

Gorski, PA, Davison, MF, and Brazelton, TB. Stages of behavioral organization in the high-risk neonate. Theoretical and clinical considerations. Seminars in Perinatology, 3:61–72, 1979.

Gottfried, AW. Environment of newborn infants in special care units. In Gottfried, AW, and Gaiter, JL (Eds.), Infant stress under intensive care: Environmental neonatology. Baltimore: University Park Press, 1985, pp. 23–54.

Grant, VJ. Pedestrian traffic in a pediatric ward. New Zealand Medical Journal, 96:91–93, 1983.

Guttentag, DNW, Albritton, WL, and Kettner, RB. Daytime television viewing by hospitalized children. Pediatrics, 68:672–676, 1981.

Hensel, H. Thermal sensations and thermoreceptors in man. Springfield, Ill.: Charles C Thomas, 1982.

Ilardo, JA. Ambiguity tolerance and disordered communication: Therapeutic aspects. Journal of Communication, 23:371–391, 1973.

Izumi, K. Perceptual factors in the design of environments for the mentally ill. Hospital and Community Psychiatry, 27: 802–806, 1976.

Katz, ER, Kellerman, J, and Siegel, SE. Behavioral distress in children with cancer undergoing medical procedures: Developmental considerations. Journal of Consulting and Clinical Psychology, 48:356–365, 1980.

Kellerman, J, Rigler, D, and Siegel, SE. Psychological responses of children to isolation in a protected environment. Journal of Behavioral Medicine, 2:263–274, 1979.

Kornfeld, DS. The hospital environment: Its impact on the patient. In Moss, RH (Ed.), Coping with physical illness. New York: Plenum Medical Book Co., 1977, pp. 237–249.

Lacy, M. Creating a safe and supportive treatment environment. Hospital and Community Psychiatry, 32:44–47, 1981.

Levine, S. Stimulation in infancy. In Greenaugh, WT (Ed.), The nature and nurture of behavior. San Francisco: WH Freeman & Co., 1973.

Linn, PL, Horowitz, FD, Buddin, BJ, Leake, JC, and Fox, HA. An ecological description of a neonatal intensive care unit. In Gottfried, AW, and Gaiter, JL (Eds.), Infant stress under intensive care: Environmental neonatology. Baltimore: University Park Press, 1985, pp. 83–111.

Long, JG, Lucey, JF, and Philip, AGS. Noise and hypoxemia in the intensive care nursery. Pediatrics, 65:143–145, 1980.

Lundberg, U, and Frankennauser, M. Psychophysiological reactions to noise as modified by personal control over noise intensity. Biological Psychology, 6:51–59, 1978.

MacLeod, P, and Stern, L. Natural variations in environmental illumination in a newborn nursery. Pediatrics, 50:131–133, 1972.

Mitchell, PH. Sensory status. In Mitchell, PH, and Loustau, A (Eds.), Concepts basic to nursing (3rd ed.). New York: McGraw-Hill, Inc., 1981, pp. 309–341.

Monshon, JA, and Van Sheyters, RC. Visual neural development. Annual Review of Psychology, *32*:477–522, 1981.

Newman, LF. Social and sensory environment of low birth weight infants in a special care nursery: An anthropological investigation. Journal of Nervous and Mental Disease, *169*: 448–455, 1981.

Nightingale, F. Notes on nursing. New York: Dover Publications, 1969.

Parmelee, AH, and Sigman, MD. Perinatal brain development and behavior. In Mussen, PH (Ed.), Handbook of child psychology (Vol. 2). Infancy and developmental psychobiology. New York: John Wiley & Sons, Inc., 1983, pp. 95–156.

Patton, HD. Audition and disturbances. In Patton, HD, Sundsten, JW, Crill, WE, and Swanson, PD (Eds.), Introduction to basic neurology. Philadelphia: WB Saunders Co., 1976.

Porter, DR. Hospital architecture. Guidelines for design and renovation. Ann Arbor, Mich.: Health Administration Press, 1982.

Rose, MH. Coping behavior of physically handicapped children. Nursing Clinics of North America, *10*:329–339, 1975.

Rose, MH. The concepts of coping and vulnerability as applied to children with chronic conditions. Issues in Comprehensive Pediatric Nursing, *7*:177–186, 11984.

Rosenweig, MR, Bennett, EL, and Diamond, MC. Chemical and anatomical plasticity of the brain: Replication and extensions. In Gaito, J (Ed.), Macromolecules and behavior (2nd ed.). New York: Appleton-Century-Crofts, 1972, pp. 205–277.

Roy, SC, and Roberts, SL. Theory construction in nursing: An adaptation model. Englewood Cliffs, N.J.: Prentice-Hall, Inc., 1981.

Sallustra, F, and Atwell, CW. Bodyrocking, head banging, and head rolling in normal children. Journal of Pediatrics, *93*:704–708, 1978.

Schaefer, M, Hatcher, RP, and Barglow, PD. Prematurity and infant stimulation: A review of research. Child Psychiatry and Human Development, *10*:199–212, 1980.

Schultz, D. Sensory restriction: Effects on behavior. New York: Academic Press, 1965.

Shelby, JP. Sensory deprivation. Image, *10*:49–55, 1978.

Smart, JL. Behavioral correlates of brain development in the rat. Developments in Neuroscience, *9*:213–215, 1980.

Tesler, M, and Savedra, M. Coping with hospitalization: a study of school-aged children. Pediatric Nursing, *2*:35–38, 1981.

Thoman, EB. Self-regulation of stimulation by prematures with a breathing blue bear. In Gallagher, JJ, and Ramey, CT (Eds.), The malleability of children. Baltimore: Paul H. Brookes Publishing Co., 1987, pp. 71–84.

Thomas, KAJ. How the NICU environment sounds to a preterm infant. MCN: American Journal of Maternal Child Nursing (in press).

Thomas, KAJ. The influence of incubator air temperature on the respiratory responses of preterm infants. Unpublished doctoral dissertation, University of Washington, Seattle, 1986b.

Verzemnieks, IL. Developmental stimulation for infants and toddlers. American Journal of Nursing, 84:749–752, 1984.

Yakovlev, PI, and Lecours, A. The myelinogenetic cycles of regional maturation of the brain. In Minkowski, A, (Ed.), Regional development of the brain in early life. Oxford, England: Blackwell Scientific Publications, Inc., 1967, pp. 3–70.

CHAPTER 18

VESTIBULAR STIMULATION

DEBRA LENERS, M.A., R.N.

Whenever a researcher investigates the subject of sensory stimulation, two major concepts are involved—sensory deprivation and sensory overload. Sensory deprivation and sensory overload are concepts that have been established historically as environmental sources of stress and have been primarily studied as external physical stressors. Since the 1960's, there has been growing recognition that although stress is inevitable in human life, it is coping that makes the difference to ultimate outcomes. Because there are important individual differences in the response to stress, researchers began to examine the possible effects of mediation, individual variables that moderate, adjust for, or negotiate different responses to stress (Lazarus and Folkman, 1984). There is a wide range of individual responses to sensory deprivation and sensory overload, reflecting a mediation of stress that is influenced by cultural and personal differences (Goldberger, 1982).

The concepts of sensory deprivation and sensory overload were researched extensively in the early 20th century; however, the outcomes of this research rarely found application in nursing interventions (Leners, 1981). This chapter explores sensory stimulation as a nursing intervention, one that could potentially be a dynamic focus for care in neonatal and pediatric populations. The focus of this chapter is on the vestibular mode of stimulation.

THEORETICAL FOUNDATION

Vestibular sources of sensory stimulation are major contributors to cortical arousal because of the location of the vestibular tract. The eighth cranial nerve is the route for directing vestibular stimulation and channeling information to the medulla and pons. Vestibular stimuli are major contributors to neurological rhythms in the body, including heart rate, respiratory rate, and neuron synapse activity. Because the vestibular nerve root is the first to be myelinated, its maturity as a channel for sensory input is more effective than other types of stimulation (Larrouche, 1966). Vestibular will be defined as pertaining to the vestibulocochlear nerve, the eighth cranial nerve, which emerges from the brain between the pons and medulla oblongata.

Vestibular stimulation has been described developmentally as the most constant form of stimulation in intrauterine life, generated by the fetus's own movements as well as by maternal position changes (Korner et al., 1975). Hospitalized children, particularly premature infants, can be deprived of weeks, perhaps even months, of vestibular stimulation presumed to be conducive to growth and development (Rice, 1977; Kramer and Pierpont, 1976; Korner et al., 1982). In infants and children, growth and development may be positively influenced by nursing interventions designed to meet vestibular stimulation needs.

Vestibular stimulation is important to the maturation of neurological tissues. Vestibular nerve reflexes are sensitive indicators of central nervous system maturity and later development (Eviatar et al., 1974; Parmelee et al., 1972; Wright, 1971; Drillen, 1970; Parmelee and Schulte, 1970; Kramer et al., 1975). Adaptive benefits of vestibular stimulation have been researched extensively with neonatal populations. The benefits include the promotion of intellectual, physiological, and psychosocial growth and development (Table 18–1). Vestibular dysfunction in children is often noted in the most severe developmental deviations. Affected children demonstrate abnormal social and perceptual behavior and often are not able to overcome these early deficits (Mitchell, 1973). It may be speculated that the use of vestibular stimulation with disabled children could improve developmental and maturational outcomes. One study shows that environmental deficits and stress impair early cognitive and psychosocial development in full-term and preterm infants (Escalona, 1982). If attention to maintenance of vestibular sensory needs leads to proportional increases in maturation of neurological tissue, maturity in intellectual and social development may follow.

Sensoridynamism

The term sensoridynamism is used to denote the state of constant individual adjustment to stimuli from the environment. Sensory overload and sensory deprivation disrupt sensoridynamism. Sensoristasis is defined by Schultz (1965) as a need for the living organism to maintain an optimal level of sensory variation. This optimal level is postulated to be within a range balanced and mediated by the ascending reticular activating system. The reticular formation can be conceived of "as a kind of barometer for both input and output [sensory] levels" in order to keep the organism from experiencing sensory overload or sensory deprivation (Lindsley, 1961, p. 176).

Sensory overload is defined as two or more sensory modalities directed simultaneously toward an organism at levels greater than normal, with the combination being introduced all at once rather than gradually (Lindsley, 1961; Goldberger, 1982). Sensory deprivation, at the other extreme, is reduction in the amount, intensity, or patterning of stimulus input (Kubzansky and Leiderman, 1961; Goldberger, 1982). "There is a common core of meaning and significance in sensory deprivation . . . and sensory overload [which] directly or indirectly implicates the reticular formation" (Lindsley, 1961, p. 175). If the reticular formation encounters a sensory imbalance, it meets with a condition that is unfamiliar; the reticular activating system then becomes adjusted or attuned to certain average thresholds of activity (Schultz, 1965). Most theorists indicate that stimulus input is transcribed into a complex code of individual perceptions and meaning, and that sensory overload or sensory deprivation disrupts this processing code (Schultz, 1965; Lindsley, 1961; Hebb, 1949; Jackson and Ellis, 1971; Maddow and Snow, 1970).

In both of the offsetting conditions, sensory overload and sensory deprivation, there is pathology which upsets the balance of the regulating system because of an intense blocking of reticular formation (Lindsley,

Table 18–1. REVIEW OF VESTIBULAR STIMULATION RESEARCH

Author	Type of Stimulation	Subjects	Outcomes
Millen/Davies (1946)	Rockerbeds	Newborns	More efficient respiration
Lee (1954)	See-saw; resuscitators	Newborns	Decreased apnea
Hasselmeyer (1963)	Manual rocking	Infants	Less crying
White/Castle (1964)	Manual rocking	Infants	More visual pursuit
Birns et al. (1966)	Manual rocking	Infants	Less crying
Freedman/Boverman (1966)	Isolette; rockerbeds	Premature infants	More relaxation; more smiling
Neal (1967)	Swinging hammocks	Premature infants	Greater visual, auditory, and motor development
Ambrose (1969)	Manual rocking	Infants	Less crying
Earle (1969)	Mechanical and manual rocking	Newborns	Greater audiovisual development
Solkoff (1969)	Manual rocking	Infants	Increased weight gain
Van den Daele (1970)	Motorized rockerbox	Newborns	Ledd crying; increased arousal
Wright (1971)	Manual rocking	Infants	Increased weight gain
Barnard (1972)	Isolette and rockerbeds	Premature infants	Increased sleep; greater maturation
Korner/Thoman (1972)	Oscillating waterbeds	Infants	Less crying; more visual pursuit
Gregg et al. (1976)	Manual rocking	Newborns	More visual pursuit
Kramer/Pierpont (1976)	Rocking waterbeds	Premature infants	Growth enhanced; increased weight
Korner et al. (1978)	Oscillating waterbeds	Premature infants	Decreased apnea
Hayes (1980)	Manual rocking	Premature infants and newborns follow-up 6 mo.	Enhanced auditory and visual recognition
Brown et al. (1980)	Manual rocking	Premature infants follow-up 9 mo.	Increased parent visitation

1961). The crucial concern with any stimulation intervention is that the client be evaluated for current individual stimulation needs and thresholds.

Human-environment interactions are the focus of nursing theorist Martha Rogers. Her model of unitary man views humans as homeodynamic and consistently interacting with, changing, and responding to the environment. Rogers illustrates how man and environment change together in order to continue their dynamic relationship (Rogers, 1980). Unitary man is not homeostatic, but involved in an evolutionary change toward more complexity. Dynamic equilibrium is rejected in favor of a constant dynamic readjustment of human and environment as the two interact with each other. Rogers (1970) defined the goal of professional nursing with this statement:

nursing seeks to promote symphonic interaction between man and environment to strengthen the conference and integrity of the human field, and to direct and redirect patterning of the human and environmental fields for realization of the maximum health potentials (p.122).

Research utilizing Rogers' theoretical principles of homeodynamic human-environment interaction have been tested primarily through stimulation research. Krieger (1979) utilized therapeutic touch, and Katz (1971) and Porter (1972) demonstrated the effects of auditory stimulation on infants. These are but two examples in which environmentally imposed stimuli have been noted to have a positive effect on growth and development. Because the human person is dynamically adjusting between sensory overload and sensory deprivation in everyday human-environment interactions, interventions aimed at the manipulation of the environment to promote unitary man's dynamic patterns could serve to operationalize Rogers' theory more precisely. In keeping with Rogers' theory of homeodynamic man, the term sensoridynamism refers to a healthy state of dynamic human-environment interaction.

Vestibular Stimulation Modalities and Efficacies

Rocking is a simple, yet ancient form of vestibular stimulation which typifies the type of movement that is inherently vestibular: swaying movement back and forth or side to side. The practice of rocking infants and children has been widely used through the ages among diverse social and cultural groups. This widespread use of rocking is said to imply the existence of a common interval need for vestibular sensation (Van den Daele, 1970). Other examples of vestibular stimulation are the motions produced by waterbeds, body rocking over large rollers, and body flotation in watertubs.

A strong interdependence exists between environmental stimulation and the ongoing abilities of the individual to respond adaptively. This interdependence is identified in psychosocial theory as person-environment fit (French et al., 1974) and as homeodynamic unitary man in Rogers' theory (1980). If sensoridynamic vestibular stimulation is not maintained at a young age, the growth and development of learning tasks that require a dynamic balance of sensory input may be impeded (Fiske and Maddi, 1961). In the neurological process of maturation, there is little myelinization at first; neurological function occurs primarily at the brainstem and spinal cord level (Klaus and Fanaroff, 1979). For example, the respiratory pattern of premature infants is irregular and unstable, becoming more regular with increased myelinization and cortical control (Parmelee et al., 1972). Vestibular stimulation via the eighth cranial nerve directs information to the medulla and pons, centers for vital rhythmic functions such as respiration and heart rate. Hyden (1959) demonstrated that vestibular stimulation of neurons from the reticular formation resulted in increased ribonucleic acid (RNA) and respiratory enzymes, enhancing neurogenic cellular maturation of the respiratory center. If vestibular stimulation provided afferent input to the respiratory centers, it would serve to promote and mature respiratory function.

Rhythmicity in Stimulation

Rogers' (1980) theory maintains that rhythmicity is a fundamental characteristic of all living systems and can be found at all levels of organization within the human organism. Sollberger (1965) stresses the organizing and regulatory importance of rhythms and indicates that in vertebrates the maturity of the nervous system is intimately connected with rhythm control. For example, a lack of exposure to environmental rhythms, such as vestibular motion, may be one primary contributing factor to the poor organization of physiological maturation in premature infants. In both premature and full-term infants, rhythmic movement is the first and most dominant means of establishing physiological and psychosocial homeostasis. Updike and colleagues (1985) suggest nurses focus on these endogenous rhythms in developing a time-based plan for assessment and intervention.

The rhythm component of movement serves to adjust an organism to a changing environment (Sollberger, 1965; Updike et al., 1985). Rocking is rhythmic vestibular stimulation which may be an appropriate way of meeting a child's need for sensoridynamism. Rhythmicity is constant in the environment of the fetus. However, upon delivery, the newborn's biological rhythms may not be synchronized with the extrauterine environment (Deters, 1980), especially if the environment is an Isolette with a nursery policy of minimal handling. Birth is an obligatory change; one major task of adapting to this change is the reorganization of endogenous rhythms (Blackburn, 1979).

Rhythmic vestibular stimulation is classified as kinesthetic in nature. Theories specifying the vestibular stimulation needs of older children are discussed within the context of adult rhythmicity theories. However, it has been theorized that infants have an instinctive stimulus hunger for kinesthetic stimulation, in particular, vestibular stimulation (Ribble, 1965; Kulka et al., 1960). These vestibular needs are probably gratified in intrauterine life, but gradual transition with compensatory vestibular sensoristasis in the postnatal period may be mandatory for healthy development (Kulka et al., 1960). Rocking by a caretaker may provide the necessary vestibular input and compensate for the premature infant's inherent inability to provide himself or herself with movement because of physiological instability.

Vestibular dysfunctions have been recognized as important in the development of childhood schizophrenia as well as the psychosocial maladaptions associated with dyslexia and multiple learning disorders (Clark et al., 1977; Eviatar et al., 1974; Frank and Levinson, 1973). Rocking, head banging, and other similar rhythmic movements are seen in infants and children with prolonged vestibular deprivation. These behaviors may be an attempt to gratify inherent kinesthetic needs (Eviatar et al., 1974; Kulka et al., 1960).

According to Rogers (1980), rhythmicity serves as a synchronizer in the human life processes. Repetitive, rhythmic actions, such as head banging, spoon banging, rocking, jumping, marching, and singing, have been noted historically as pleasurable to children. The ability to initiate such rhythmic activities may or may not be in the power of an infant or child, depending on their health and developmental status. Rhythms are classified according to cycle, origin, and patterning in order to examine and promote the ability of an individual to synchronize their own rhythms (Table 18–2). For example, when rocking a child, the rhythmic motion could pattern that of a familiar song or nursery rhyme. Rhythmic vestibular stimulation interventions tailored to human sensoridynamic needs promote the dynamic realization of maximum health potential and facilitate person-environment fit (French et al., 1974; Rogers, 1980).

ASSESSMENT

Infants and children who require sensoridynamic vestibular stimulation as a nursing

Table 18–2. RHYTHMICITY

Categories	Examples
Cycles	
Circadian = 24 hours	Body temperature
	Enzyme levels
	Nervous system activity
Ultradian <24 hours	Respiratory patterns
	Infant sleep-rest cycles
Infradian >24 hours	Monthly menstrual cycles
Origins	
Exogenous rhythms	External stimuli; from outside the body
Endogenous rhythms	Internal stimuli; with or without external correlates
Patterns	
Microrapid rate, duration < 1 hour, regulatory in nature	Heart rate Respiratory rate
Macroslow rate, duration 1 hour to 1 week	Renal function Blood platelet counts
Long term > 1 week	Mood swings

intervention are those diagnosed with sensory-perceptual alteration. Antecedent conditions evolve from experiences that could serve to alter sensoridynamism. Four potential etiologies are designated by Kim and Moritz (1982): (1) altered environmental stimuli (from excess to deprivation); (2) alterations in the individual's ability to receive, transmit, or integrate stimulation; (3) chemical alterations that are due to fluid and electrolyte imbalances or drug actions; and (4) psychological stressors leading to a lack of person-environment fit. It is imperative that prior to the initiation of stimulation in any form, accurate assessment must be made to ascertain (1) the normal sensory environment for the individual, (2) the current individual sensoridynamic balance, and (3) individual stimulation thresholds.

The crucial step of carefully assessing data to determine what type and degree of stimulation dynamically supports the individual's interaction with the environment cannot be overemphasized. In a newborn, for example, the nurse considers the intrauterine environment and may attempt to approximate that sensoridynamism by rocking the infant at a rate approximating the average maternal heartbeat. Maternal information regarding typical daily activities during pregnancy, the pattern of fetal movements during gestation, and impressions of the infant's needs will be most valuable to a sensory needs assessment. For infants and children, data should be gathered from parents about the amount, type, and frequency of vestibular stimulation, such as rocking, provided in the home environment.

Defining characteristics of an overload of vestibular stimuli in infants include irritability, hyper-reactivity, hypertonicity, irregular respirations, apnea, irregular heart rates, poor feeding behavior, and increased frequency of stooling or emesis (Leners, 1981). Defining characteristics that indicate possible sensory deprivation include lethargy, lack of response to cuddling, lack of orienting behavior, extension, poor feeding, irregular heart rate, irregular respiratory rate, and increased frequency of stooling or emesis (Leners, 1981). The overlap of behaviors that characterize both extremes makes it difficult to specify an accurate diagnosis. The lack of specific tools to adequately assess sensoridynamism is a serious problem which needs to be addressed.

One tool available for use with premature infants is the Assessment of Premature Infant Behavior (APIB) developed by Als (Als et al., 1983). The tool evaluates and validates developmental cues, physiological stability, and stimulus thresholds. The APIB is an extention of the Brazelton Neonatal Behavior Assessment Scale and is fairly novel to most neonatal practice settings. Professional use of the APIB requires special training and practice because of the complex nature of the instrument. Initial training requires individual instruction with the manual and working with at least five infants for exposure to the assessment methodology (Als et al., 1982). After assessment of another 20 to 25 infants in the work setting, the trainee returns for further supervised practice and to establish inter-rater reliability.

The APIB identifies five subsystems of functioning: (1) the autonomic, (2) the motor, (3) the state-organizational, (4) the attentional-interactive, and (5) the self-regulatory balancing subsystems. Theoretically, the infant negotiates the integration and differentiation of these subsystems in dynamic interaction with the environment. Signals of stress and signals of self-regulation can be assessed at each level.

The APIB sequences increasingly vigorous environmental inputs, moving from distal stimulation presented during sleep to mild tactile stimulation. Next, medium tactile stimulation is paired with vestibular stimulation. Finally, more massive tactile stimulation is paired with vestibular stimulation. A social-interactive-attentional portion of the tool is administered whenever the infant's behavioral organization indicates readiness. The systems sheet assesses which tasks are tolerated easily by the infant, which stress the infant, and which tasks are inappropriate for the infant. From these data, developmentally appropriate goals can be formulated without overtaxing or under-challenging the premature infant. The goal is to reduce stress signals and enhance stabilization signals.

Unfortunately, few of the vestibular stimulation researchers have examined infant or child readiness for vestibular interventions. Stimulus inputs can produce pathological changes if not modulated according to the child's sensoridynamic threshold. The APIB provides assessment data and cues about this readiness in premature infants. However, similar tools are needed that will adjust for age and developmental stage.

INTERVENTION STRATEGIES

Stimulation, if inappropriately timed or inappropriate in quality and intensity, will cause the organism to move away from it and protect itself. Stimulation if appropriately timed or appropriate in quality and intensity will cause the organism to seek it out and move towards it while maintaining a balanced level.

Als, 1982, pp. 238–239

This statement illustrates the importance of basing nursing interventions on observations of individual behavioral responses to stimuli and the current environment. When planning vestibular stimulation, the nurse must carefully determine the need for stimulation, the type and quality of stimulation to use, the frequency of the intervention, the intensity and quantity of time to spend on the intervention, and the rhythmicity of the intervals in relationship to the child's activities of daily living. The last item, rhythmic timing of stimulation, represents an attempt on the part of nurses to provide synchrony of care. For example, waterbed therapy may be identified as a need for an infant or child based on the observation of immediate relaxation of large muscle groups with wavelike flotation on the water mattress. With this ability to relax, pain tolerence may be increased for the child. In order to synchronize this stimulus with the individual need, the nurse needs to carefully plan flotation intervention before or after painful procedures and to specify the length and intensity of the flotation movement, the interval frequency at which to place the child on the moving mattress, and behaviors indicating the potential for sensory overload versus deprivation. Outcome measurements might include changes in frequency of requests for pain medication, observed behaviors, or individual statements in response to therapy. The individuality of the child's response to vestibular stimulation is imperative knowledge for the nurse in planning vestibular sensory interventions. Vestibular stimulation must be synchronized with individual rhythms in order to promote a positive person-environment fit.

Infant and pediatric stimulation programs

provide guidelines for planning and implementing specific stimulation interventions. Through the use of a planned program, such as the Infant-Interaction Standards of Care (Denver Children's Hospital, 1986), vestibular stimulation can be designed to respond to the child's behavior. Volunteers, parents, and other caregivers can be educated to observe the child and respond to behavioral cues. The caregiver is specifically taught to provide time out when avoidance behaviors are demonstrated and to support and enhance approach behaviors. Examples of assessment tools, documentation of infant behavior, and care plans are available in the literature (Cole, 1985; Als et al., 1982; Denver Children's Hospital, 1986).

Implementation of the program plan is best accomplished using caregiving guidelines. Vestibular stimulation should be provided as a single additional sensory experience. Interventions need to be tailored to the amount of stimulation the child can handle. For example, the nurse should allow the child to adapt to a rocking stimulus prior to simultaneously adding other sensory modes such as music, stroking, or visual stimulation. In this way, interaction with a caregiver is gradual and less likely to produce sensory imbalance. The nurse should observe and document the sensory threshold and behavioral responses to each stimulus.

Next, the nurse should use vestibular stimulation strategies to attempt to normalize or dynamically balance the patient's environment rather than exaggerate the intervention to the extremes of deprivation or overload. Normalizing includes adjusting the amount, frequency, and velocity of vestibular movements to the child's changing needs, physiological tolerance, behavioral cues, and development. A toddler who has recently experienced painful procedures, a loss of environmental control, or iatrogenic regression may be supported with minimal stimulation such as simple holding without rocking, stroking, or auditory or visual stimuli. In an attempt to achieve sensoridynamism for this child, the caregiver could overcompensate or enhance sensory imbalances by simultaneously initiating all of the sensory modalities at once. In order to effect sensoridynamism, the potential for deprivation or overload needs to be considered.

Finally, interventions should seek to incorporate and solicit the involvement of the family or other caregivers. Parents can be taught their infant's unique behavioral cues and responses to interventions. When they are directly involved in the planning of care, parents can take an immediate role in caregiving activities. Volunteer cuddler programs and parent interaction and bonding programs seek to utilize parents and ancillary caregivers under the supervision of the nurse. Vestibular stimulation methods can also be coordinated with ancillary personnel such as occupational therapists and physical therapists. Vestibular stimulation has long been used in these specialties to promote large muscle movement and coordination.

Various creative methods and equipment have been utilized to provide vestibular stimulation to children. Historically, research has investigated rocking intervention methods primarily in the premature and newborn age groups (see Table 18–1). There has been little research with older children. However, pediatric nurses have traditionally used waterbeds, swings, rolling balls, wagons, strollers, infant carriers, hammocks, cradles, wheelchairs, and rocking chairs. Nurses intuitively feel the movement provided by these methods sooth and comfort children.

Although all of the equipment described provides vestibular sensation, it appears that waterbeds, swings, rocking chairs, hammocks, cradles, and rolling balls have been used to provide the rocking movement researched extensively in the neonatal populations. When providing vestibular stimulation with this equipment, the pediatric nurse needs to carefully plan specific parameters beyond simply rocking the infant. For instance, the speed with which an infant is rocked, the time of day, how long the infant is rocked, and the frequency of rocking periods are all important parameters to consider. Following the guidelines provided from rocking research with neonates, the goal should be to intervene with planned parameters of rocking, being continually alert to signs of stress or stabilization. When using vestibular stimulation, the nurse seeks to reduce stress signals and enhance stabilization signals. Just what these signals are must be established via diligent research. However, the nurse can increase awareness of potential signs of deprivation versus overload by providing a specific rationale for initiating a rocking intervention, anticipating what behaviors the child might use as signals of stress or stabilization, and observing individual responses during the intervention. Too often an agitated, crying child is simply placed into a swing to keep him occupied or to provide distraction in order to sooth the child without forethought or observation as to the rationale for the intervention and the specific responses to the intervention.

Equipment that provides vestibular motion includes wagons, strollers, infant carriers, and wheelchairs. Pediatric nurses have noticed since Nightingale's era that children provided this type of movement respond positively by becoming more aware and interested in their environment and are soothed or comforted by this activity. Is the change in behavior due to distraction or the movement per se, or a combination of the two? Only research can provide these answers. However, caution is again recommended when providing an intervention along these lines. Assessment of potential stimulation needs with a specified rationale for the use of vestibular stimulation is important in order to determine what individual behaviors will be designated as stress signals and which will be designated as stabilization signals. Again, the goal should be to reduce stress signals and enhance stabilization signals in order to support sensoridynamism.

EVALUATION

Behaviors and other indications of stability or sensoridynamism are as follows:

1. *Autonomic-visceral*: smooth respirations; good, stable color and stable digestion.

2. *Motoric*: smooth, well-modulated posture; well-regulated tone; synchronous movements, with hand clasping, foot clasping, finger folding; hand-to-mouth grasping; suck searching; sucking; handholding; and tucking-in posture.

3. *State-related*: clear sleep states; rhythmic, lusty crying; effective self-quieting; focused, shiny-eyed alertness; animated facial expressions of frowning, cheek softening, mouth pursing to ooh shape, cooing, and attentional smiling (Als et al., 1982).

The behaviors and other indicators that characterize sensory imbalance include the following:

1. *Autonomic-visceral*: seizures, respiratory irregularities, color changes, gagging, hiccuping, straining, tremors, startle reaction, coughing, sneezing, and yawning and sighing

2. *Motoric*: flaccidity of trunk, extremities, and facies; hypertonicity with hyperextensions of legs or arms; trunk arching; finger splaying; facial grimacing; tongue extension; and protective maneuvers such as flailing of fists, guarding and arm protection, and frantic or diffuse activity

3. *State-related*: eye floating, sleep and awake states with whimpering, glassy-eyed staring, strained fussing or crying, active averting, panicked alertness, rapid state oscillation, crying, and irritability (Als et al., 1982).

These stress behaviors should alert the nurse to alter the plan to accommodate the sensoridynamic needs of the individual. Evaluation is crucial to protecting the infant from overload or deprivation. Ideally, vestibular stimulation strategies should seek to provide an optimal match between the environment and the infant's ability to respond to the environment. A one-size-fits-all approach to stimulation intervention strategies typifies an ignorance with regard to individuation in human care interventions and does not promote person-environment fit. Infants and children communicate through their behavioral cues. As nurses learn to be sensitive observers of these individual cues and integrate this information into nursing care, the appropriate interventions may become obvious.

Case Studies

CHRISTY

Christy was at risk for abnormal neurological development because of intensive care environmental stimuli that were not tailored to promote individual person-environment fit. The physically stable 30-week premature infant was housed in a neonatal intensive care unit in an Isolette. The infant experienced frequent apnea primarily during the day shift and demonstrated persistent limb extension with stress behaviors. The observed stress behaviors were tongue thrusts, gagging, facial grimaces, and overall irritability whenever she was held. The infant was assessed with the APIB tool. The outcome indicated behavior consistent with infants experiencing sensory imbalance. A nursing diagnosis of *Sensory perceptual alteration* was made. Because of the physiological maturity of the vestibular system, interventions focusing upon the vestibular mode were chosen. Christy was placed on a waterbed and positioned with her limbs in flexion whenever possible. Als (1982) has noted that this position is conducive to stress reduction. Whenever Christy experienced startle reflexes or spontaneous body movement, the waterbed was oscillated for a few seconds. All other forms of sensory input, such as extraneous room noise, handling, music, stroking, and visual stimuli, were minimized whenever possible. Medical management by attending physicians was held constant during this nursing intervention. Apnea spells were reduced by 36% within 48 hours. The APIB criteria were used to evaluate behavioral responses. After the first eight hours of intervention, Christy was able to tolerate programmed oscillations at a frequency and rhythmicity that matched her mother's average heart rate and activities of daily living experienced while in utero. Long-term evaluation outcomes documented were reduced apnea, more even respiratory patterns, weight gain, and increased visual attentiveness.

NOAH

Noah, a two year old, was discharged from the hospital after an acute epiglottitis experience. The pediatric home health nurse observed that the toddler had spasmodic, crouplike coughing followed by lethargy and listlessness. Noah would not cuddle with caretakers or demonstrate flexion upon being held. Noah's parents anxiously sat at his bedside without rest, frustrated by their inability to comfort their son. Noting that dehydration and sepsis were ruled out, a nursing diagnosis of *Sensory perceptual alteration* due to psychological and physiological stressors was made. Noah had been a very cuddly child prior to his illness, constantly desiring to be held. During his hospitalization, Noah was in an oxygen tent and had not been held during the entire experience. Not only was he terrified of the hospital environment and painful procedures but he was also unable to receive the normal cuddling that was a significant part of his previous life. Upon discharge, Noah's parents, afraid of bothering him and unable to understand his lethargy, were reluctant to try to return to their normal interactions with their son. Noah's parents were taught to provide vestibular stimulation by rocking Noah every two hours for 15 minutes. Within six hours, Noah was anticipating the rocking, demonstrating flexion of limbs when held, and beginning to cuddle into his parents' arms. The frequency and quality of the crouplike cough remained unchanged; however, the depression behaviors gradually disappeared over the next 24 hours.

RESEARCH IMPLICATIONS

The culmination of the research in the area of vestibular sensoridynamism has provided some important principles to consider in neonatal nursing: (1) weight gains achieved by premature infants who are rocked closely match expected fetal weight gains of full-term pregnancies; (2) the more active and distressed an infant, the more effective the rocking; and (3) when using rocking, a 60-per-minute cycle appears to be most effective in soothing infants. However, research is seriously lacking in information regarding the use of vestibular stimulation. Unfortunately, an inherent assumption in the majority of vestibular stimulation research is that patients were experiencing sensory deprivation. Given the typical hospital environment with the bright lights, constant interruptions, and painful procedures, it is more likely that patients were experiencing sensory overload, yet needing sensory stimulation that would more closely resemble that in their normal, everyday lives. Too often nurses have relied on intuition to determine stimulation needs. These intuitive thoughts must be addressed as research topics in today's age of nursing science.

Infants and children up to the age of ten years have been postulated to be sensory augmenters: that is, individuals who inherently tend to increase the intensity of any stimulus to promote growth and development (Buchsbaum, 1976).

Opening the sensory floodgates helps satisfy the augmenters' craving for sensation, but can have adverse effects if they become overloaded . . . thus excessively or inappropriately applied, [stimuli] could theoretically lead to or exacerbate . . . illness.

Buchsbaum, 1978, p. 100

The effects of vestibular stimulation interventions on the neurological development and maturation of children with developmental disabilities, physical handicaps, or other conditions which limit mobility and movement is another area where research is needed. These are areas where nursing research could open avenues for the development and testing of novel nursing interventions.

Current attention to the personhood of the patient through ethical caring interventions requires that nurses do not simply make assumptions about the patient's sensory status. Specific, individualized interventions based on assessment of the child's behavioral cues are necessary. Perhaps the wrong research questions have been asked because of this oversight. Identification of specific behaviors that indicate vestibular sensory imbalance is imperative for accurate diagnosis. Only then can interventions be tested systematically. Identified behavior that demonstrates sensoridynamism is also crucial. Increased awareness of the environment and normal individual vestibular sensory patterning is important as histories are taken and families are consulted for input. Further development and refinement of tools that help to qualitatively and quantitatively measure vestibular sensoridynamism are desperately needed. As the science of caring, nursing must determine how to facilitate the establishment of interventions which promote a dynamic, harmonious human-environment interaction within the realm of sensoridynamism.

References

Als, H. Toward a synactive theory of development: Premise for the assessment and support of infant individuality. Infant Mental Health Journal, 3:229–243, 1982.

Als, H, Lester, BM, Tronick, EC, and Brazelton, TB. Towards a research instrument for the assessment of preterm infants' behavior (APIB) and Manual for the assessment of preterm infant's behavior (APIB). In Fitzgerald, HE, Lester, BM, and Yogman, MW (Eds.), Theory and research in behavioral pediatrics (Vol. 1). New York: Plenum Press, 1982, pp. 35–132.

Ambrose, JA. Stimulation in early infancy. New York: Academic Press, 1969.

Barnard, KA. The effect of stimulation on the duration and amount of sleep and wakefulness in the premature infant. Unpublished doctoral dissertation, University of Washington, Seattle, 1972.

Beckwith, L, and Cohen, SE. Preterm birth. Infant Behavioral Development, 1:403–411, 1978.

Birns, B, Blank, M, and Bridger, WH. The effectiveness of various soothing techniques on human neonates. Psychosomatic Medicine, 28:316–322, 1966.

Blackburn, ST. The effects of caregiving abilities in the neonatal intensive care unit on the behavior and development of premature infants. Unpublished doctoral dissertation, University of Washington, Seattle, 1979.

Brown, JV, LaRossa, M, and Aylward, G. Nursery-based intervention with prematurely born babies and their mothers: Are there effects? Journal of Pediatrics, 97:487–491, 1980.

Buchsbaum, MS. Self-regulation of stimulus intensity: Augmenting/reducing and the average evoked response. In Schwartz, G, and Shapiro, D (Eds.), Consciousness and self regulation (Vol. 1). Advances in research. San Francisco: Plenum Publishing Corp, 1976, pp. 101–135.

Buchsbaum, MS. The sensoristat in the brain. Psychology Today, 11:96–104, 1978.

Clark, D, Kreutzberg, J, and Chee, F. Vestibular stimulation influence on motor development in infants. Science, 196:1228–1229, 1977.

Cole, JG. Infant stimulation reexamined: An environmental and behavioral based approach. Neonatal Network, 3:24–31, 1985.

Denver Children's Hospital. Unpublished standards of care. Denver: 1986.

Deters, G. Circadian rhythm phenomenon. MCN: American Journal of Maternal Child Nursing, 5:249–251, 1980.

Drillen, CM. Fresh approaches to prospective studies of high risk infants. Pediatrics, 45:7–8, 1970.

Earle, AM. The effect of supplementary post-natal kinesthetic stimulation on the developmental behavior of the normal female newborn. Unpublished doctoral dissertation, New York University, New York, 1969.

Escalona, SK. Babies at double hazard: Early development of infants at biologic and social risk. Journal of Pediatrics, 70:670–676, 1982.

Eviatar, L, Eviatar, A, and Naray, I. Maturation of neurovestibular responses in infants. Developmental Medicine and Child Neurology, 16:435–466, 1974.

Fiske, D, and Maddi, S. Function of varied experience. Homewood, Ill: The Dorsey Press, 1961.

Frank, J, and Levinson, H. Dysmetric dyslexia and dyspraxia. American Academy of Child Psychiatry Journal, 12:690–701, 1973.

Freedman, D, and Boverman, H. The effects of kinesthetic stimulation on certain aspects of development in premature infants. American Journal of Orthopsychiatry, 36:223–224, 1966.

French, J, Rodgers, W, and Cobb, S. Adjustment as person-environment fit. In Coelho, G, Hamburg, DA, and Adams, JE (Eds.), Coping and adaptation. New York: Basic Books, Inc., 1974, pp. 316–333.

Goldberger, L. Sensory deprivation and overload. In Goldberger, L, and Breznitz, S (Eds.), Handbook of stress. New York: Free Press, 1982, pp. 1–60.

Gregg, C, Haffner, ME, and Korner, A. The relative efficacy of vestibular proprioceptive stimulation and the upright position in enhancing visual pursuit in neonates. Child Development, 47:309–314, 1976.

Hasselmeyer, E. Handling and premature infant behavior. Unpublished doctoral dissertation, New York University, New York, 1963.

Hayes, J. Premature infant development: The relationships of neonatal stimulation, birth condition, and home environment. Pediatric Nursing, 6:33–36, 1980.

Hebb, D. The organization of behavior. New York: John Wiley & Sons, Inc., 1949.

Hellmuth, J. Exceptional infant studies in abnormalities (Vol. 2). New York: Brunner/Mazel, 1971.

Hyden, H. Quantitative assay of compounds in isolated, fresh nerve cells and glial cells from control and stimulated animals. Nature, 8:433–435, 1959.

Jackson, CW, and Ellis, R. Sensory deprivation as a field of study. Nursing Research, 20:46–54, 1971.

Katz, V. Auditory stimulation and developmental behavior of the premature infant. Nursing Research, 20:196–201, 1971.

Kim, MJ, and Moritz, DA. Classification of nursing diagnosis: Proceedings of the third and fourth national conferences. New York: McGraw-Hill, Inc., 1982.

Klaus, M, and Fanaroff, A. Care of the high-risk neonate. Philadelphia: WB Saunders Co., 1979.

Korner, A, Guilleminault, C, Van den Hoed, J, and Baldwin, R. Reduction of sleep apnea and bradycardia in preterm infants on oscillating waterbeds: A controlled polygraphic study. Pediatrics, 61:528–533, 1978.

Korner, A, Kraemer, H, Haffner, E, and Casper, L. Effects of waterbed flotation on premature infants: A pilot study. Pediatrics, 56:361–367, 1975.

Korner, A, and Thoman, E. The relative efficacy of contact and vestibular-proprioceptive stimulation in soothing neonates. Child Development, 43:443–453, 1972.

Korner, A, Ruppel, E, and Rho, J. Effects of waterbeds on the sleep and motility of theophylline treated preterm infants. Pediatrics, 70:864–869, 1982.

Kramer, M, Chamorro, I, Green, D, and Krudtson, F. Extra tactile stimulation of the premature infant. Nursing Research, 24:324–334, 1975.

Kramer, B, and Pierpont, ME. Rocking waterbeds and auditory stimuli to enhance growth of preterm infants. Journal of Pediatrics, 88:297–299, 1976.

Krieger, D. The therapeutic touch. Englewood Cliffs, N.J.: Prentice-Hall, Inc., 1979.

Kubzansky, P, and Leiderman, PH. Sensory deprivation: An overview. Cambridge, Mass.: Harvard University Press, 1961.

Kulka, A, Fry, C, and Goldstein, FJ. Kinesthetic needs in infancy. American Journal of Orthopsychiatry, 30:562–571, 1960.

Larrouche, JC. The development of the central nervous system during intrauterine life. In Falkner, F (Ed.), Human development. Philadelphia: WB Saunders Co., 1966, pp. 257–276.

Lazarus, RS, and Folkman, S. Stress, appraisal, and coping. New York: Springer Publishing Co., 1984.

Lee, H. A rocking bed respirator for use with premature infants in incubators. Journal of Pediatrics, 44:570–573, 1954.

Leners, D. A survey of rocking interventions utilized by Iowa nurses in the care of premature infants. Unpublished master's thesis, University of Iowa, Iowa City, Iowa, 1981.

Lindsley, D. Common factors in sensory deprivation, sensory distortion, and sensory overload. In Solomon, P (Ed.), Sensory deprivation. Cambridge, Mass: Harvard University Press, 1961, pp. 174–195.

Maddow, L, and Snow, L. The psychodynamic implications of physiological studies on sensory deprivation. Springfield, Ill.: Charles C Thomas, 1970.

Millen, R, and Davies, J. See-saw resuscitator for the treatment of asphyxia in the newborn. American Journal of Obstetrics and Gynecology, 52:508–509, 1946.

Mitchell, P. Concepts basic to nursing. New York: McGraw-Hill, Inc., 1973.

Mitchell, R, and Berger, A. Neural regulation respiration. American Review of Respiratory Disease, 111:206–224, 1975.

Neal, M. The relationship between a regiment of vestibular stimulation and developmental behavior of the premature infant. Unpublished doctoral dissertation, New York University, New York, 1967.

Parmelee, A, Stern, E, and Harris, M. Maturation of respiration in prematures and young infants. Neuropediatrie, 3:294–304, 1972.

Parmelee, AH, and Schulte, FJ. Developmental testing of preterm and small-for-date infants. Pediatrics, 45:23–28, 1970.

Porter, LS. The impact of physical-physiological activity on infant growth and development. Nursing Research 21:210–219, 1972.

Ribble, M. The rights of infants. New York: Columbia University Press, 1965.

Rice, RD. Neurophysiological development in premature infants following stimulation. Developmental Psychology, 13:69–76, 1977.

Rogers, M. An introduction to the theoretical basis of nursing. Philadelphia: FA Davis Co., 1970.

Rogers, M. Nursing: A science of unitary man. In Richland, JP, and Roy, C (Eds.), Conceptual models for nursing practice (2nd ed.). New York: Appleton-Century Crofts, 1980, pp. 329–337.

Schultz, D. Sensory restriction: Effects on behavior. New York: Academic Press, 1965.

Solkoff, N. Effects of handling on the subsequent development of premature infants. Developmental Psychology, 1:765–768, 1969.

Sollberger, A. Biological rhythm research. New York: Elsevier Science Publishing Co., 1965.

Solomon, P (Ed.). Sensory deprivation. Cambridge, Mass: Harvard University Press, 1961.

Strang, LB. Neonatal respiration: Physiological and clinical studies. Oxford, England: Blackwell Scientific Publications, 1977.

Updike, P, Accurso, F, and Jones, R. Physiological circadian rhythmicity in preterm infants. Nursing Research, 34:160–163, 1985.

Van den Daele, L. Modification of infant state by treatment in a rockerbox. Journal of Psychology, 74:161–165, 1970.

White, B, and Castle, P. Visual exploratory behavior following postnatal handling of human infants. Perceptual and Motor Skills, 18:497–502, 1964.

Wright, L. The theoretical research base for a program of early stimulation and training of premature infants. In Hellmuth, J (Ed.), Exceptional infant studies in abnormalties, (Vol. 2). New York: Brunner/Mazel, 1971.

CHAPTER 19

SLEEP PROMOTION

KATHY D. SCHIBLER, M.S.N., C.P.N.P., R.N.,
and SUSAN A. FAY, M.S.N., R.N.

Sleep is one of the basic needs of the human organism. It is necessary for the maintenance of life and the restoration of health. Sleeping and waking states together form the framework within which all living organisms conduct their daily lives. Humans spend approximately one third of their lives sleeping. Nurses who work with infants and children know that sleep difficulties in infants from birth to three years have become one of the most common problems in pediatric practice (Ferber, 1985). Salzarulo and Chevalier (1983) found that children who experience disorders of sleep-wake rhythm early in life are more likely to have associated sleep problems later in childhood, and recovery is difficult.

The purpose of this chapter is to discuss strategies to promote regular sleep patterns in infants and young children who are hospitalized. The theoretical framework for this intervention has been drawn from the literature on the development of sleep patterns in children and disruption of sleep-wake rhythm as related to physiological, psychosocial, and environmental factors.

THEORETICAL FOUNDATION

An understanding of normal sleep patterns is important in order to assess, diagnose, and treat actual or potential sleep pattern disturbances. Sleep has been defined as "a natural, recurring state of altered consciousness that provides rest for the body, mind, and spirit, and is terminated by intrinsic or extrinsic stimuli" (Barndt-Maglio, 1986, p. 342). Theories describing the need of living organisms for sleep have not been empirically proven, although it is believed that sleep is essential for both physical and emotional well-being. Oswald (1970) postulates that deep sleep is necessary for growth and renewal of basic tissue. In addition, Lamberg (1984) reports that deep sleep appears to be necessary to restore energy, provide relaxation, and stimulate growth hormone secretion. These factors facilitate general physical growth and wound healing during sleep. Other theories postulate that sleep is necessary for emotional well-being. Lamberg (1984) states that "sleep is part of a perpetual cycle and is the most powerful organizer in our lives" (p. 9).

Consequences of prolonged sleep deprivation are variable. Studies conducted on rats demonstrated that sleep serves a vital function: rats kept awake continuously became scrawny and weak, then died within a few days (Lamberg, 1984). Baker (1985) found that rats deprived of sleep exhibited increased aggressiveness, increased sexual drive, and learning difficulties. Chronic fatigue leads to both mental and physical difficulties in humans, such as difficulty concentrating, decreased fine motor skill performance, and irritability (Lamberg, 1984).

Current understanding of sleep relates back to the discovery of the physiological phenomenon of rapid eye movement (REM) sleep in the 1950's (Aserinsky and Kleitman, 1953; Dement and Kleitman, 1957). Prior to that time, sleep was thought to be one single state. Sleep is now recognized as two distinct states of central nervous system (CNS) activity, REM and non-REM sleep states, which are described in Table 19–1. Both states occur cyclically and are controlled by separate neurophysiological and biochemical regulators. Dopamine neurons in the pons act as the control mechanism for REM state, and serotonergic neurons in the forebrain act as the control mechanism for the non-REM state (Anders and Keener, 1983). The non-REM state, or quiet sleep, is considered important for restorative (anabolic metabolism) function whereas the REM state, or active sleep, is important for mental restoration, information processing, and memory (Denenberg and Thoman, 1981). In clinical research, sleep activity is monitored by polygraphic recordings, including electroencephalograms, electro-oculograms, and electromyograms, which demonstrate distinct wave patterns during each stage of sleep.

In addition to knowledge of the characteristics of sleep stages outlined in Table 19–1, knowledge of general sleep patterns is important to understand the etiology of various sleep disorders and intervention strategies to promote sleep. Beginning at about three months of age, the non-REM state develops into four distinct stages and a single nighttime sleep pattern becomes established. In general, the length of sleep cycles and the amount of REM and of non-REM Stage IV change with maturation (Table 19–2). A complete sleep cycle length increases from about 50 minutes in the full-term infant to 90 minutes by adolescence. The duration of Stage IV decreases as the total amount of sleep decreases through childhood, and the total amount and percent of the REM state decrease throughout adolescence and stabilize during adulthood (Ferber, 1985).

The characteristics of a night's sleep can best be understood using an illustration of sleep patterns (see Table 19–1). After about three months of age, a child enters non-REM sleep immediately after falling asleep and progresses to Stage IV within about ten minutes (Ferber, 1985). During the initial Stage IV sleeping time, the child is in an especially deep sleep and is almost impossible to arouse. The child may stay in this deep sleep for approximately one hour, then progress back to Stage I and even awaken briefly. During these periods of arousal, which may occur eight to nine times per night, the child may exhibit a wide range of behaviors. Common behaviors may include rubbing the eyes, staring blankly, speaking unintelligibly, or sleepwalking. Other less common behaviors may include sleep terrors, confused thrashing, or bed-wetting. According to Ferber (1985), these behaviors are not stimulated by dreams.

An arousal which occurs early in the night may be followed by a brief REM phase of five to ten minutes. The child may then return to deep sleep. As the night progresses, the child spends less time in deep sleep and more time in Stage II sleep. Overall, more time is spent in deep sleep early in the night; light sleep and dreaming occur during the remainder of the night (approximately seven hours total), although a short episode of deep sleep is experienced again prior to awakening (Ferber, 1985). According to Ferber

Table 19–1. DESCRIPTION OF SLEEP STAGES*

Non-REM Sleep

Stage I
 Relaxed and dreamy state; may have some imagery
 Somewhat aware of the environment
 May awaken and rub eyes
 Lasts a few seconds
 EEG appears low voltage, 4–6 cycles/second
Stage II
 Progresses to deeper level of sleep
 Unaware of surroundings
 Easily awakened (often by a jerk of a leg or body)
 EEG appears high voltage with sleep spindles, 13–15 cycles/second; large K-Complexes
Stage III
 Muscles relax
 Pulse rate slows
 Temperature drops
 Blood pressure lowers
 Remains easily arousable
 EEG appears as slow-wave delta, 1–4 cycles/second
Stage IV
 Pulse and blood pressure regular, muscles relaxed; profuse sweating may occur
 Confused if awakened (children may experience sleep terrors, sleep walking, and confused thrashing if abruptly
  awakened)
 Need is greater after a day of exertion
 People generally judge sleep adequacy based on this stage
 Occurs about 40 minutes after entering stage I
 Decreases as REM sleep increases progressively with each cycle (in adults, 4–5 cycles/night, 90–100 minutes
  long)
 Growth hormone, which facilitates wound healing, is secreted during this stage
 EEG appears as slow-wave delta
 Present in proportionally large amounts during afternoon naps

REM Sleep

 Important for memory, learning, and psychosocial adaptation
 Day's events are reviewed, categorized, and integrated for storage
 Problems may be solved during this stage and new perspectives gained
 If psychological stress is occurring, the need for REM sleep is greater
 Deprivation can lead to psychotic episodes
 Dreams occur during REM sleep, but may not be remembered upon awakening
 Dreams may contain the illusion of paralysis (such as inability to run from a pursuer)
 Present in proportionately large amounts during morning naps
 Impaired temperature regulation (will not shiver or sweat)
 If awakened, able to alert quickly and may report dreaming
 Heart rate, respiratory rate, and blood pressure increases
 Poor muscle tone, especially head and neck
 Twitching of hands, legs, and face

*Adapted with permission from Barndt-Maglio, B. Sleep pattern disturbance. Dimensions of Critical Care Nursing, 5:342–349, 1986.
 Abbreviations: REM, Rapid eye movement; EEG, electroencephalogram.

(1985), the difficulty experienced in transferring from Stage IV non-REM sleep to an alert state accounts for night terrors and sleepwalking as well as for the confused thrashing demonstrated when children are awakened abruptly. The complex body movements of sleepwalking and night terrors cannot occur during REM sleep because this stage is characterized by poor muscle tone, especially of the head and neck.

The organization of sleep stage cycles from neonate to adult occurs along a developmental continuum. In utero, active REM sleep of the fetus can be recorded by six to seven months' gestation; non-REM sleep can be recorded by seven to eight months, and both are well established by eight months. Anders and Keener (1983), who have studied the development of sleep patterns, reported that significant changes occur from neonate to adult. The most substantial change is the ratio of REM to non-REM sleep. REM sleep predominates in the immature infant and declines with maturation. Thus, sleep begins

Table 19–2. COMPARISON OF INFANT AND ADULT SLEEP PATTERNS*

Characteristics of Sleep	Infant	Adult
Sleep state proportions of REM/Non-REM (%)	50/50	20/80
Periodicity of sleep states	50–60 min. REM/Non-REM cycle	90–100 min. REM/Non-REM cycle
Sleep onset state	REM sleep onset	Non-REM sleep onset
Temporal organization of sleep states	REM/Non-REM cycles equally throughout sleep period	Non-REM Stages III–V predominant in first third of night REM state predominant in last third of night
Maturation of EEG patterns	LVF pattern HVS pattern 1 Non-REM EEG stage	K-Complexes Delta waves 4 Non-REM EEG stages

*Adapted with permission from Anders, T, and Keener, M. Sleep-wake state development and disorders of sleep in infants, children, and adolescents. In Levine, MD, Carey, WB, Crocker, AC, and Gross, RT (eds): Developmental-Behavioral Pediatrics. Philadelphia, WB Saunders Co, 1983, p 598.

Abbreviations: REM, Rapid eye movement; EEG, electroencephalogram; LVF, low-voltage fast (awake/REM); HVS, high-voltage slow (sleep).

with the REM state during early life and gradually changes to non-REM as the first sleep state. This change from the predominance of REM to non-REM sleep explains the findings that young infants, especially premature infants, experience an immature organization of sleep, called indeterminate sleep. All infants, especially immature infants, exhibit indeterminate sleep (Milner, 1982).

The length of a normal sleep cycle and the amount of REM and non-REM sleep vary with age (Table 19–3). Infants spend 50% of sleep time in REM sleep and start each period of sleep in active REM. In the newborn, the REM state can be observed by eye movement, twitching, and an occasional smile. It is during REM sleep that newborns receive stimulation necessary for higher brain center development. This phenomenon appears to decrease as the child requires less intrinsic stimulation (Castiglio, 1987).

The development of a diurnal pattern of sleep and wakefulness in the infant occurs as short sleep episodes are consolidated into longer periods with a shift to nighttime hours. The major developmental changes occurring in sleep are dramatic. Consider that the amount of time in REM sleep decreases from 50% in the full-term infant to 33% in the three year old and 25% in the adolescent. The duration of a typical sleep cycle increases from 50 minutes in the full-term newborn to 90 minutes in the adolescent and adult (Ferber, 1985).

Circadian rhythms guide sleep patterns. In Latin, *circa* means approximately and *dies* means day. Circadian rhythms include patterns of sleep-wake states, activity-rest, hunger-eating, temperature fluctuations, and hormone release. All of these rhythms are important for a sense of well-being and influence the ability to fall asleep and stay asleep. During a typical cycle, a person falls asleep as the body temperature decreases and awakens as the temperature reaches its peak. In addition, the cortisol level decreases upon falling asleep and increases upon awakening. Studies indicate that internal circadian rhythms naturally follow a 25-hour schedule. That is, in the absence of external influences, humans begin to sleep one hour later each evening and awaken one hour later each day (Ferber; 1985; Lamberg, 1984).

The development of a diurnal sleep-wake pattern is dependent upon maturation of the CNS as well as the infant's ability to become entrained by environmental cues. Indicators of environmental time, called zeitgebers, include the 24-hour light-dark cycle, the timing of meals, and social contacts (Okawa and Sasaki, 1987; Czeisler et al., 1981; Goetz et al., 1976; Wever, 1979; Vernikos-Danellis and Winget, 1979).

Common Sleep Problems

A helpful way to view sleep problems in children is from a developmental framework. Maturation is known to influence sleep structure, the development of a diurnal pattern, the length of sleep episodes, and

Table 19–3. SLEEP CYCLES OF CHILDREN*

Full-term infants	Sleep time ranges between 10 and 23 hours per day (average 17 hours)
	Usually sleep in periods of 3–4 hours
	Night awakenings common through first year
	Non-REM sleep is not differentiated into stages
	May progress from wakefulness directly into REM sleep
	50%–95% of total sleep time (TST) is spent in REM sleep
	Usually begin to sleep through the night at 6–8 months
1 year olds	Sleep about 12 hours per night with a morning and afternoon nap
	Non-REM sleep begins to be differentiated into stages
	Sleep cycles are 45–60 minutes in length
	30%–40% of TST spent in REM sleep
	Sleep about 10–13 hours per night
2 to 5 year olds	Begin experiencing nightmares
	Decrease in nap time to elimination after age 5
	Sleep cycles are 45–60 minutes in length
	Boys require more TST than girls
	REM sleep time increases while time in Stages III and IV decreases
8 to 12 year olds	Sleep between 8.5 and 10 hours per night
	Generally play hard and sleep soundly
	The 90-minute adult sleep cycle is firmly in place
12 to 14 year olds	Sleep time is about 8.5–9 hours per night
	Hormonal changes with growth spurts increase the need for sleep
	REM sleep is 20% of TST
15 year olds	Sleep time is 7–8.5 hours per night
	Adult sleep cycle fixated
	Stage I is 5% of TST
	Stage II is 50% of TST
	Stage III is 10% of TST
	Stage IV is 10% of TST
	REM sleep is 20–25% of TST

*Adapted with permission from Barndt-Maglio, B. Sleep pattern disturbance. Dimensions of Critical Care Nursing, 5:342–349, 1986.

the total amount of time asleep (Richman, 1987). The prevalence of sleep difficulties also shows developmental trends.

Barnard (1974) has established the following criteria to identify sleep problems: (1) the inability to maintain an eight-hour sleep duration after three months of age; (2) recurring problems (more than three times a week) of getting to sleep for naps or night sleep; or (3) parental perception that there is a sleep problem (p. 145). For infants, sleep problems relate to the time of getting to sleep and nighttime awakenings. Both of these problems are related to establishing a sleep routine since sleep needs and patterns change during this period.

The toddler experiences several sleep-related problems, including increased difficulty in getting to sleep. At this age, the child frequently demands parental presence at bedtime; therefore, consistent routines are important. Changes in these routines are likely to cause increased difficulties in going

to sleep. Night awakenings are common at three years of age (Barnard, 1974). During the preschool years, enuresis is common, and during the school-aged years, nightmares are common. Anxiety-provoking events may precipitate nighttime fears, dreams, or nightmares at any age.

Longitudinal studies of children who had sleep pattern disturbances in the first year of life revealed persistent sleep problems into the toddler and preschool years (Jenkins et al., 1984; Bernal, 1973; Blurton-Jones et al., 1978). Results regarding the persistence of problems of night awakenings vary; however, correlates for waking problems at different ages are reportedly low in school-aged children. Infants who were described as irritable slept little and cried frequently; they were also more likely to be poor sleepers during the second year of life (Bernal, 1973; Blurton-Jones et al., 1978). Richman (1987), in a review of studies related to persistent wakers aged one to five years, concluded that "persistent wakers could be particularly susceptible to irregular sleep patterns because of neurophysiological or temperamental factors" (p. 124).

A common cause of sleep disturbances in infants and young toddlers is a prolonged need for feedings in the middle of the night (Schmitt, 1981). This need is far more common in breast-fed babies, who become accustomed to small, frequent feedings. These infants become hungry every three to four hours and are unable to maintain the eight- to ten-hour fast that nighttime sleep demands (Schmitt, 1985). Many parents introduce solid foods at the last evening feeding to help the young child sleep through the night; however, the literature contains no evidence to support the practice of giving solid foods to prolong nighttime sleep intervals (Beal, 1969).

Individual differences in temperament have also been demonstrated to affect sleep-wake patterns. Weissbluth and colleagues (1985) found that poor adaptability, high intensity, and negative mood were all related to decreased total sleep duration. At age three, children who were more adaptable, mild, and positive in mood tended to have longer total sleep durations. The sensitive infant may have difficulty filtering out or habituating to external environmental stimuli and thus may arouse easily. An intense child may have difficulty relaxing and falling asleep.

Variables which influence sleep patterns of hospitalized children can be divided into three clusters: (1) physiological, (2) psychological, and (3) environmental. Physiological variables include pain, sensory impairment, medications, feedings, CNS dysfunction, or internal biological rhythms such as hormone levels and body temperature. Psychological factors include individual differences in temperament, separation from family, change or loss of routines and rituals during hospitalization, fears regarding self-mutilation, and even the fear of death. Pre-existing psychological stressors create excessive anxiety and worry in the child who is in a strange setting. A child may be admitted to the hospital with a sleep pattern disturbance which has been reinforced by parental mismanagement at home.

Psychological stress that is due to hospitalization and illness contributes significantly to sleep-wake pattern disturbances.

The child's separation from parents and anxiety related to the presence of unfamiliar persons and surroundings interfere with the latency period, and frequent awakenings throughout the night are common (Monroe, 1967). The most likely etiology for fearful night crying is separation anxiety (Breziz et al., 1980). In addition, the absence of or alteration in sleep rituals may prolong the latency period and result in nighttime awakenings. Bedtime rituals serve as cues to sleep for the child and also provide a sense of security and relaxation.

Pre-existing psychosocial stressors, including parental discord, financial stress, or chronic illness, also contribute to sleep pattern difficulties. A child may be able to suppress worries during wakeful periods, but they come to awareness as defenses relax during sleep states. These worries may be so intense that they prevent the child from falling asleep or cause fearful nighttime awakenings. Fears of self-mutilation and death and the inability to accurately mentally process treatments performed on other children in the hospital are also contributory because "young children in particular possess little knowledge or past experience that facilitate their understanding of events that resemble nightmares" (Barndt-Maglio, 1986, p. 345).

An interruption in circadian rhythm may also result in a sleep pattern disturbance. This biological cycle affects body temperature and cortisol levels. Both drop off early in the night and rise to higher levels just prior to awakening in the morning. If the child is requested to awaken when these levels are still low, difficulty in arousal results. Similarly, difficulty in falling asleep results if body temperature remains elevated. The inherent length of the circadian cycle is 25 hours, and it must be "reset" every day through consistent mealtimes, bedtime, and time of arousal. If disrupted through poor scheduling or procedures, the child may sleep poorly at night and experience behavior difficulties during the day (Ferber, 1985).

Ferber (1985) has noted that all children learn to associate certain conditions with falling asleep. These conditions include lying in a particular position with the noise or lighting at a particular level, holding a favorite toy or blanket, or taking other preferred comfort measures. If children awaken during the night and the conditions are the same, they are likely to return to sleep. Unfortunately, some sleep associations a child develops can result in difficulty in returning to sleep when the conditions are absent upon awakening. Such associations include being held or rocked to sleep, having a back rub until sleep is achieved, falling asleep while being fed, or falling asleep while an adult is in bed with the child. If the child awakens and the conditions have changed, arousal to a heightened state occurs.

The hospital environment itself poses sleep hazards. Environmental conditions which adversely affect normal sleep-wake patterns during hospitalization include poorly established light-dark differences, the continuous noise of monitors and staff conversation, exposure to activities or treatments on other patients, and treatment protocols which mandate frequent interruption of sleep. However, the impact that each of these has upon a child is extremely variable. Desynchronization of circadian rhythms is an intense, commonly occurring phenomenon in critical care units. Critical care personnel use the term ICU psychosis to describe the symptomatology of desynchronization and behavior disturbances resulting from frequent interruption of sleep. Symptoms of this disorder include disorientation, irritability, fear, and paranoia. Nursing care contributes significantly to frequent disruptions of sleep of hospitalized children. Korones (1976) noted that "it is by accident rather than by intent, that infants (hospitalized in the NICU [neononatal intensive care unit]) are left at rest." Duxbury and colleagues (1984) state, "Nurses are the caregivers who can best intervene to promote rest and sleep by minimal interference of the naturally occurring state cycles" (p. 147).

Sleep pattern disturbance is a frequent side effect of drugs prescribed for pain relief (Barndt-Maglio, 1986). Barbiturates, which are commonly used for sedation and pain relief in postoperative patients, tend to decrease REM sleep (Schmitt, 1985). Both meperidine (Demerol) and morphine decrease REM sleep (Kales and Kales, 1970), whereas diazepam (Valium) decreases REM as well as Stage III and IV non-REM sleep (Kleitman, 1972). It is important to note that these drugs may have a paradoxical effect of increasing excitability and restlessness in children.

Sedatives are not effective when used alone in the management of sleep pattern disturbances if parents continue to reinforce poor sleep habits; however, they may be helpful when used in conjunction with behavioral management or environmental manipulation. Chloral hydrate is a useful sedative because it facilitates relaxation and eases sleep stage transitions with minimal effect on REM sleep (Barndt-Maglio, 1986).

Drugs used for treatment of specific conditions may also interfere with normal sleep cycles. Conversely, the internal circadian rhythm may affect the metabolism of some drugs in the system. For example, aspirin taken at 7:00 a.m. remains in the system 22 hours; however, when taken at 7:00 p.m., aspirin is used up five hours sooner (Lamberg, 1984). A documented side effect of digoxin is violent nightmares (Breziz et al., 1980). Drugs used to treat reactive airway disease, such as theophylline and metaproterenol (Alupent), are stimulants which may interfere with sleep. Sometimes the drug itself may not be the cause, but the liquid base acts as a stimulant (Ferber, 1987b). Studies on the effects of methylphenidate (Ritalin) on sleep have been inconclusive; however, when given late in the day, Ritalin has been noted to cause a prolonged latency phase in sleep (Ferber, 1987b).

Sleep difficulties may be more common in selected populations, such as children with juvenile rheumatoid arthritis, who awaken frequently because of the pain experienced when changing sleep positions, or children with obstructive sleep apnea, who experience sleep fragmentation (Weissbluth et al., 1983). Postoperatively, children may have difficulty falling asleep because of pain and stiffness. Further, the incision may inhibit them from assuming their normal sleep position (Barndt-Maglio, 1986). Newborn infants with jaundice and those born to diabetic mothers have been noted to sleep significantly more than normal infants (Duxbury et al., 1984).

Children with central nervous system disorders, such as mental retardation and cerebral palsy, often have disturbed sleep patterns exhibited by disordered sleep-wake rhythm, sleep apnea, delirium, insomnia, or hypersomnia (Ferber, 1985; Okawa and Sasaki, 1987). Irregular sleep-wake rhythms have been observed in some children with Down syndrome, severe mental retardation, and autism. These symptoms are attributed to dysfunction or destruction of specific areas of the brain responsible for generating sleep and sleep-wake rhythms (Ferber, 1985).

ASSESSMENT

Assessing established sleep habits during the initial phases of hospitalization can assist the nurse in planning care which will promote adequate rest and sleep and minimize the negative effects of hospitalization. Data gathered should result in a well-defined data base which describes the child's normal sleep-wake cycle and sleep routine and provides a statement regarding the child's chronological age and expectations for sleep. The optimal time to gather this information is during the admission process. Most often, questions related to sleep habits focus on the usual bedtime, time of morning arousal, and frequency of naps. Specific information relative to the schedule and length of naps, bedtime rituals, the occurrence of nighttime awakenings, and parental management of sleep behavior is often not obtained. The following questions, adapted from Barndt-Maglio (1986), serve as a general guideline for assessing sleep patterns; this information needs to be documented in the admission history and can then serve as a reference point for comparison of the child's sleep-wake cycle during hospitalization.

1. What time does your child usually go to bed at night?
2. What time does your child usually arise in the morning?
3. What is your child's usual routine before retiring for the night?
4. Does your child have a special blanket or toy that he/she usually takes to bed?
5. How long does it usually take for your child to get to sleep?
6. In what position does your child usually sleep?
7. Does your child often wake up and have difficulty falling asleep? If so, how many times per night, per week?
8. What helps your child return to sleep once awake?
9. How well would you say your child sleeps at night?
10. Does your child take naps? If so, at what time of day?

Research has demonstrated that change in sleep-wake cycles occurs as the result of neurological maturation; age-based norms have been established. Therefore, the admission history should also include a statement about the child's sleep habits compared with others of his age. This process allows for early identification of a sleep pattern disturbance so that intervention can be planned at the outset of hospitalization. A reference chart which lists the norms according to age should be available on the nursing unit for all nurses. In this way, reinforcement of norms and awareness of these norms by all nurses can be increased.

An assessment tool to document a child's sleep pattern is the Nursing Child Assessment Sleep Activity record (NCASA) developed by Barnard (1979). This tool (Fig. 19–1) allows the nurse to objectively record a child's sleep-wake behavior over a period of seven days. From these data, patterns of sleep behavior emerge, the child's response to intervention can be consistently recorded, and caregivers can begin to look more objectively at their responses to the child. A seven-day recording is used to describe average sleep behavior. Symbols are used to indicate those activities which are being monitored. The record begins at noon so that the nighttime hours are presented in an uninterrupted manner. The afternoon-evening period is on the left of the chart, the nighttime hours in the middle, and the morning hours on the right. This order facilitates comparison of morning, afternoon-evening, and nighttime activities of the child. The five columns on the right side of the chart can be used to record 24-hour summaries, such as total amount of sleep, duration of longest night sleep, duration of longest day sleep, how many times intervention was required by the caregiver to get the child back to sleep, and so on. Drugs administered to the child should also be recorded to look for possible effects on sleep-wake patterns. The results obtained within each section can be summarized to describe typical sleep behavior and compare the sleep patterns with age-based norms (Ferber, 1985). In addition to identifying actual periods of sleep, it is also important to record the length of time it takes the child to fall asleep once he is placed in bed. The NCASA is useful to monitor the child's response to intervention, allowing for a systematic, consistent approach to documentation.

CAREGIVERS USUAL BEDTIME _11 PM_
CAREGIVERS USUAL AWAKENING _6 30AM_

CHILD'S NAME _SMITH   JOE_
LAST NAME   FIRST NAME
BIRTH DATE _1-8-84_
DATE OF RECORDING _7-13 → 15 -87_

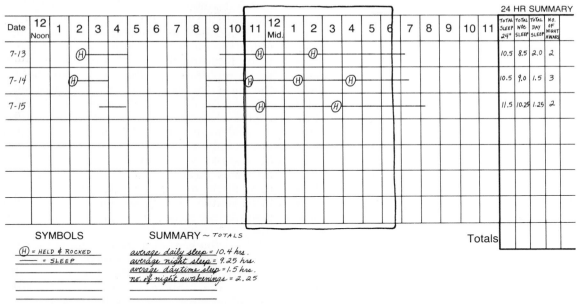

Date	12 Noon	1	2	3	4	5	6	7	8	9	10	11	12 Mid.	1	2	3	4	5	6	7	8	9	10	11	TOTAL SLEEP 24°	TOTAL NOC SLEEP	TOTAL DAY SLEEP	NO. OF NIGHT AWAKS
7-13			Ⓗ										Ⓗ		Ⓗ										10.5	8.5	2.0	2
7-14		Ⓗ											Ⓗ		Ⓗ		Ⓗ								10.5	9.0	1.5	3
7-15													Ⓗ			Ⓗ									11.5	10.25	1.25	2

SYMBOLS

Ⓗ = HELD & ROCKED
—— = SLEEP

SUMMARY ~ _TOTALS_

average daily sleep = 10.4 hrs.
average night sleep = 9.25 hrs.
average daytime sleep = 1.5 hrs.
no. of night awakenings = 2.25

Totals

Developed by the University of Washington, School of Nursing NCAP Project.

Figure 19–1. Nursing Child Assessment Sleep Activity record. (Copyright © Kathryn Barnard. From the Nursing Child Assessment Satellite Training Program developed by Dr. Kathryn Barnard, University of Washington School of Nursing, 1979.)

Data obtained from the NCASA can be used to determine if defining characteristics for the nursing diagnosis of *Sleep pattern disturbance* exist. Kim et al. (1984) list some defining characteristics that are appropriate for infants and young children. These characteristics include interrupted sleep, awakening earlier or later than desired, increased irritability, restlessness, disorientation, listlessness, frequent yawning, and dark circles under eyes. However, these characteristics may require increased specificity for children, and this specificity is offered in the NCASA. Criteria from the defining characteristics of sleep pattern disturbance and the NCASA can also be used to evaluate the effectiveness of the intervention of sleep promotion.

The primary goal of the nurse in promoting sleep is establishment of a regular sleep pattern as is indicated by (1) a sleep-wake cycle that is consistent with the child's normal lifestyle, (2) a sleep-wake pattern that is appropriate for the child's chronological age, and (3) an established sleep routine.

INTERVENTION STRATEGIES

Once a data base has been established and an actual or potential sleep pattern disturbance has been diagnosed, the nurse can then initiate intervention strategies aimed at maintaining or restoring the normal sleep pattern. The NCASA or other evaluation tools can be utilized to document the child's response to the intervention. Necessary alterations in the plan can then be introduced and the response again documented.

Establishing and Maintaining a Sleep Pattern

If the initial assessment indicates the absence of a sleep disturbance, the nurse needs to maintain the child's daily routine to prevent the development of a sleep disturbance that is due to the stresses inherent in the hospital environment and expected routine changes. Routine sleep pattern maintenance can be accomplished by posting a daily schedule at the child's bedside and documenting it in the nursing care plan. All members of the health team as well as parents should be informed of this schedule and should participate in its implementation. This schedule provides a sense of order to hospitalization, which can be fairly chaotic. If the child requires procedures or medications, these should be scheduled between the child's normal periods of sleep. For the seriously ill child who requires frequent or continuous monitoring of vital signs or procedures, these activities should be planned in clusters to reduce the number of sleep disruptions. When possible, 60- to 90-minute sleep intervals should be scheduled to allow for completion of one sleep cycle (Barndt-Maglio, 1986). The child's need for sleep should be maintained as a priority.

The plan of care should include increasing the awareness of parents and other health care providers about the importance of adhering to established routines, special sleep difficulties which may result from the child's condition, and methods to promote relaxation. Their assistance in promoting the child's sleep is a necessary adjunct to nursing care.

Social contacts, particularly the presence of parents, are critical for the maintenance of a child's normal daily routines during hospitalization. Meaningful parental activities, such as bathing the child, reading to the child, or simulating home activities with the child, offer cues to the child as to time of day and provide a sense of order. Typical hospital activities, laboratory tests, x-rays, or physical assessment are unfamiliar to the child and frequently occur haphazardly. They offer no structure or cues to synchronize sleep-wake patterns. Because of these problems, hospitalized children may experience sleep deprivation or incomplete sleep cycles that affect health restoration. For example, shortened REM or minimal deep sleep may adversely affect healing and recovery. Therefore, the importance of synchronizing the external environment with a child's normal routines is especially important during hospitalization.

A special population of children who may pose a unique pattern of sleep disturbance are those children who require continued nutrition through the night. These children include the failure-to-thrive population, who consume inadequate calories during the normal daytime hours, and children with short-gut syndrome, who require continuous gastric infusion of formula. The latter group may be able to maintain a continued sleep state despite the infusion of formula, provided the nurse is quiet and does not physically interrupt the child's sleep as the feeding is monitored. In the former population, the need for increased calories must take priority over the child's need for uninterrupted sleep, but a plan should be implemented to minimize the length and degree of disruption. The volume of daytime feedings can be increased so that a smaller volume may be consumed during the night. A nasogastric tube can be placed during the last evening feeding so that the nighttime feedings are given through the tube while the child sleeps.

When the goal of a feeding program is to establish improved oral intake, this should be accomplished while the child is normally awake; oral intake during the nighttime should be minimized. For the infant who is admitted with frequent nighttime awakenings for feedings, the nurse can instruct the parents to begin increasing daytime feeding intervals to four hours or more, thereby conditioning the infant to prolong the sensation of hunger and tolerate increased volumes of formula (Schmitt, 1985). During the day, demands for feeding can be decreased by use of a pacifier, extra holding, and rocking. Once daytime feeding intervals are normalized, the night feedings can be phased out by decreasing the volume of formula by one ounce every few nights until the infant no longer awakens for a nighttime feeding.

For infants and children experiencing pain, the incorporation of analgesics or comfort measures to minimize pain facilitates sleep. If at all possible, intravenous lines should be placed in areas which will minimize abnormal positioning. This is especially important for the young child who routinely self-comforts through thumb or finger sucking.

Other positioning strategies can be used to decrease sleep interruptions from pain. For the child with limited mobility or who is confined to bed rest, the nurse should decrease skin irritation and positional discomfort by padding the bed with an eggcrate-like pad. Assisting the child into a comfortable or normal sleep position through the use of pillows for support or bracing of painful areas will also facilitate comfort and subsequent sleep.

Children with vision or hearing problems have special needs. Maintenance of daily routines utilizing activity and auditory cues is of prime importance for the visually impaired child, who cannot rely on light and dark differences to enhance sleeping habits; therefore, morning arousals, mealtimes, and sleep routines must be firmly maintained. In addition, because of the keen olfactory and hearing senses of these children, noxious stimuli should be avoided. The nurse should turn monitor alarms to a low volume and place the child in a private or semiprivate room away from the nurses' station and other areas where noise levels are high. For the hearing-impaired child, use of visual and activity cues to enhance sleep should be incorporated into daily routines. Dimming of lights, screening the child from viewing painful procedures done on other children, and avoiding excessive visual stimulation through bright pictures and television near bedtime should be considered. Soothing activities which facilitate relaxation should be incorporated into the bedtime ritual.

Children with neurological disorders such as mental retardation and autism often have disturbed sleep-wake rhythms (White et al., 1983). Factors which may contribute to the disturbance must be examined carefully before appropriate intervention can be initiated. These factors include parental overprotection with resulting poor sleep associations, reinforcement of night awakenings, and medications the child may be taking. The nurse should not assume that the sleep disturbance is part of the neurological disorder and is, therefore, not treatable because it may be a separate entity which can be managed in the same way as sleep disturbances in other children. However, "in a number of children, the brain damage is in itself the cause of the sleep problem" (Ferber, 1985, p. 97). Minimal improvement may be obtained through restructuring daily routines and altering parental response so that nighttime awakenings are not reinforced. Sedative medications such as chloral hydrate, when used in conjunction with behavioral therapy, may result in more satisfactory sleep habits. The need for this must be clearly documented, and careful monitoring of the child's response to any medication is mandatory to justify its continued use. Parents of children with brain damage should be taught about the need to maintain consistency in daily routines and methods to minimize reinforcement of nighttime awakenings. In addition, the nurse should refer the parents for consultation with an expert if the child's sleep difficulties continue to be disruptive and interfere with family functioning.

Facilitating Sleep

Since common causes for distress and sleep disturbances in the hospitalized child are separation from parents, deviation from normal routines, and anxiety related to fears of death and mutilation, nursing intervention must be directed towards the psychological needs of the child to facilitate rest and sleep (White et al., 1983). "Restful sleep cannot be achieved until the need for security is met" (Barndt-Maglio, 1986, p. 343). The child's optimal adjustment to hospitalization will occur if the parent is able to room-in and offer the child emotional support. However, this is not always possible, and alternate forms of support must be utilized. The nurse needs to assess the child's developmental age to identify other types of support that would be most effective.

For infants and young children, security can be offered in the form of being held close and rocked during the day and evening. The use of a blanket, a stuffed animal which the child can hold, or a familiar lullaby may ease the stress of separation. For the preschooler and school-aged child, opportunities to express fears and act out feelings about the hospital experience can be provided. This expression can occur through imaginary doll play; use of puppets; drawings; or through direct, supportive interviews with the child. If parents are unable to stay with the child, they should be encouraged to leave pictures of themselves and siblings or friends, familiar toys, and familiar clothes so that the child may maintain some sense of contact with home. The use of these transitional objects assists the child in feeling relaxed and helps the child to rest and fall asleep more readily.

The use of a tape-recorded story which can be played at the child's bedside each evening may also minimize separation anxiety and resultant sleep difficulties. Several authors (Wear, 1974; Hennessy, 1976) have suggested the use of telephone calls or tape-recorded messages by the parents to decrease separation anxiety. White and colleagues (1983) found playing of a story tape-recorded by a parent appeared to have a soothing effect on children, helping them to fall asleep and maintain a longer sleep duration than those children who did not have a story read. The children who had heard the story also demonstrated increased self-consoling behaviors as an apparent means to cope with separation and the hospital experience.

If at all possible, any painful or anxiety-producing treatments should be avoided prior to scheduled sleep or rest periods. Painful procedures create excessive anxiety in children, which does not end with the experience. The child may begin to associate the pain with sleep and may become afraid to fall asleep. This same anxiety and fear may result if the child witnesses a procedure used to treat a neighboring hospital patient. Curtains should be drawn or the child removed from the room to avoid exposure to the treatments of others. In addition, the child's bed should remain "safe" for the child, with all painful procedures conducted in a separate treatment room.

Sleep rituals deserve special attention, as they are of paramount importance in treating sleep disturbances. A bedtime ritual may be defined as the activities in which the child normally engages to facilitate sleep. These activities serve as cues as the child learns to associate them with sleep. During hospitalization, the child's bedtime rituals need to be maintained. If the parents have not utilized a bedtime ritual for the child prior to hospitalization, the nurse can teach parents about the importance of this and work with the parents to develop an acceptable routine to be followed during hospitalization. Parents should also be informed that although rocking a child and offering a bottle as part of the ritual is an acceptable practice, the child should be placed in the bed awake and without a bottle so that he learns to rely on himself to actually fall asleep. If the child then awakens during the night, he is more likely to be able to get himself back to sleep without relying on rocking or the bottle. The nurse also needs to teach parents about using calming behaviors within the nightly ritual and avoiding activities which increase stimulation to the child such as tickling, wrestling, and watching television.

For the child who is very sensitive to environmental stimuli and slow to adapt to change, the nurse needs to manipulate the environment to minimize stimulation and maintain firm adherence to routines for the child. Placing the child in a private or semi-private room where the noise level and lighting is minimal is recommended. The nurse should anticipate the child's awakening during the night and be available to offer reassurance so that a quick return to sleep can be achieved. The nurse should avoid picking up the child or offering any form of reinforcement which may also bring the child to a more alert state, prolonging the waking interval. As these children may also have negative moods, the nurse needs to allow for adequate rest to prevent fatigue, which increases irritability.

Light and dark differences which coincide with daytime and nighttime routines should be provided for all hospitalized children. Lights should be turned on and dimmed at the same time each day, and the volume of alarms and staff conversation should be decreased at night. If a 24-hour parent visitation policy is allowed, parents should be informed of the importance of visiting at consistent times during the day or evening and avoiding visits when the child has gone to sleep at night. If several parents are rooming-in with their children in open wards, they should all be encouraged to keep their late-evening and nightly conversations to a minimum. Television should be curtailed at an early evening hour for preschoolers, and violent programs should be restricted. For school-aged children and adolescents, television may be incorporated into the bedtime ritual. However, violent or anxiety-producing programs should be avoided. If parents wish to view late-night television, they should do this in a separate parent's lounge.

For the child who has emotional difficulties and a secondary sleep disturbance, the nurse needs to assess the nature of the emotional problems and enlist appropriate resources for management of these problems. Childhood depression is often manifested as sleep problems in the form of a prolonged latency period and frequent night awakenings. The child may have difficulty sleeping because of worry about a variety of stressors at home. Again, these need to be assessed further and intervention directed toward the primary problem, because sleep disturbance may be only a symptom of another problem.

Behavior Management Strategies

Traditional methods to resolve sleep disturbance problems have included establishment of consistent bedtime routines; firm limit setting at settling-in times, with physical separation from the parent; use of transitional objects; use of behavior modification techniques; administration of sleep-inducing medications; and parental counseling (Schumann, 1981). Hagemann (1981) conducted a descriptive study of 34 preschool and early school-aged children to address sleep duration and sleep disruption in hospitalized children. Results indicated children lost one fifth to one fourth of their usual sleep time while hospitalized. Delay in sleep onset produced the greatest loss of sleep. The study cited the absence of established presleep routines and the lack of deliberate comfort measures by nurses, which could have facilitated the children's ability to sleep.

Some children may prolong the latency phase of sleep by getting out of bed and requesting a drink of water or additional attention by the caretaker. The caretaker should calmly place the child back into bed and tell him that he must stay in bed or the curtains will be pulled around his bed or the door will be shut. If the child gets out of bed again, the caretaker needs to follow through in pulling the curtains or shutting the door and leaving the child's room. If after one minute the child remains in bed, the door or curtain can be opened. This sequence needs to be repeated if the child gets out of bed again, increasing the door or curtain closure to two minutes, then three minutes, and up to a five-minute maximum. The child needs to learn that persistence in getting up does not pay off in terms of getting what is desired. The caretaker needs to remain calm and nonthreatening to the child during this process. Threats or scoldings may result in a power struggle and increased anxiety in the child, which may further exacerbate the problem.

A reward system can be used alone or in conjunction with the above process. The child can obtain stars or stickers which are placed on a poster at the child's bedside for compliance with the bedtime routine. A bigger reward, such as an additional story at bedtime or one-to-one attention for a special game or play activity, may be earned by the child who receives five stars. This reward system needs to be highly individualized since what is rewarding to one child may not be to another. Such a strategy allows the nurse to learn more about the child's interests and gives the child some control in the hospital setting.

For the child who awakens during the night, the nurse should go to the bedside to make sure the child is not experiencing any pain or discomfort and offer calm reassurance to help the child return to sleep. If the nurse picks the child up or spends an extended period of time talking or playing with him or her, nighttime awakenings are inadvertently reinforced and are more likely to recur. The nurse should also instruct the parents in how to manage these nighttime awakenings.

If a child awakens with nightmares or complains of fears while trying to go to sleep, the nurse should offer calm reassurance and comfort to dispel the child's fears. Occasional nightmares are common in all children and reflect emotional conflicts the child experiences during developmental transitions or unresolved feelings related to frightening or threatening events. In the hospitalized child, nightmares are apt to occur more frequently than in the normal population because the child is exposed to many frightening or threatening procedures, many of which occur while the child is in bed. Intervention by the nurse depends upon the child's age but always involves measures which offer reassurance. The toddler or infant will respond best to physical comforting, such as being held and calmly rocked. The child under two years of age has no conception of what a dream is, so that he or she will not respond to verbal explanations of the event. For the older toddler, reassuring words and physical comfort should be used. The nurse should listen sympathetically as the child describes his or her dreams or fears. By age three or four, the child can be reminded that it was only a dream and not an actual event, but the child's fear still needs to be treated with reassurance and empathy. Opportunities which allow the child to express fears and aggression during daily play activities should be provided. For more pervasive fears which result in continual or frequent nightmares, the nurse should recommend that professional counseling for the child be obtained.

The nurse needs to determine if the child is experiencing a nightmare or a night terror (Ferber, 1985). The nurse should avoid waking the child who is experiencing a night terror; she should avoid asking the child to describe this "dream." Instead, the nurse ought to allow the episode to run its course, anticipating that the child will soon return to sleep. The child may respond aggressively if the nurse interferes with the episode. If a child is frequently experiencing night terrors, the physician should be informed because, although temporal lobe epilepsy is a rare occurrence, night terrors may be a manifestation of this type of pathology (Guilleminault, 1987).

Relaxation

The unfamiliar surroundings of the hospital coupled with the effects of illness and surgery increase the amount of sleep needed, yet also provide an environment less conducive to sleep. Techniques to induce sleep by promoting neuromuscular relaxation continue to be studied. Beardslee (1976) found that touch provides comfort and relaxation which promote sleep. A biochemical explanation of how muscular relaxation promotes sleep has been introduced. According to the monoaminergic theory proposed by Jouvet (1974), elevated levels of serotonin appear as a result of an increased breakdown of neurotransmitters (monoamines), which occurs with muscle relaxation. The increased levels of serotonin are believed to lower brain cell activity, which subsequently decreases stimulation of the CNS and promotes sleep.

Based on these findings, a step-by-step plan to induce relaxation and sleep by touch is described by Schumann (1981). The first step is to create an environment conducive to relaxation. Measures to consider include reducing noise level and lighting, maintaining a constant temperature, providing nonrestrictive clothing and fluids to quench thirst, and making sure the child has an empty bladder. The child then needs 15 minutes to settle down. Activities such as looking at a book, listening to music, or talking to a doll assist in reducing muscle tension. Nurses should be positive, patient, and persistent in encouraging relaxation. Also, a key word can be chosen to convey relaxation to the child; suggested words include *heavy, slow, droopy, easy,* or *loose.* The nurse should use one word or phrase to show or tell the child what to expect; the nurse can say, for example, "you will feel so heavy that you can't move your legs." The nurse should use the same example consistently.

The relaxation process begins by stretching the body from head to toe while arching the back. The child next takes a cleansing breath by inhaling deeply through the nose and exhaling through the mouth while assuming a comfortable position. Using a quiet, even voice with few inflections, the nurse begins to help the child relax each part of the body. Repeatedly, about six to eight times, the nurse states that the body part is "heavy." At the same time, the nurse strokes the body part firmly with two hands, beginning with the toes and proceeding through the following sequence: toes, feet, legs, back or stomach, fingers, hands, arms, shoulders, neck, eyes, lips, and chin. Each muscle group is examined for tenseness. When the nurse is moving from one area to another, the child is reminded to keep previously relaxed areas feeling heavy. The nurse's words convey positive reinforcement and are said in a monotone. Once the body has been sequenced, the child is likely to be in the early stages of sleep. The nurse should stay by the bedside for two to three minutes to ensure the child will not awaken. If the child is drowsy or awake at the end of the sequence, the nurse should repeat the routine without touching each body part. In general, the younger the child, the more important is the use of touch.

Discharge Planning

A discharge plan incorporating potential sleep-wake pattern disturbance is important given the disruption hospitalization causes in the life of a child and family. The crisis of hospitalization for the child coupled with the heightened anxiety of the parents regarding the child's well-being makes the transition to home difficult.

Although no studies reviewed documented sleep-wake disturbances following hospital discharge, health care providers are becoming aware of this potential, given the difference between hospitalization and established sleep routines of home. Salzarulo and Chevalier (1983) conducted a retrospective study of 218 children, ages two to 15 years, who had experienced disorders of sleep-wake rhythms of at least three months' duration. Results indicated that children experienced significantly more night wakings and enuresis from two to five years of age; nightmares occurred more frequently in children six to ten years. Parental anxiety related to the child's illness and hospitalization also contributed to the potential for sleep-wake rhythm disturbances of the child. According to Ferber (1985), "If the parents fail to recognize and respond properly to the child's signals of an emerging circadian rhythm, or if they fail to provide regular input by which the child can adapt, significant sleep disturbances may appear" (pp. 165–166). Parents anxious about providing home care for the child who has just been discharged may subtly reinforce maladaptive sleep patterns or inappropriate sleep associations. The parents may be so worried about the child's medical condition and related treatments that they misinterpret the origin of the sleep problem.

Aspects of the child's illness itself, prescribed medications, common sleep problems associated with various ages, and pre-existing psychosocial and emotional problems in the home may also contribute to sleep-wake disturbances. Green (1984) found that sleep problems were commonly characteristic of the vulnerable child syndrome. The parent unwittingly keeps the child awake each night through a series of visual, auditory, and tactile stimuli that arouse the child, thus reassuring the parent that the child is alive.

The discharge plan should include information about normal sleep patterns at specific chronological ages and common sleep problems of different age levels, strategies for establishing a consistent sleep routine for the child, a review of appropriate sleep associations to fit the lifestyle of the child and family, descriptions of prescribed medications which may interfere with or promote sleep, discussion of aspects of the illness which may affect sleep, and strategies to alleviate sleep disturbances. It is important to reassure parents that sleep-wake disturbances are not uncommon during childhood following a change in established routines. In fact, parents should anticipate sleep disturbances in children who are experiencing a change in their health, daily routine, or environment.

EVALUATION

Evaluation of intervention strategies to treat sleep disturbances is an integral part of the treatment plan. Evaluation data not only ascertain the effectiveness of the intervention but also are the basis of recommendations to continue, modify, or discontinue care. Reaching the outcome goals may require time; therefore, daily monitoring and recording of sleep behavior and related variables using a tool such as the NCASA will show small behavior changes that may not be evident otherwise. Such information gives nurses and parents evidence of progress, however slow, and movement toward the outcome goals. This is encouraging to parents who may need support while working to modify their child's sleep pattern.

Sleep disturbances are usually the result of a unique combination of factors, requiring individualized planning and treatment for each child and family situation. Therefore, evaluation needs to take into account the special needs or health problems of the child, his or her developmental level, the etiology of the problem, the family situation, and the individualized care plan. When a combination of strategies is used, it may be difficult to evaluate whether success or failure of the treatment plan was due to one specific strategy or a combination of strategies. In a research setting, it may be possible to isolate strategies to determine which strategy most likely produced the desired effect or if the best outcome was achieved from two or more strategies in combination. However, this process is time-consuming and may not be practical in a clinical or home setting where prompt treatment is necessary to reverse a sleep problem that is disruptive to the health of the child or the functioning of the family.

CASE STUDY

Adam was a three year old admitted to the pediatric intensive care unit following an emergency appendectomy. His postoperative course was complicated by peritonitis and infection of the surgical incision, which were treated by intravenous antibiotics and dressing changes four times a day. Postoperative pain was managed with intravenous Demerol every four to six hours.

By the fifth postoperative day Adam was irritable and difficult to comfort. His sleep-wake patterns were poorly organized, characterized by frequent daytime naps and multiple nighttime awakenings.

Review of assessment data collected from his mother upon admission indicated no sleep problems. Information regarding normal hours of sleep, bedtime routines, and the length and times of daily naps was unavailable in the history. The primary nurse gathered data about Adam's regular sleep patterns prior to hospitalization. Adam had reportedly been sleeping from 9:00 p.m. to 7:00 a.m. without waking during the night. He occasionally took a one-hour midafternoon nap. He was accustomed to sleeping with a stuffed bear and night light. This history indicated a consistent sleep routine and no sleep pattern disturbances prior to hospitalization.

The nurse next gathered data relevant to Adam's current sleep disturbances to determine the etiology of this hospital-related problem. The nurse began a four-day recording of Adam's sleep-wake activities using the NCASA, documenting periods of sleep, the administration of medications, dressing changes, and parent visitation. She also summarized the nurses' responses to Adam's nighttime awakenings. Results from the NCASA indicated multiple interruptions of Adam's nightly sleep for procedures, including dressing changes, monitoring vital signs, and administering medications. There were minimal day-night differences in sleep patterns. No bedtime routines had been initiated to facilitate night sleep. Parental visitation usually occurred from midafternoon through early evening and was restricted to 30 minutes every other hour. None of Adam's toys, including his favorite bear, was available to him. Documentation of the nurses' response to his nighttime awakenings indicated that analgesics were administered routinely because his awakenings and crying were interpreted as being due to pain. No sedatives or behavioral techniques to facilitate relaxation had been instituted. The nurses had spent time talking with Adam to offer emotional support and reassurance during and following procedures. Assessment of environmental factors indicated that the lights were dimmed at the same time (9:00 p.m.) every evening and turned back up at 6:00 a.m. However, monitor alarms remained at the same volume, and the level of activity and staff conversation remained fairly consistent across the 24-hour period.

A nursing diagnosis of *Sleep pattern disturbance* was made after review of assessment data. It appeared that the etiology of Adam's sleep-wake pattern disturbance was a combination of physiological, psychological, and environmental factors. Contributing physiological factors included interference with Adam's circadian rhythm, continued use of narcotic analgesics, and abdominal pain. Psychological factors included the stress of hospitalization, Adam's separation from his parents and familiar routines, and the absence of established sleep routines. Environmentally, very few day-night differences in noise and activity levels were noted, and Adam's sleep was repeatedly interrupted for procedures and caretaking activities.

To manage Adam's sleep-wake pattern disturbance, the nurse worked with Adam's mother to establish an acceptable daily routine which would allow for periods of uninterrupted sleep and clear differences in his day-night activities. This schedule was posted at his bedside. Monitor volumes were turned down when the lights were dimmed each evening; bedtime routines, consisting of a story read by his mother while Adam held his favorite bear, were established. The mother was also encouraged to bring in some of Adam's toys and family pictures which he could look at in his parents' absence. Dressing changes, vital sign checks, and administration of medications were decreased to one time each night to allow for only one necessary interruption of Adam's sleep. A minimum interval of 90 minutes between interruptions was attempted if Adam needed to be awakened. If he awakened between times, the nurse was instructed to offer physical and emotional reassurance while the lights remained off, encouraging Adam to return to his former sleep state. An order for choral hydrate was requested to promote sleep and was alternated with Demerol every four hours as needed to relieve pain and fatigue. In addition, the primary nurse reviewed the neuromuscular relaxation technique with Adam's mother; both the staff and parents were encouraged to implement this strategy when Adam experienced difficulty getting to sleep.

Documentation of Adam's response to these interventions heightened the awareness of the nursing staff and parents of Adam's gradual improved sleep pattern. Adam became less irritable and more relaxed, and complained of less pain over the course of a few days. He became more cooperative when his nighttime ritual was initiated and settled in more easily for sleep. The need for medication to facilitate sleep and ease pain was reduced within two days of these interventions. After several days, the defining characteristics for the diagnosis reversed, indicating the effectiveness of the intervention.

RESEARCH IMPLICATIONS

A review of studies on sleep problems reveals numerous difficulties in collecting reliable, valid data and comparable results. It is important to note that there seems to be an absence of consensus of what constitutes a sleep problem and how this varies with age. One difficulty which exists is measuring duration and frequency of sleep problems over time; much of our current data rest upon retrospective parental report. Anders (1978) found parents underreported night awakenings in the young children. This problem may also exist for older children, who are able to self-console and thus may not report night awakenings to the parents. Other factors which enter into parental report variability include parental expectations of what is normal as well as social, cultural, and family influences. Cultural differences in sleep habits are important to note. In Japan, a mother and her children sleep in one room and the father in another, whereas in India the family sleeps together on one large mat. As the children near school age, they are suddenly thrust into sleeping alone, with a period of emotional readjustment ensuing. These factors must be considered when comparing rates of sleep difficulties in different cultures (Brazleton et al., 1987).

According to Richman (1987), information about social expectations and norms related to sleep patterns or sleep problems is minimal. In addition, children who participate in specialized sleep clinics may differ from those in the general population in terms of both family and social characteristics since middle-class families who can afford the costs are more likely to attend these clinics.

The limitations of existing reports on sleep problems are also found in the few studies that have been done on hospitalized children. Further, most studies are retrospective in design and dependent upon parental report (Richman, 1987). Similarly, sleep difficulties at home following hospital discharge may be underreported by parents as these difficulties may seem expected or less important when compared with the life-threatening illnesses children have experienced while hospitalized.

Examples of research questions to ask include the following:

1. Do parents, in fact, overlook sleep problems because of worry over the child's health status?

2. Are sleep-wake disturbances expected during hospitalization, and, therefore, not reported when the disturbance continues after discharge?

3. What nursing strategies to promote sleep and rest during hospitalization are needed for clinical practice?

4. Does sleep occur simply by chance in populations of other ages, as reported by Korones (1976) in the neonatal population?

5. What intervention strategies do nurses employ, perhaps unknowingly, to promote sleep?

In addition, nurses need to know the influence of several variables on sleep: (1) Aside from sleep deprivation and sleep-wake pattern disturbance which have been recorded during hospitalization, what are other common sleep problems specific to developmental age, disease condition, immobility, or treatment?; (2) Which of these are amenable to nursing intervention?; and (3) What impact does length of hospitalization or severity of disease have upon the development of sleep difficulties?

Finally, also lacking are research studies that test intervention strategies designed to promote sleep in children, comparing what strategies are effective at different age levels. Studies of interventions that are specific to special populations of children, for example, children with specific physiological or psychiatric disorders and children treated with medications that have the potential of altering sleep patterns, would be particularly helpful to nurses in their clinical practice. Knowledge of strategies that promote sleep in infants and children is also essential to counsel parents in preventing as well as treating sleep disturbances in children. Such empirical data are the foundation of nursing practice; information that is vital as the nursing profession matures and more clearly articulates its methods of promoting sleep in children. Since there is so little known about sleep in the hospitalized child, nurses have an opportunity to contribute to the knowledge base in this area through research.

References

Anders, T. Home recorded sleep in two- and nine-month-old infants. Journal of the Academy of Child Psychiatry, 17:421–432, 1978.

Anders, T, and Keener, M. Developmental course of nighttime sleep-wake patterns in full-term and premature infants during the first year of life. Sleep, 8:173–192, 1985.

Anders, TF, and Keener, MK. Sleep-wake state development and disorders of sleep in infants, children and adolescents. In Levine, M, Carly, W, Crocker, A, and Gross, R (Eds.), Developmental-behavioral pediatrics. Philadelphia: WB Saunders Co., 1983, pp. 596–606.

Aserinsky, E, and Kleitman, N. Regularly occurring periods of eye motility and concomitant phenomena during sleep. Science, 118:243–274, 1953.

Baker, T. Introduction to sleep and sleep disorders. Medical Clinics of North America, 69:1123–1152, 1985.

Barnard, KE (Ed.). Nursing child assessment training (NCAT) sleep activity manual. Seattle: The University of Washington School of Nursing, 1979.

Barnard, KE. Sleep patterns. In Barnard, KE, and Douglas, HB (Eds.), Child health assessment, Part I: A literature review. Bethesda, U.S. Dept of HEW, 1974, pp. 137–148.

Barndt-Maglio, B. Sleep pattern disturbance. Dimensions of Critical Care Nursing, 5:342–349, 1986.

Beal, VA. Termination of night feeding in infancy. Journal of Pediatrics. 75:690–691, 1969.

Beardslee, C. The sleep-wakefulness pattern of young hospitalized children during naptime. Maternal-Child Nursing Journal, 5:15–24, 1976.

Bernal, J. Night wakings in infants during the first fourteen months. Developmental Medicine and Child Neurology, 15:760–769, 1973.

Blurton-Jones, N, Rosetti-Ferreira, MC, Farquar-Brown, M, and McDonald, L. The association between perinatal factors and later night-waking. Developmental Medicine and Child Neurology, 20:427–434, 1978.

Brazleton, TB, Johnson, CD, and Wood, S. Ain't mis-behavin': Supporting the developing needs of young families. Presentation at Methodist Hospital of Indiana, Indianapolis, 1987.

Breziz, M, Michaelis, J, and Hamburger, R. Nightmares from digoxin. Annals of Internal Medicine, 93:639–640, 1980.

Castiglia, P. Growth and development. Journal of Pediatric Health Care, 1:48–49, 1987.

Czeisler, CA, Richardson, GS, Zimmerman, JC, Moore-Ede, MC, and Weitzman, ED. Entrainment of human circadian rhythms by light-dark cycles: A reassessment. Photochemistry and Photobiology, 34:239–247, 1981.

Dement, W, and Kleitman, N. Cyclic variations in EEG during sleep and their relationships to eye movements, body motility, and dreaming. Electroencephalography and Clinical Neurophysiology, 9:673–690, 1957.

Denenberg, V, and Thoman, E. Evidence for a functional role for active (REM) sleep in infancy. Sleep, 4:185–191, 1981.

Duxbury, ML, Broz, L, and Wachdorf, C. Caregiver disruptions and sleep of high-risk infants. Heart and Lung, 13:141–147, 1984.

Ferber, R. Solve your child's sleep problems. New York: Simon and Schuster, Inc., 1985.

Ferber, R. Circadian rhythym and schedule disturbances. In Guilleminault, C (Ed.), Sleep and its disorders in children. New York: Raven Press, 1987a, pp. 165–174.

Ferber, R. The sleepless child. In Guilleminault, C (Ed.), Sleep and its disorders in children. New York: Raven Press, 1987b, pp. 141–163.

Goetz, F, Bishop, J, and Halberg, F, et al. Timing of single daily meal influences relations among human circadian rhythms in urinary cyclic AMP and hemic glucagon, insulin and iron. Experientia, 32:1081–1084, 1976.

Green, M. Sleep disorders. In Green, M, and Haggerty, R. (Eds.), Ambulatory pediatrics (Vol. 3). Philadelphia: WB Saunders Co., 1984, pp. 249–252.

Guilleminault, C. Disorders of arousal in children: Somnambulism and night terrors. In Guilleminault, C (Ed.), Sleep and its disorders in children. New York: Raven Press, 1987, pp. 243–252.

Hagemann, V. Night sleep of children in a hospital, Part I: Sleep duration. Maternal-Child Nursing Journal, 10:1–13, 1981.

Hennessy, J. Hospitalized toddlers' responses to mothers' tape recording during brief separation. Maternal-Child Nursing Journal, 5:69–91, 1976.

Jenkins, S, Owen, C, Bax, M, and Hart, H. Continuities of common behavior problems in preschool children. Journal of Child Psychology and Psychiatry, 25:75–89, 1984.

Jouvet, M. The role of monoaminergic neurons in the regulation and function of sleep. In Petre-Quadens, O, and Schlag, JD (Eds.), Basic sleep mechanisms. New York: Academic Press, Inc., 1974, pp. 207–236.

Kales, A, and Kales, J. Evaluation, diagnosis and treatment of clinical conditions relative to sleep. Journal of the American Medical Association, 213:2229–2235, 1970.

Kim, MJ, McFarland, GK, and McLane, AM. Pocket guide to nursing diagnosis. St. Louis: CV Mosby Co., 1984.

Kleitman, N. Sleep and wakefulness. Chicago: University of Chicago Press, 1972.

Korones, SB. Disturbance and infants' rest: Iatrogenic problems in neonatal intensive care. Report on the Sixty-ninth Ross Conference on Pediatric Research. Columbus: Ross Laboratories, 1976.

Lamberg, L. The American Medical Association: Guide to better sleep. New York: Random House, Inc., 1984.

Lozoff, B, Wolf, A, and Davis, N. Sleep problems seen in pediatric practice. Pediatrics, 75:477–483, 1985.

Milner, J. Management of infant sleeping problems. Midwife, Health Visitor and Community Nurse, 18:98–100, 1982.

Monroe, LJ. Psychology of good and poor sleepers. Journal of Abnormal Psychology, 12:255–264, 1967.

Nagera, H. Sleep and its disturbances approached developmentally. The Psychoanalytic Study of the Child, 21:393–447, 1966.

Okawa, M, and Sasaki, H. Sleep disorders in mentally retarded and brain-impaired children. In Guilleminault, C (Ed.), Sleep and its disorders in children. New York: Raven Press, 1987, pp. 269–290.

Oswald, I. Sleep, the great restorer. New Scientist, 23:170–172, 1970.

Parmelee, AH, and Stern, E. Development of states in infants. In Clemente, C, Parpuro, D, and Mayer, F (Eds.), Sleep and the maturing nervous system. New York: Academic Press, Inc., 1972, pp. 199–228

Richman, N. Surveys of sleep disorders in children in a general population. In Guilleminault, C (Ed.), Sleep and its disorders in children. New York: Raven Press, 1987, pp. 115–125.

Salzarulo, P, and Chevalier, A. Sleep problems in children and their relationships with early disturbances of the waking sleeping rhythms. Sleep, 6:47–50, 1983.

Schmitt, BD. Infants who do not sleep through the night. Journal of Developmental and Behavioral Pediatrics, 2:20–23, 1981.

Schmitt, BD. When baby just won't sleep. Contemporary Pediatrics, 2:38–52, 1985.

Schumann, MJ. Neuromuscular relaxation: A method for inducing sleep in young children. Pediatric Nursing, 7:9–13, 1981.

Vernikos-Danellis, J, and Winget, CM. The importance of light, postural and social cues in the regulation of the plasma cortisol rhythms in man. In Reinberg, A, and Halberg, F (Eds.), Chrenopharmacology. New York: Pergamon Press, Inc., 1979, pp. 101–106.

Wear, E. Separation anxiety reconsidered: Nursing implications. Maternal-Child Nursing Journal, 3:9–18, 1974.

Weissbluth, M. Sleep duration, temperament, and Conners' rating of three-year-old children. Developmental and Behavioral Pediatrics, 5:120–123, 1984.

Weissbluth, M, Hunt, CE, Brouillette, R, Hanson, D, David, R, and Stein, I. Respiratory patterns during sleep and temperament ratings in normal infants. Journal of Pediatrics, 106:688–690, 1985.

Weissbluth, M, Davis, AT, Poncher, J, and Reiff, J. Signs of airway obstruction during sleep and behavioral, developmental, and academic problems. Developmental and Behavioral Pediatrics, 4:119–121, 1983.

Wever, RA. The circadian system of man: Results of experiments under temporal isolation. New York: Springer-Verlag, New York, Inc., 1979.

White, MA, Wear, E, and Stephenson, G. A computer compatible method for observing falling asleep behavior of hospitalized children. Research in Nursing and Health, 6:191–198, 1983.

CHAPTER 20

PAIN MANAGEMENT

MARILYN SAVEDRA, D.N.S., R.N.,
JOANN M. ELAND, Ph.D., R.N., and
MARY TESLER, M.S., R.N.

Pain is part of the life experience of almost all children. For some, as in the case of children who suffer from sickle cell disease, pain may dominate much of life, with one sickle cell crisis following another. For others, pain is a prevailing factor for an extended time during treatment of a major burn or cancer. Most children have brief, intermittent episodes of pain that are associated with everyday bumps and bruises, common childhood illnesses, routine immunizations, or a surgical procedure. And then there are those who experience loss, uncertainty, doubts, and fear and equate the feelings engendered by these experiences with pain.

This chapter addresses pain from the perspective of children. Theories of pain are presented, with implications for assessment and intervention. A case presentation high-

lights the factors that influence how pain is experienced and demonstrates strategies for assessing and intervening when pain is part of illness and treatment. Although children may equate pain with an emotional state, this chapter will focus on pain associated with a physical injury.

THEORETICAL FOUNDATION

Definition of Pain

There is no one definition of pain. The most widely accepted definition is that proposed by the International Association for the Study of Pain, which states that pain "is an unpleasant sensory and emotional experience associated with actual or potential tissue damage or described in terms of such damage" (Merskey, 1979, p. 249). This definition acknowledges that pain is more than a physical sensation and is undesirable. Although few would challenge the idea that pain is unpleasant, it is only in recent years that the emotional or affective component of the pain experience has been taken into consideration.

From a nursing perspective, McCaffery's definition that "pain is whatever the experiencing person says it is, existing whenever he says it does" (McCaffery, 1979, p. 11) acknowledges that pain exists for a child if he or she says it does even when a physical cause cannot be identified. This definition does not, however, take into consideration the situation of infants and young children, who cannot verbally communicate the experience of pain.

Associated with the definition of pain are three terms that are closely related: (1) pain threshold: the lowest stimulus value producing the report of pain; (2) pain tolerance level: the lowest stimulus level producing the report of no longer being able to tolerate pain in duration or intensity; and (3) sensation threshold: the lowest stimulus value at which a sensation is felt (Melzack and Wall, 1982). Although sensation threshold is uniform in adults, there are marked differences in pain threshold and tolerance levels (Melzack and Wall, 1982). Ethical consideration prohibits controlled tests of pain threshold and tolerance in children, yet empirical evidence seems to point to a range of threshold and tolerance levels for pain. Haslam's findings (1969) from a study of pain tolerance in 115 school children, ages five to 18 years, suggest that pain threshold increases with age.

Pain is also defined as acute or chronic. Acute pain is of shorter duration and is associated with trauma, surgery, diagnostic tests, treatments, and pathology of a specific condition, such as a ruptured appendix. Chronic pain extends over a time period greater than six months and may lead to a state of disability.

Theories of Pain

Understanding how pain is transmitted is important to the diagnosis and management of pain. New discoveries are constantly expanding knowledge of pain and changing some commonly held beliefs. The earliest belief that specific pain receptors, fibers, and tracts relayed pain sensations to specific pain centers in the brain is no longer a tenable theory. The existence of phantom limb pain following surgical intervention is a prime example that demonstrates that this simple stimulus-response theory does not provide an adequate explanation. In contrast to the specificity theory, pattern theory states that pain is caused by excessive stimulation of nonspecific fibers that produces a pattern of nerve impulses interpreted as pain. This theory, too, has been refuted by research that indicates there is a high degree of receptor and fiber specialization.

The gate control theory first proposed by Melzack and Wall in 1965 is currently the theory most widely accepted to explain the perception and transmission of pain and the mechanisms behind the effectiveness of intervention strategies for pain relief. This theory takes into account physiological specialization, temporal and spatial patterning in information transmission, and the influence of psychological processes. It proposes that mechanisms in the dorsal horns of the spinal cord act as a gate, permitting or inhibiting the flow of nerve impulses from the peripheral fibers to the central nervous system, depending on the extent to which the gate is open. When the gate is closed, pain impulses cannot be transmitted to the brain. More specifically, the gate control model proposes that cells in the gelatinous substance of the spinal column (the gating site) act on the signals transmitted by the large-diameter (A-beta) and small-diameter (a-delta and C) fibers and modulate the input before it is acted upon by the transmission (T) cells. The gating mechanisms are influenced by the relative activity in the sensory fibers, with input from the large fibers closing the gate and input from the small fibers opening the gate. The output of the T cells must reach a certain level before the message of pain can be transmitted to the brain. Additionally, structures in the brain, thalamus, brain stem, and cerebral cortex, which control cognitive processes such as attention, emotion, and memory, influence the gating mechanism and thus have an impact on the T cells and the consequent transmission of pain (Fig. 20–1). This theory provides a conceptual basis for pain in the

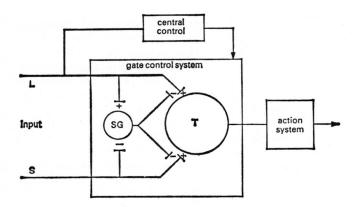

Figure 20–1. The gate control theory: Mark II. (From Melzack, R., and Wall, P. D. *The challenge of pain*. New York, Basic Books, Inc., 1982. Reprinted by permission.)

presence of injury (gate opened by small fiber stimulation) or the absence of injury (gate opened by cognitive processes), as well as in the relief of pain (rubbing an injured part activates large-fiber activity, which diminishes the ability of small-fiber activity to open the gate).

Shortly after the gate control theory was proposed, it was demonstrated that stimulation of the periaqueductal gray matter of the brain stem of the rat produced analgesia (Reynolds, 1969) and, subsequently, that opiate receptors exist in several areas of the human body. This led to the search for and discovery of narcotic-like substances, the endogenous opiates, that are produced in the body and may be responsible for altering pain perception. Research in this area is ongoing.

Pain Dimensions: Tools and Strategies

Pain measurement in the infant and child has always been a difficult task. Because of the personal nature of the experience, another can never fully know what is felt by the child. A determination of the child's pain is colored by the nurse's personal experiences with pain. Yet measurement is critical to establish the diagnosis of pain and intervene effectively.

Four dimensions of pain must be considered in the assessment process: intensity, quality, location, and chronology. Additionally, answers must be sought to the questions of what aggravates or eases the pain and what factors are present that may influence how the pain is perceived by the child.

Location

For the child who can understand and who is suspected of having pain, the first step is to tell the child to "show me where it hurts." The directive to "show me" versus "tell me" is useful in avoiding the possibility that the young child may not give the correct location because the proper terminology is not known. Even a toddler can point to a place that hurts. The body outline, a tool used with adults (Melzack, 1983; Margolis et al., 1986) has potential for use with children. Research has shown that children as young as six years can mark the location of internal body parts (Porter, 1974). Building on the work of Eland (Eland and Anderson, 1977), Savedra and colleagues (in press) have evaluated the reliability of a body outline to assist hospitalized children eight to 17 years old to communicate the location of their pain. Findings indicate that children accurately mark the location of pain they report. Although some tools use figures with hair and clothing (Varni, personal correspondence), children have no problems when these are omitted and are provided with figures similar to those on the McGill Pain Questionnaire but developmentally proportional to a child's body. It is important to provide a front and back and to note right and left sides since young children may find it difficult to visualize right and left body sides. Children should be encouraged to shade in the area of the body that has pain.

Eland (1973) provided children with eight crayons. Children were asked to select crayons that represented different amounts of pain and to use the appropriate crayons to show on a body outline where they hurt. Information provided by the children related to pain intensity as well as location. It is not unusual for a child asked to mark his or her pain on a body outline to mark several sites (Eland, 1986a; Savedra et al., in press). This process may provide a more complete listing than when a child is asked to point to where it hurts. When children are too young to show where it hurts or to mark an outline, behavioral indications such as tugging or rubbing a part may be the only indication of where the pain is felt.

Intensity

After the location of pain has been noted, information about the intensity of the pain is sought, such as whether the pain is mild, moderate, severe, or unbearable. Since intensity is subjective, the most valid assessment should include the child's report. Several tools have been used with children, including the Hester Poker Chip Tool (Hester, 1979), in which one chip represents a "little bit" of hurt and four chips the most hurt the child can have; the Pain Ladder (Jeans and Johnston, 1985), in which the first of nine rungs represents the least pain; the Oucher (Beyer and Aradine, 1986), in which a series of faces showing pain gradations is correlated with a numerical scale (Fig. 20–2); and the Molsberry Hurt Thermometer (Molsberry, 1979).

There are several types of scales for assessing pain intensity, including the visual analogue scale (VAS), graphic rating scales, numerical scales, and color scales. The simple descriptive tool devised by Keele (1948) uses words, including such words as absent, mild, moderate, and severe, and numbers (a scale of zero through ten). Adaptations for children are the Hester Poker Chip Tool and the Oucher just mentioned.

A simple descriptive tool is easy to administer and interpret and is understood by young children once the concept of small versus large has been acquired. The major disadvantage is that responses are limited to the number of choices presented. When words are used, they must be appropriate for the age of the child. For example, the young school-aged child may not understand the term moderate but would be more likely to understand the term medium. Chips, figures, and faces are more concrete than words or numbers and allow the child to use sensory and motor skills in addition to cognitive skills.

The VAS is a straight line with a marker at both ends representing no pain and the worst pain possible. Varni and colleagues (1987) have adapted the scale by placing a sad face at one end and a happy face at the other end. Compared with the simple descriptive scale, this scale is more sensitive, allowing the child to mark at any point on the ten centimeter line. The scale may be horizontal or vertical. For accurate measurement, the child must place a perpendicular mark on the line. Children aged five and over can usually manage this type of scale (Scott et al., 1977). Savedra et al. (1987), in a study of 958 children and adolescents, reported that eight to 17 year olds had no difficulty using the VAS and that there was a high degree of correlation between VAS markings and markings on four other commonly used scales. The children indicated, however, that of the five scales, this was the least preferred and hardest to use.

Graphic rating scales use a 10-centimeter (cm) line but are divided by markers or words. The Pain Ladder and the Molsberry Hurt Thermometer are adaptions of this type of tool for use with children. The authors have found that even when hospitalized, school-aged children are able to easily use this type of scale (Savedra et al., 1988a; Abu-Saad and Holzemer, 1981). Compared with simple descriptive scales, graphic rating scales have greater sensitivity, but they are less sensitive than the VAS.

Color scales use a gradation of colors or encourage children to assign colors to pain. Eland (Eland and Anderson, 1977) has employed this latter technique, whereas Savedra et al. (in press) have evaluated a scale similar to the Stewart Color Scale (Stewart, 1977). The colors range from yellow to bright red, yellow being a color rarely associated with pain and red being the color most frequently associated with pain (Savedra et al., 1982; Abu-Saad, 1984b, 1984c, 1984d). Nonhospitalized children reported that this scale was the most preferred and easiest to use of the five scales presented; hospitalized children, when given a choice of five scales, in most instances selected a word-graphic rating scale (Savedra et al., 1987).

Repeated markings over time on any scale produce a pain profile. In addition to being used to assess pain per se, they may be used to assess the amount of distress associated with pain or to assess the effectiveness of pain-relieving measures.

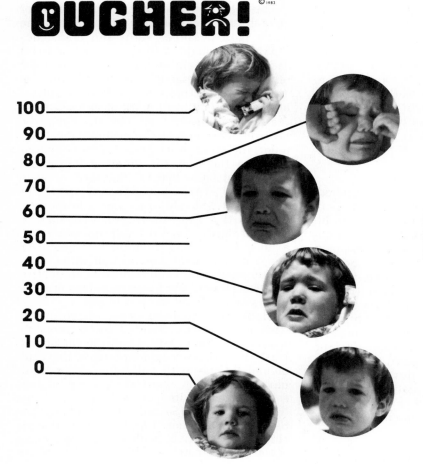

Figure 20–2. The Oucher. (Copyright © Judy Beyer. From The University of Virginia Alumni Foundation, 1983.)

Quality

The quality or nature of pain and the pain experience is assessed by listening to the words the child uses to describe his or her pain. The McGill Pain Questionnaire includes 78 words that describe sensory qualities in terms of temporal, spatial, pressure, thermal, and other properties; affective qualities in terms of tension, fear, and autonomic properties that are part of the pain experience; and the subjective overall intensity of the total pain experience with evaluative words (Melzack, 1975). The tool has been used with adolescents but is not developmentally appropriate for younger children. A word list appropriate for children eight through 17 has been developed and tested (Tesler et al., 1987). Word lists are particularly useful for children who are less articulate. Word recognition is greater than word usage. Word lists also may help children to use words that have been recently acquired.

Chronology

Observing and recording pain in relation to time is important to establish a chronology of pain. Chronology involves assessing the onset and duration of pain and factors that precipitate or alleviate the pain. It is important to establish when the pain began and to identify factors related to the possible cause of the pain. In assessing the duration of the pain, consideration is given to when the pain first occurred and how long a given episode of the pain lasts. That is, is the pain continuous or intermittent? If the child is able to verbally communicate, this information is best gathered by asking questions. Older children are able to indicate what they do to relieve pain (Tesler et al., 1981).

Myths and Beliefs about Pain

Inaccurate beliefs about pain in children often hamper the process of identifying and determining the nature of pain. Foremost is the myth that children do not experience pain with the intensity of an adult because of an immature nervous system. At the extreme is the belief that infants do not feel pain. Current research on responses of the infant to a pain stimulus refute this belief (Owens and Todt, 1984; Johnston and Strada, 1986; Dale, 1986).

A second myth that children cannot communicate accurately about the nature and location of their pain may result in not seeking the child's input about this subjective experience. Savedra et al. (1988a), conducting a study of children eight to 17 years of age who were experiencing pain, have found that the children could mark their pain on a body outline accurately, indicate the intensity on a scale, and provide words to describe the nature of their pain. Ross and Ross (1983), in a study of 944 children five to 12 years old, reported that children *were* able to describe pain they felt, often using graphic words to describe the nature of the pain.

A third myth, that children do not remember pain, although related more specifically to the intervention phase of the nursing process, may affect assessment as well. The need to identify the affective and evaluative components of pain may be viewed as unnecessary if the pain experience is expected to be soon forgotten. Levy's (1960) finding that fear is displayed by previously inoculated infants as young as six months of age at the sight of a needle and syringe during preparation for an inoculation suggests that the very young have a memory for pain. Nine to 12 year old children reporting what had caused them pain in some instances indicated that the painful experience had occurred when they were much younger (Savedra et al., 1981).

The belief that pain exists because an adequate stimulus is present may cause the nurse to disregard pain for which no stimulus is noted. A myth that is more applicable to adults and older children than to the very young is that it is possible to identify the person who is faking pain from the person who is a true pain sufferer.

Problems Related to Pain Measurement

Aside from the myths that exist, there are several problems that influence the measurement of pain. The primary problem is the limited potential for accurately assessing the intensity of pain in children who cannot talk or whose language is limited. The tools available are untested, and operational definitions of the behaviors need refining (Craig et al., 1984; McGrath et al., 1985). Some strategies require special equipment and are time-consuming, making them more appropriate for research than clinical practice (Levine and Gordon, 1982; Johnston and Strada, 1986). Exciting approaches to this problem are found in the works of Oster (1972) and Izard and colleagues (1980; 1982), who have explored the configuration of facial movements to assess pain in infants. For children who can verbalize, it is possible to tell what they experience only to the extent they are willing to share it with others. Some children view pain-relieving injections as more frightening than the pain itself. The inability to determine if behavioral and physiological changes are due to pain alone or are the result of fear and anxiety is troublesome. Although fear and anxiety may occur in the absence of pain, severe pain is almost always accompanied by distress.

ASSESSMENT

The nurse's role in making a diagnosis of *Altered comfort* or *Pain* is to gather physiological and behavioral data that are related to pain. Depending upon the circumstances and setting, the nurse may be involved in compiling a detailed pain history or may focus only on gathering data related to the four dimensions of pain. The assessment and measurement of pain is an ongoing process that precedes and follows intervention to relieve or eliminate pain.

Physiological responses, more common with acute than with chronic pain, include increased blood pressure; tachycardia; skin color changes, such as flushing or pallor; diaphoresis; hyperventilation; pupil dilation; and nausea and vomiting. The unfamiliar and unexpected sensation triggers the fight-or-flight reaction, resulting in blood shifts from viscera and superficial vessels to organs essential for muscular exertion. Heart contractions are increased, bronchioles dilate, and gastric secretions are inhibited (Cannon, 1929).

Behavioral responses to pain include crying; moaning; screaming; verbalizations such as "owie" and "it hurts"; and facial expressions including a tense or worried look, frowning, and squinting. Body expressions may provide evidence for a specific location of pain, as when a child clutches or rubs a body part or keeps a specific body part still. The child may make every effort to prevent a painful area from being touched or manipulated. General inactivity or restlessness, or inappropriate or unexplained body movement may also signal the presence of localized or diffuse pain.

Behavior observation tools focus on behaviors specific to pain and provide information on the total pain experience. Examples of such scales are the Inventory of Pain Indicants (Smith, 1976) for use with preschoolers; the Pediatric Pain Inventory (Lollar et al., 1982), designed to measure pain perception in children four to 19 years of age; the Children's Hospital of Eastern Ontario Pain Scale (CHEOPS) (McGrath et al., 1985), which measures pain behaviors in children one to five years; and the Procedure Behavioral Rating Scale (Katz et al., 1980) for children eight months to 17 years. Drawings have also been used to better understand how pain is experienced by children, as noted by Denehy in Chapter 8 (Jerrett, 1985; Kurylyszyn et al., 1987).

The determination of the existence of pain seems to be most problematic when assessing infants and young children. In making a nursing diagnosis of pain, factors that influence a child's response to pain must be considered, including developmental stage, gender, ethnicity, and situational variables. With increasing age, pain behaviors are learned, and children become cognitively aware of the implications of specific responses as well as of the meaning of pain in terms of health and activity level. For example, children learn that pain may excuse them from chores or may prevent them from attending special events. Adolescents more than younger children equate pain with a psychological cause such as feelings of loss or incompetency (Savedra et al., 1988b). In a study of 39 children with juvenile rheu-

matoid arthritis, younger children reported the same sensations as the older children but not the unpleasant feelings (Beales et al., 1983).

Although little is reported in the literature on gender differences, the findings of Savedra et al. (1982) suggest possible sex differences in the feelings experienced while in pain. In a study of 214 children between the ages of nine and 12, girls more than boys stated that when in pain they felt like crying and actually cried, like crying but did not cry, sick to their stomach, embarrassed, or nervous.

Cross-cultural studies of pain in children are limited. Abu-Saad (1984a, 1984b), using an adaptation of a pain questionnaire (Tesler et al., 1983), studied what a limited number of Asian-American and Arab-American children said caused pain, the words they used to describe pain, the colors they ascribed to pain, the feelings they experienced when in pain, how they coped with pain, and what they said was good about pain. The findings were not that different from studies in which similar questions were asked of American children (Schultz, 1971; Tesler et al., 1981; Savedra et al., 1981, 1982). Although Zborowski's (1969) classic study of cultural differences of adults in pain suggests marked response differences, more research is needed to determine how ethnicity affects the responses of children to pain.

Several other factors related to pain, including the severity, duration, location, cause, degree of immobility imposed, and the body part involved, influence a child's reaction to pain and should be considered in the assessment process. The presence or absence of family may be an important factor in a child's response to pain. Having the mother or father close by may help the child to handle pain in a more controlled manner or may provide freedom to openly express feelings of distress.

THE INTERVENTION

Pain in children is most commonly caused by injury; disease; medical treatment; or nonspecific disease states such as migraine, abdominal pain, and limb pain (Varni et al., 1982). Despite the varying etiologies, almost all pain is amenable to and treatable by two interventions: (1) the use of nonpharmacological strategies, including sensory stimulation and cognitive-psychological measures, and (2) the use of drugs, which is the pharmacological approach (Melzack and Wall, 1982; McCaffery, 1979). The rationale for the use and effectiveness of drugs is based on the gate control theory; they either interrupt the transmission of the pain sensory impulse to the brain or alter the perception of the pain sensation by the brain.

More than one approach from each intervention may be used; that is, two nonpharmacological approaches, such as relaxation and distraction, could be combined. Also, pharmacological and nonpharmacological interventions could be combined; for example, heat, cold, or distraction could be used in conjunction with medication. Although parents, children, and nurses are aware of the effectiveness of many of the nonpharmacological interventions to pain relief and use them daily, these interventions have not been subjected to rigorous testing with children, and the literature in this area is scant. Some work is that of Jay and colleagues (1985). They tested the effects of a combined package of interventions: breathing exercises, reinforcement, imagery and distraction, behavior rehearsal, and filmed modeling on children's distress and reported pain during bone marrow aspirations. They reported that this multicomponent approach was significantly more effective than minimal treatment attention.

Nonpharmacological Strategies

The most common nonpharmacological approaches for acute pain relief are distraction, cutaneous stimulation, relaxation, and guided imagery (McCaffery, 1979). The last approach is akin to hypnosis; however, special training is required for hypnosis. Elements of these approaches often overlap, and one approach may include aspects of other strategies.

Relaxation

The goal of this strategy is to reduce the muscle tension that usually accompanies pain and to achieve a tension-free physical and mental state. McCaffery (1979) identifies several benefits that can arise from relaxation: stress reduction, decreased anxiety

level, distraction from pain, alleviation of muscle tension that causes pain, reduced fatigue, and facilitation of sleep. Regardless of the approach, there are four basic requirements for its success: (1) a distraction-free, quiet environment; (2) a position of comfort; (3) a point to concentrate upon; and (4) a passive attitude (Donovan, 1980, 1982; Benson et al., 1977; McCaffery, 1979; Jeans and Johnston, 1985). The approach also has been used successfully in dental treatment (Nocella and Kaplan, 1982).

Benson et al. (1977) suggest a simple approach for use by busy individuals or on a busy unit. They advise the nurse to ask the child to (1) close his or her eyes and sit comfortably and quietly; (2) deeply relax all muscles, starting at the feet and continuing to slowly relax the muscles as he or she moves up to the face; and (3) breathe through the nose saying "one" while breathing out. They recommend continuing the procedure for 20 minutes, but that may be too long for most children. Jay and colleagues (1985) instruct children to pretend they are a tire, to fill the tire with air by taking a deep breath, and then to slowly let the air out. The children are asked to repeat this breathing exercise. This approach is part of a group of interventions that are applied as a whole package of the activities described earlier.

Children can be taught relaxation techniques. The nurse should give simple instructions such as, "make your legs and arms like a rag doll" and then practice breathing techniques with young children to help them relax. Infants can be wrapped snugly in blankets and rocked. This reduces the painful stimuli and provides a comfortable position. Holding and rocking is also useful for toddlers. Older children can try more sophisticated methods, such as biofeedback and meditation. The relaxation approach is often combined with other interventions, such as distraction or guided imagery.

Distraction

This approach is described as focusing on any object, thought, or event inside or outside the body other than pain. Any concentrated effort that mentally blocks the pain stimulus and moves the perception of pain away from the center of awareness can be considered a distraction. Children are very resourceful in identifying distractions. Playing—alone, with other children, or with pets—watching television, playing games, reading, and visiting with other children and with family members are useful distraction approaches (Tesler et al. 1981). Other techniques include talking on the telephone and playing video, mental, or card games. Distraction techniques are often self-initiated by children. Younger children may suck their thumbs, play with favorite toys, or rock in their beds. Patients may also focus on physiological strategies such as slow, rhythmic breathing or rubbing parts of the body other than the pain site.

Distraction is a valuable tool for use with infants and young children, whose short attention span readily makes them able to concentrate on other interesting events and activities. Infants can be picked up, talked to, and moved about the room. Providing a pacifier may distract them. Toddlers can play simple games, such as saying "choo-choo-choo-choo" like a train or playing peekaboo. Preschoolers can sing simple songs and recite familiar nursery rhymes. School-aged children and adolescents are easily distracted by games or by stories they can read themselves. Because of the wide variety of choices available to the nurse and child, distraction is one of the most effective strategies for short-term or long-term pain relief of mild to moderate pain. It is important to remember, however, that the complexity of the distraction needs to be increased as the intensity of the pain increases (McCaffery, 1979; Jeans and Johnston, 1985). For example, although counting out loud could be a simple distraction, counting by twos or threes offers a more complex task. Venham and colleagues (1981) demonstrated its successful use in young dental patients.

Nurses need to be alert, however, to the fallacy of the common myth that because children are playing they are not in pain. In the absence of adequate assessment and appropriate treatment, distraction may be the only way children have of helping themselves. The nurse must consistently keep in mind the projected pattern of pain resulting from a specific therapy or condition and continually make assessments and provide needed medication in addition to encouraging distraction.

Guided Imagery

This approach focuses on the memory or visualization of a pleasant experience to re-duce pain intensity, distress, or fear. It differs from distraction in that imagery depends on mental rather than internal or external physical stimuli. Here the stimuli exist primarily in the mind. There is a fine line between this approach and biofeedback, relaxation, and hypnosis, for they share many common features. Unlike hypnosis, however, this process does not include altering the state of consciousness. The child is asked to concentrate on a pleasant memory or experience and is guided through the experience by the nurse or coach. Several helpful references provide descriptions of how to utilize guided imagery (McCaffery, 1979; Donovan, 1980; Chaves and Barber, 1974).

A simple example of guided imagery is asking the child to think of a place or an activity that is associated with pleasant memories. The nurse then engages the child in a description of going to the place (say, the beach or a ball game) and vividly describes what they see and do along the way or when they get there. Other activities include guiding the child through the mental experience of decorating a Christmas tree or baking cookies.

Some children are unable to implement these strategies for fear of losing control. The relaxation response may cause problems for children with cardiac or respiratory problems, since it reduces respiratory rates; its use should be carefully evaluated in these populations. Because of their active imaginations, children are especially adept at using guided imagery and, when carefully guided, can benefit from the interaction. However, both distraction and guided imagery may have to be simplified if a child is fatigued and has difficulty concentrating.

Hypnosis

Although not in the realm of routine nursing care, hypnosis has been found to be a useful tool in reducing pain in children. In fact, Zelter and LeBaron (1982) found it was more effective than distraction and self-control efforts in reducing the pain during bone marrow aspirations. Hilgard and LeBaron (1982) described the successful use of hypnosis with pediatric cancer patients. However, this strategy requires additional knowledge and skills on the part of the nurse, which indicates the need for special preparation.

Cutaneous Stimulation

The theoretical basis for the multiple approaches to pain relief under this category is not clear. It is believed that stimulation of the large A-beta and A-alpha fibers in the skin and muscles inhibits the input of the small A-delta and C pain fiber afferents in the dorsal horn of the spinal cord, similar to the T cell proposed by Melzack and Wall (1965). A second explanation is that the production of a counter pain stimulates endogenous opiate release. The placebo response also cannot be ruled out. Whatever the mechanism, cutaneous stimulation inhibits or reduces the pain stimulus transmission to the higher brain center (Melzack and Wall, 1982; Bishop, 1980; Wyke, 1985; Yaksh and Hammond, 1982; Fields, 1987).

Cutaneous stimulation includes a large category of measures that serve to stimulate or irritate other nerves, sometimes producing a counter pain and altering the transmission of the pain impulse. Research on the use of these approaches in children is not available, but adaptations from adult research for several measures appear to apply to children. The most common strategies for use with children include the use of massage, applying pressure, and the use of heat or cold. Eland (1986b) has reported the successful use of transcutaneous electrical nerve stimulators (TENS) with children undergoing bone marrow aspirations. Transcutaneous electrical stimulation is produced by placing small electrodes on selected areas of the body. The electrodes are attached to a small power source and, when activated, stimulate the areas under the electrodes, exciting large-fiber activity and reducing the stimulus transmission.

Rubbing over the painful area with long strokes or in circles has been known to reduce the intensity of the pain. If the painful area cannot be rubbed directly, the surrounding area, the contralateral area, or any other available area can be rubbed. Massaging can include the skin as well as the deeper tissues, depending on the location of the pain. The use of warm lubricants, lotions, or powder can reduce the friction between the hands and the skin. The effectiveness of this strategy is influenced by the emotional component associated with the intervention. Rubbing or massaging most often includes the ministering presence of another person whose actions can be seen as nurturing and caring and thus affects the emotional component of the pain perception.

Parents use cutaneous stimulation readily with infants and young children when dealing with the daily falls and scrapes of childhood. Picking up the child and rubbing his or her back, arm, or legs while talking to the child is often all that is needed to reduce the intensity of the discomfort. Older children often massage sore muscles resulting from athletic or active play activities, or to relieve stiff muscles from being in one position too long. The traditional back rub can reduce muscle stiffness and help a child sleep (McCaffery, 1977, 1979).

Heat and Cold

Hot compresses, hot water bottles, and heating pads are the most common ways to apply topical heat for the reduction of pain. Heat is believed to reduce pain associated with bruises, torn muscles, and arthritis by increasing the circulation to the area. The increased circulation augments the supply of the reparative nutrients needed and carries away the products of tissue damage. Another belief, likewise untested, is that heat can stimulate nerve impulses that stop the transmission of pain at the dorsal horn. Heat is also believed to increase the extensibility of collagen tissue and when combined with physical therapy can be helpful in the treatment of contractures and the associated pain (Melzack and Wall, 1982; Lehmann et al., 1974).

Many parents have helped relieve their child's pain by placing the child in a warm bath or applying a hot water bottle to the abdomen for stomachaches or to the head for earaches. Adolescent girls frequently relieve the intensity of their menstrual pain with heat. Also, both boys and girls find heat comforting for strained muscles and ligaments.

Cold, likewise, reduces pain intensity and is believed to work by reducing the rate at which the pain impulses are transmitted. Cold decreases the inflammatory response and edema. Both cold and heat reduce muscle spasms and decrease the intensity of the pain (Melzack and Wall, 1982; Lehmann et al., 1974). Eland (1981) successfully reduced the intensity of the pain associated with intramuscular injections for immunization in preschool children by spraying the area with a cooling agent prior to the injection. However, the application of both heat and cold must be used with great caution when children are concerned. Both therapies can cause burns, and when used with children who are unable to communicate their pain, the nurse needs to be doubly vigilant and monitor the patient frequently and carefully.

Preparatory Information

This intervention has been used extensively with children to reduce stress associated with hospitalization and procedures (see Chapter 6). Its use to reduce pain perception is based on its potential for reducing anxiety and fear that are concomitants of and increase pain in children. When children who have limited experience and preparation for pain encounter it, their response is often disproportionate to the event (Stoddard, 1982). Unless their anxiety is extremely high, children, with the exception of infants, need information about their illness and what they can expect. They need to know about the treatments: why they are needed and how they will be done, as well as a description of the sensory experiences, including any pain they will feel. The information, although it needs to be honest, should provide only relevant information and not overwhelm the child.

Johnson and colleagues (1975) demonstrated the effectiveness of providing both procedural and sensory information to children undergoing cast removal. This group showed significantly less distress than the control group, who received only procedural information. Siegel and Peterson (1980) used a similar preparatory program with similar results for children undergoing dental care. Filmed modeling using either a mastery or a coping approach has been described by Melamed et al. (1975) and Macher and Johnson (1974). Therapeutic play using medical equipment has been in practice for many years and is an important preparation because fear of needles still is one of the major concerns of children (Kassowitz, 1958; Lewis, 1978; Taylor and Williams, 1980). Fernald and Corry (1981) described two approaches, an empathetic and a directive approach, to prepare children for needles. The empathetic approach produced less distress. A helpful guide for age-specific approaches

has been prepared by Hansen and Evans (1981).

As more knowledge about children's responses to painful situations and a better understanding of children's coping has become available, measures that combine both information and strategies for children to help them cope with painful experiences have been developed. Wolfer and Visintainer (1975) reported a stress point preparation that described what was going to happen and what the child's role in the procedure was to be. Jay and colleagues (1985) have developed a specific procedural package for helping children cope with the pain of bone marrow aspiration. Using a preventive approach, Ross and Ross (1985) taught a group of third and fourth graders about pain, needle procedures, hospitalizations and training in cognitive coping strategies. Pretest and post-test scores showed that children's knowledge about pain could be significantly improved. They also describe a novel strategy of "thought stopping" as one of the methods of stress reduction in leukemic children. Thought stopping is a process that can help a child cope with impending painful procedures. With adult help, the child recalls previous similar procedures and lists all the positive facts about it that can be remembered: "The doctor can do it; the needle goes in fast; the needle is small." Next, all information about what the child can do is listed: "I can ask for a specific doctor; I can hold the nurse's hand; I can move my feet." These facts are summarized on a card and when the child starts thinking of the impending painful procedure, he stops and reads aloud or subvocally the positive and reassuring facts previously listed. The child then resumes normal activity and repeats the process if the upsetting thoughts reoccur. This strategy helps the child focus on the positive aspects of the situation (Ross and Ross, 1984).

Operant Conditioning

The chronic pain experience, unlike acute pain, is the result of a complex interaction of the neurophysiological experience, the subjective responses of children, and the pain behaviors of individuals as they interact with the cultural and environmental behaviors of others. Crying, moaning, asking for medication, withdrawing from role functions, and other pain behaviors elicit responses from others in the environment that can either reinforce or eradicate the pain behaviors (Masek et al., 1984; Melamed and Siegel, 1980). Fordyce and colleagues (1973) labeled these pain behaviors as operant behaviors and developed a program of behavior modification in which the environmental reinforcers of pain behaviors were eliminated and nonpain behaviors (decreased reports of pain, carrying out of roles, and decreased medication demands) were reinforced. Parental guidelines for managing the symptoms included encouraging normal behavior, discouraging pain behavior, and administering pain medication on a schedule rather than a *pro re nata* (p.r.n.) basis (Gross and Gardner, 1980; Masek et al., 1984). The environmental modification can be combined with self-regulation therapies (relaxation, biofeedback, and imagery) for the most comprehensive approach.

Pharmacological Management of Pain in Children

Pharmacological management of children's pain is predominantly achieved by the use of two classes of drugs: the opioids and the nonsteroidal anti-inflammatory drugs (NSAIDs). The first have their major mode of action in the central nervous system, and the second act peripherally in the body. Guidelines similar to those for adults for the use of these drugs, with smaller parameters of safety, apply to children. General guidelines restrict the use of narcotics to severe pain and recommend treating other pain with NSAIDs. Although both classes of drugs relieve pain, their modes of action and thus their administration and monitoring of both desired and undesired effects are different. NSAIDs provide excellent analgesia without the untoward effects of tolerance and dependence associated with narcotics.

The opioids, a term that encompasses the natural products of opium (morphine and codeine), the semisynthetic derivatives (heroin, hydromorphone, oxymorphone, oxycodone), and the purely synthetic compounds (meperedine, methadone, and levorphanol among others), are believed to achieve analgesia by binding to specific opiate receptors. These receptors are found in many parts of the central nervous system but are especially concentrated in the periaqueductal gray matter, hypothalamus, and specifically laminae one, two, and three of the dorsal horn. Outside the central nervous system, opiate receptors are found in the gut (Bishop, 1980; Fields, 1987; Basbaum and Fields, 1984; Fields and Levine, 1984; Inturrisi and Foley, 1984).

The major mechanism of action of NSAIDs and acetaminophen appears to take place at the site of injury. The salicylates (aspirin and related products) interfere with the synthesis of prostaglandins, which influence the pain stimulus at the site of local tissue damage. Aspirin is also believed to have central action on pain control by reducing the sensation of pain in the hypothalamus. Acetaminophen (Tylenol) is probably the most frequently used drug for the relief of minor to moderate pain in children. It is reputed to be less toxic than aspirin. Its mode of action is unclear. It is thought to have both peripheral and central action but is believed to be less effective than aspirin on peripheral prostaglandin synthesis (Szigeti and Sachse, 1979).

A number of new NSAIDs are now available for pain relief. It is of special importance to remember that for unknown reasons, some of these drugs appear to have a ceiling analgesic effect, which has not been ascertained for individual drugs. After the ceiling has been reached, additional medication will not provide increased analgesia, but instead risks toxicity (Kantor, 1984).

How well drugs relieve pain is determined by their concentration in the fluid surrounding the receptors. This is influenced by the absorption, distribution, metabolism, and finally excretion of the drug. These drug kinetics are in turn influenced by the child's developmental stage, physiological functions, and disease processes.

Intervention Modifiers

Development

Developmental immaturity of significant organs puts the infant, both full-term and preterm, at increased risk for alterations in drug kinetics. Absorption of drugs from the infant stomach is increased by the low gastric acidity of the stomach and by the increased permeability of the gastrointestinal membrane in the period immediately following birth. Absorption is also increased through the neonate's skin and eyes. On the other hand, the small muscle mass of the newborn makes the absorption of intramuscular drugs more difficult for neonates, though the absorption of most antibiotics is adequate. Distribution of drugs is influenced by the larger total body water of the infant, causing the drug to be distributed in a larger pool. Distribution to the central nervous system is affected by the incomplete glial development of both premature and full-term infants. This increases the permeability of the blood-brain barrier and causes drugs such as morphine to concentrate in the brain (Russell, 1980).

The metabolism of drugs into more useful compounds is largely a function of the liver. Immature liver function in premature infants and newborns may result in higher drug concentrations in the gut and less drug available for use, and dosages may need to be adjusted. Lastly, drug excretion is again influenced by lower renal blood flow and limited glomerular filtration (Russell, 1980).

These narrowed physiological parameters require that medication doses for the young be carefully calculated, that appropriate routes of administration be used, and that both the desired and untoward actions of drugs be carefully monitored. In the management of pain, the actions of narcotics and other adjunct drugs should be routinely and carefully evaluated. The nurse needs a knowledge of peak levels and duration of action of drugs.

Development includes cognitive and psychosocial development as well as physiological maturation. The influence of these developmental variables on nonpharmacological approaches to pain management has been incorporated as age-appropriate interventions in the discussion of individual strategies.

Physiological and Psychological Status

PHYSIOLOGICAL FUNCTION

Normal physiological function has a direct impact on drug treatment. The first-pass drug destruction by the liver can adversely limit the drug available for use. It accounts for the 1:6 ratio for single doses of parenteral to oral morphine. Repeated doses have different ratios. Normal blood flow to the area likewise influences absorption from the area. The deltoid muscle has more rapid absorption than do the vastus lateralis and the gluteal muscles and could influence site selections for intramuscular drugs (Russell, 1980).

Fatigue is a concomitant part of the hospitalization experience resulting from sleep deprivation, increased vigilance, surgical and diagnostic trauma, hunger, boredom, and the healing process, but most significantly resulting from pain itself. Pain can be very fatiguing, sapping limited stores of strength. Interventions are less likely to succeed when the child is exhausted. A tired child has neither the interest nor the ability to participate in self-management approaches of pain control. Nursing actions to prevent fatigue should be part of all nursing care. Controlling a child's pain by routine rather than p.r.n. medications is one of these important measures.

PSYCHOLOGICAL FUNCTIONS

Distress and anxiety are important variables that both influence and are influenced by pain. Behavioral assessment tools of children's pain assess distress behaviors; the question is often raised whether the tool is measuring distress or pain (Shacham and Daut, 1981). This is not a relevant management issue because the pain experience includes both, and reducing one often reduces the other.

Anxiety and distress are concomitants of acute pain; depression is frequently associated with chronic pain. There is a circular relationship between pain and anxiety. They tend to increase each other when the child's pain remains unrelieved. The level of anxiety can adversely influence the child's ability to utilize nonpharmacological approaches as well as his or her response to analgesic treatment. Nonpharmacological approaches should be rehearsed before the child is in pain. The nurse has an important role in supporting both the child and family to keep anxiety at a minimum and to medicate on a round-the-clock rather than a p.r.n. basis to keep the pain manageable.

DISEASE PROCESSES

Various disease states alter body function in ways that influence drug kinetics. Absorption from the gut is influenced by diarrhea and inflammation. Absorption from intramuscular and subcutaneous routes is influenced by the amount of scar tissue at those sites, reduced blood flow resulting from hypovolemic shock, compromised cardiac status, or destruction of vessels and tissue by burns or trauma. Absorption of intramuscular drugs can be assisted by the application of heat or rubbing the area.

Meningitis, brain tumors, and head trauma increase blood-brain barrier permeability. Hepatitis and obstructive jaundice influence drug metabolism, and renal disease can adversely influence drug excretion (Cook, 1976; Gregory, 1983; Russell, 1980). Trang and colleagues (1984) provide an excellent discussion of pharmacokinetics.

Family Influences

The family's impact on the child's response to pain can be a cause of concern for the nurse on a busy ward. Research in this area is scant and inconclusive (Shaw and Routh, 1982; Hallstrom, 1968). Clinical reports that children are more upset and require more medication when parents are present are frequently offered by many nurses. Hallstrom (1968), however, reported that children held by their mothers during immunizations demonstrated significantly less distress. Shaw and Routh (1982) also studied the responses of children to injections with mothers present or absent and found that separation fears were reduced by the presence of the mother but that behavior was more negative. Although this latter study appears to reflect a negative impact of parental presence, the effect may be just the opposite. Mather and Mackie (1983) reported that children tend to just lie there when in pain. Children who do not ask for pain medication when their parents are not there may not know how to ask or may be afraid or too exhausted to ask for pain relief. The increased demand for medication when the mother is present may result from the mother's ability to read the subtle pain cues the child is manifesting, or it may be that when the mother is present, the child may feel more free to express feelings. In those rare situations in which the mother's anxiety and fears influence her ability to support her child, the nurse needs to assess the mother's needs and concerns and provide appropriate

help for her because the presence of parents is generally considered helpful to children and should be encouraged and supported (see Chapter 4).

The Nature of Acute and Chronic Pain

ACUTE PAIN

The management of acute and chronic pain presents different problems for the nurse. The management of acute pain resulting from trauma, surgical or diagnostic interventions, or acute infection should achieve total relief for the patient.

The best-studied approach to the management of acute pain in children has been with postoperative pain (O'Hara et al., 1987; Dilworth and MacKellar, 1987; Kay, 1974; Smith and Jones, 1982; Lau, 1984; Bray, 1983; Dahlstrom et al., 1978). Bray (1983) and Dahlstrom et al. (1978) studied the impact of intravenous morphine during and after surgery on the pain responses of infants and children. Bray compared the pain relief provided to postoperative children by a loading dose of morphine and a continuous infusion dose with that of children receiving intramuscular morphine every four hours. Children who received the continuous morphine had better pain control. He did find that three children under six months developed irregular breathing patterns. Breathing returned to normal after the infusion was stopped; however, he stopped using morphine infusions with this age population. Other institutions, however, continue to give intravenous morphine to infants by increasing the time between administrations and report success with it. Dilworth and MacKellar (1987) reported on the use of regional analgesia, intermittent intramuscular injections, and variable rate continuous intravenous narcotic infusions. O'Hara et al. (1987) compared the use of oral morphine and intramuscular meperidine (Demerol) to relieve orthopedic surgery pain. They found that morphine was more effective. These studies have provided important data regarding narcotic protocols for the management of pediatric pain.

Work in this area points to the desirability of maintaining a therapeutic blood level of the drug by continuous infusion or by round-the-clock administration, thus avoiding the peaks and valleys that are associated with interval drug administration. It is important to avoid p.r.n. administration that attempts, often unsuccessfully, to provide relief when the patient's pain has gotten out of control. This practice results in the administration of more narcotics rather than less. Work with adults has demonstrated that patient-controlled analgesia (PCA) in postoperative patients in which the patient administered his or her own pain medication resulted in higher dosages the first two days and then a drop, resulting in less total medication administered (Tamsen et al., 1979). Patient-controlled analgesia with children is not widely reported on, but Webb et al. (1987) studied the experiences of 15 children, 11 to 18 years old, who had undergone a variety of surgical procedures with PCA. Protocols for the monitoring of pain status and vital signs were established and carried out every two hours during the day and every four hours at night. They reported success with the program. As in the adult reports, children administered higher doses of morphine during the first 24 to 48 hours; then medication use dropped dramatically by 72 hours after surgery. Both children and families were pleased with how the pain was managed and the control the children had over their pain. Nurses also reported that the patients had better pain control. Minor problems related only to technical difficulties of moving the machine around when the child was up. That unit now has two machines that are used with select populations. Tyler (1987) reported the successful use of PCA using morphine with postoperative adolescents who achieved good pain relief without side effects.

Another medication challenge is pain relief for the trauma patient. Although most sources recommend against the use of narcotics for the trauma patient, Lord (1983) advises their use with caution and with specific recommendations, especially in head injury cases. His recommendations for the treatment of the emergency patient are valuable and may be novel to practice in this country. Beckmeyer and Bahr (1980), Green and Haggerty (1984), and Reece (1984) described the slow dripping of a local anesthetic such as lidocaine (Xylocaine) into a wound and then infiltrating the wound edges with the drug using a 26 gauge needle to provide analgesia for suturing the wound. The use of local analgesics can be deleteri-

ous, however; unless they are administered carefully, they burn severely for several minutes and cause severe pain until the analgesia takes effect. By that time, the child may have lost all trust and control.

Besides emergency treatments, children are often exposed to the pain that is associated with treatments, diagnostic tests, and other painful procedures. Because they are not as formalized procedures as surgery, children often don't have the support they need to deal with their considerable pain.

CHRONIC PAIN

Unlike acute pain, total relief of chronic pain as experienced in sickle-cell disease, juvenile rheumatoid arthritis, hemophilia, and terminal cancer is not a realistic goal. The best the patient and caretaker can hope for is a balance between reduced pain and ability to function (Newburger and Sallan, 1981).

While the incidence of chronic pain is not as significant in children as it is in adults, it is detrimental to the child's growth and to family function (Hodges et al., 1985). There is also evidence that children with chronic pain are more likely to experience chronic pain as adults (Merskey and Spear, 1967). Thus, adequate management of pediatric chronic pain is desirable not only from a humanitarian stance but also from a preventive health point of view. Chronic pain in children results from (1) specific disease entities such as hemophilia, sickle-cell disease, and juvenile rheumatoid arthritis and (2) conditions that are less distinct but are recurring such as abdominal pain, headaches, and limb pain. Oster (1972) reported that abdominal pain was found in 15%, headache in 21%, and limb pain in 16% of children from six to 19 years. All three were more common in girls.

Treatment of pain associated with specific disease entities most often combines both pharmacological and nonpharmacological measures. Sickle-cell pain, for example, is treated by both low-potency drugs for mild pain and narcotics for severe pain. They are often used in conjunction with hydration and oxygen therapy to treat the underlying problem. A major concern about analgesic treatment for these patients is the professional and public fear of addiction. The sickle-cell crisis lasts anywhere from several hours to five to seven days, and during this time the child will need adequate analgesia. It is believed that addiction does not occur when medication is given for existing pain, but it may occur if given or taken for the avoidance of pain. Although some therapists are employing hypnosis, biofeedback, and guided imagery for sickle-cell pain, these have not been tested (Rozzell et al., 1983).

Treatment of nonspecific pain situations has included many behavioral approaches that have helped reduce the amount of medication a child is taking. Reduction of headache pain behaviors has been reported by Mehegan et al. (1987), who used electromyographic (EMG) feedback, relaxation, and operant conditioning in children seven to 12 years old. Results indicated that pain behaviors decreased and remained so for most of the children at the six and 12 month followups. Shinnar and D'Souza (1981) described a comprehensive approach to the management of migraine headaches using both drug and behavior therapies.

Feuerstein et al. (1982) report that in a study comparing children with recurrent abdominal pain (RAP) with a control group, the RAP children responded similarly to control groups and did not manifest signs of autonomic system deficit or increased subjective pain response. Miller and Kratochwill (1979) reported a case of a ten year old girl whose frequent complaints of stomachache were reduced by a time-out strategy. The child's pain behavior was handled by her being put in bed to rest for the remainder of the day with no special attention. The pain behaviors gradually decreased. Varni et al. (1981) used self regulation techniques to reduce pain in a hemophelic child. Masek et al. (1984) have provided an excellent guide to behavioral management strategies, Newburger and Sallan (1981) have outlined an excellent list of management principles, and Schechter (1984) has developed a useful overview and approach. Definitive strategies are described in the section on operant conditioning.

Barriers to Successful Pain Management

Realistic constraints to successful pediatric pain management are those identified by Eland and Anderson (1977) in the seminal work related to professional attitudes regarding pain in children. They cited numerous myths, "old nurses' tales," relating to children's responses to pain and to narcotics that influenced nurses' medication decisions and practices. Although most of these myths have been dispelled, the parsimonious approach to medicating children for pain still exists. Another source of constraints were those identified by Strauss and Fagerhaugh (1977), who identified the problem of nonaccountability for pain management among the health care team.

These problems have led to the findings that children's pain is poorly managed in hospitals. Although initially reported by Eland in 1977, the number of medications administered to infants and children in hospitals compared with adults with similar diagnoses remains still disproportionately low. Eland reported that a comparison of 25 children and 18 adults with similar diagnoses revealed that adults received 24 times more analgesics than children. Beyer et al. (1983) compared the number and dosage of analgesics and antipyretics that had been ordered and administered to a randomly selected sample of children and adults who had undergone open heart surgery. They found that six children had had no analgesics ordered, 12 had received no analgesics during the first three days, and there were significant differences between the proportion of adults and children who had orders for morphine and codeine. Adults received 564 (70%) and children 237 (30%) of the doses of analgesics.

Mather and Mackie (1983) studied the postoperative pain management of 170 children. Postoperative analgesics, both narcotic and non-narcotic, were ordered for 84%, and where both narcotic and non-narcotic were ordered, 29% were given only the non-narcotic drug. Only 25% had no pain the first day, but 13% reported severe pain regardless of the treatment. Another study focusing on burn patients surveyed the pain management practices in 151 burn facilities (Perry and Heidrich, 1982). Although narcotics in varying doses were preferred for adults, more respondents preferred no analgesics for children, despite the fact the most frequent pain rating, moderate, was the same for both adults and children. An interesting finding was that nurses' tenure in the institution (five years or less) appeared to lead to the higher pain ratings they gave to the tubbing procedure than nurses who had longer service. Burokas (1985) studied pediatric nurses' practices relating to pain management and reviewed charts of a select population for narcotic medications prescribed and administered. Although a statistically significant number of nurses chose to medicate the patients, 21% selected a non-narcotic and 11% selected an analgesic at the lower dosage range; only 32% chose the highest dosage ordered. The unit the nurse worked on influenced the strength and kind of analgesic chosen. Pediatric intensive care unit and surgical unit nurses selected more and higher doses of narcotics. Nurse attitude about inflicted pain was not a significant concern, as 84% reported that it did not stop them from administering an intramuscular injection.

EVALUATION

Assessment data are also helpful in determining the absence of pain following intervention. That is, following intervention, the defining characteristics of pain should be reduced or gone. There appear to be no formal evaluations of pain management, and chart audits supported the lack of documentation of the results of medication administration for pain. Measuring outcomes of interventions is the weakest component of pain management on pediatric units today. Even though advances are slowly being made for implementing pain reduction measures, changing the attitudes of health professionals about pain assessment and management and the documentation of the effectiveness of these measures is lacking. Flow sheets monitor the time and dosage of drugs administered but not the effects of the drug. It is not unusual to find a scenario in which four days into narcotic therapy, nurses are concerned about administering too much drug, the child is still in pain, and no one knows how effective the drug regimen has been.

In addition to problems with evaluation, variables affecting pain response are understudied. It is usually not known how preparation affected the child's ability to cope with the pain of an intrusive procedure. An evaluation tool that asks the following questions should provide information necessary to determine the effectiveness of interventions: (1) Was the dosage of the drug adequate? (2) Was the frequency of administration appropriate? (3) Were there side effects to the drugs administered? (4) Did the drug reduce the pain? and (5) How effectively was the pain reduced, and for how long? Meinhart and McCaffery (1983) provide a useful flow sheet that can help both the nurse and physician monitor the effectiveness of pain relief drug therapy. Another important criterion to be considered is both client and family satisfaction with the pain management.

Case Study

Chad was a six year old who had been recently diagnosed as having an inoperable Wilms' tumor and was undergoing radiation and chemotherapy to shrink the tumor. The areas being irradiated included his kidneys, stomach, and lower abdomen. He left his room once a day to undergo radiation treatments but at all other times he remained in bed.

His medical orders included appropriate doses of Demerol and promethazine HCl (Phenergan) for pain and nausea. The nursing staff had been administering both drugs around the clock, but this approach had not provided adequate pain relief or controlled his nausea. Chad became extremely irritable to all stimuli.

To assess his pain, the nurse asked him to color his pain using the Eland Color Tool. He intensely colored his entire lower abdomen with red, the color he chose to represent worst pain. Additionally, he colored the inner aspect of both of his lower legs red. He said that his abdomen hurt most of the time but his leg hurt came and went. When asked if the leg pain was sharp like a knife (nerve involvement) or if it felt like his heart beating in his leg (ischemic pain), he could not say. He looked very tired and so did his mother. When asked how long it had been since either of them had had a good night's sleep, the mother replied, "Two months." Data that are supportive of the nursing diagnosis *Alteration in comfort: acute pain* are listed in Tables 20–1 and 20–2.

After some initial research in the library, three important facts that directly related to Chad were discovered:

1. Demerol has a metabolite called normeperidine that causes irritability, restlessness, and central nervous system excitation, which can eventually lead to seizures (Kaiko et al., 1983; McCaffery, 1984).

2. Demerol and Phenergan are antagonists and, although this has been known since 1961, it is still common practice to administer both drugs together (Moore and Dundee, 1961).

3. Chad was in overwhelming pain. According to Twycross and Lack (1983), a potent analgesic

Table 20–1. DATA SUPPORTIVE OF THE NURSING DIAGNOSIS OF ALTERATION IN COMFORT: *ACUTE PAIN*

Subjective
Red coloring over area of tumor and legs

Objective
Compression of tissue
Obstruction of a ureter
Displacement of bowel by tumor
Radiation of tumor
Tense affect
Narrowed focus of attention
Facial mask of pain
Guarded movements
Nausea and vomiting*
Tachycardia*
Increased respiratory rate*
Diaphoresis*
Pupillary dilatation*

*May be directly caused by tumor.

would be required to allow him to sleep and bring his pain under control.

The following morning, the nurse shared the articles with the resident physician in charge of Chad. He studied the information and stated, "I bet it's the Demerol that's making him so crabby. Let's give him morphine instead and hydroxyzine HCl [Vistaril] for nausea and anxiety-related pain." When the nurse showed him Chad's coloring, his immediate response was, "That's a dermatome. I bet he has a damaged nerve in his back from the tumor. Shrinking the tumor will probably take care of that pain, but I sure didn't have any idea he hurt there. I just thought he hurt all over."

The nursing staff agreed to administer the morphine round-the-clock to maintain a therapeutic blood level of the analgesic. His nurses explained to Chad's parents that Chad was going to be receiving a different drug for his pain that should bring his pain under control, and when his pain was relieved he would probably sleep for two or three days because he had not slept for so long. Further, his parents were reminded that when Chad was awakened for medicine, he would act like a normal sleepy child and probably go back to sleep. The nurse explained that morphine was important to stop Chad's pain, but after the pain was under control and the tumor reduced with

Table 20–2. DEFINING CHARACTERISTICS OF COMFORT, ALTERED: *CHRONIC PAIN*

Evidence of pain for more than six months
Physical and social withdrawal
Anorexia*
Weight changes*
Changes in sleep pattern
Facial masks
Guarded movement

*May be directly caused by tumor.

radiation and chemotherapy, a non-narcotic might be effective. There were also several other options available, such as relaxation, imagery, distraction, and TENS ("magic boxes") that were available for Chad to use, but first his pain must be brought under control with potent narcotics and he must catch up on his sleep.

After the first two doses of morphine, Chad slept soundly; three days later, Chad and his mother reported the best sleep they had experienced in two months. Chad continued to sleep most of the following two days, and his vomiting stopped, leading the primary nurse to believe that pain had played a significant role in Chad's mood and temperament. Three days later, a well-rested Chad told his mother (much to her amazement) that he wanted to go to the playroom and then outdoors. Chad continued to sleep well and act more like his old self during the daylight hours. He was fatigued from the chemotherapy and radiation, but the overall success with pain relief was expressed by Chad's mother when she said, "This is our Chad, the Chad we haven't seen in months!" The tumor responded well to the medical treatment, but it would take months for it to shrink and be surgically resectable. Chad was dismissed from the hospital with a supply of slow-release morphine.

RESEARCH IMPLICATIONS

The report of the Consensus Development Conference at the National Institutes of Health in May 1986 (National Institute of Health, 1987) addressed the difficulties in assessing children's pain and the undertreatment of children's pain. The conference participants recommended the development of innovative assessment tools specific to children and others who are handicapped by language barriers and thus cannot readily report their pain.

Stevens and colleagues (1987), in a provocative and thoughtful summary of the dilemmas surrounding the theoretical, practice, and research issues concerning pediatric pain, made ten practice and seven research recommendations that address many of the problems identified in this chapter. The ten practice recommendations are: (1) recognize that all children are capable of feeling pain; (2) recognize that children's pain can be expressed in many and conflicting ways; (3) realize that a child's coping behaviors, such as sleeping or playing, do not necessarily mean he or she is pain-free; (4) consider the verbal cues and behaviors of children and parental input when assessing children's pain, but do not make the parents totally responsible for pain management decisions; (5) assess pain and record the assessment at regular intervals after diagnostic or therapeutic measures; (6) plan for both pharmacological and nonpharmacological measures to manage or prevent pain; (7) teach and encourage parents to participate in pain reporting and relief measures; (8) obtain needed information regarding drug side effects rather than withhold medication; (9) learn and utilize nonpharmacological approaches; and (10) analyze one's own feelings and beliefs regarding pain and its treatment.

The seven major research issues are (1) the continued exploration of the pain phenomenon in children, (2) the development of a bank of reliable and valid assessment tools for assessing pain across all developmental stages, (3) careful study of nurses' beliefs about pain and its treatment, (4) development of administrative protocols that assign responsibility for pain management, (5) rigorous appraisal of interventions that are used and measurement of their efficacy in reducing pain, (6) careful examination of the educational preparation of health team members in pain management, and (7) the study of the long-term effects of children's pain. Once a bank of valid and reliable tools has been developed, clinical trials of nursing interventions need to be implemented. The adaptation of adult interventions needs to be tested with children across developmental stages. These are valid concerns, for although ethical issues place constraints on much pain research in children, clinical practice provides ample opportunities to evaluate many problems in common practice.

References

Abu-Saad, H. Assessing children's responses to pain. Pain, 19:163–171, 1984a.

Abu-Saad, H. Cultural components of pain: The Arab-American child. Issues in Comprehensive Pediatric Nursing, 7:91–99, 1984b.

Abu-Saad, H. Cultural components of pain: The Asian-American child. Children's Health Care, 13:11–14, 1984c.

Abu-Saad, H. Cultural group indicators of pain in children. Maternal-Child Nursing Journal, 13:187–196, 1984d.

Abu-Saad, H, and Holzemer, WL. Measuring children's self-assessment of pain. Issues in Comprehensive Pediatric Nursing, 5:337–349, 1981.

Basbaum, AI, and Fields, HL. Endogenous pain control systems: Brainstem spinal pathways and endorphin circuitry. Annual Review of Neuroscience, 7:309–338, 1984.

Beales, JG, Keen, JH, and Holt, PJL. The child's perception of the disease and the experience of pain in juvenile chronic arthritis. Journal of Rheumatology, 10:61–65, 1983.

Beckmeyer, P, and Bahr, JE. Helping toddlers and preschoolers cope while suturing their minor lacerations. Maternal-Child Nursing Journal, 5:326–330, 1980.

Benson, H, Kotch, JB, and Crossweller, KD. The relaxation response: A bridge between psychiatry and medicine. Medical Clinics of North America, 61:929–939, 1977.

Beyer, JE, and Aradine, CR. Content validity of an instrument to measure young children's perceptions of the intensity of their pain. Journal of Pediatric Nursing, 1:386–395, 1986.

Beyer, JE, DeGood, DE, Ashley, LC, and Russell, GA. Patterns of postoperative analgesic use with adults and children following cardiac surgery. Pain, 17:71–81, 1983.

Bishop, B. Pain: Its physiology and rationale for management. Part I: Neuroanatomical substrate of pain. Physical Therapy, 60:13–27, 1980.

Bray, RJ. Postoperative analgesia provided by morphine infusion in children. Anaesthesia, 38:1075–1078, 1983.

Burokas, LB. Factors affecting nurses' decisions to medicate pediatric patients after surgery. Heart and Lung, 14:373–379, 1985.

Cannon, WB. Bodily changes in pain, hunger, fear and rage (2nd ed.). New York: D. Appleton-Century, 1929.

Chaves, JF, and Barber, TX. Cognitive strategies, experimenter modeling, and expectation in the attenuation of pain. Journal of Abnormal Psychology, 83:356–363, 1974.

Cook, DR. Pediatric Anaesthesia: Pharmacological considerations. Drugs, 12:212–221, 1976.

Craig, KD, McMahon, RJ, Morison, JD, and Zaskow, C. Developmental changes in infant pain expression during immunization injections. Social Science and Medicine, 19:1331–1337, 1984.

Dahlstrom, B, Bolme, P, Feychting, H, Noack, G, and Paalzow, L. Morphine kinetics in children. Clinical Pharmacology and Therapeutics, 26:354–365, 1978.

Dale, JC. A multidimensional study of infants' responses to painful stimuli. Pediatric Nursing, 12:27–31, 1986.

Dilworth, NM, and MacKellar, A. Pain relief for the pediatric surgical patient. Journal of Pediatric Surgery, 22:264–266, 1987.

Donovan, M. Relaxation with guided imagery: A useful technique. Cancer Nursing, 3:27–32, 1980.

Donovan, M. Cancer pain: You can help! Nursing Clinics of North America, 17:713–728, 1982.

Eland, JM. Eland Color Tool interview protocol. University of Iowa, Iowa City, 1973.

Eland, JM. Minimizing pain associated with prekindergarten intramuscular injections. Issues in Comprehensive Pediatric Nursing, 5:361–372, 1981.

Eland, JM. The assessment of pain in children. Paper presented at the Consensus Development Conference, National Institutes of Health, Washington, D.C. 1986a.

Eland, JM. The use of TENS (transcutaneous electrical nerve stimulation) with pediatric oncology patients.

Paper presented at the Consensus Development Conference, National Institutes of Health, Washington, DC, 1986b.

Eland, JM, and Anderson, JE. The experience of pain in children. In Jacox, AK (Ed.), Pain: A source book for nurses and other health professionals. Boston: Little, Brown and Co. Inc., 1977, pp. 453–476.

Fernald, CD, and Corry, JJ. Empathic versus directive preparation of children for needles. Children's Health Care, 10:44–47, 1981.

Feuerstein, M, Barr, RG, Francoeur, TE, Houle, M, and Rafman, S. Potential biobehavioral mechanisms of recurrent abdominal pain in children. Pain, 13:287–298, 1982.

Fields, HL. Pain. New York: McGraw-Hill Book Co. 1987.

Fields, HL, & Levine, JD. Pain: Mechanisms and management. The Western Journal of Medicine, 141:347–357, 1984.

Fordyce, WE, Fowles, RS, Lehman, JF, de Lateur, BJ, Sand, PL, and Frieschmann, RB. Operant conditioning in the treatment of chronic pain. Archives of Physical Medicine and Rehabilitation, 54:399–408, 1973.

Green, M, and Haggerty, RJ. Ambulatory pediatrics (Vol. 3). Philadelphia: WB Saunders Co., 1984.

Gregory, GA. Pharmacology. In Gregory, GA (Ed.), Pediatric anesthesia. New York: Churchill Livingstone, Inc., 1983.

Gross, SC, and Gardner, GG. Child pain: Treatment approaches. In Smith, WL, Merskey, H, and Gross, SC (Eds.), Pain: Meaning and management. New York: SP Medical & Scientific Books, 1980.

Hallstrom, BJ. Contract comfort: Its application to immunization injections. Nursing Research, 17:130–134, 1968.

Hansen, BD, and Evans, ML. Preparing a child for procedures. Maternal-Child Nursing Journal, 6:392–397, 1981.

Haslam, DR. Age and the perception of pain. Psychonomic Science, 15:86–87, 1969.

Hester, NK. The preoperational child's reaction to immunization. Nursing Research, 28:250–255, 1979.

Hilgard, JR, and LeBaron, S. Relief of anxiety and pain in children and adolescents with cancer: Quantitative measures and clinical observations. International Journal of Clinical and Experimental Hypnosis, 30:417–442, 1982.

Hodges, K., Kline, JJ, Barbero, G, and Flanery, R. Depressive symptoms in children with recurrent abdominal pain and their families. Journal of Pediatrics, 107:622–626, 1985.

Inturrisi, CE, and Foley, KM. Narcotic analgesics in the management of pain. In Kuhar, M, and Pasternak, G (Eds.), Analgesics: Neurochemical, behavioral, and clinical perspectives. New York: Raven Press, 1984.

Izard, CE, and Dougherty, LM. Two complementary systems for measuring facial expressions in infants and children. In Izard, CE (Ed.), Measuring emotions in infants and children. New York: Cambridge University Press, 1982.

Izard, CE, Huebner, RR, Risser, D, McGinnes, GC, and Dougherty, LM. The young infant's ability to produce discrete emotion expressions. Developmental Psychology, 16:132–140, 1980.

Jay, SM, Elliott, CH, Ozolins, M, Olson, RA, and Pruitt, SD. Behavioral management of children's distress during painful medical procedures. Behavior Research Therapy, 5:513–520, 1985.

Jay, SM, Elliott, CH, Katz, ER, and Siegel, SE. Cognitive behavioral interventions for children undergoing painful medical procedures: Final results of a treatment outcome study. In Varni, JW (Chair). Comprehensive assessment of acute and chronic pain in children. Symposium conducted at the annual meeting of Association for Advancement of Behavior Therapy, Houston, 1985.

Jeans, ME, and Johnston, CC. Pain in children: Assessment and management. In Lipton, S, and Miles, J (Eds.), Persistent pain: Modern methods of treatment (Vol. 5). London: Grune & Stratton, Inc., 1985, pp. 111–127.

Jerrett, MD. Children and their pain experience. Children's Health Care, 14:83–89, 1985.

Johnson, JE, Kirchoff, KT, and Endress, MP. Altering children's distress behavior during orthopedic cast removal. Nursing Research, 24:404–410, 1975.

Johnston, CC, and Strada, ME. Acute pain response in infants: A multi-dimensional description. Pain, 24:373–382, 1986.

Kaiko, RF, Foley, KM, Grabinski, PY, Heidrich, G, Rogers AG, Intrussi, CE, and Reidenberg, MM. Central nervous system excitatory effects of meperidine in cancer patients. Annals of Neurology, 13:180–185, 1983.

Kantor, TG. Peripherally acting analgesics. In Kuhar, M, and Pasternak, G (Eds.), Analgesics: Neurochemical, behavioral, and clinical perspectives. New York: Raven Press, 1984.

Kassowitz, KE. Psychodynamic reactions of children to the use of hypodermic needles. American Journal of Diseases of Children, 95:253–257, 1958.

Katz, ER, Kellerman, J, and Siegel, SE. Behavioral distress in children with cancer undergoing medical procedures: Developmental considerations. Journal of Consulting and Clinical Psychology, 48:356–365, 1980.

Kay, B. Caudal block for post-operative pain relief in children. Anesthesia, 29:610–611, 1974.

Keele, KD. Pain chart. Lancet, 2:6–8, 1948.

Kurylyszyn, N, McGrath, PJ, Cappelli, M, and Humphreys, P. Children's drawings: What can they tell us about intensity of pain? Clinical Journal of Pain, 2:155–158, 1987.

Lau, JTK. Penile block for pain relief after circumcision in children. Annals of Surgery, 147:797–799, 1984.

Lehmann, JF, Warren, CG, and Scham, SM. Therapeutic heat and cold. Clinical Orthopedics and Related Research, 99:207–212, 1974.

Levine, JD, and Gordon, NC. Pain in prelingual children and its evaluation by pain-induced vocalization. Pain, 14:85–93, 1982.

Levy, DM. The infant's earliest memory of inoculation: A contribution to public health procedures. Journal of Genetic Psychology, 96:3–46, 1960.

Lewis, N. The needle like an animal: How children view injections. Children Today, 7:18–21, 1978.

Lollar, DJ, Smits, SJ, and Patterson, DL. Assessment of pediatric pain: An empirical perspective. Journal of Pediatric Psychology, 7:267–277, 1982.

Lord, SM. Relief of pain after accidents or in emergencies. In Lipton, S, and Miles, J (Eds.), Persistent pain: Modern methods of treatment (Vol. 4). London: Grune & Stratton, Inc., 1983, pp. 133–144.

Macher, JB, and Johnson, R. Desensitization, model-learning and the dental behavior of children. Journal of Dental Research, 53:83–87, 1974.

Margolis, RB, Tait, RC, and Krause, SJ. A rating system

for use with patients with pain drawings. Pain, 24:57–65, 1986.

Masek, BJ, Russo, DC, and Varni, JW. Behavioral approaches to the management of chronic pain in children. Pediatric Clinics of North America, 31:1113–1131, 1984.

Mather, L, and Mackie, J. The incidence of postoperative pain in children. Pain, 15:271–282, 1983.

McCaffery, M. Pain relief for the child: Problem areas and selected nonpharmacological methods. Pediatric Nursing, 3:11–16, 1977.

McCaffery, M. Nursing management of the patient with pain. Philadelphia: JB Lippincott Co., 1979.

McCaffery, M. Problems with meperidine. American Journal of Nursing, 84:525–526, 1984.

McGrath, P, Johnson, G, Goodman, JT, Schillinger, J, Dunn, J, and Chapman, JA. CHEOPS: A behavioral scale for rating postoperative pain in children. Advances in Pain Research and Therapy, 9:387–402, 1985.

Mehegan, JE, Masek, BJ, Harrison, RH, Russo, DC, and Leviton, A. A multicomponent behavioral treatment for pediatric migraine. Clinical Journal of Pain, 2:191–196, 1987.

Meinhart, NJ, and McCaffery, M. Pain: A nursing approach to assessment and analysis. Norwalk, Conn.: Appleton-Century-Crofts, 1983.

Melamed, B, Hawes, RR, Heiby, E, and Glick, J. Use of filmed modeling to reduce uncooperative behavior of children during dental treatment. Journal of Dental Research, 54:979–981, 1975.

Melamed, BG, and Siegel, LJ. Behavioral medicine: Practical applications in health care. New York: Springer Publishing Co., Inc., 1980.

Melzack, R. The McGill Pain Questionnaire: Major properties and scoring methods. Pain, 1:277–299, 1975.

Melzack, R. The McGill Pain Questionnaire. In Melzack, R (Ed.), Pain measurement and assessment. New York: Raven Press, 1983, pp. 41–47.

Melzack, R, and Wall, PD. Pain mechanisms: A new theory. Science, 150:971, 1965.

Melzack, R, and Wall, P. The challenge of pain. New York: Basic Books, Inc., 1982.

Merskey, H, and the International Association for the Study of Pain Subcommittee on Taxonomy. Pain terms: A list with definitions and notes on usage. Pain, 6:249–252, 1979.

Merskey, H, and Spear, FG. Pain: Psychological and psychiatric aspects. London: Bailliere Tindall & Cassell, 1967.

Miller, AJ, and Kratochwill, TR. Reduction of frequent stomachache complaints by time out. Behavior Therapy, 10:211–218, 1979.

Molsberry, D. Young children's subjective qualifications of pain following surgery. Unpublished master's thesis, University of Iowa, Iowa City, 1979.

Moore, J, and Dundee, JW. Alterations in response to somatic pain associated with anaesthesia. VII: The effects of nine phenothiazine derivatives. British Journal of Anaesthesia, 33:422–431, 1961.

National Institutes of Health. Consensus Development Conference, 1986. Journal of Pain and Symptom Management, 2:35–44, 1987.

Newburger, PE, and Sallan, SE. Chronic pain: Principles of management. Journal of Pediatrics, 98:180–189, 1981.

Nocella, J, and Kaplan, RM. Training children to cope with dental treatment. Journal of Pediatric Psychology, 7:175–178, 1982.

O'Hara, M, McGrath, PJ, D'Astous, J, and Vair, CA. Oral morphine versus injected meperidine (Demerol) for pain relief in children after orthopedic surgery. Journal of Pediatric Orthopedics, 7:78–-82, 1987.

Oster, J. Recurrent abdominal pain, headache, and limb pain in children and adolescents. Pediatrics, 50:129–136, 1972.

Owens, ME, and Todt, EH. Pain in infancy: Neonatal reaction to a heel lance. Pain, 20:77–86, 1984.

Perry, S, and Heidrich, G. Management of pain during debridement: A survey of U.S. burn units. Pain, 13:267–280, 1982.

Porter, CS. Grade school children's perceptions of their internal body parts. Nursing Research, 23:384–391, 1974.

Reece, RM. Manual of emergency pediatrics (3rd ed.). Philadelphia: WB Saunders Co., 1984.

Reynolds, DV. Surgery in the rat during electrical analgesia induced by focal stimulation. Science, 164:444–445, 1969.

Ross, DM, and Ross, SA. Childhood pain: The school-aged child's viewpoint. Pain, 20:179–191, 1983.

Ross, DM, and Ross, SA. Stress reduction procedures for school-age hospitalized leukemic child. Pediatric Nursing, 10:393–395, 1984.

Ross, DM, and Ross, SA. Pain instruction with third- and fourth-grade children: A pilot study. Journal of Pediatric Psychology, 10:55–63, 1985.

Rozzell, MS, Hijazi, M, and Pack, B. The painful episode. Nursing Clinics of North America, 18:185–199, 1983.

Russell, H. Developmental aspects of drug response. In Russell, H (Ed.) Pediatric drugs and nursing intervention. New York: McGraw-Hill, Inc., 1980.

Savedra, M, Gibbons, P, Tesler, M, Ward, J, and Wegner, C. How do children describe pain? A tentative assessment. Pain, 14:95–104, 1982.

Savedra, M, Tesler, M, Ward, J, Wegner, C, and Gibbons, P. Description of the pain experience: A study of school-age children. Issues in Comprehensive Pediatric Nursing, 5:373–380, 1981.

Savedra, M, Tesler, M, Ward, J, Holzemer, W, and Wilkie, D. Children's preference for pain intensity scales. Paper presented at the Vth World Congress on Pain, Hamburg, West Germany, 1987.

Savedra, MC, Tesler, MD, Holzmer, WL, Wilkie, DJ, and Ward, JA. Advances in pain research and therapy. Proceedings of the First International Symposium on Pain. Seattle, July 1988a.

Savedra, MC, Tesler, MD, Ward, JA, and Wegner, C. How adolescents describe pain. Journal of Adolescent Health Care 9:315–320, 1988b.

Savedra, MC, Tesler MD, Holzemer, WL, Wilkie, DJ, and Ward, JA. Pain location. Validity and reliability of body outline markings by hospitalized children and adolescents. Research in Nursing and Health (in press).

Schechter, NL. Recurrent pain in children: An overview and an approach. Pediatric Clinics of North America, 31:949–968, 1984.

Schultz, NV. How children perceive pain. Nursing Research, 19:670–673, 1971.

Scott, J, Ansell, BM, and Huskisson, EC. The measurement of pain in juvenile chronic polyarthritis. Annals of Rheumatic Disease, 37:186–187, 1977.

Shacham, S, and Daut, R. Anxiety or pain: What does the scale measure? Journal of Consulting and Clinical Psychology, 49:468–469, 1981.

Shaw, EG, and Routh, DK. Effect of mother presence

on children's reactions to aversive procedures. Journal of Pediatric Psychology, 7:1, 33–42, 1982.

Shinnar, S, and D'Souza, BJ. The diagnosis and management of headaches in childhood. Pediatric Clinics of North America, 29:79–94, 1981.

Siegel, LJ, and Peterson, L. Stress reduction in young dental patients through coping skills and sensory information. Journal of Consulting and Clinical Psychology, 48:785–787, 1980.

Smith, BAC, and Jones, SEF. Analgesia after herniotomy in a pediatric day care unit. British Medical Journal, 285:1466, 1982.

Smith, ME. The preschooler and pain. In Brandt, PA, Chinn, PL, and Smith, ME (Eds.), Current practice in pediatric nursing. St Louis: CV Mosby Co., 1976.

Stevens, B, Hunsberger, M, and Browne, G. Pain in children: Theoretical, practical and research dilemmas. Journal of Pediatric Nursing, 12:154–165, 1987.

Stewart, ML. Measurement of clinical pain. In Jacox, AV (Ed.), Pain: A source book for nurses and other health professionals. Boston: Little, Brown & Co., 1977, pp. 107–138.

Stoddard, FJ. Coping with pain: A developmental approach to treatment of burned children. American Journal of Psychiatry, 139:736–740, 1982.

Strauss, A, and Fagerhaugh, SY. Politics of pain management: Staff-patient interaction. Menlo Park, Calif.: Addison-Wesley Publishing Co., Inc., 1977.

Szigeti, E, and Sachse, M. Pain. In Wiener, M, Pepper, G, Kerhn-Weisman, G, and Romano, J (Eds.), Clinical pharmacology and therapeutics in nursing. New York: McGraw-Hill, Inc., 1979.

Tamsen, A, Hatvig, P, Dahlstrom, B, Lindstrom, B, and Holmdahl, MH. Patient controlled analgesic therapy in the early post-operative period. Acta Anaesthesiologica Scandinavica, 23:462–470, 1979.

Taylor, MM, and Williams, HA. Use of therapeutic play in the ambulatory pediatric hematology clinic. Cancer Nursing, 3:433–437, 1980.

Tesler, MD, Wegner, C, Savedra, M, Gibbons, P, and Ward, J. Coping strategies of children in pain. Issues in Comprehensive Pediatric Nursing, 5:351–359, 1981.

Tesler, MD, Ward, J, Savedra, M, Wegner, C, and Gibbons, P. Developing an instrument for eliciting children's description of pain. Perceptual and Motor Skills, 56:315–321, 1983.

Tesler, MD, Savedra, M, Ward, J, Holzemer, W, and Wilkie, D. Children's language of pain. Paper presented at the Vth World Congress on Pain, Hamburg, West Germany, 1987.

Trang, JM, Kluza, RB, and Kearns, GL. Pharmacokinetics for pediatric nurses. Pediatric Nursing, 10:267–274, 1984.

Tyler, DC. Patient controlled analgesia in adolescents (Abstract 437). Pain, Supplement 4, 1987.

Twycross, RC, and Lack, SA. Symptom control in far-advanced cancer. London: Pitman, 1983.

Varni, JW. The Varni/Thompson Pediatric Pain Questionnaire. Personal correspondence, 1986.

Varni, JW, Gilbert, A, and Dietrich, SL. Behavioral medicine in pain and analgesia management for the hemophilic child with factor VIII inhibitor. Pain, 11:121–126, 1981.

Varni, JW, Katz, E, and Dash, J. Behavioral and neurochemical aspects of pediatric pain. In Russo, D, and Varni, J (Eds.), Behavioral pediatrics. New York: Plenum Publishing Corp., 1982, pp. 177–224.

Varni, JW, Thompson, KL, and Hanson, V. The Varni/ Thompson Pediatric Pain Questionnaire: 1. Chronic musculoskeletal pain in juvenile rheumatoid arthritis. Pain, 28:27–38, 1987.

Venham, LL, Goldstein, M, Gaulin-Kremer, E, Peteros, K, Cohan, J, and Fairbanks, J. Effectiveness of a distraction technique in managing young dental patients. Pediatric Dentistry, 3:7–11, 1981.

Webb, C, Rodgers, B, and Stergios, D. Patient controlled analgesia in a pediatric population. Personal communication, 1987.

Wolfer, J, and Visintainer, M. Psychological preparation for surgical pediatric patients: The effects on children's and parents' stress responses and adjustments. Pediatrics, 58:187–202, 1975.

Wyke, BD. Neurological aspects of pain therapy: A review of some current concepts. In Swerdlow, CM (Ed.), The therapy of pain. Philadelphia: JB Lippincott Co., 1985.

Yaksh, T, and Hammond, D. Peripheral and central substrates involved in the rostrad transmission of nociceptive information. Pain, 13:1–85, 1982.

Zborowski, M. People in pain. San Francisco: Jossey-Bass, Inc., 1969.

Zelter, L, and LeBaron, S. Hypnosis and nonhypnotic techniques for reduction of pain and anxiety during painful procedures in children and adolescents with cancer. Journal of Pediatrics, 101:1032–1035, 1982.

CHAPTER 21

NUTRITIONAL SUPPORT

MARTHA J. CRAFT, Ph.D., R.N.

While the term nutritional support is sometimes used in reference to supplemental avenues of nutritional sources, such as hyperalimentation, nutritional support will be used throughout this discussion to refer to the nursing intervention of enhancing nutritional status for infants and children with nutritional deficits through specified strategies. These strategies change the cause, or antecedents, of nutritional deficits in some instances. In other instances, nursing strategies change the modifiers, or intervening variables, affecting nutritional status.

The total arena of nursing practice provides numerous opportunities for utilization of the nutritional support intervention. Community and ambulatory care nurses have access to clients and their families over a period of time, providing opportunities for assessment, intervention, and evaluation. Similarly, nurses in acute care settings have contact with clients and families 24 hours a day. Thus, these nurses can intervene directly through strategies that support nutritional status, as well as prepare patients and families for continued nutritional habits that restore and maintain health after their return to the community.

Clearly, nurses have a crucial and unique role in nutritional support. Their use of this intervention is ubiquitous because of the connection between nutrition and human survival. Human survival is contingent upon an adequate supply of energy to the cell. Indeed, a supply of glucose to the cell is the cornerstone of life.

THEORETICAL FOUNDATION

Glucose and Cellular Life

All cells require energy for the transport of substances across the cell membrane and for the synthesis of substances within the cell. In addition, specialized cells require energy in order to perform mechanical and electrical work. The form of energy utilized by the cell is adenosine triphosphate (ATP), which is a nucleotide composed of adenine, a nitrogen base, ribose, a sugar, and three phosphate radicals (Alberts et al., 1983). The formation of ATP begins with ingestion of nutrients. From these nutrients, cellular energy is derived.

The Derivation of Cellular Energy

Nutrition for life begins largely in the form of proteins, lipids, and polysaccharides, which must be broken down into smaller molecules before cells can use them. The catabolism, or enzymatic breakdown, of these molecules follows a systematic process that can be conceptualized in three phases.

The first phase occurs when these large polymeric molecules are broken down into their monomeric subunits through a process of digestion. Digestion, of course, occurs outside the cells through the action of secreted enzymes, which convert proteins into amino acids, polysaccharides into sugars, and fats into fatty acids and glycerol.

In the next phase, the small molecules derived from digestion enter cells and are further processed in the cellular cytoplasm. Most of the carbon and hydrogen atoms of sugars are converted into pyruvate, which is then converted into the acetylcoenzyme A (acetyl-CoA). Like ATP, acetyl-CoA is a chemically reactive compound that releases a great deal of energy when it is hydrolyzed. Fatty acids also produce major portions of acetyl-CoA (Alberts et al., 1983). Further, amino acids are converted initially to acetoacetic acids, which are then also converted into acetyl-CoA, as summarized in Figure 21–1.

The formation of acetyl-CoA from the three basic nutrients makes it possible for the power unit of the cell, the mitochondrion, to utilize the nutrients to derive cellular energy, which is the last phase in the derivation of cellular energy. The mitochondria are active organelles of the cell that are changing shape constantly. They are especially active and numerous in highly metabolic tissue, such as the liver. A hypothetical mitochondrion with components, as it might appear enlarged thousands of times under an electronic microscope, is sketched in Figure 21–2.

Mitochrondria are crucial to human survival because they contain enzymes of the Krebs cycle along with the enzymes and cellular respiratory pigments that form the electron transport chain (Shekleton, 1979). Hydrogen atoms and electrons are transferred via a series of oxidation-reduction reactions along the electron transport chain to oxygen, the final acceptor, to form water (Fig. 21–1). During these reactions the importance of oxygen becomes apparent, because oxygen is required for inorganic phosphate to become coupled with adenosine diphosphate (ADP) to form ATP, a process called oxidative phosphorylation (Shekleton, 1979). Most of the ATP is generated during this last phase of catabolism and cellular energy derivation, as acetyl-CoA is completely degraded to carbon dioxide and water (Fig. 21–1).

Thus, through oxidative phosphorylation, energy originally present in glucose is transformed into ATP energy. Approximately 10^9 (ten to the ninth power) molecules of ATP are in solution throughout the intracellular space in a typical cell, where their formation, as well as energetically favorable hydrolysis back to ADP and phosphate, provides the driving energy for a variety of reactions (Alberts et al., 1983). It is thought that 70% of the energy in food becomes heat energy in the formation and coupling of ATP (Shekleton, 1979).

It can be seen readily that sound nutrition is absolutely essential for cellular life. Further, oxygen cannot be utilized by the cell without the presence of glucose, even though many nurses believe that oxygen is more crucial than glucose for survival. Fortunately, the fact that glucose can be stored in the form of glycogen in older infants and children facilitates its use for cellular energy as needed in states of health and illness.

However, the effects of prematurity, congenital anomalies, and injury or illness are likely to impede the supply of glucose to the cell because of disruptions in normal nutritional intake, digestive and absorptive prob-

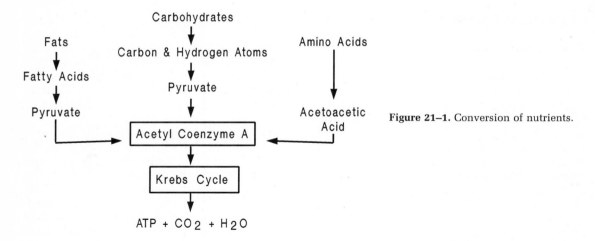

Figure 21-1. Conversion of nutrients.

lems, nutritional loss from vomiting and diarrhea, and increased metabolic and cellular demands. Thus, a paradox arises: a situation is present in which there are existing demands for increased nutrients to maintain the relatively high metabolic rate and growth for infants and children. Then, these demands are increased by even higher nutrient needs that are imposed by injury or illness at the same time the supply of nutrients is likely to be reduced.

INCREASED NUTRITIONAL DEMANDS ASSOCIATED WITH INJURY AND ILLNESS

Disabilities from prematurity, congenital anomalies, injury, and illness, therefore, present a supply and demand problem. Just when the demand for nutrients is increased, the supply is decreased. The increase for

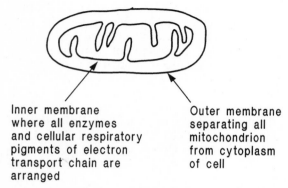

Inner membrane where all enzymes and cellular respiratory pigments of electron transport chain are arranged

Outer membrane separating all mitochondrion from cytoplasm of cell

Figure 21-2. Sketch of mitchondria with components.

nutrients occurs largely through the metabolic response. Energy and protein needs can be estimated by indirect calorimetry. The estimated metabolic response to injury and illness measured thusly has shown that the Basal Energy Expenditure (Harris and Benedict, 1919) increases by a multiple of factors. For example, the Basal Energy Expenditure must be multiplied by a factor of 1.2 during confinement to bed. The same factor of 1.2 is used when determining energy and protein needs for an infant or child who has experienced a minor operation. However, the Basal Energy Expenditure must be multiplied by a higher factor for sepsis ($\times$ 1.6) and severe thermal burns ($\times$ 2.1) (Long et al., 1979). Similarly, Blackburn and colleagues (1977) have shown that major surgery and severe sepsis increase the rates of hypermetabolism as measured by urine nitrogen excretion (Fig. 21-3). However, these factors have not been studied and reported in children.

As Blackburn and associates (1977) have noted, amino acids are used for calorie, or energy, expenditure during infection, major injury, or sepsis. However, even though this conversion of amino acids to energy during periods of high metabolic demand or starvation is a normal homeostatic mechanism, it is inefficient and a threat to health restoration. It is inefficient because protein used for energy is unavailable for cellular repair. Also, protein is unavailable for the hormonal, enzymatic, and buffer demands in stress, immune response healing, and hypermetabolism processes.

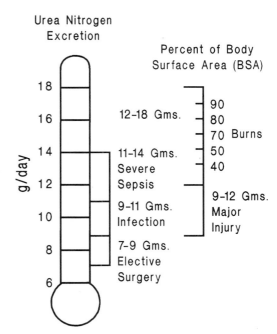

Figure 21–3. Hypermetabolism as measured by urine nitrogen excretion.

Stress

The psychological stress experienced by hospitalized infants and children has been well documented and reviewed (Thompson, 1985). However, the effects of stress upon their nutritional status have received less attention. Stress-induced acceleration of the autonomic nervous system produces epinephrine release from the adrenal medulla and norepinephrine release from peripheral nerve endings. In turn, epinephrine release increases blood glucose simultaneously with the catabolism of protein and fats. Norepinephrine release stimulates the liver also to increase blood glucose, along with protein and fat catabolism (Axelrod, 1985). At the same time that the autonomic nervous system is accelerated, the anterior pituitary gland produces increased amounts of adrenocorticotropic hormone (ACTH) that stimulate the adrenal cortex to increase aldosterone and cortisol release. Aldosterone release increases sodium retention, which is accompanied by water retention, while cortisol release also increases blood glucose, protein, and fat catabolism (Burns and Carlson, 1985).

It is apparent, then, that both the autonomic nervous system response and the anterior pituitary response to stress foster increased demands for glucose, protein, and fat. Further, the retention of sodium and water results from the combined actions of ACTH and aldosterone.

Immunocompetence

Since disability, injury, and illness are associated with altered immunocompetence, it is important to consider the relationship of nutrition to the efficiency of the immunological system. The normal immunodeficiencies of the preterm infant and neonate place babies at especially high risk, but all infants and children need increased nutrients for the demands that occur from rapid cellular proliferation in the lymphoid organs and cell-mediated immunity.

Immunoglobulins are composed of heavy and light chain amino acids. Further, the active binding site of the antibody molecule is part of a region of amino acid composition that gives the antibody its specificity. That is, glycoproteins are opsonins that coat microbes in such a way that microbes are recognized as foreign, or as antigens. This process of coating, or opsonization, is thought to be essential for mitogen binding and cell proliferation. The mitogens normally cause DNA synthesis, blast transformation, and lymphoctye division (Shekleton, 1979, p. 95; Lahita, et al., 1984).

Preterm infants normally do not have reserves of immunoglobulins, primarily immunoglobulin G (IgG), which are stored for the last weeks of gestation. Further, immunoglobulin A (IgA), which plays a major role in defense against viral infections, and immunoglobulin M (IgM), which is important in defense of gram-negative organisms, are not transferred to fetuses, placing infants at risk for infection from these organisms. In addition, neonates have a less effective circulation and phagocytic capacity in their leukocytes. Also, they suffer from decreased monocytic function, a low level of complement, and diminished opsonic ability (Savilahti, et al., 1983; Hay, 1985; Pereira and Barbosa, 1986). Adding to these problems is a hypofunctioning adrenal gland, with only a minimal anti-inflammatory response to antigens (Sammons and Lewis, 1985).

However, Locke has written that the critical factors in the stress-adaptation-immunity relationship are the duration and proximity of the stressor, the adaptive capacity of the individual, and the differential effects of certain stressors on immune components (Locke, 1982; Kiecolt-Glaser, Garner, et al., 1984; Kiecolt-Glaser, Ricker, et al., 1984). Thus, while the challenge to the immune system imposed by illness and injury, plus stress resulting from changing physiological status, a new setting, and new caretakers, may seem overwhelming, nurses can intervene to enhance the adaptive capacity of infants and children through enhancing nutritional status.

Cellular and Tissue Repair

Stress and immunocompetence are prevalent concerns during acute and chronic illness. In addition, nutritional needs increase when actual cellular injury and damage occur from accidents, surgery, or burns. For cellular and tissue repair to restore and maintain health, a greater supply of all of the major nutrients, including specific vitamins and minerals, is required.

Protein and nucleic acids are the two most vital macromolecules of the cell. They make up approximately two thirds of its dry weight. Therefore their presence is crucial for cellular repair and growth. The amino acids of methionine, cystine, and lysine have been reported to be especially important in wound healing for premature and newborn infants (Levenson et al., 1979). In addition, the amino acids that are not used for biosynthesis can be oxidized to generate metabolic energy (Alberts et al., 1983).

Approximately 52% to 60% of total protein is albumin, a protein formed in the liver that is needed for transport of blood constituents, such as ions, pigments, bilirubin, hormones, fatty acids, enzymes, and certain drugs. The remaining portion of protein is globulin, which functions in antibody formation and in the development of fibrinogen and prothrombin, required for coagulation (Fischbach, 1984).

During illness and injury, protein intake is often reduced. If supplemental protein is not supplied, the need for protein can only be met by catabolism of the body mass, thus reducing the protein available for repair and regeneration (Temple et al., 1975; Irvin, 1978). If carbohydrates and fats are insufficient for cellular energy, protein is also catabolized to replace the energy derived from them.

The fat nutrient is important because fats are also components of cellular membranes and cellular structures. Linoleic, linolenic, and arachidonic acids, essential fatty acids, are needed for healing of impaired cells immediately after an injury occurs. There is no time for synthesis of these fatty acids. Therefore, individuals who lack stores of these acids, such as premature infants, neonates, or cachectic children, are at risk for inadequate healing.

Fats play a very consequential role in cellular repair. In addition, they affect the inflammatory processes and circulation of oxygen to damaged tissue, because fats are a part of prostaglandin. Prostaglandins are lipid-like substances that have been shown to play a role in a number of processes, including cell membrane interactions and smooth muscle contractility. Prostaglandin alters the permeability occurring in cell membrane during inflammation through the release of histamine. Further, the effect of prostaglandin on smooth muscle contractility has an impact on the circulation of oxygen to damaged cells.

Vitamins C, A, D, B, and K are thought to be important in cellular and tissue repair. Vitamin C is important (1) as a reducing agent for conversion of oxygen to superoxide, which slows bacterial action at the site of cellular injury; (2) in the formation of fibroblasts, which are necessary for collagen formation; and (3) for the hydroxylation of proline and lysine to form collagen (Pollack, 1979). The metabolic demands for vitamin C increase during infection and wound healing. Thus, in the severe cellular injury that occurs from burns and severe wounds, vitamin C may need to be supplemented (Levenson et al., 1979).

Vitamin A is important in healing. As with vitamin C, an adequate supply of vitamin A is crucial for collagen formation. However, vitamin A is needed in addition for epithelialization and capillary budding. It has been found useful in counteracting the anti-inflammatory processes of long-term corticosteroid medications (Hunt et al., 1969).

The importance of vitamins D and K is well known. Vitamin D is crucial for the absorption of calcium, needed for bone healing or growth and many enzyme systems, including collagenases (Stotts, 1986), and vitamin K is needed for blood coagulation. Unlike vitamins D and K, vitamin B is water-soluble, so all of the vitamin B family must be provided daily except for vitamin B12. Vitamin B acts as a co-factor in enzymatic reactions utilized during the healing process. Similarly, certain minerals are crucial to the healing process.

If serum zinc levels are below normal ranges, zinc must be supplemented to bring cellular and tissue repair up to the normal rate, although supplemental zinc will not increase healing of individuals with normal serum levels (Lee et al., 1976). Similarly, iron is needed for collagen formation and must be within normal ranges in order for the nucleus of the hemoglobin molecule to carry oxygen that is crucial for cellular repair (Levenson et al., 1979).

Fluid and Acid-Base Balance

As noted previously, the importance of protein in the stress, immunological, and healing responses cannot be exaggerated. Equally important, however, is the role protein plays in maintaining fluid and acid-base balance. The albumin component of protein is essential for the maintenance of colloidal osmotic pressure and normal distribution of body water, whereas globulins function primarily as an immunological agent. However, serum globulins also play a part in fluid balance when the albumin supply is diminished owing to changing cell permeability. Normally, capillary walls are impermeable to plasma protein. If, however, cell permeability shifts and albumin can "seep through," the larger globulin molecules remain within the blood stream and fulfill the role usually assumed by albumin, that of maintaining osmotic pressure. Because of the difference in the globulin and albumin molecules, globulin fulfills this role to a lesser extent, meaning that fluid shifts are likely to occur (Fischbach, 1984).

Proteins are also powerful buffers. They act as one of several main buffering systems—carbonic acid, bicarbonate, phosphate, and respiratory—that function together to maintain a blood pH that is compatible with life. Proteins are versatile buffers as they can act as acid or base, depending on the homeostatic demand. Further, they function intracellularly as well as extracellularly. Within the cell it is the hemoglobin, with the globin acting as a protein of the erythrocyte, that provides the majority of the chemical buffering power of bodily fluids (Forlaw, 1983).

Growth and Metabolic Demands

The increased nutritional demands imposed by injury and illness apply to people of all ages; however, infants and children have additional needs that arise from their higher metabolic rate, growth, and developing immunocompetence. Metabolic needs of preterm and newborn infants are especially high, gradually lowering throughout childhood and adolescence. This phenomenon is illustrated by the changes occurring in secretion of the thyroid gland, which influences metabolic rate. For example, thyronine concentration (in mg/dl) decreases from a mean of 12.5 in full-term neonates of 120 hours of age, to 10.3 in infants of six weeks of age, to 9.3 in children five to ten years of age, to 8.4 in male adolescents in Stage V of the Tanner Scale, and to 8.3 in adults 21 to 45 years of age. The concentrations of triiodothyronine and thyroid-stimulating hormone follow a similar downward trend (Kay et al., 1966; Spencer, 1970; Hung, 1974).

In addition, the increased secretion of testosterone in male adolescents at puberty enhances muscle tissue deposition and anabolism. Increased testosterone secretion plus the enlarging body surface area contributes to the higher metabolic rate for adolescent males than for young women.

The rapid growth period of infancy, in which infants triple their birth rate by one year of age, is similar to the pace of growth in adolescents, in which literally every part of the body changes. It is not surprising that caloric needs are very high for preterm (100 to 150 cal/kg in 24 hours) and newborn infants (100 cal/kg in 24 hours) and for adolescents (2800 to 3000 cal/day for boys and 2100 to 2400 cal/day for girls (National Academy of Sciences, 1980).

The interruptions in nutritional intake that occur frequently during injury and illness commonly affect growth, which seems to have lower priority, temporarily, than metabolic demands and the other demands on nutrition noted earlier. Therefore, delayed physical development often accompanies illness and injury (Manser, 1984).

Decreased Supply of Nutrients

For people of all ages, the changes imposed by illness and injury carry the potential for decreased nutritional intake. However, infants and children have several unique problems. First, preterm infants often lack adequate suck, swallow, and gag reflexes to take in nutrients. Further, their immature gastrointestinal systems cannot digest and absorb the volume of nutrients required for health restoration and growth in many instances.

Second, congenital anomalies of the neonate are barriers to nutritional intake. For example, newborn infants who are well nourished from placental infusions in utero will soon have nutritional problems if a severe cleft palate exists. Similarly, neonates who have been well oxygenated from a sound supply of placental oxygen will become hypoxic and have difficulty eating after placental separation if they have cyanotic heart disease.

Third, the immature cognitive development in children may interfere with their understanding of the importance of eating and drinking to improve their health. Thus, young children present challenges in motivation to gain their cooperation. Last, the knowledge and vocabulary of young children may present the communication of their preferences and needs. They may have difficulty telling nurses what food or drink

they prefer, that they are nauseated, or that they are experiencing abdominal cramping.

In summary, the characteristics of infants and children with a diversity of pathology present many barriers to nutritional intake, including difficulties in communication, because of varied cognitive development and immature knowledge and vocabulary related to body parts and their function (Denehy, 1984).

ASSESSMENT

The data collected upon first contact with the infant, child, and family can be used to determine the need for intervention. Even though all writers on nursing diagnosis have identified selected defining characteristics for altered nutritional status, applicability to infants and children has not been tested. Therefore, it is helpful to recognize additional data indicating altered nutritional status.

A diet history provides a portrait of daily nutritional intake. Parents and children are asked to list the food and liquids eaten and drunk in a typical 24 hour day. The nature of the nutrients taken, as well as the patterns of eating and any eating problems, is important to assess. For example, if a baby routinely ingests 240 cc at a feeding but vomits 60 cc, a nutritional deficit will be observed.

Diet history data will also suggest the level of nutrient storage that can be used to predict response to illness. An infant or child with a diet history of prolonged patterns of decreased protein intake will have an increased probability of slow wound healing. Several guidelines for obtaining diet histories are available in the literature, such as that proposed by Foman and colleagues (1977). Other tools to assess nutritional status include the use of various growth charts, which will be mentioned only briefly in this discussion. The gestational assessment measures are helpful because they provide a means of assessing the nutritional status of preterm and full-term infants (Ballard et al., 1979). Thus, a preterm infant who is born small for gestational age has a higher probability for nutritional deficits than a preterm infant who is assessed to be appropriate for gestational age. Similarly, all pediatric growth charts offer a rapid and practical method of preliminary nutritional assessment. They are the first step in making a decision about nutritional status. Even though abnormal findings may indicate problems without a nutritional basis, growth chart entries are often the first indication that further exploration is needed (Hamill et al., 1979).

One type of growth chart for adolescents that is often overlooked is the Tanner Scale of secondary sex characteristics (Marshall and Tanner, 1969; Marshall and Tanner, 1970), even though the developmental pattern of secondary sex characteristics indicates nutritional status. For example, a developmental delay of secondary sex characteristics in adolescent girls may be related to altered nutritional status from anorexia nervosa or bulimia. Thus, nurses need to be alert to the fact that the physiological changes occurring at puberty are associated with nutritional as well as endocrine status.

The weight and dietary intake of infants and children admitted to an acute care facility need to be monitored throughout their health restoration period as one measure of nutritional status. Weight changes of 100 gm/day cause concern in neonates and young infants. For older children and adolescents, percentages of weight loss greater than these parameters are of concern: (1) 2% over one week's duration; (2) 5% over one month's duration; (3) 7.5% over a period of three months; and (4) 10% over a period of six months (Blackburn et al., 1977).

The monitoring of weight, dietary intake, and fluid balance is an additional method of collecting data to determine the need for nutritional support. Nurses monitor data regarding daily caloric intake with some global measures, such as the portion of food eaten or the number of cubic centimeters of formula, juice, or milk taken. It is also possible to derive caloric intake through conversions from fluid ounce to calories per ounce (usually 20 calories per formula ounce, or 24 calories per ounce in premature infant formula). Conversions from ingestion of grams of protein (4 cal/gm), carbohydrate (4 cal/gm), and fat (9 cal/gm) also can be made. It is possible to be very precise in calculation of nutritional intake if warranted by the pathological condition.

The calculation of precise output is not quite so easy. When older children and adolescents use emesis basins, urinals, and bedpans appropriately, the calculations are

not difficult. However, the accurate measurement of emesis, urine, and stool for infants and toddlers is a challenge.

The most accurate measures of emesis output are obtained when it is possible to predict those infants who are most likely to vomit. For them, spit cloths are preweighed and that amount subtracted from the total weight of a used spit cloth. However, problems arise when the emesis is unexpected and must be estimated visually. The author and a colleague, Dr. Jean Moss, have studied the difficulties in accurate determinations of fluid volumes using visual perception. Two studies have been conducted and a third is in progress. The first study used a psychophysical theoretical framework with the premise that visual perceptions of volume would increase in accuracy with subject feedback. Nursing students observed 100 slides of emesis in different configurations and made judgments as to the amount. Subjects in the experimental group received feedback as to their accuracy, whereas subjects in the control group received no feedback. The results showed that accuracy did increase during the process of observing and recording volume for the experimental group. However, this difference between the experimental and control group faded in the post test that immediately followed the slide presentation (Moss and Craft, 1989). Several colleagues suggested that experienced nurses be included in the subject pool for another study. The purpose of the second study, which included experienced nurses and used realistic emesis displays rather than slides, was to determine accuracy and variables related to accuracy. Unexpectedly, the data from the second study showed that experienced nurses were no more likely to be accurate than student nurses and that error was prevalent. The variables that accounted for a significant proportion of variance in accuracy were the method taught, the nursing status (student versus staff), and the nature of experience. That is, the nurses who practiced in a sick infant unit had less error. Nurses who were taught to use a mental frame of reference from which they subtracted when they observed the emesis were more accurate. Further, accuracy was increased when weight was assessed in addition to vision (Craft and Moss, in review). Since the method learned initially for estimating fluid volume was a significant factor, this method will be studied and compared with other methods in a current study.

Perhaps the most important conclusion of the research at this point is that decisions and judgments made using visual perception data should be viewed with skepticism, and that some error must be assumed. Thus, it is best to avoid measurement using only visual perception whenever possible. When it is necessary, the documentation needs to be clear that the amount recorded was an estimation, rather than a precise measure.

While assessing accurate intake and output is an important measure of nutritional status, other indicators of nutritional status are used commonly in clinic and acute care settings. These include determinations of levels of serum blood sugar, hemoglobin, total protein as well as albumin/globulin ratio, creatinine, cholesterol, lymphocytes, and nitrogen balance, and anthropomorphic measurements. Their application for appraisal of nutritional status is summarized in Table 21–1.

As noted earlier, the defining characteristics presented for *Altered nutritional status: Less than body requirements* include more global indicators that will apply to all age groups. These indicators include (1) loss of weight with adequate food intake; (2) body weight 20% or more under the ideal weight for height and frame; (3) reported inadequate food intake of less than the recommended daily allowance (RDA); (4) weakness of muscles required for swallowing or mastication; (5) reported or evidence of lack of food intake; (6) lack of interest in food; (7) excessive loss of hair; and (8) poor muscle tone (Kim et al., 1984).

THE INTERVENTION

The possibility of a deficit in nutritional status exists for every infant and child with an injury, illness, or disability. Throughout the following discussion the strategies used by nurses to implement nutritional support will be directed toward the cause or a modifying variable affecting the diagnosis. Strategies will be appropriate for various age groups, with the discussion beginning with the first stage of life, infancy.

Non-nutritive Sucking

Pacifiers have been used to promote sucking during nasogastric and gastrostomy feedings for decades. The rationale for the use of non-nutritive sucking often included the need to quiet infants during feedings to prevent contracting abdominal muscles that supply negative pressure against a feeding flowing by gravity. An additional reason was the importance of sucking to emotional development and the development of normal eating ability later in infancy.

However, the seminal research of Measel and Anderson (1979) revealed that non-nutritive sucking had significance in other areas. These investigators found that preterm infants receiving non-nutritive sucking during every tube feeding and for five minutes after the feeding had significantly different increases in weight and reduced days of hospitalization. This investigation fostered the study of non-nutritive sucking by other researchers (Caple, 1982; Field et al., 1982; Bernbaum et al., 1983; Schwartz et al., 1987), whose work has been combined in a meta-analysis of critical outcome variables. The analysis showed the outcome variable yielding the most significant results was days of hospitalization. On the average, non-nutritive sucking reduced hospitalization by 6.3 days (Schwartz et al., 1987).

Thus, this strategy has important ramifications for nutritional status and needs to become a part of daily care for preterm infants who do not use their suck reflex for eating. For preterm and full term infants who have a weak suck reflex, nursing strategies to structure the suck reflex can make the difference between those infants who can take nutrients orally and those who will require tube feedings.

Structuring the Suck Reflex

The sleepy, full-term newborn infant, the baby who is breast feeding, and the baby who is waking from surgical anesthesia all present temporary challenges for increasing oral intake. However, for preterm infants or those who have congenital facial anomalies, feeding problems are long-term and are likely to alter nutritional status. Therefore, strategies are needed that increase oral intake. A strategy that is effective in structuring the suck reflex often will make the difference between oral feeding and the need to be fed via nasogastric tube or gastrostomy. The strategy is based upon the principle of

Table 21–1. INDICATORS FOR NUTRITIONAL SUPPORT

Nutritional Measure	Normal Values	Importance During Injury or Illness
Serum glucose	80–120 mg/dl	Indicates whether glucose is available for use by the cell. Cells of the cardiac muscle and brain cannot tolerate reduced glucose. Further, preterm and newborn infants have no glycogen stores.
Hemoglobin in gm/dl	Neonate: 14–20 2 mo: 9–14 6–12 yr: 11.5–15.5 12–18 yr: Males: 13.0–16.0 Females: 12.0–16.0	Globin is composed of amino acids. Lower cellular protein is reflected in a lower hemoglobin.
Total blood protein in gm/dl	Preterm infant: 4.3–7.6 Neonate: 4.6–7.4 3–5 yr: 6.7–8.0 6–8 yr: 5.9–7.9 12–16 yr: 6.3–8.8	Reduced total protein indicates inadequate supply for cellular maintenance and repair.
Albumin	Preterm infant: 3.0–4.2 Neonate: 3.6–5.4 3–5 yr: 2.9–5.2 6–8 yr: 3.3–4.9 12–16 yr: 3.1–5.3	Reduced albumin suggests the possibility of fluid shifts due to altered colloidal osmotic pressure.
Globulin* Alpha-1	Preterm infant: 0.25–0.66 Neonate: 0.08–0.43 3–5 yr: 0.08–0.40 6–8 yr: 0.09–0.45 12–16 yr: 0.09–0.32	Alpha-1 globulin includes alpha-1 lipoproteins, antitrypsins, glycoproteins, and thyroxine-binding globulin.
Alpha-2	Preterm infant: 0.44–0.94 Neonate: 0.40–1.13 3–5 yr: 0.43–0.99 6–8 yr: 0.50–0.83 12–16 yr: 0.50–0.97	Nine alpha-2 globulins are necessary for growth factor activity, for binding insulin fats, especially triglycerides, for binding iron, and for hydrolyzing acetylcholine and prothrombin.
Beta	Preterm: 0.42–1.56 Neonate: 0.39–1.4 3–5 yr: 0.47–1.1 6–8 yr: 0.45–0.93 12–16 yr: 0.48–0.88	Needed for lipid and iron transport, phagocyte properties, and lysis of fibrin in blood clots, as well as development of fibrinogen.
Gamma	Preterm: 0.81–1.61 Neonate: 0.25–1.05 3–5 yr: 0.54–1.66 6–8 yr: 0.70–1.95 12–16 yr: 1.08–1.96	Immunoglobulin G: antibody effective against viruses, bacterial toxins, Rh antibodies, nuclear antibodies, anti-insulin, and ragweed antibodies. Immunoglobulin A: antibodies for antibacterial agglutinins, and is the predominant immunoglobulin in body fluids and secretions. Immunoglobulin M: includes antibodies for ABO isoagglutinins to gram-negative bacteria. Immunoglobulins D and E: functions unknown at the time of writing.
Creatinine	Serum: 0.7–1.4 mg/dl	Assuming normal kidney function, this measure can be used to determine muscle mass breakdown, which occurs during starvation: elevation may mean protein catabolism, and decrease may mean inadequate intake.
Lymphocytes	1000–4000 cu mm	Reflect protein/caloric intake
Nitrogen balance	10–20 (blood urea nitrogen [BUN] in mg/dl)	Nitrogen is the end product of protein catabolism. Assuming normal renal function and hydration, elevation means a negative nitrogen balance exists.
Anthropometric measures, using triceps (given in mm)	See Foman (1977) and Hamill (1979) for technique and normative data	Used to distinguish between excess muscle and excess fat when attempting to determine whether an overweight child is simply muscular or has extra fat.

*Normative data are taken from Ellis and Robbins (1978) and Fischbach (1984).

supporting or maximizing the existing suck reflex.

Correct placement of the bottle nipple is the first step in this strategy. A soft nipple, especially manufactured for preterm infants, must be placed on top of the tongue. This process is not always easy in a preterm infant, whose tongue has little cartilage and falls easily to the top of the palate. Therefore, the baby's body and head position must be changed slowly to get the tongue to drop down to the floor of the mouth. Next, the fifth or little finger of the nurse is placed beneath the tip of the mandible or chin, with the thumb supporting one side and the index finger supporting the other side of the baby's mandible. The result of this finger placement is full support of the mandible at the tip and on both sides plus support of the muscular stratum of the cheeks. This strategy is modified somewhat for the baby with anomalies that interfere with the suck reflex, such as cleft lip or palate. However, the principle is identical—that is, the existing suck reflex is enhanced through placement of the bottle nipple and support of the suck.

The existence of a cleft lip presents only few problems in oral intake, provided that some upper lip that contains the necessary muscle to supply suction remains intact. In these instances a soft nipple or a lamb's nipple is placed between the intact upper and lower lips on top of the tongue.

When babies have a cleft palate as well, the placement of the lamb's nipple will vary depending on the location of the cleft. If the cleft is in the soft palate, the nurse can avoid placing the nipple in the cleft and use the existing hard palate to provide the suction and negative pressure. In contrast, when the cleft is in the hard palate for which a complete surface exists, the nipple is placed in the cleft to facilitate use of the hard palate in the supply of negative pressure.

In both these instances, suck restructuring is based upon a combination of preferences of the baby plus the knowledge and skill of the nurse. Thus, the nurse carefully determines the suck and swallow patterns of the infant and then modifies the structuring to reach a goal of increased oral intake.

Positioning

While it is obvious that the anatomy of humans is such that nutritional intake is enhanced by the flow of gravity from the posterior nasopharynx to the gastric and duodenal areas of the gastrointestinal tract, this anatomical structure is ignored commonly as infants or children are fed and positioned after a feeding. Nurses can increase the digestion and absorption of nutrients as well as diminish gastric reflux by body positioning.

First, the head should be upright during feeding for two reasons. As noted earlier, the swallow and gravity flow of nutrients is enhanced through head elevation. Of equal importance, however, is the increase in the exchange of oxygen and carbon dioxide at the alveolar level due to the potential for increased lung expansion. That is, the stomach lies against the lower lobes of the lungs when an infant or child is lying flat or with the head elevated only slightly. This position impedes lung expansion.

Next, the flow of nutrients from the stomach to the duodenum following a period of eating is increased by body positioning on the right side. Such a position facilitates movement of gastric air above the lesser curvature of the stomach into the region of the fundus, which removes the air from the greater curvature, so that air does not interfere with the gastric flow of nutrients into the pyloric canal, through the pylorus, and into the duodenum.

The flow of nutrients from the stomach to the duodenum is reduced for reasons other than body position in some instances. One of the more common reasons is a reflux or regurgitation of nutrients due to a cardiac sphincter with inadequate cartilage development. In these instances placement with the head elevated after eating will decrease reflux up the esophagus because the reflux will have a gravitational barrier.

Maintain Normal Body Temperature

Changing body temperature results in a hypermetabolic state that increases the demand for nutrients. A preterm infant who is unable to maintain normal body temperature responds to hypothermia with an elevated metabolic rate. In older children, the hypermetabolic state is related to the reverse—an elevated body temperature—with an additional 12% caloric requirement for every temperature elevation of 1°C (Hardy, 1980).

It is important to maintain body temperature through nursing actions including retention of body heat, control of environmental temperature, temperature control of solutions entering the body, appropriate clothing, and measures to reduce elevated body temperature.

Retention of body heat is accomplished by prevention of heat loss through radiation, conduction, convection, and evaporation (Arshavskii, 1976). The amount of heat lost by radiation from the skin varies as needed by dilatation of surface blood vessels when a heat elevation occurs and by vasoconstriction when heat loss needs to be decreased. Heat radiates from the body surface to nearby objects that are cooler than the skin and radiates to the skin from those that are warmer than the skin. Heat conduction occurs when heat is transferred to any substance actually in contact with the body, such as clothing or linens. Heat loss by convection occurs when body heat is aided by surrounding currents from ambient air. Thus, the placement of infants close to air conditioning outlets should be avoided. They should be transported in a unit with solid sides that will prevent air currents from reaching them.

Evaporation also accounts for a major source of body heat loss. Newly born infants are covered with amniotic fluid. Exposure to the cold temperatures in the delivery room fosters evaporation, so their hair and skin need to be dried rapidly before they are wrapped in a warm towel and placed in a warm environment. Similarly, an infant with an unstable body temperature should not be bathed until the body temperature is normal. Further loss of body heat from evaporation can be retarded through use of humidity.

The control of environmental temperature must be complete for preterm infants, which necessitates the use of incubators with thermostatic control through feedback from abdominal skin probes for the smallest preterm infants. Similarly, full term newborn infants may require the use of a warmer-bed until their body temperature has stabilized when they are wrapped in warm blankets. However, it must be noted that environmental temperature needs to be monitored and controlled for all infants and children. Similarly, all fluids that enter infants and children should be as close to body temperature as possible. These fluids include formula, food, blood, or enema solutions. Each solution can be warmed or cooled to body temperature before use.

The selection of clothing that will maintain normal body temperature for infants and children is difficult, because it is impossible to predict to what extent a modification in clothing will alter body temperature. For example, preterm infants who are hypothermic and wear a warm, knitted hat will probably respond with an elevation in body temperature. However, it is impossible to predict how much their temperature will rise. Therefore, modifications in clothing must be accompanied by careful monitoring of body temperature.

When body temperature is elevated, reverse strategies can be used to lower temperature. Evaporation that occurs with sponging will reduce body temperature, and heat loss will result from radiation to a cooler surface, such as a cooling blanket, as well as from conduction to cooler bed clothing and convection provided by a fan. Altered body temperatures change metabolic demands for nutrients. These demands can slowed by maintaining body temperature.

Increasing Energy and Oxygenation for Eating

Even though nutrient demands are elevated during prematurity, injury, and illness, increasing the time to feed in an attempt to increase food intake at the expense of caloric use during eating is ill advised. It is not wise to continue urging an exhausted infant or child to eat, because the calories used in this expenditure of energy beyond reasonable expectations can be greater than the calories obtained from eating. In addition, aspiration becomes a danger with patient exhaustion. Therefore, the time interval during eating should be monitored and the patient watched closely for signs of decreasing energy that suggest the need to rest.

Infants and children who are debilitated from prolonged illness also require rest before eating. This required rest is usually a part of sleeping patterns for infants (see the chapter on sleep). However, planned resting or sleeping periods before meals need to be implemented for older children.

Rest prior to eating will provide energy to eat, and rest periods during eating are often helpful for exhausted or hypoxic clients. Food can be left in the room while older children take a brief rest during meals, and their food can be rewarmed when they are ready to eat. Similarly, the formula of infants can be refrigerated while they rest during feedings and then rewarmed as indicated when they are rested and ready to eat.

The energy required to eat is available only when an adequate supply of glucose and oxygen to cells exists, which is problematic in some instances. As stated earlier in this discussion, oxygenation for all infants and children during eating is enhanced by head elevation. When altered nutritional status is apparent in hypoxic children, it is necessary to supply additional oxygen during feedings or meals in order to increase their nutritional intake.

Prevent Vomiting

Vomiting should be prevented whenever possible, because of the loss of nutrients as well as the danger of aspiration. Since nausea is a subjectively experienced phenomenon, older children can be questioned in a manner studied by Rhodes and associates (1984, 1985) for use with adults, to determine whether they are nauseated. Nausea assessment measures for younger children need to be developed. Strategies that can be used to prevent vomiting include the appropriate spacing and nature of food intake, behavior management decreasing rumination or self-induced vomiting, use of both pharmacological and nonpharmacolgical antiemetics, and use of deep breathing and distraction.

Spacing of Food Intake

Because the stomach empties only when peristalsis in the small and large intestine permits it to empty, food intake must be timed according to stomach-emptying capacity. This principle applies to patients of every developmental stage, but the strategies used to space food appropriately will differ.

Spacing of food intake is important because the stomach has a limited capacity. When that capacity is exceeded, vomiting is more likely to occur. In small, preterm infants, the capacity of the stomach is tested by tube aspiration prior to the administration of a nasogastric feeding. If a large portion of a feeding given prior to the aspiration still remains, the portion is returned to the stomach and the volume amount aspirated subtracted from the feeding to be given. If a high percentage of the prior feeding remains, it may be necessary to omit one feeding.

In very small preterm infants, continuous drip nasogastric feedings have two advantages. First, the amount infused is never large and stomach capacity is not exceeded. Second, the supply of nutrients is continuous, which facilitates weight gain. For these reasons, this is often the preferential method of nutritional intake for well preterm infants weighing less than 1250 gm at birth (Toce et al. 1987).

Similar principles apply for patients being fed by gastrostomy. That is, the presence of a large reflux in the gastrostomy tubing and syringe indicates that the stomach is unable to accept more. Therefore, the syringe and tubing are elevated to use gravity for increasing the flow of contents into the stomach. If the contents do not proceed downward, either the tubing is plugged or the stomach is full. In either case, adding more fluid is inappropriate.

Spacing of food intake for toddlers can be challenging, because of their developmentally appropriate dislike for sitting long enough to eat. For these children, small nutritious snacks are suggested that can be eaten while they are involved in other activities.

Older children and adolescents can verbalize a sensation of hunger or satiation when they are conscious. They are usually reliable sources of data regarding the readiness of their stomach to receive increased content and should be listened to carefully. The two exceptions to this statement are teens with either anorexia nervosa, who are likely to underestimate their nutritional needs, and those with bulimia, who are likely to binge eat before vomiting or purging (Comerci et al., 1985).

Modify the Nature of Food Intake

Nausea and vomiting require a succession of nursing actions that modify the nature of food intake. They are commonly used but have received very little systematic study. They are all directed toward placing the gastrointestinal tract at complete rest or diminished activity until inflammation or other pathology is corrected.

When nausea or vomiting occurs, the absence of any oral intake is recommended for at least 20 minutes, sometimes longer. Following rest, the first nutrients introduced are clear liquids, which take the form of oral electrolyte solutions for infants. However, older children and teens also need clear liquids that will supply needed potassium and nutrients. Therefore, these solutions should be chosen carefully.

If the gastrointestinal tract can manage oral electrolyte solutions and clear liquids, formula that is diluted to one-half strength for infants and soft foods for older children are recommended. The last step is the return to the usual diet.

In each of these steps individual preferences should be identified and respected, since nausea and vomiting produce different nutritional needs. Thus, children receiving chemotherapy who crave salty, spicy foods should be provided with those foods because of their need for added salt.

Whenever possible, oral rehydration is recommended rather than the use of parenteral fluids. However, prolonged lack of intake mandates the use of intravenous fluids for fluid intake. Further, when the lack of intake begins to affect nutritional status, total parenteral nutritional supplements are indicated; these involve another set of nursing actions, discussed in most basic nursing textbooks.

Behavior Management

Vomiting is self-induced in some instances, and strategies are needed to prevent this from happening. Self-induced vomiting occurs in infant rumination and bulimia. Infant self-induced vomiting is seen most frequently in chronic illness requiring months of hospitalization. These months of hospitalization are too often accompanied by a lack of a consistent caretaker, lack of attachment, and sensory deprivation or overload. Thus, it is hypothesized that infants who ruminate are using self-stimulation when they put their fingers in the back of their throat, gag themselves, and vomit. The vomiting, then, is accompanied by increased attention by a caretaker, which is thought to be a reinforcement of the vomiting behavior. Whenever possible, this type of behavior

should be prevented by insuring that infants with chronic illness have consistent caretakers and receive stimulation that is comparable to that received by an infant in the home. However, when rumination occurs, a behavior management plan is needed that will be implemented consistently to prevent vomiting.

Vomiting can be prevented through two steps. First, stop the finger from going into the mouth through the use of soft restraints or clothing that prevents arm extension for young infants. In addition, older infants will understand if "No, no" is said every time their fingers go up to their mouths and then their hands are guided gently away. Second, increased stimulation, cuddling, and attention should be supplied by someone on an intensive basis.

Nonpharmacological Strategies

While nurses give antiemetics frequently to prevent nausea and vomiting, nonpharmacological strategies are of equal importance. These strategies include the use of certain foods, distraction, and deep breathing. Women have used pickles and crackers to deal with the nausea and vomiting of pregnancy for generations. It is interesting that salty foods like chips and popcorn seem to help nausea and vomiting from other causes, such as the side effects of chemotherapy. Foods that diminish the changing taste from chemotherapy, such as gum or hard candy, also can be used during chemotherapy administration to decrease nausea.

Distraction can be effective in early nausea. The distraction can be provided by verbal exchange or by the use of imagery, although both of these strategies need to be studied. As noted in the chapter on pain, hypnosis is effective in providing comfort; similarly, it is an effective measure in the prevention of nausea and vomiting.

The encouragement and modeling of deep breathing is also effective in the prevention of vomiting. Although the reason for this effectiveness is often attributed to relaxation, a sound physiological basis is involved. That is, abdominal muscles must contract for vomiting to occur. On inspiration of air the diaphragm falls and prevents abdominal muscles from contracting. Thus, vomiting is prevented (Norris, 1979).

A sensation of coolness has long been used by nurses to manage vomiting. It is provided through a cold cloth on the forehead in some instances. Nurses also use a cool cloth or ice on the abdomen. The rationale is unknown at this point, and further research in this area is indicated.

Maximize Nutritional Contributions of Intake

Infants and children who are experiencing stress, an altered immune system, and cellular and tissue damage need increased intake of calories, protein, vitamins C and B and the mineral zinc. These increases are supplied in various manners. For infants there appears to be no substitute for breast milk from their own mothers (Foman et al., 1977; Hambraeus, 1977; Gross et al., 1981).

Human milk has a biological adaptation to meet the needs of preterm infants. Milk of the mothers of preterm infants has been demonstrated to be more suited to the specific needs of their preterm infants than is pooled breast milk (Foman et al., 1977; Atkinson et al., 1980). Preterm infants require more protein per kilogram to support rapid growth. Breast milk contains increased cysteine and taurine, amino acids that are needed for body and brain growth. These two amino acids may be essential for infants, especially preterm infants (Hambraeus, 1977; Lawrence, 1980).

Human milk fat is more easily digestible than cow milk fat. It forms smaller globules and is more easily emulsified than cow milk (Foman, 1974). It is also high in protein and has an increased ratio of lactalbumin to casein. Fresh human milk protects against a variety of bacterial and viral infections. The most important factors are secretory IgA, milk leukocytes, lysozyme, and lactoferrin (Lawrence, 1980; Yu et al., 1981; May, 1984). IgA is the principal immunoglobulin that is present in greater concentrations in milk of mothers of preterm infants (Gross et al., 1981), and it is crucial for controlling the microbial environment of the intestinal tract. Breast milk can be supplied through breast feeding, even for preterm infants under 1500 grams (Meier and Anderson, 1987). However, when infants do not have adequate suck, gag, and swallow reflexes or are simply too weak to suck and swallow, breast milk from the mother can be supplied through nasogastric feedings.

Mothers can be encouraged to supply their sick infants with their own milk either directly, through breast feeding, or indirectly, through teaching them how to express breast milk manually or through the use of a pump. Mothers who return home before their infants are discharged need to be taught how to store their milk at home and bring it to the hospital, where it can be stored and used to feed their babies (Bell, 1987).

Increased supplies of calories for preterm infants are provided by formulas containing more calories and medium chain triglycerides. This type of fat is digested and metabolized readily and offers a source of energy for small infants. Providing increased nutrients for health restoration for infants is convenient, since breast milk and formulas contain these nutrients or can be modified readily to supply them.

Supplying therapeutic nutrients for toddlers and older children is more challenging. The most important principle to remember in meeting this challenge is that all food and liquids that sick children take should provide nutrients needed for health restoration. When children are fussy and selective about food, nurses can begin by finding *something* they will eat and drink. Then, nurses should attempt to compromise by adding a nutritional component. For example, if a child with little appetite is willing to eat a piece of toast, an attempt can be made to get the child to take some butter or peanut butter on it as well. If there are no contraindications, a child can be encouraged to drink milk instead of a carbonated beverage, which will fill the stomach but add few needed nutrients.

Role Modeling and Socialization

Infants and children who are not eating will sometimes eat when they see others eating. In these cases, role modeling and socialization promote nutritional intake. Role modeling is suggested for those infants who have never learned to eat. Infants must see eating to know what is expected, so they should be with other children who are eating and also go to meals with nurses. Similarly, older children with a poor intake will benefit from eating with other children rather than in a room by themselves. If group dining is not possible, children can bring their trays into other rooms when there are no contraindications.

Some infants and children benefit from the company of others, but others are distracted by the stimulation. Distracted or overstimulated infants and children will benefit by a quiet, private environment during mealtime. Currently, our lack of research makes it impossible to predict the optimal environment for each child. Therefore, role modeling and socialization are manipulated to increase nutritional status individually.

EVALUATION

The aforementioned defining characteristics and other indicators are used to determine whether the intervention of nutritional support is needed and to evaluate the outcome. If nutritional status rises, the intervention was effective.

Case Study

Jess was an 11 month old boy who had been born prematurely. He also had jejunal atresia that necessitated surgery, followed by prolonged nutritional support with hyperalimentation. At this time he was on gastrostomy feedings and had a tracheostomy. He had never been home, and his family lived a great distance from the hospital. They came to see him approximately once a month. The longer he was in the hospital, the less frequent were the family visits.

During the last week, nurses had documented spontaneous vomiting unrelated to eating. Nurses would find emesis on Jess' clothing when he was out in the hall, in the swing, or in the playpen. His weight began to drop in spite of adequate intake of calories. The nursing diagnosis of Nutrition, *alterations in: less than body requirements* was made.

The primary nurse for Jess called a meeting to ask for very close observation to determine the cause of his vomiting, Radiographs were negative. After two days of careful observation, a pattern began to emerge. Jess placed the fingers of his right hand into his mouth, gagged himself, and vomited whenever he was left alone for a lengthy period during the day. He did not vomit at night because he slept through the night.

Using these data, the primary nurse developed a plan to manage, or decrease, this behavior. Increased attention and stimulation were to be given to Jess, plus teaching him that his behavior was not acceptable before a vomiting episode. Thus, all the nurses agreed to say "No, no" to Jess whenever he began to move his right hand to his mouth. Then, they were to move his hand away gently and praise him for keeping it away from his mouth.

The increased attention and stimulation took the form of scheduled play three times daily, plus a daily trip to the playroom to watch other children play and take part in the morning music therapy. The nurses had always hugged and cuddled Jess, but this process was also increased. Further, he was old enough to teach how to "kiss," and he was encouraged to kiss his nurses, who kissed him back.

Within two weeks the vomiting episodes decreased, and they disappeared within a month. His weight began to increase and the desired intervention goal was reached.

RESEARCH IMPLICATIONS

Though the area of nutrition has been studied by scientists from other disciplines, nursing has a short history of investigation in this area. The work of Rhodes, Watson, and Johnson (1984, 1985) represents beginning work on nausea and vomiting assessment for adults. As noted previously, selected research questions have been studied, such as the effects of non-nutritive sucking or techniques and methods in nasogastric feedings, but few research programs have been established to investigate the manipulation of the modifying or intervening variables on nutritional status.

For this reason, the intervention strategies discussed previously are largely unstudied and need testing by nursing researchers. The strategy of body positioning, for instance, is logical from an anatomical perspective, but systematic demonstration of the effectiveness is needed. Similarly, the strategies of body temperature maintenance, increasing energy, and oxygenation and the strategies used to prevent vomiting by nurses have not been studied.

The technology needed to answer some of our basic nursing questions is becoming more accessible. For instance, if a nurse wished to investigate the relationship of body positioning during feeding to oxygenation, continuous oxygen readings from oximeters or transcutaneous monitors are now possible. If a nurse wanted to investigate the effects of body positioning after feeding on esophageal reflux, the use of esophageal pH probes and continuous monitoring is now possible.

The reason that nutrition is an understudied area in nursing research could be related to the difficulty of these questions as they appear in humans. Perhaps more investigators will need to follow the example of Heitkemper and Marotta (1985), who began their studies with rats and lower primates and then expanded their studies to humans. More drastic manipulation of variables would be possible with animals. Thus, heating pads could be used to alter body temperature, keeping intake constant, in order to investigate effects on nutritional status. Or the nature of the environment could be manipulated to investigate effects on animals. For example, the effects of rest and stress on nutritional status can be studied in the animal model.

This is not to say that nutritional nursing research on humans is impossible. Instead, descriptive studies are badly needed to generate hypotheses, and data collection in clinical settings might be a sound beginning. Nurses can collect longitudinal data to determine variable relationships as they exist in homogeneous clinical populations. If it could be demonstrated, for example, that a significant association exists between crying frequency in babies and weight gain, the effects of a touch or comfort intervention strategy on nutritional status could be studied. Similarly, if a significant association could be found between rest after eating and weight gain, then rest as nutritional intervention strategy could be studied in an experimental design.

It is important for nurses to test nutritional inventions strategies to identify those that are the most useful. However, it is also important to determine the appropriateness of their use. Take, for instance, the use of distraction with nausea to prevent vomiting. Nurses have observed that this intervention strategy is not effective if delayed. Thus, indicators for and the timing of intervention strategy use would be helpful to identify and test. The basis for their identification could also begin with nursing observation and documentation on clinical units with homogenic populations.

In summary, the area of nutritional nursing research has received very little attention in spite of the importance of nursing care to nutritional status. Nurses interested in clinical research will make a contribution through descriptive studies that generate testable hypotheses. Nurses interested in physiological research will make contributions through animal model research that provides hypotheses for study of humans. These hypotheses can be tested by clinical nurse researchers. Nutritional research has always been important, but the importance has gained added attention as the relationship between nutrition and health has become more visible. Because the nursing profession is grounded in the goals of health promotion and restoration, the research area of nutritional strategies to restore health should be a high priority for nursing scientists.

REFERENCES

Alberts, B, Bray, D, Lewis, J, Raff M, Roberts, K, and Watson J. Molecular biology of the cell. New York: Garland Publishing Co., Inc., 1983.

Arshavskii, ID. Physiological analysis of physical development with special reference to the newborn infant. Human Physiology, 5:169–180, 1976.

Atkinson, SA, Anderson, GH, and Bryen, NH. Human milk: Comparison of the nitrogen composition in milk from mothers of premature and fullterm infants. Journal of Clinical Nutrition, 33:811–815, 1980.

Axelrod L. Adrenal cortex. In Smith, LH Jr., and Thier, SO (Eds.). Pathophysiology: The biological principles of disease, 2nd ed. Philadelphia: WB Saunders Co, 1985.

Ballard, JL, Novak KK, and Driver, M. A simplified score for assessment of fetal maturation of newly born infants. Journal of Pediatrics, 95:769–774, 1979.

Bell, E. Expression and storage of breast milk. Unpublished paper, The University of Iowa, 1987.

Bernbaum, JC, Pereira, GR, Watkins, JB, and Perkins, GJ. Nonnutritive sucking during gavage feeding enhances growth and maturation in premature infants, Pediatrics, 71:41–45, 1983.

Blackburn, G, Bistrian, B, Maini, B, Schlamm, H, and Smith, M. Nutritional and metabolic assessment of the hospitalized patient. Journal of Parenteral and Enteral Nutrition, 1:11–21, 1977.

Burns, TW, and Carlson, HE. Endocrinology. In Sodeman, WA, and Sodeman, TM (Eds.). Pathologic physiology, 7th ed. Philadephia: WB Saunders Co., 1985.

Caple, JIH. The effect of nonnutritive suckling on the clinical course of tube-fed premature infants. Unpublished master's thesis, Houston Baptist University, Houston, 1982.

Comerci, GD, Kilbourne, K, and Carroll, AE. Eating disorders in the young; Anorexia nervosa and bulima: Part II. New York: Year Book Medical Publishers, 1985.

Craft, MJ, and Moss, J. Variables related to accuracy in visual perceptual skills, in review.

Denehy, J. What do school-aged children know about their bodies? Pediatric Nursing, 10:290–292, 1984.

Dodge, PR, Prensky, AL, and Feigin, RD. Nutrition and the developing nervous system. St. Louis: CV Mosby Co., 1975, p. 1.

Ellis, EF, and Robbins, JB. Relation of serum protein levels to age. In Children are different: Developmental physiology, 2nd ed. Columbus: Ross Laboratories, 1978, p. 188.

Field, T, Ignatoff, E, Stringer, S, Brennan, J, Greenberg, R, Widemayer, S, and Anderson, GC. Nonnutritive sucking during tube feedings: Effects on preterm neonates in an intensive care unit. Pediatrics, 70:381–384, 1982.

Fischbach, FT. A manual of laboratory diagnosic tests, 2nd ed. Philadelphia: JB Lippincott, 1984.

Foman, SJ. Infant nutrition, 2nd ed.. Philadelphia: WB Saunders Co., 1974.

Foman, SJ. Nutritional disorders of children. Washington, D.C.: US Department of Health, Education and Welfare, PHS Publication No. (HSA) 75–5612, 1977.

Foman, SJ, Ziegler, EF, and Vasques, HD. Human milk and the small premature infant. American Journal of Diseases in Children, 131:463–467, 1977.

Forlaw, L. The critically ill patient: Nutritional implications. Nursing Clinics of North America, 18:111–117, 1983.

Groer, ME. Pathophysiology; Causes by cellular deviation. In Groer, ME, and Shekleton, ME (Eds.). Basic pathophysiology. St. Louis: CV Mosby Co., 1979.

Gross, SJ, Buckley, SS, Wakel, DC, McAllister, RJ, Faix, D, and Faix, RG. Elevated IgA concentration in milk produced by mothers delivered of preterm infants. Journal of Pediatrics, 99:389–393, 1981.

Hambraeus, L. Proprietary milk versus human breast milk in infant feeding. A critical appraisal from the nutritional point of view. Pediatric Clinics of North America, 24:17–36, 1977.

Hamill, PVV, Drizd, TA, Johnson, CL, Reed, RB, Roche, AF, and Moore, WM. Physical growth: National Center for Health Statistics percentiles. American Journal of Clinical Nutrition, 32:607–629, 1979.

Hamilton, WJ, Boyd, JD, and Mossman, HW. Human embryology, 3rd ed. Cambridge: W. Heffer & Sons, 1962, p. 1.

Hardy, JD. Body temperature regulation. In Mountcastle, VD (Ed.). Medical physiology, 14th ed. (Vol. 2). St. Louis: CV Mosby Co., 1980.

Harris, JA, Benedict, FG. A biometric study of basal metabolism in man. Washington, D.C.: Carnegie Institute of Washington, Publication No. 279, 1919.

Hay, WW. Nutritional requirements and recommended feeding for premature infants. Pediatric Basics, 42:4–11, 1985.

Heitkemper, MM, Marotta, SF. Role of diets in modifying gastrointestinal neurotransmitter enzyme activity. Nursing Research, 34:19–23, 1985.

Hung, W. Growth and development of the thyroid. In Davis, JA, and Dobbing, J (Eds.). Scientific Foundations of Paediatrics. Philadephia: WB Saunders Co, 1974, p. 514.

Hunt, TK, Ehrlich, HP, Garcia, JA, and Dunphy, JE. Effect of vitamin A on reversing the inhibitory effect of cortisone on healing in open wounds in animals and man. Annals of Surgery, 170:633–641, 1969.

Irvin, TT. Effects of malnutrition and hyperalimentation on wound healing. Surgical and Gynecological Obstetrics, 146:33–37, 1978.

Kay C, Abrahams S, and Molcina, P. The weight of normal thyroid glands in children. Archives of Pathology, 82:329, 1966.

Kiecolt-Glaser, J, Garner, W, Speicher, C, Penn, G, Holliday, J, and Glaser, R. Psychosocial modifiers of immunocompetence in medical students. Psychosomatic Medicine, 46:7–14, 1984.

Kiecolt-Glaser, J, Ricker, D, George, J, Messick, G. Specher, C, Garner, W, and Glaser, R. Urinary cortisol levels, cellular immunocompetency, and loneliness in psychiatry inpatients. Psychosomatic Medicine, 46:15–23, 1984.

Kim, MJ, McFarland, GK, McLane, AM. Nursing diagnosis. St. Louis: CV Mosby Co., 1984.

Lahita, R, Levy, J, Weksler, M, Perrie, B, Hausman, P, and Schwab, R. Effects of sex hormones, nutrition, and aging on the immune response. In Stites D, Stobo, J, Fudenberg H, Wells, J (Eds.). Basic and clinical immunology, 5th ed. Los Altos, Calif., Lange Medical Publishing Co., 1984, pp. 288–311.

Lawrence, RA. Breast-feeding: A guide for the medical profession. St. Louis: CV Mosby Co., 1980.

Lee, PWR, Green, MA, Long, WB III, and Gill, W. Zinc and wound healing. Surgery, Gynecology, and Obstetrics 143:549–554, 1976.

Levenson, S, Seifer, E, and Van Winkle, W Jr. Nutrition. In Hunt, TK, Dunphy, JE (Eds.). Fundamentals of wound management. Norwalk, Conn., Appleton-Century-Crofts, 1979, p. 308.

Linn, M, Linn, B, and Jensen J. Stressful events, dysphoric mood, and immune responsiveness. Psychological Reports, 54:219–222, 1984.

Locke, S. Stress, adaptation and immunity: Studies in humans. General Hospital Psychiatry, 4:49–58, 1982.

Long, CL, Schaffel, N, Geiger, JW, Schiller, WR, and Blakemore, WS. Metabolic response to injury and illness: Estimation of energy and protein needs from indirect calorimetry and nitrogen balance. Journal of Parenteral and Enteral Nutrition, 3:452–456, 1979.

Manser, JI. Growth in the high risk infant. Clinical Perinatology, 11:19, 1984.

Marshall, WA, and Tanner, JM. Variation in the pattern of pubertal changes in girls. Archives of Diseases in Children, 44:291, 1969.

Marshall, WA, and Tanner, JM. Variation in the pattern of pubertal changes in boys. Archives of Diseases in Children, 45:13, 1970.

May, JT. Antimicrobal properties and microbial contaminants of breast milk—an update. Australian Paediatric Journal, 20:265–269, 1984.

Measel, CP, and Anderson, GC. Nonnutritive sucking during tube feedings: Effect on clinical course in premature infants. Journal of Obstetrical and Gynecologic Nursing, 8:265–272, 1979.

Meier, P, and Anderson, GC. Responses of small preterm infants to bottle and breast feeding. Maternal-Child Nursing Journal, 12:97–105, 1987.

Moss, J, and Craft, MJ. Accuracy in visual estimation of infant emesis volume. Western Journal of Nursing Research, 11:352–360, 1989.

National Academy of Sciences, Food and Nutrition Board. Recommended dietary allowances. Washington, DC: National Research Council, 1980.

Norris, C. An adjustment model of nausea and vomiting. Presented at a conference on concept clarification on the campus of The University of Iowa, Iowa City, 1979.

Pereira, GR, and Barbosa, MM. Controversies in neonatal nutrition. Pediatric Clinics of North America, 33:65–89, 1986.

Pollack, SV. Wound healing: A review. III. Nutritional factors affecting wound healing. Journal of Dermatological and Surgical Oncology, 5:615–619, 1979

Rhodes, VA, Watson, PM, and Johnson, MH. Development of reliable and valid measuress of nausea and vomiting. Career Nursing, 7:33–41, 1984.

Rhodes, VA, Watson, PM, and Johnson, MH. Patterns of nausea and vomiting in chemotherapy patients: A preliminary study. Oncology Nursing Forum, 12:42–48, 1985.

Riscalla, L. The influence of psychological factors on the immune system. Medical Hypotheses, 9:331–335, 1982.

Sammons, WAH, and Lewis, JM. Premature babies: A different beginning. St. Louis: CV Mosby Co., 1985.

Savilahti, E, Jarvenpaa, A, and Raiha, NCR. Serum immunoglobulins in preterm infants: Comparison of human milk and formula feeding. Pediatrics, 72:312–316, 1983.

Schwartz, R, Moody, L, Yarandi, H, and Anderson, GC. A meta-analysis of critical outcome variables in non-nutritive sucking in preterm infants. Nursing Research, 36:292–295,1987.

Shekleton, ME. Oxygenation and cellular metabolism. In Groer, ME, and Shekleton, ME. Basic pathophysiology: A conceptual approach. St. Louis: CV Mosby Co., 1979.

Spencer, RP, and Banever, C. Human thyroid growth: A scan study. Investigations in Radiology, 5:111, 1970.

Stotts, NA. Impaired wound healing. In Carrieri, VK, Lindsey, AM, and West, CM (Eds.). Pathophysiological phenomena in nursing—Human responses to illness. Philadelphia: WB Saunders Co., 1986.

Temple, WJ, Voitak AJ, Snelling, CFT, and Crispin, JS. Effect of nutrition, diet and suture material on long-term wound healing. Annals of Surgery, 182:93–97, 1975.

Thompson R. Psychosocial research on pediatric hospitalization and health care: A review of the literature. Springfield, Ill., Charles C Thomas, 1985.

Toce, SS, Keenan, WJ, and Homan, SH. Enteral feeding in very-low-birthweight infants. A comparison of two nasogastric methods. American Journal of Diseases in Children, 141:439–444, 1987.

Udelman, D. Stress and immunity. Psychotherapy and Psychosomatics, 37:176–184.

Yu, VYH, Jamieson, J, and Bajuk, B. Breast milk feeding in very low birth weight infants. Australian Paediatric Journal, 17:186–190, 1981.

CHAPTER 22

CEREBRAL EDEMA MANAGEMENT

ROJANN ALPERS, M.S., R.N.,
and VICKY L. HERTIG, M.A., R.N.

While the term *increased intracranial pressure* is familiar to most nurses, additional knowledge has made it possible to increase the precision of that term. That is, knowing that pressure produces cerebral cellular edema enables nurses to describe the pathology more accurately. Thus, the term *cerebral edema* has replaced increased intracranial pressure in much of the literature. Until recently, the role of nursing in working with patients with cerebral edema was essentially that of monitoring, with most of the literature addressing this phenomenon devoted to medical therapies to alleviate or mitigate pressure changes. Only a few studies have directly or indirectly examined the role of nursing in management of cerebral edema.

Although nursing care activities may not alter major pathological processes, knowledge of nursing management that can affect cerebral edema and devastating neurological sequelae from prolonged edema is essential for nurses. Further, shaping nursing care around this knowledge can reduce significantly the possibility of transient or sustained increases in cerebral edema.

Normal pressure is maintained by a homeostatic balance of brain tissue, blood, and cerebrospinal fluid. Any increase in one of these components will result in increased cerebral pressure. Normally, small increases in one intracranial component are compensated for by a comparable decrease in another volume, rendering the total intracranial volume unchanged (Hanlon, 1977).

345

However, once these homeostatic mechanisms are utilized to their capacity, even small changes in intracranial volume cause large changes in pressure.

Cerebral edema can result from a number of pathological conditions and lead to devastating sequelae. In certain instances edema can impair cerebral perfusion and metabolism, resulting in an ischemic process that can damage vital cranial structures. The goal of nursing care is to direct and control factors that might further increase intracranial volume, pressure, and edema, thus leading to herniation or cerebral ischemia or both (Hanlon, 1977).

The purpose of this chapter is to discuss nursing strategies to reduce the rate of pathological changes influencing edema and to enhance homeostatic mechanisms. The intervention of cerebral edema management is directed toward stabilizing fluid volumes, reducing cerebral changes, and increasing patient tolerance of cerebral edema. Appropriate nursing strategies to manage cerebral edema are indicated by several antecedents, presenting data, and nursing diagnoses.

THEORETICAL FOUNDATION

Source of Change in Cerebral Edema

The most common antecedents of cerebral edema in infants and children can be grouped into three categories: (1) brain mass changes; (2) blood volume changes; and (3) cerebrospinal fluid changes.

Brain Mass Changes

Brain mass expansion is most frequently the result of generalized brain swelling; it is an immediate vasogenic response to injury and is actually a severe hyperemia of the brain. Tornheim and McLaurin (1981) state that the actual mechanical force generated as the brain tissue strikes the cranium is sufficient to elicit the subsequent brain swelling. However, Penn (1980) believes that the trauma contributes to loss of cerebral blood flow and autoregulation, thereby allowing systemic blood pressure changes to dilate cerebral capillaries and lead to leakage of proteins and fluids.

Vasogenic edema is the most predominant type of cerebral edema seen clinically (Sherman and Easton, 1980). The disruption of the blood-brain barrier allows the passage of proteins from the intravascular space through the capillary wall into the extracellular space. This vascular damage results in increased permeability of the capillary wall and increased outflow of plasma proteins, followed by an influx of water into the brain parenchyma. While this process starts in the area of injury, it spreads rapidly to adjacent tissues (Baethmann and Schmiedek, 1973).

The precise mechanism by which this increase in permeability takes place is unknown. However, it is postulated that biogenic amines, which constitute the tight junction of endothelial and glial cells and surround the capillary wall, might be important elements in this process (Brightman et al., 1970).

With blood-brain barrier damage, proteins and other large molecular substances from the vascular system enter the brain. The protein escape into the extracellular space increases the osmolality outside the blood-brain barrier. Through osmosis, water follows these proteins into the extracellular space, leading to an increase in brain water volume and subsequent cerebral edema (Arabi and Long, 1979).

Agents believed to cause disruption in the blood-brain barrier and to be responsible for early development of cerebral edema are serotonin and prostaglandin E. Prostaglandin E is a potentiator of serotonin; both these elements are released from disintegrated platelets in the traumatized region of the brain (Mohanty et al., 1979).

Cytotoxic cerebral edema is a less understood response, but it is known to be due to a particular toxic factor that directly affects the cellular elements of the blood-brain barrier and brain parenchyma (Speers, 1981). Cytotoxic cerebral edema is characterized by intracellular swelling (Hochwald et al., 1976). A precipitating event known to cause this type of cerebral edema is acute oxygen deficiency with carbon dioxide retention, as seen in cardiac arrest, asphyxia, anoxia, and diabetic coma. In addition, cytotoxic cerebral edema is associated with acute hyponatremia with inappropriate secretion of antidiuretic hormone (ADH) and with general hyponatremia, water intoxication, and Reye's syndrome. Cytotoxic edema may augment vasogenic edema.

Cytotoxic cerebral edema involves damage

to cell metabolism—specifically, to the adenosine triphosphate–dependent sodium pump, which is responsible for the normal distribution of electrolytes and water across the cell membrane (Sherman and Easton, 1980). Initially, there is a loss of potassium from the cortical neurons and a greater gain of sodium and chloride by the cells in the extracellular space. Water follows by osmosis to maintain osmotic equilibrium. This mechanism results in swelling of the cells, a shrinking of the extracellular space, and an increase in tissue osmolarity.

The third type of cerebral edema, ischemic edema, is classified as a separate entity because it is not exclusively vasogenic or cytotoxic but contains components of both. Ischemic edema is confined to the intracellular compartment and is believed to result from failure of the homeostatic mechanisms secondary to oxygen deficiency. In ischemic edema, intracellular sodium and water increase, while potassium moves outward into the intercellular space. Thus, the cells increase in size, expanding the brain mass volume. If ischemia continues, necrosis of the brain cells occurs, which results in changes in the pressure gradient. At this time, it is thought that proteins are transported across the endothelium and the extracellular space re-expands because of increasing blood-brain barrier permeability (Fenstermacher and Patlak, 1976). The evolution from cytotoxic to vasogenic edema occurs hours and even days after the onset of ischemia. With this type of edema, ischemia appears to be the result of cerebral infarction (Speers, 1981).

The last type of cerebral edema is interstitial edema. This edema develops when the outflow of cerebrospinal fluid becomes obstructed and the intraventricular pressure increases. This problem results in the movement of sodium and water across the ventricular wall into the extracellular space (Sherman and Easton, 1980). According to Speers (1981), interstitial edema is seen most frequently as obstructive hydrocephalus resulting from tumor growth.

Blood Volume Changes

Normally, cerebral blood pressure and flow are maintained at a constant level from 50 to 170 mm Hg, despite fluctuations in mean arterial pressure. This phenomenon is the result of an autoregulatory mechanism, or an automatic alteration in the diameter of the resistance vessels to maintain constant blood flow during changes in perfusion pressure (Mauss and Mitchell, 1976). Autoregulation is lost in damaged brain tissue and at moderate levels of intracranial hypertension. The result of this lost autoregulation is that cerebral blood flow and volume vary passively with systemic blood pressure changes. Increases in systemic blood pressure, which normally would have no effect on cerebral pressure, are now reflected directly in the increasing edema of the damaged brain.

Vasodilation of cerebral arteries is another factor that increases cerebral blood flow. Carbon dioxide is the most potent vasodilating substance known. The relationship between changes in partial pressure of carbon dioxide ($PaCO_2$) and cerebral blood flow is almost linear; therefore, any increases in $PaCO_2$ can serve to increase cerebral blood flow and lead to increased edema. For example, accumulation of tracheobronchial secretions can lead to hypercapnia ($PaCO_2$ greater than 42 mm Hg) owing to a lack of CO_2 expiration, thus leading to increased cerebral edema. Other agents known to cause vasodilation and contribute to increased cerebral blood flow are volatile anesthetics such as halothane and nitrous oxide, as well as drugs such as ketamine and histamine (Mauss and Mitchell, 1976).

Any condition that acts to decrease or interrupt venous outflow may serve to increase cerebral blood by leaving more blood in the cranial cavity. The major portion of venous outflow is via the internal jugular vein, with a smaller portion leaving through the basal cerebral venous system. Compression of the internal jugular and vertebrobasilar venous system can occur with head and neck positioning. Thus, flexion-extension-rotation of the neck during position changes and suctioning are examples of activities that may alter venous outflow. Similarly, venous outflow also can be decreased by an increase in intrathoracic or intra-abdominal pressure. Because the venous system has no valves, an increase in pressure in any portion of the system will be transmitted throughout the system. The Valsalva maneuver is an example of an activity that increases intrathoracic and intra-abdominal pressure, leading to increased cerebral pressure. Also, positive end-expiratory pressure used with assisted ventilation has been associated with increased intracranial pressure in some patients (Mitchell, 1980).

Changes in Cerebrospinal Fluid

Cerebrospinal fluid production and absorption are major factors involved in compensating for volumetric changes within the cranium. The spatial alteration ability of cerebrospinal fluid is the homeostatic mechanism responsible for the maintenance of normal cerebral pressure in spite of volume changes (McNamara and Quinn, 1981). The success of this cerebrospinal fluid buffer system is dependent on the patency of the subarachnoid space and ventricular outflow tracts. With free flow possible between the spinal subarachnoid space and arachnoid villi, rapid outflow of cerebrospinal fluid can occur, resulting in minimal change in intracranial pressure (Bruce, 1978).

Under the conditions of an obstruction or occlusion of the cerebrospinal fluid pathways, cerebrospinal fluid is an antecedent to increased pressure. An obstruction of the cerebrospinal fluid, because of reduced absorption or altered or blocked flow, results in a sudden decrease in spatial altering capacity, or movement through the ventricles and the spinal cord. Hence, previously tolerated volume changes now may lead to critical increases in pressure and edema (Bruce, 1978).

Cerebrospinal fluid reabsorption is dependent on the difference in hydrostatic pressure between the subarachnoid space and the dural sinuses. When the brain begins to swell, the subarachnoid spaces are compressed, cerebrospinal fluid is progressively lost through osmosis, and a point is reached at which the subarachnoid space is effectively collapsed because of pressure. When this process occurs, little or no residual cerebrospinal fluid is being produced. Then, no outflow can occur and the edematous condition worsens (Bruce, 1978).

ASSESSMENT

Data indicating the possible presence of cerebral edema are first detected in the history. If suspected, the following areas need to be explored: (1) history of substance use or overdose; (2) poisoning; (3) ingestion of toxic substances; (4) head trauma; (5) loss of consciousness; (6) seizures; and (7) neurological or infectious disease. Data should include the rate of symptom onset as well as the past history. For example, a history in younger children might include sudden short episodes of dizziness and frequent early morning headache, characterized by rubbing or shaking of the head, increased irritability; and inconsolable crying. In older children, alteration or loss of speech, episodes of syncope, and ataxia are significant. Progressive changes in mental status, increasingly short attention span, confusion, lethargy, agitation, drowsiness, motor function deficits, focal or generalized muscle weakness, unsteady gait, temporary paresthesia, or paralysis should be noted. Changes in visual acuity, loss of part of the visual field, eye deviation, the presence of nausea, projectile vomiting, and a high-pitched cry in infants are also significant. Information concerning hypertension, obesity, diabetes mellitus, and heart and vascular disease should also be elicited.

The scope of the assessment must be adjusted to the condition of the patient. Ideally, a systematic assessment includes vital signs, level of consciousness, pupil checks, motor function, presence of injuries, and skin condition. If a client is unstable, priority assessment is done, which includes only vital signs, level of consciousness, and pupil checks.

Vital sign assessment should begin with the observation of respiratory status. After it is determined that the airway is clear, the respiratory rate is observed for depression of the respiratory center, which is controlled by the motor cortex–medullary center. A decreasing respiratory rate, irregular breathing patterns and depth, and the presence of apnea are indications of respiratory center involvement. Monitoring of blood pressure will tell the nurse whether an increase in systolic pressure and a widening pulse pressure are present.

Other vital signs are also important. The temperature is regulated in the hypothalamus. Therefore, an unstable temperature indicates hypothalamic pathology. Apical pulse is also reliant upon a functioning hypothalamus, as well as functioning of the tenth cranial nerve and sympathetic ganglion (Mitchell et al., 1984).

After vital signs have been assessed, the

level of consciousness is observed. The assessment of the level of consciousness of infants and children requires knowledge of normal growth and development. Notations are made of responses to questions and commands, plus the ability to speak clearly and appropriately in older children. Infants are assessed for normal crying patterns, pitch of the cry, and methods of expressing their needs. Further, their reaction to separation from parents produces important data. Irritability, restlessness, and sleepiness are primary discriminators of increasing cerebral pressure and edema. In addition, in infants, increased head circumference, bulging tense fontanels, and distended scalp are indications of increasing intracranial pressure (Hausman, 1981).

Assessment continues with noting pupillary changes, pupil size, response to light, and symmetry of pupil size and response. Increased edema will be reflected in either bilateral or unilateral fixed dilated pupils. Also important to note are the presence of side-to-side eye deviation, papilledema, or doll or sunset eyes (Mitchell et al., 1984).

The recognition and interpretation of the data reflecting cerebral edema are primary nursing responsibilities. The ability of nurses to establish baseline data and note and interpret subtle changes and deviations from the baseline has a significant bearing on the outcome.

There is no question that it is a nursing responsibility and prerogative to diagnose increasing cerebral edema. The nursing diagnosis suggested is decreased adaptive capacity due to (1) pathological changes exceeding compensatory mechanisms, including tumors, hemorrhage, or brain swelling; (2) blood volume changes, including vasodilation and interrupted venous outflow; and (3) cerebrospinal fluid changes, including overproduction, obstruction, or interference in reabsorption.

THE INTERVENTION

Variables related to cerebral edema can be controlled by nurses. The intervening variables related to edema that nursing can best affect through intervention are (1) anxiety; (2) stimulation; (3) hypercapnia and hypoxia; (4) inappropriate fluid loads; (5) pressure shifts; (6) intrathoracic and intra-abdominal pressure; and (7) spacing of rest intervals.

Lowering Anxiety

Because of the evidence that stress and anxiety stimulate the sympathetic autonomic nervous system, anxiety should be controlled to minimize cerebral edema. Anxiety is a subjectively experienced feeling of apprehension. It is often accompanied by muscle tension, nausea, an increase in pulse and respiratory rate, and tremors, all of which can contribute to transient increases in pressure and edema. Nursing strategies that reduce anxiety and promote comfort and, therefore, minimize cerebral edema are developmentally appropriate communication, mobilization of support systems, and maintenance of appropriate environment.

Communication at the child's developmental level promotes trust and comfort, thereby reducing anxiety and agitation and their effect on cerebral edema. The developmental stage and culture of the child determine the nature of information and avenues of communication (see chapters on therapeutic play, touch, drawings, cross-cultural communication, and psychological preparation). For example, children generally respond more to the tone of voice than to the content. For this reason it is helpful to speak in a slow, low-pitched, calm voice. In addition, tactile as well as verbal communication is suggested with children of all ages. Toddlers and infants respond especially well to touch, holding, and rocking (Walleck, 1982; Mitchell et al., 1985). (See chapter on touch.)

Nurses use their awareness of each stage of the unique relationship of the child and family, as discussed in Section I of this book (see chapter on family integrity). Infants, young children, and adolescents are physically, emotionally, and legally dependent on their families to varying degrees.

Parents are the most important support system to the child, and mobilization of their influence can be used to reduce anxiety (Hertig, 1985; Hendrickson, 1987). Parents support the child in at least two ways: they are sensitive to cues indicating anxiety, and they function to reduce anxiety. Because families have a great influence on children, parents are indispensable in detecting anxiety in their child as well as providing comfort and distraction.

In addition, parents assist in maintaining daily routines of hygiene, play, and rest. This is important, because to a certain extent anxiety can be contained by predictability. Also, families are helpful by participating in necessary care, such as maintaining fluid restrictions, monitoring intake and output, observing intravenous infusions for irritation and infiltration, administering oral medications, and performing passive range-of-motion exercises. Parental involvement in these activities decreases anxiety. Therefore, parents should be encouraged to stay with their children, as discussed previously in the chapter on family integrity.

When it is not possible for parents to stay with their children, nurses can make several adjustments. Parents can record favorite stories or poems for the child to play. Parents can bring special articles that the child will recognize as his or her own (Pollack and Goldstein, 1981). Consistency in caregivers is important when the parents are absent. If possible, the primary nurses assigned to the child should interact with the parents in the child's presence before the parents depart.

Other nursing measures to decrease unnecessary anxiety are possible. When entering the child's room and approaching the bed, begin speaking quietly and in a soothing manner to avoid a startle reaction. Nurses present at the bedside during physician visits and examinations can provide support and clarification to patients and parents. Also, they can encourage conversations directed *to* the patient, as opposed to *about* the child. Mitchell and Mauss (1978) found a significant difference in intracranial pressure changes when conversations included the patient.

Nurses can encourage parents to bring safe, favorite, and "different-feeling" toys from home, such as toys that are fuzzy, smooth, cool, squeezable, and mushy. Further, room temperature should be constant, with slight coolness preferable to a warm temperature. Restraints must be used only when absolutely necessary, as they frequently cause fear and apprehension, which often results in combative and crying behaviors that increase cerebral edema.

Environmental Manipulation

The environment may be a source of anxiety and fear as well as inappropriate stimulation, all of which can elicit agitated behaviors that can have a profound impact on cerebral pressure. The environment should communicate child-centeredness, while providing appropriate stimulation and safety (see chapter on environmental manipulation).

Stimulation and safety needs can be provided for the child simultaneously by padding side rails with softly colored quilts, pillowcases, and blankets. Alert toddlers and older children can be encouraged to draw pictures with washable ink pens on solid-color pillowcases used for padding. Colorful pictures, mobiles, and pictures of parents, friends, and siblings can be attached to cribs and beds. The room should be slightly darkened; indirect lighting is preferred. Equipment, tubing, and monitoring cords should be kept out of sight and reach of infants and young children. In addition, nurses can wear patterned or colored blouses to avoid the association of white clothing with fear. Animal clip-ons and pins on uniforms are useful as communication initiators and distractors. Movements within the child's line of vision should be executed slowly and with prior explanation. Also, necessary care should be organized and carried out in smooth and quiet way.

Music should be used carefully. Some types of music are soothing—for example, soft, quiet music, or a parent's recording of favorite lullabies. Television and radio should be used judiciously. Stories and poems provide auditory stimulation. Simultaneously, they override noxious or loud sounds intrinsic in any hospital setting. In a study by Wincek, reviewed by Wong (1988), it was found that controlled auditory stimulation such as soothing, quiet music promoted physiological relaxation and lowered intracranial pressure in children.

Control of Hypoxia and Hypercapnia

Hypoxia and hypercapnia can be responsible for increasing intracranial pressure. That is, a reduction of partial pressure of oxygen (PaO_2) less than 50 mm Hg or an increase in partial pressure of carbon dioxide ($PaCO_2$) greater than 42 mm Hg leads to vasodilation and increased cerebral blood volume.

In many instances, nurses can control the amount of hypoxia. One such example is the transient hypoxia occurring during endotracheal suctioning, which can be reduced by hyperinflating the lungs prior to suctioning (Naigow and Powaser, 1977). Fell and Cheney (1971) determined that partial pressure of oxygen (PaO_2) greater than 65 mm Hg during endotracheal suctioning is most effectively achieved by hyperinflating the lungs for one minute with 100% oxygen prior to suction and limiting suction to fifteen seconds. However, this process can create a danger for increasing intrathoracic and intra-abdominal pressure, which leads to increases in cerebral edema. Therefore, suctioning should be used cautiously and be based on evaluation of breath sounds and arterial blood gases (Mitchell, 1980).

The potential for hypoxia should always be considered when caring for a patient with suspected neurological pathology. Thus, a victim of head injury should have blood gas determinations for several reasons, including the possibility that any existing hypoxia will contribute to increasing cerebral edema.

Control of Fluids

Clinical dehydration and the administration of hypertonic solutions have long been advocated in the treatment of cerebral edema. When a hypertonic solution, such as mannitol, urea, or glycerol, is added to plasma, it will directly affect brain volume by draining fluid from the brain into the vascular compartment through the creation of an osmotic gradient.

While the reduction of cerebral edema is desirable, other problems may arise, such as fluid overload. Fluid overload may occur because an osmotic diuretic pulls tissue fluid into the blood vessels, increasing blood volume. Therefore, observation for signs and symptoms of fluid overload is essential. Nurses should monitor the central venous pressure (CVP), keeping in mind that an increased CVP inhibits venous outflow from the brain, exacerbating the cerebral pressure (Burgess, 1985).

Both hypertonic fluid administration and fluid restrictions necessitate that nurses keep meticulously and evaluate fluid intake and output records, as well as closely monitor electrolytes, blood urea nitrogen (BUN), and serum osmolarity for indications of dehydration (Burgess, 1985). Clinical data on hydra-

tional status should be reported, recorded, and followed carefully.

It is important to note that the aforementioned practices regarding fluid management may be changing. Some authorities have suggested that fluid restriction enhances increased intracranial pressure by causing hypovolemia and thereby further reducing cerebral perfusion. In addition, compensatory blood volume mechanisms are elicited (Burgess, 1985).

Proper Body Positioning

Certain head and body positions have been shown to decrease venous outflow and exacerbate cerebral edema (Lipe and Mitchell, 1980). These positions include (1) neck flexion, (2) neck extension, (3) head rotation to the right, (4) left lateral body positioning, (5) flat supine, and (6) prone. When body position changes cannot be avoided, the effects on cerebral pressure and edema need to be monitored. Body positioning should include elevating the head of the bed to a thirty-degree angle. Older, responsive children can be instructed to avoid turning their heads during conversation. Several measures can help maintain appropriate body positions. For example, nurses can place items, such as tissues or water, in front of the child rather than to the side. Food trays, articles used for diversional activities, and even the television set should be placed directly in front of the child.

Position changes are often indicated, and they are hazardous for the patient with increased cerebral pressure. Therefore, passive position changes by nurses must be preceded by instructions to the child to exhale during turning to prevent isometric contractions and the Valsalva maneuver. Pillows should be used to stabilize the head and neck and to maintain the body in the same direction of the head during turning.

Reduction of Intrathoracic and Intra-abdominal Pressure

Venous return from the brain can be impeded by increases in intrathoracic and intra-abdominal pressure produced by coughing, sneezing, chewing, hiccuping, crying, abdominal distention, straining at stool, and rectal manipulation (Bruya, 1981; Boortz-Marx, 1985).

Nurses can use many strategies to control intrathoracic and intra-abdominal pressure. For instance, the frequency of coughing and sneezing can be reduced by avoiding use of perfumed lotions, soaps, and powders during hygiene care. Also, a nasogastric tube should be manipulated only when necessary. Fewer tube changes are recommended, when possible, to reduce the cough and gag reflex associated with tube placement. Frequent nasal care around the tube is essential as this reduces irritation and secretion accumulation that often leads to sneezing. Pressures generated by chewing and hiccuping can be minimized by providing soft, puréed, or full-liquid diets for those patients capable of oral intake. Infants should be burped frequently during feedings; older children should not be permitted to chew gum or to drink carbonated beverages.

Bowel programs will prevent or alleviate constipation and the need for straining at stool (see chapter on bowel and bladder maintenance) (Speers, 1981). Rectal manipulations are avoided by eliminating rectal temperatures, suppositories, and enemas.

Activity Spacing

Mitchell, Ozuna, and Lipe (1981) reported a steady increase in cerebral pressure when care activities are spaced only 15 minutes apart. In fact, activities that were spaced only 15 minutes apart created cumulative pressure increases; that is, the starting pressure at the time of the second activity was close to the ending pressure of the preceding one, without a return to the pre-activity baseline. However, no increase in intracranial pressure was noted when the same activities were spaced one hour apart.

This finding suggests that nursing interventions, such as suctioning, position changes, patient hygiene, and meals, ought to be planned well in advance to allow for adequate rest periods (Hertig, 1985). These plans must also take into account scheduled laboratory tests, other therapies, quiet play, and physician visits. It is suggested that each infant and child have a written schedule of activities on the nursing care plan that indicates the sequence of activities and the time frame in which they are to be initiated

and completed. The care plan should also indicate when tests, visits, and procedures would be best scheduled in terms of needed rest periods.

It is evident that a number of variables can have a range of subtle-to-profound impact on cerebral edema. And it is the diverse and integrated knowledge base of nurses that makes it possible to identify those biophysical and psychosocial variables operating in the infant and child who may develop or may have cerebral edema. That knowledge base also enhances individualized strategies to be planned and implemented for management of cerebral edema.

EVALUATION

Outcome is measured by a reversal of defining characteristics, or data obtained upon assessment. A decreasing pulse pressure, respiratory regularity, and apical pulse regularity indicate decreasing cerebral edema.

Case Study

David, 3½ years old, has a concussion from falling from a tree. The nursing diagnosis is disorientation due to cerebral edema. The following observations were noted: (1) he was alert and oriented to place and person; (2) he moved all extremities spontaneously and to command; (3) his pupils were equal and reactive to light; and (4) his vital signs were stable.

When the nurse made rounds at 7:30 A.M., she found David lying on his stomach, crying loudly and screaming when approached. The side rail made a slight squeak when it was put down, and David grimaced and held his head. The nurse talked quietly and soothingly to him. When he began to calm down and answer some questions, it was discovered he did not remember climbing the tree or being in the hospital. He continued to move all extremities spontaneously and to command. His pupils were equal and reacted briskly to light; his vital signs remained stable.

As his change in level of consciousness was obvious, the nurse turned David on his back, elevated the head of his bed 30 degrees, and notified his physician, while continuing observations every 15 minutes. The overhead lights were dimmed, and quiet play with puppets was initiated. The nurse continued to calm him, while reassuring him that she would stay with him.

If the increase in edema was transient and due to his positioning and anxiety, David would gradually remember the tree climbing and fall. If the nurse's talking and quiet play helped reduce David's anxiety, he would allow greater physical contact and become more compliant with care and assessment. However, if he continued to fuss and refused to stay positioned on his back with the head elevated, his edema would continue to rise. That is, the nurse would begin to see signs of early deterioration, such as a rapid decrease in movement and weakness in grips and pushes, plus a change in level of orientation as manifested by decreased ability to play.

Happily, David's loss of memory was the only adverse sign noted. As he relaxed, the memory of the fall returned so that he could tell the physician upon arrival. The rapid, effective strategies of his nurse prevented worsening cerebral edema.

RESEARCH IMPLICATIONS

A search of the literature on increased intracranial pressure, or cerebral edema, revealed that a large part of nursing practice may be based on a somewhat outdated medical perspective. The few medical and nursing articles that are current suggest that systematic exploration of increased intracranial pressure and the factors that influence it is needed. Strategies to guide patient care are offered in the research of Mitchell and her colleagues.

The assumptions upon which these preceding strategies are based is that a relationship exists between psychological and physiological well-being, care activities, and cerebral edema, and that cerebral edema is an appropriate topic for nursing investigation. However, it is not surprising that little systematic work has been done, given the small number of nurses prepared in pediatric neuroscience and research methodologies.

It is encouraging to note that nursing-focused research on cerebral pressure is beginning, perhaps because of increasing nursing autonomy, responsibility, specialization, and research preparation. Certainly, the pioneering work done by Mitchell on neuroassessment and the relationship between nursing activities and cerebral pressure has laid a substantive foundation from which to build a program of research. Important research topics are the mechanisms underlying cerebral pressure response to position change, the relative influence of neck position and blood pressure on increased cerebral pressure, and the cumulative effect on cerebral pressure of grouping care activities (Mitchell, 1980). Questions that need exploration are, do flotation mattresses provide as much skin pressure relief as position change? How is anxiety related to cerebral pressure? Do certain colors and patterns in nurses' clothing reduce children's anxieties? Do specific rhythmic sounds have a calming effect, and if so, how are these related to cerebral pressure? The validation and refinement of nursing diagnosis is also a topic for exploration and research.

References

Arabi, B, and Long, DM. Dynamics of cerebral edema. Journal of Neurosurgery, 51:779–784, 1979.

Baethmann, A, and Schmiedek, P. Pathophysiology of cerebral edema: Chemical aspects. In Schurmann, K, Brock, M, Reulen, JH, and Voth, D (Eds.), Brain edema: Pathophysiology and therapy. New York: Springer-Verlag, 1973.

Boortz-Marx, R. Factors affecting intracranial pressure: A descriptive study. Journal of Neurosurgical Nursing, 17:89–90, 1985.

Brightman, MW, Klatzo, I, Olsson, Y, and Reese, TS. The blood-brain barrier to proteins under normal and pathological conditions. Journal of Neurological Science, 10:215–239, 1970.

Bruce, DA. The pathophysiology of increased intracranial pressure. New York: The Upjohn Company, Scope Publication, 1978.

Bruya, MA. Planned periods of rest in the intensive care unit: Nursing care activities and intracranial pressure. Journal of Neurosurgical Nursing, 13:184–193, 1981.

Burgess, KE. Inside increased intracranial pressure. Nursing Life, March/April, 1985.

Fell, T, and Cheney, FW. Prevention of hypoxia during endotracheal suction. Annals of Surgery, 174:24–28, 1971.

Fenstermacher, JD, and Patlak, CS. The movement of water and solutes in the brain of mammals. In Pappius, HM, and Feindel, W (Eds.), Dynamics of brain edema. New York: Springer-Verlag, 1976.

Hanlon, K. Intracranial compliance, Interpretation and clinical application. Journal of Neurosurgical Nursing, 9:34–40, 1977.

Hausman, KA. Nursing care of the patient with hydrocephalus. Journal of Neurosurgical Nursing, 13:326–332, 1981.

Hendrickson, SL. Intracranial pressure changes and family practice. Journal of Neurosurgical Nursing, 19:14–17, 1987.

Hertig, V. The effects of nursing care activities on intracranial pressure. Master's Thesis, University of Iowa, 1985.

Hochwald, GM, Marlin, AE, Wald, A, and Malham, C. Movement of water between blood, brain, and CSF in cerebral edema. In Pappius, HM, and Feindel, W (Eds.), Dynamics of brain edema. New York: Springer-Verlag, 1976.

Lipe, HP, and Mitchell, PH. Positioning the patient with intracranial hypertension: How turning and rotation affect the internal jugular vein. Heart and Lung, 9:1031–1037, 1980.

Mauss, NK, and Mitchell, PH. Increased intracranial pressure: An update. Heart and Lung, 5:919–926, 1976.

McNamara, M, and Quinn, C. Epidural intracranial pressure monitoring: Theory and clinical application. Journal of Neurosurgical Nursing, 13:267–281, 1981.

Mitchell, PH. Intracranial hypertension: Implication of research for nursing. The Journal of Neurosurgical Nurses, 12: 145–154, 1980.

Mitchell, PH, Cammermeyer, M, Ozuna, J, and Woods, NF. Neurological assessment. Reston, Va: Prentice-Hall Company, 1984.

Mitchell, PH, Haberman-Little, B, Johnson, F, Van Inwegen-Scott, D, and Tyler, D. Critically ill children: The importance of touch in a high-technology environment. Nursing Administration Quarterly, Summer, 1985:38–46.

Mitchell, PH, and Mauss, NK. Relationships of patient-nurse activity to intracranial pressure variations: A pilot study. Nursing Research, 27:4–10, 1978.

Mitchell, PH, Ozuna, J, and Lipe, HP. Moving the patient in bed: Effects on intracranial pressure. Nursing Research, 30:212–218, 1981.

Mohanty, S, Sey, PK, and Ray, AH. The role of serotonin in cerebral edema. Indian Journal of Medical Research, 69:1001–1007, 1979.

Naigow, D, and Powaser, M. The effect of different endotracheal suction procedures on arterial blood gases: A controlled experimental model. Heart and Lung, 6:808–816, 1977.

Penn, RD. Cerebral edema and neurological function in human beings. Neurosurgery, 6:249–254, 1980.

Pollack, LD, and Goldstein, GW. Lowering of intracranial pressure in Reye's syndrome by sensory stimulation (letter). New England Journal of Medicine, 304:732, 1981.

Sherman, DG, and Easton, JD. Cerebral edema in stroke. Postgraduate Medicine, 68:107–120, 1980.

Speers, I. Cerebral edema. Journal of Neurosurgical Nursing, 13:102–115, 1981.

Tornheim, PA, and McLaurin, RL. Acute changes in regional brain water content following experimental closed head injury. Journal of Neurosurgery, 55:407–413, 1981.

Walleck, CA. The effects of purposeful touch on intracranial pressure. Master's Thesis, University of Maryland, 1982.

Wong, D. Changing what children hear in the ICU can lower intracranial pressure. American Journal of Nursing, 88:279–280, 1988.

Zeidelman, C. Increased intracranial pressure in the pediatric patient: Nursing assessment and intervention. Journal of Neurosurgical Nursing, 12:7–10, 1980.

CHAPTER 23

BOWEL AND BLADDER MAINTENANCE

PATRICIA A. SMIGIELSKI, M.S., R.N., C.P.N.P.,
and JANET R. MAPEL, B.S.N., R.N., C.P.N.P.

Bowel and bladder habits, generally considered to be normal body functions, are frequently altered in children with developmental disabilities. Whether due to decreased activity level or central nervous system pathology, alterations in bowel and bladder maintenance occur frequently in this population and become an area of major concern for disabled children and their parents. Bowel and bladder maintenance is defined as the ability to maintain the optimal bowel and bladder continence possible for each child's developmental level and extent of pathology. Implicit in this definition are the goals for independent management of elimination needs and the prevention of illness.

Children with a physical disability that is characterized by a sensory or motor impairment are at risk for altered health states related to elimination as well as for incontinence. Because of the private nature of waste elimination and associated embarrassment, problems in bowel and bladder maintenance are particularly stigmatizing to a child already regarded as "different." Bowel and bladder continence becomes an important issue when the physically disabled child enters the social environment of school and is exposed to the expectations of nondisabled peers. Because most disabled children are now mainstreamed into public schools, school personnel are required to provide assistance with bowel and bladder management during school hours. Clean intermittent catheterization is considered a special education–related service; therefore, it is each school's responsibility to implement the catheterization program (Stauffer, 1984). Because of this requirement, nurses in schools and other community settings are frequently confronted with problems in bowel and bladder maintenance. Nurses can intervene to minimize these problems by helping to normalize elimination as much as possible. This intervention, in turn, may reduce family stress, enhance the child's self-esteem, and facilitate integration into a society of peers.

This chapter will discuss indications for nursing interventions, the interventions themselves, and outcome criteria for bowel and bladder maintenance. The discussion will focus on physically disabled children, regardless of the presence of mental disability. Alterations of bowel and bladder maintenance due to cognitive limitations alone, such as toilet training for the mentally retarded child, will not be discussed. Much of this chapter will focus on children with myelodysplasia, since they are the population of disabled children in which alterations in bowel and bladder maintenance occur most frequently.

THEORETICAL FOUNDATION

Becker's health belief model provides a useful conceptual framework for explaining the health behavior of disabled children and their parents in the area of bowel and bladder management. The health belief model applies psychological theories of decision-making to an individual's choice of health behaviors. In other words, for people to take preventive health action, they need to believe that (1) they are personally susceptible to a negative health state, (2) the negative health state would have some degree of severity, and (3) taking action would be beneficial despite the disadvantages of doing so (Becker, 1974). Becker described sick role behavior in relationship to compliance with a prescribed regimen when a person has a chronic condition. Sick role behavior includes the element of re-susceptibility or the likelihood of the recurrence of the negative health state.

If a child is teased or shunned by peers

when incontinent or becomes ill with a bladder infection, compliance with a recommended program of catheterizations may be enhanced. If, on the other hand, a child receives no negative feedback for being incontinent or has an asymptomatic urinary tract infection, catheterizations may not be perceived as beneficial and will not be done. This is especially true if the child thinks the disadvantages of catheterizing, such as interrupting play or missing a favorite television program, are severe. There is some evidence to support the hypothesis that children's health behaviors reflect the health beliefs of their parents (Becker et al., 1977). In planning nursing interventions for bowel and bladder maintenance, therefore, it is wise to consider the experiences and perceptions of the parents as well as the child, given the known demographic and sociopsychological factors.

Fecal Incontinence

Toilet training is a developmental milestone that is accomplished by a physically and mentally normal child somewhere between one and one-half and four years of age. The acquisition of toileting skills depends upon neurological maturation and cooperation from the child. When a child has a neurological deficit, such as meningomyelocele, toilet training cannot be achieved in the usual manner, and bowel and bladder maintenance becomes a significant and lifelong part of a child's daily health care regimen. Hendry and Geddes (1978) reported that in their clinical myelodysplasia practice bowel and bladder maintenance was the area of greatest parental concern because of the social ramifications of incontinence. The children suffered peer ridicule because of the odor and wetness of incontinence, and family social activities were often severely restricted because of a fear of possible bowel or bladder accidents.

In a study conducted by Hunt (1981), 100 children with meningomyelocele were assessed to determine the implications of their disability on their education and school adjustment. Half these children were incontinent of feces during school hours, which was distressing to the child, teacher, and classmates. Whatever method was used to control incontinence, most of the children were wet, smelly, or dirty from time to time. Professional expertise is needed to assist a child and parents to manage issues of bowel and bladder maintenance. It has been estimated that 90% of all children with meningomyelocele have neurogenic bowel dysfunction, resulting in some degree of constipation or incontinence (Shurtleff, 1980). A neurogenic bowel results from impaired innervation at or above the sacral level, since intact sacral nerve roots are needed for normal external sphincter control, internal reflex sphincter relaxation, rectal sensation, and, in part, colonic motility (Hesz and Wolraich, 1987). A child with a neurogenic bowel, therefore, may experience any or all of the following difficulties: (1) inability to evacuate stool, (2) lack of sensation of a full rectum, (3) inability to retain stool voluntarily leading to incontinence, and (4) constipation due to inefficient peristalsis, resulting in bowel impaction.

Constipation is the most common alteration in bowel elimination among children with a physical disability. Constipation can be defined as "a nonpathological condition in which the individual exhibits infrequent bowel movements or the absence of stool" (Duespohl, 1986). Constipation in physically disabled children is usually a direct result of their underlying neuromuscular impairment. Therefore, children with a neuromuscular impairment that is either static, as in cerebral palsy, or progressive, as in muscular dystrophy, are at risk for becoming constipated. Likewise, children who have a degree of paralysis resulting from spinal cord trauma or a congenital or acquired spinal cord lesion frequently become constipated. Gastrointestinal peristalsis may be decreased owing to overall central nervous system damage, as in the spastic quadriplegic form of cerebral palsy, or to a neurogenic bowel, as in meningomyelocele. Secondary conditions resulting from neurologic deficits that may predispose a child to constipation include immobility, weak abdominal muscles, and less than adequate dietary bulk and fluids.

Dietary factors, such as inadequate roughage, contribute to constipation. This problem is accounted for, in part, by the permissiveness exhibited by some parents in the area of nutrition. Attitudes held by such parents imply that if children have few choices in other avenues of life because of a disability, they should at least be able to eat what they like. Acquiescence to the desires of children is often an easier solution than struggling with children who refuse to eat important but not necessarily desirable foods such as fruits and vegetables. A second factor for the child with cerebral palsy who has oral-motor involvement may be the inability to handle some of the more advanced food textures found in "roughage" foods. Feeding difficulties also preclude adequate hydration to maintain soft stools. Children with severe central nervous system damage resulting from birth asphyxia or intrauterine infection may sometimes receive less than 10 ounces of fluids by mouth each day. Despite optimal efforts of caretakers, dehydration may also result from weak suck, poor suck-swallow coordination, or hyperexcitable gag reflex. Medications, such as some antacids used in gastrostomy-fed children or anticholinergics used to increase bladder capacity in children with spina bifida, can be constipating.

For those children dependent on the assistance of others for toileting, constipation can result if a consistent toileting program is not established and followed each day. Furthermore, if children are not positioned correctly for toileting, with a firm foot base and arm rest, they may be unable to exert enough intra-abdominal pressure for a full bowel evacuation, contributing to constipation. Noncompliance with an established program of laxative use can also result in constipation. Although some parents may terminate the use of cathartics because of a fear that their child will become dependent on medication, certain children, especially those with meningomyelocele, often require long-term intervention of this type to prevent constipation. Without intervention, the adverse effects of constipation, including irritability, decreased appetite, abdominal discomfort, and possible bowel obstruction, create further management difficulties for caretakers.

Several investigators (Hesz and Wolraich, 1987; Henderson and Synhorst, 1977; Sullivan-Bolyai et al., 1984) have outlined bowel management programs for children with meningomyelocele which include regular evacuation through scheduled toileting and the prevention of constipation by increased fluids, high-fiber diets, and the use of stool softeners. White and Shaker (1974) have suggested that the sooner evacuation programs are established for these children, the more likely it is that continence will be achieved. They stated that the children with the most success at remaining continent had begun their toileting program at an average age of 3.3 years, whereas those who were less successful had no bowel training program until an average age of 6.6 years.

Fecal incontinence is a common problem among disabled children and results from neuromuscular/sensorimotor impairment or cognitive limitations. Fecal incontinence is defined as "a condition in which the individual is unable to control the passage of stool" (Duespohl, 1986). The primary pathophysiological cause of fecal incontinence in disabled children is a neurogenic bowel found in those children with spinal cord damage due to a congenital abnormality such as meningomyelocele, infection involving the central nervous system, or a traumatic spinal cord injury. Bowel continence is not a major concern for the very young child, but at school age (five to seven years of age), the social ramifications of "messy pants" necessitate interventions to achieve continence.

Nonphysiological causes of fecal incontinence in disabled children with and without neurogenic bowels are due to situational or maturational factors. Children with physical disabilities are often dependent on others for their toileting and need a regular toileting schedule to avoid incontinence. If timely assistance is unavailable to take the child to the bathroom, undress and position the child on the toilet, then reverse this procedure, incontinence may result. This also means that adequate bathroom facilities must be available whether the child is at the shopping mall, school, or an interstate highway service station. Toileting must be done at regular and consistent times despite family activities since irregular evacuation times may lead to accidents. Some children are susceptible to even slight alterations in their gastrointestinal homeostasis resulting from certain dietary changes such as eating spicy food like tacos. Illness may also predispose an otherwise continent child to bowel accidents. Similarly, overuse or overdosage of laxatives often causes loose stools resulting in some degree of fecal incontinence.

Other causes of bowel incontinence include cognitive limitations, speech and language deficits, and behavior problems. Mentally retarded children may be expected to be toilet trained before they are cognitively ready and therefore have frequent episodes of incontinence. Retarded children or children with speech and language deficits, such as nonverbal children with cerebral palsy, are often unable to express their toileting needs and therefore remain incontinent. Incontinence can result from behavioral resistance to toileting, causing an encopresis-like state.

Studies have shown that biofeedback techniques using anorectal manometry can also be effective in managing the fecal incontinence of some children with meningomyelocele (Wald, 1981; Whitehead et al., 1981). Factors that increase success with biofeedback therapy include (1) cognitive development that facilitates understanding and cooperation; (2) presence of some rectal sensation as documented by anorectal manometry; (3) sufficient abdominal muscle strength to learn to push; (4) sufficient strength and coordination of lower back and gluteal muscles to learn to squeeze; and (5) neural deficit at the level of the fifth lumbar vertebra or lower, minimal physical and functional disability, and sufficient motivation (Richardson et al., 1985). The biofeedback conditioning consists of teaching children to voluntarily contract the external anal sphincter in response to various degrees of rectal distention, using balloons filled with progressively larger amounts of air inserted into the rectum. The balloons are attached to a polygraph tracing, which gives children immediate visual feedback of their sphincter contraction efforts.

Neurogenic Bladders

The majority of the literature that discusses neurogenic bladders relates to children with meningomyelocele. Children with other disabilities, however, also have neurogenic bladders. One study (McNeal et al., 1983) reported the incidence of symptomatic neurogenic bladders in a cerebral palsy population. Of the 50 patients screened, 13 were referred for urological evaluation because of symptoms such as dribbling or stress incontinence; four were found to have a neurogenic bladder. Subjects with neurogenic bladders were successfully treated with anticholinergic medication.

Children with physical disabilities are at greater risk than other children for acquiring urinary tract infections resulting from urinary retention. Disabled children who are most likely to experience urinary tract infections are those with an underlying sensorimotor or neuromuscular impairment that predisposes them to structural and physiological abnormalities of the renal system. Nearly all children with meningomyelocele have a neurogenic bladder because voluntary control of the bladder muscle wall/urinary sphincter depends on intact sensation at the second to third sacral vertebra (S2-S3) cord level. Sensorimotor impairment of the majority of children with meningomyelocele occurs at the S2 level or above. A neurogenic bladder, therefore, can be defined as "a bladder disturbance due to dysfunctions related to lack of neural control of voiding" (Brunner and Suddarth, 1986, p. 539). A neurogenic bladder frequently entails both a lack of sensation of bladder fullness and the inability to control the bladder muscle and sphincter.

Neurogenic bladders can be spastic, flaccid, or a combination of the two. A spastic bladder (hypertonic) is the most common type and results from an upper motor neuron lesion causing a loss of conscious sensations and cerebral motor control. The bladder behaves in a reflex fashion, resulting in spontaneous, uncontrolled voidings. The result is reduced bladder capacity and marked hypertrophy of the bladder wall, which may lead to vesicoureteral reflux and hydronephrosis. On the other hand, a flaccid (hypotonic) bladder is caused by a lower motor neuron lesion. The bladder continues to fill until it becomes very distended; there are no forceful contractions. When pressure reaches a breakthrough point, small amounts of urine dribble from the urethra as the bladder continues to fill, resulting in overflow incontinence. Extensive bladder distention may cause urinary tract infection from pooling of stagnant urine; pyelonephritis is caused by the backward pressure, or reflux, of urine.

Most children with neurogenic bladders are started on programs of clean, intermittent catheterizations (CIC) to prevent infections and preserve renal function. Even with a CIC program, urinary tract infections may still occur if catheterizations are carried out improperly. Poor catheterization technique by the child, parent, or caretaker may result from a variety of causes, including poor motivation, lack of knowledge and understanding, carelessness, behavioral rebellion, developmental immaturity, contaminated equipment, and fine motor difficulties. Urinary tract infections are also common if medications, such as prophylactic antibiotics or urinary antiseptic bladder instillations, are not administered as prescribed.

Disabled children with normal kidney and bladder function may also experience urinary tract infections resulting from infrequent bladder emptying, inadequate fluid intake, poor hygiene, immobility, or extreme constipation. Each time a disabled child is seen for a health assessment, information should be obtained about voiding patterns, characteristics of the urine, and any symptoms of urinary tract infection. Urinary incontinence is more prevalent among children with disabilities than is bowel incontinence. Urinary incontinence is defined as a condition in which the individual is unable to control the passage of urine. As with bowel incontinence, urinary incontinence results from either neuromuscular/sensorimotor impairment or cognitive limitations. The most frequent physiological cause of urinary incontinence in the disabled population is neurogenic bladder.

For children with a neurogenic bladder who utilize an artificial means of urinary elimination such as clean intermittent catheterization, an artificial sphincter, or an external collection device, incontinence may continue to be a problem. Children or their parents may not comply with the recommended program, the procedure may be carried out improperly, or the equipment may be faulty. If medications are used to increase bladder capacity and resistance to outflow, incontinence may continue to occur if the type of drug, dose, and time of administration are not carefully monitored.

Children with neuromuscular disorders, such as cerebral palsy, may have voluntary control over their bladders but experience urinary incontinence for other reasons. Physically disabled children who are not independent in toileting need prompt and regular assistance for this task. Bathrooms must be accessible; the child may need help to use a urinal or transfer to the toilet, remove braces and clothing, and reverse this process. This can be time consuming, and children are not always toileted fast enough to prevent incontinence. Children also need a means of communicating their toileting needs, particularly if they cannot communicate orally because of oral-motor dysfunction. Incontinence can be avoided in certain nonverbal children by establishing an appropriate communication system.

Stress incontinence is occasionally seen in these children. This is characterized by incontinence in situations that are stressful, such as school examinations or when extra intra-abdominal pressure is exerted in laughter or coughing. Incontinence also results when a cognitive deficit is present and toilet conditioning cannot be accomplished with the child.

For children with neurogenic bladders due to myelodysplasia, two noninvasive methods exist for emptying the bladder and collecting urine. The first method is suprapubic bladder expression or the Credé method. This method is not necessarily routine care for all infants with meningomyelocele because many can empty their bladders completely without intervention. Credé should be used with caution and is indicated only in the absence of vesicoureteral reflux. If suprapubic expression is performed on a child with reflux, high intravesical pressure is transmitted directly to the kidney (Action Committee, 1979). External urinary collection devices are helpful in achieving social continence for some boys. These devices usually consist of a condom-type appliance attached to a leg bag that is emptied at regular intervals. Some appliances are designed to press against the suprapubic area, which assists in emptying the bladder and prevents leakage. These devices are recommended for the boy with a small bladder, small residual volume, and low resistance to outflow (Action Committee, 1979). No effective external collective device has been developed for females.

Clean intermittent catheterization (CIC) is the preferred therapeutic management for neurogenic bladders among the meningomyelocele population (Lapides et al., 1972). Studies have clearly demonstrated that clean intermittent catheterization is a safer intervention over time than urinary diversion. In one study, 80% of children with urinary diversions (ileal conduits) experienced deterioration of the upper tracts, 40% experienced pyelonephritis, but only 17% of chil-

dren on CIC had further deterioration of the upper tracts (Crooks and Enrile, 1983). Ehrlich and Brem (1982) compared urine cultures of children on CIC with those who had ileal loop diversions and concluded that although the short-term morbidity associated with both forms of treatment is similar, there is significantly less asymptomatic bacteriuria in children maintained on CIC. However, Brem and colleagues (1987) found that bacteriuria and reflux did not appear to correlate with decreasing renal function. They concluded that it is not the method of intervention but the character of the bladder that is the crucial factor in ultimate renal deterioration.

Problems associated with ileal diversions include odor, skin irritation, and lack of adherence of the ostomy appliance, resulting in leakage of urine. For these reasons, urinary diversion has virtually been replaced by CIC as a treatment modality and is only used as a last resort when there is bladder deterioration, permanent hydronephrosis, or insufficient compliance with other methods. Undiversion, or the reanastomosis of the ureters to the bladder, can sometimes be accomplished, but it is often difficult to predict bladder function afterward. This surgery is most effective when done on children in whom overflow incontinence, reasonable bladder capacity, and adequate outflow resistance were present before diversion (Action Committee, 1979).

Clean intermittent catheterization, however, is not without problems. It has been estimated that only 26% of children on CIC become continent (Hesz and Wolraich, 1987). Those who remain incontinent have a small bladder capacity and poor resistance to outflow of urine. Continence can be increased by anticholinergic medication, such as oxybutynin or Ditropan, which increases bladder capacity by inhibiting bladder contractions, or alpha-adrenergic agents, such as phenylpropanolamine, which increase resistance to outflow. Among 44 patients on CIC, 77% achieved urinary continence using such medications (Mulcahy and James, 1979). In another study, 49% of children on CIC who were using oxybutynin or phenylpropanolamine or both became completely continent, and 100% showed improved continence (Wolraich et al., 1983).

Clean intermittent catheterization is performed by a parent or other caretaker until the child is developmentally capable of self-catheterization. Several studies have reported success in teaching self-catheterization to school-aged children 6 to 12 years old (Hardy et al., 1975; Lyon et al., 1975; Mulcahy et al., 1977). Hannigan (1979) suggested that preschool children can be taught the procedure with some success. Of four five year olds, two children had remained independent in performing self-catheterization through first grade. Hannigan cautioned, however, that preschoolers must have sufficient cognitive skills, manual dexterity, and motivation for successful instruction. Data on bacteriuria among these children were not reported.

Improper catheterization technique can lead to asymptomatic urinary tract infections, the long-term effects of which are still unknown. The use of antibiotic bladder irrigations or instillations of 1:1000 silver nitrate solution have resulted in significantly less asymptomatic bacteriuria (Mulcahy and James, 1979; Wolraich et al., 1983).

Over the last decade, the artificial urinary sphincter (AUS) has been used with increased frequency to treat urinary incontinence in children with neurogenic bladders. The artificial sphincter is a silicone device that is surgically implanted, consisting of a cuff, pressure-regulating balloon, and control pump (Fig. 23–1). When the pump is activated, the cuff occludes the urethra by exerting sufficient pressure to obstruct urine flow without impairing urethral blood supply (Faller and Vinson, 1985).

Much of the research on artificial sphincters has been done using adult subjects. Barrett and Furlow (1982) implanted artificial sphincters in 24 subjects with meningomyelocele aged 7 to 56 years. Although urinary control was achieved in 92% of the subjects, no longitudinal data were available on long-term effectiveness. The researchers cautioned that selection of patients must be done carefully, since the longevity of the device and the long-term effect on the upper urinary tract are as yet unknown.

In another study (Gonzales and Sheldon, 1982), artificial sphincters were implanted in ten boys and five girls aged 5 to 17 years who had neurogenic bladders. Nine boys were continent, whereas only one girl was continent. Sphincter failure was attributed to erosion of the bladder neck, mechanical malfunction, or bladder spasticity. Others (Moore, 1985; Gonzales and Sheldon, 1982; Barrett and Furlow, 1982; Faller and Vinson, 1985) agree on patient selection criteria for implanting an artificial sphincter; criteria include absence of residual urine, normal renal function and normal upper tracts, absence of vesicoureteral reflux, sufficient manual dexterity to operate the pump independently, and sufficient motivation to manage this therapy. The complications and failure rate of the AUS in many medical centers is high and seems to increase with time. The

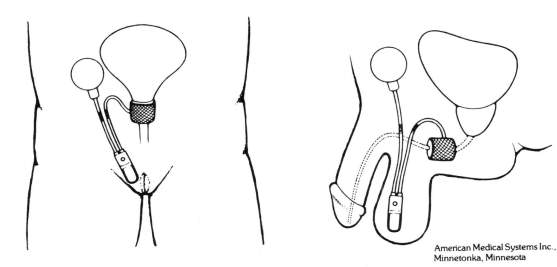

American Medical Systems Inc.,
Minnetonka, Minnesota

Figure 23–1. The artificial sphincter. (Copyright © University of Iowa, 1985.)

American Academy of Pediatrics suggests that caution and restraint should be exercised when recommending the artificial sphincter for children (Action Committee, 1979).

ASSESSMENT

Alterations in bowel and bladder maintenance that occur commonly among developmentally disabled children can be grouped under four nursing diagnoses: (1) *Alterations in bowel elimination: Constipation;* (2) *Alterations in bowel elimination: Incontinence;* (3) *Alterations in patterns of urinary elimination related to urinary retention;* and (4) *Alterations in patterns of urinary elimination related to incontinence.* Each diagnosis will be discussed in relation to its antecedent conditions, assessment strategies, defining characteristics, and planning for implementation of intervention.

The defining characteristics of constipation include hard, formed stool; decreased frequency of the bowel evacuation; palpable stool mass in colon; presence of hard stool in rectal ampule; decreasing bowel sounds; straining at stool; less than the usual amount of stool; and anal fissures or streaks of fresh blood in the stool. Bowel incontinence is the involuntary passage of stool, which can be described as a bowel movement or fecal smear in diapers or underwear after five years of age.

THE INTERVENTION

A major goal is to increase the independence of both children and their parents in managing the child's bowel and bladder maintenance program. This goal is accomplished by providing information and practice that will enable the parents and child, when developmentally appropriate, to be knowledgeable and self-confident enough to make modifications in the therapeutic program independently.

Decreasing Constipation

The goals of nursing strategies for decreasing constipation are to reduce present symptomatology and promote adequate and regular bowel function. When a child presents with severe constipation, interventions are initiated to cleanse the gastrointestinal tract of stool. This usually involves a combination of enemas, digital removal of stool, and suppositories. The rationale for each intervention must be carefully explained to the parent and child; emotional support should be provided to the child during these invasive and uncomfortable procedures.

Fortunately, anticipatory guidance can often prevent severe constipation and the need for such procedures. Constipation due to prolonged transit time usually can be prevented by increasing fluids, dietary manipulation, and the use of stool softeners. Counseling related to potential bowel problems and preventive measures should begin during infancy whether or not constipation is a current issue. Although there appears to be a positive correlation between severity of physical disability and degree of constipation, most physically disabled young children have problems with hard stool.

Management of constipation in an infant or young child begins with increasing fluid intake and diet manipulation. Infants under the age of six months may benefit from adding one to two teaspoons to one tablespoon of dark Karo syrup to their formula or supplementary bottles of water. The amount of Karo syrup needed to produce soft stools is often greater for disabled children than for non-disabled children. Glycerin suppositories may also be used intermittently. Once an infant is taking solid foods, dietary changes may be all that is required to soften stools. Dilute juices, including apple juice and prune juice, as well as strained fruits often act as stool softeners. Barley or blenderized bran can be added to baby cereals but must be accompanied by increased fluids. Milk intake should be limited to 1 quart a day unless needs for growth necessitate a greater volume. Foods that may be constipating and should be limited to one serving a day include rice cereal, applesauce, bananas, and highly refined carbohydrate foods such as infant desserts.

As the child matures, there will be more opportunities to make dietary changes. Prune juice is seldom acceptable to children in its natural form but can be made more palatable by mixing it with other strong-flavored juices such as grape juice, cranberry juice, or apple cider. Prune juice also can be frozen into popsicles, making it more appealing to many children. Likewise, bran muffins or cookies will be consumed more readily than bran cereals. Dried or fresh fruits, particularly those with the skin or peel left on, and raw vegetables make excellent snacks for children who are able to handle textured foods. A good variety of fruits and vegetables, salads, and whole wheat bread products should be offered.

Cultural variables and parental preferences strongly influence the extent to which the nurse can influence the family diet. In a family for whom meat, potatoes, and white bread are the main staples, drastic dietary recommendations often go unheeded. In such cases, it' is generally more effective to make one dietary change at a time. Dietary instruction should be given routinely to all cognitively intact school-aged children and adolescents as they begin to assume responsibility for their own health.

When constipation persists, despite attempts to increase fluids and change diet, consideration is given to the use of stool softeners or stimulants. The number of stool softeners and laxatives currently marketed is extensive (Table 23–1), but not all these products work as effectively in physically disabled children as they do in the normal population. Some experimentation may be necessary to find an effective stool softener for any given child. Senna-based products work well with few side effects in children with cerebral palsy and meningomyelocele. Senna is available over-the-counter in gran-

Table 23–1. LAXATIVES
AND FECAL MODIFIERS*

Irritant Stimulants	Cascara sagrada
	Castor oil
	Phenolphthalein
	Bisocodyl
	Senna
Saline Cathartics	Milk of magnesia
	Magnesium citrate
	Magnesium sulfate
	Sodium phosphate
	Potassium phosphate
Bulk-Forming Agents	Methylcellulose
	Psyllium hydrophilic muciloid
	Bran
Lubricant	Mineral oil
Wetting Agents	Dioctyl sodium sulfosuccinate

*From Henderson, M, and Synhorst, D. Bladder and bowl management in the child with myelomeningocele. Pediatric Nursing, 3:24–31, 1977.

ule or tablet form. The granules can be dissolved in a liquid such as milk or water for easier administration. In the experience of the authors, commercially prepared liquid senna is less stable than either the granule or tablet forms. Certain children respond better to other types of preparations, including bulk-forming agents, wetting agents, saline cathartics, malt or barley extracts, or a combination of these agents.

When recommending any type of stool softener or laxative, it is important to emphasize giving the medication preventively on a daily basis rather than episodically when constipation occurs. Parents are often concerned that their child will become dependent upon laxatives and therefore are hesitant to initiate their use. A careful review of the pathophysiology of their child's disability and the complications of constipation will help alleviate their anxiety. When given a stool softener or laxative regularly, children with cerebral palsy seldom need suppositories or enemas. Children with neurogenic bowels due to meningomyelocele, however, sometimes require the stimulation of a suppository to produce a complete bowel evacuation. This is particularly true for children with thoracic level lesions who lack the abdominal muscles to produce a Valsalva maneuver. Children with higher level spinal lesions frequently need suppositories, enemas or manual removal of stool on a regular basis. A glycerin suppository can be used initially; if not effective, it may be replaced by a bisocodyl sodium (Dulcolax) suppository, which has greater stimulant action. Occasionally, both types of suppositories "piggybacked" together are most effective. Parents are instructed to lubricate the suppository with water-soluble lubricant, insert it high in the rectum, and wait 15 to 20 minutes before toileting the child. It is often difficult to keep suppositories in the rectum of children with poor anal sphincter tone. The child can be put in a prone position with pillows underneath the hips to take advantage of gravity; the buttocks can be held together manually or with masking tape to prevent expulsion of the suppository. Most young children will protest these procedures, but television, books, and toys help provide diversion until the suppository has taken effect.

Some parents have difficulty with these "messier" aspects of bowel training and need encouragement and support. As children become older, they can be taught to insert suppositories or digitally remove stool. Unfortunately, children who require this type of management are often those whose physical limitations prevent them from achieving such independence. Periodic review of pathophysiology and goals of intervention helps enhance the level of compliance with any bowel management program. Consideration needs to be given to the acceptability of the intervention used and to the value placed on bowel management for each family. A mother who has four children to get off to school and is under financial and emotional stress may not be able to manage inserting a suppository each morning. A schedule change or the assistance of a school nurse or public health nurse will help achieve the desired goal. Therefore, each nursing intervention needs to be evaluated at regular intervals and modifications made as indicated.

Controlling Bowel Incontinence

The goals of nursing intervention for bowel incontinence are to reduce episodes of incontinence and to promote social continence. As children reach the ages of four to six years and enter school, bowel continence becomes significant for the purpose of fostering social relationships. Although wearing diapers is often acceptable for children in preschool, peer criticism becomes harsher as children mature. Having bowel accidents at school is likely to result in extreme social distress for children. It is therefore important to begin a bowel training program when the child first exhibits developmental readiness so that some degree of social continence is achieved by school age.

A bowel training program consists of regular stool evacuation and scheduled toileting. Readiness to begin toileting needs to be assessed individually, since many children with physical disabilities are also developmentally delayed. Toilet training usually begins when a child has reached a developmental age of two to three years. Criteria for initiating such a program include (1) the ability to sit; (2) the necessary support to sit (proper positioning on potty chair); and (3) the level of cooperation or attention span to sit on a potty chair for 3 to 5 minutes.

The assistance of an occupational or physical therapist may be needed to obtain or create an appropriate potty chair for individual children. In general, children with physical disabilities require a sturdy potty chair with a solid back, arm rests, and foot support. A lap belt may be added for extra security. Children with poor trunk control or spasticity need additional positioning modifications to maximize their balance and stability and minimize extensor muscle tone. The child is scheduled to sit on the potty chair after every meal for 3 to 5 minutes; this time is gradually increased. Sitting after meals takes advantage of the body's gastrocolic reflex. Additional scheduling times are added if the child already has a predictable time of stool evacuation. Children with cerebral palsy or other disabilities in which bowel innervation is intact can be encouraged to indicate their need for toileting. Children with speech disorders may not be able to verbalize toileting needs. Consultation from a speech-language pathologist is helpful to develop a non-oral means of communication for the child.

A thorough understanding of each child's physical limitations is needed to establish goals for independence in toileting. Over time, children can be taught to transfer to and from the potty chair/toilet, unfasten and refasten clothing, and wipe themselves if physically capable of doing these tasks. Special adaptations, such as Velcro closures on slacks, may assist the child in becoming more independent. An evaluation form for toilet training is presented in Figure 23–2.

Children with meningomyelocele do not have the urge to defecate and therefore will not be "toilet trained" in the usual manner. Parents should be reminded not to overreact if their child does not have a bowel movement while on the potty chair. Rather, their child deserves to be praised for just sitting on the potty chair. Although the sitting position increases intra-abdominal pressure, the child can be taught to perform the Valsalva maneuver by grunting, blowing up a balloon, or blowing at a pinwheel.

If a child with meningomyelocele is already taking a stool softener or laxative, the stool pattern is often one of frequent soft or formed stools. Suppositories can be used to regulate bowel evacuation times and to stimulate a full evacuation of the colon and rectum on a daily basis. The times of admin-

Name _____ Date _____

Age _____ Evaluator _____

Current status of continence _____
_____

Trunk control:

   regular toilet _____   regular toilet with special equipment _____

   potty chair _____   potty chair with special equipment _____

Communication:

   verbal _____   special words _____

   nonverbal _____   gestures _____

   ability to understand verbal requests: yes _____   no _____

Appropriate clothing for toilet training: yes _____   no _____

Comments _____
_____

Scheduled toileting:

   frequency _____

   dry between toileting: daytime: yes _____   no _____

                   nighttime: yes _____   no _____

Does child respond to adult's inquiry about toileting needs? yes _____ no _____

Does child voluntarily indicate need to urinate? yes _____ no _____

                   have bowel movements? yes _____ no _____

Ability to wipe self after toileting: yes _____ no _____

Comments _____
_____
_____

Recommendations _____
_____

Figure 23–2. Toilet-training evaluation. (From the Nursing Department, Division of Developmental Disabilities, University Hospital School, University of Iowa.)

istration of both the stool softener or laxative and the suppository can be adjusted so that the suppository is given at the time of peak action for the laxative. In other words, if a stool softener is given at bedtime and expected to reach its full effect in 6 to 12 hours, a suppository can be administered after breakfast the following morning. The administration times can be adjusted to coordinate with the family schedule in order to enhance compliance.

Close telephone contact is advised when the child is beginning a bowel training program. Parents need much encouragement and emotional support when dealing with such a long-term and often frustrating process. It is, after all, much easier to change a diaper than to remove braces, insert a suppository, and sit with the child for 20 minutes before putting her or him on the potty chair.

Periodic revisions in the bowel training program are necessary. There is no standard bowel regime for all children, and achieving maximum bowel continence can be a lengthy process. Parents should also be aware that diet, illness, surgery, and emotional stress all can exacerbate bowel incontinence. The chances of achieving reasonable continence are enhanced if there is coordination of routine between home and school. The nurse or health aide assigned to the child's school needs to be informed about the bowel management routine. In most cases, administration of laxatives and suppositories can occur outside of school hours, but scheduled toileting should continue at school. The nurse who is primarily responsible for initiating and managing the bowel program should establish a channel of communication with the school. Appropriate health teaching needs to be provided to teachers, health aides, and nurses. It is not uncommon to find school nurses who have had little experience with disabled children. In order to maintain continuity of approach, an appropriate potty chair needs to be present at school as well as home.

For the older, more independent child, bathroom facilities need to be accessible. A change of clothing should be kept at school in case of accidents. Children should not be sent home for having a bowel accident since this is punishing them for something that is out of their control. The health aide or nurse can assist in monitoring and documenting stool patterns and bowel accidents. This information is essential in order to make modifications in the program.

Bowel accidents at school are often quite distressing to children, their peers, and teachers. The incontinent child cannot always perceive the odor of feces, which leads to further social ostracism. If teachers are fully informed about the medical problem, often they can intervene to alleviate some of the public embarrassment and allow the child to participate fully in school activities.

Many children with meningomyelocele have been excluded from school swim programs because of their bowel incontinence. However, a study conducted by Schott (1978) showed that fecal coliform bacteria introduced into swimming pool water by children with meningomyelocele did not exceed the amount of bacteria introduced by non-disabled subjects. Shott concluded that in a chlorinated pool, children with meningomyelocele who are on a bowel training program and wear diapers and rubber pants do not present a health hazard to other swimmers and should not be excluded from swim class. All attempts should be made to minimize bowel accidents and normalize the child's schedule of activities.

Reducing Urinary Retention

The goals of nursing strategies are to reduce urinary retention, prevent further urinary tract infections and promote renal function. When urinary tract infections result from urinary retention, it is imperative to find the source of the infection. This is easier to accomplish when the child has a disability, such as meningomyelocele, and therefore is presumed to have neurogenic bladder.

When children with cerebral palsy or other types of physical disability present with a urinary tract infection, one must evaluate such factors as fluid intake, toileting schedule, and perineal hygiene and then make appropriate recommendations. Children with severe spastic quadriplegia often have limitations in hip abduction that make perineal hygiene extremely difficult, resulting in a bladder infection. For such children, a referral to an orthopedic surgeon is indicated. If infections are recurrent or if incontinence is a problem, a urological referral is indicated to evaluate the structure and function of the urinary tract. All urinary tract infections are treated with an appropriate antibiotic followed by a repeat urinalysis.

Children with meningomyelocele should receive routine urological evaluation from the time of their birth. Urinalyses are done about every six months and also when the child is ill or experiences symptoms of a urinary tract infection. If an infection occurs, the child is treated with an antibiotic; radiographic studies are done to determine the presence of vesicoureteral reflux, hydronephrosis, bladder irregularities, or a high bladder pressure. These procedures may include an intravenous pyelogram (IVP), delayed cystogram, cystometrogram, renal ultrasound, and nuclear studies. The nurse assists with these studies by explaining the purpose and procedure to the parents and children and interpreting the results.

Clean intermittent catheterization is the usual recommended treatment for urinary tract infections in children with meningomyelocele. This is especially true if there are recurrent infections, vesicoureteral reflux, a flaccid bladder, or a bladder pressure of greater than 40 mm. These problems most often appear during infancy or early childhood at a time when the child is not yet capable of self-catheterization. The parents or other caretakers, therefore, must assume responsibility for catheterizing the child. A teaching session is conducted by the nurse to instruct parents or other caretakers how to perform CIC. Sensitivity toward the caretaker's apprehension about this new procedure is crucial. Reminding parents that CIC is not painful because of decreased sensation may help alleviate some of their anxiety. A quiet, private room is required to provide careful and thorough instruction without interruption. One to two hours is needed to teach a parent or other caretaker how to catheterize the child. It is important that parents realize that the purpose of catheterizations is to establish complete and regular emptying of the bladder, which will prevent infections and preserve renal function. The instruction session should include a discussion of the purpose, supplies, method, and schedule of catheterizations as well as a demonstration and practice by each of the adults present. Instructional materials about intermittent catheterization are available to parents upon request from the authors.

Individual assessments are made to determine the size and type of catheter used. Following each catheterization, the catheter should be washed and flushed with cool, soapy water. Catheters need to be boiled in water for ten minutes prior to reuse. They can be packaged individually in plastic sandwich bags to remain clean until reused. With proper care, both urinary catheters and feeding tubes will last at least six months. They should be replaced when the plastic or rubber begins to deteriorate or when mineral deposits begin to clog the lumen. Periodically boiling them in 0.25% acetic acid (vinegar) solution will help to reduce mineral deposits.

A mild and nonirritating liquid or bar soap should be used to cleanse the genitalia prior to insertion of the catheter. Cleansing with cotton balls prevents recontamination. Moist towelettes can replace soap and cotton balls for the sake of convenience during travel. The towelettes, however, should contain benzalkonium chloride or another antiseptic ingredient; and parents should be instructed to fold over the towelette after each cleansing wipe to prevent recontamination.

Catheterization supplies should be kept together in a plastic shoe box, food storage container, or other convenient storage place. Parents are encouraged to obtain a small purse or makeup or shaving kit to carry supplies while traveling. Most kits of this type also have a zippered pocket in which to store dirty catheters. Kits like these are a convenient and socially attractive way for the child to carry catheterization supplies to school.

A catheterization schedule that is medically acceptable and convenient for the family is decided upon at the initial teaching session. In most cases, the bladder needs to be emptied every four hours, which means approximately four catheterizations a day. The child should be catheterized upon awakening in the morning and every four hours thereafter. Catheterizations do not need to be done during the night, but the nighttime interval between catheterizations should not exceed 12 hours. A recommended catheterization schedule might be 8 A.M., 12 noon, 4 P.M, and 8 P.M. Parents need some flexibility in this schedule. They do not need to rush home from shopping at 4 P.M., but should do a catheterization when they return home. On the other hand, parents need to know that catheterizations must continue over the family's summer vacation and while visiting grandparents.

All caretakers should learn to catheterize the child to provide maximum flexibility for the parents. This includes grandparents, day-care workers, baby sitters, and, when appropriate, older siblings. Parents can instruct these other persons in CIC if they are comfortable doing so, or they can be brought to the clinic for a teaching session. If a child attends school, a workable catheterization schedule should be agreed upon between parents, teachers, and school nurse. As part of the teaching sessions, persons performing CIC are taught to assess the color, odor, and clarity of urine. Whenever the urine is odoriferous or cloudy, appears to have blood in it, or is otherwise unusual in character, a urinalysis should be obtained. Parents need to know that urine can look dark first thing in the morning or when fluid intake is low, and that food and medication may alter its appearance. If these changes persist, however, medical evaluation is warranted.

When a urinary tract infection is diagnosed, a reassessment is made of catheterization technique, care of supplies, and catheterization schedule. Breaks in catheterization technique by parents tend to be related to incomplete emptying of the bladder. Parents need to be instructed to roll the child from side to side, sit the child upright, withdraw the catheter slightly, have the child cough, or gently aspirate urine from the bladder using a syringe in order to ensure full emptying. An observation of catheterization technique should be done routinely in the clinic setting. Parents can be likewise encouraged to observe the technique of the baby sitter, grandparents, health aide, and other caretakers. Among children, breaks in technique are seen at any and in some cases every step of the catheterization process. This includes not washing hands or genitalia, improper washing of genitalia, not holding the labia open or allowing the penis to fall against the body, letting the end of the catheter fall into the toilet bowl, and incomplete bladder emptying. Breaks in catheterization techniques should always be explained and corrected. Improper care and storage of catheters and supplies is another common source of infection; this needs to be periodically reviewed with families. Finally, the catheterization schedule should be reviewed to ensure that the bladder is emptied every four hours. If no other breaks in technique or cleanliness are discovered, a fifth catheterization time can be added to shorten the nighttime interval between catheterizations. It is never desirable to have parents awaken during the night to do a catheterization, but they can accomplish this before they go to bed, even if the child is already asleep. If infections persist in spite of these modifications, further urological evaluation is indicated.

Controlling Urinary Incontinence

The goals of nursing intervention are to reduce urinary incontinence and promote social continence. Social continence means staying dry to the extent that a child is socially acceptable. A urinalysis should be done when a child is incontinent to rule out a bacterial infection. The child's developmental level should be determined prior to setting any expectations for urinary continence. Motivation to stay dry also should be assessed, since wetness may not be perceived as a problem by the child. If there are environmental obstacles to toileting, modifications can be made to enable the child to be toileted at appropriate intervals. For example, if a child is unable to be independent in toileting at school because he or she has braces or is nonambulatory, consultation with school officials is warranted to obtain assistance from a health aide. Scheduled voiding times should be established, and fluid intake may need to be limited. If the source of incontinence is a neurogenic bladder, consideration should be given to a method of establishing social continence when the child reaches school age.

External Urinary Collection Devices

External urinary collection devices can be used in male children without evidence of urinary tract infection. When properly utilized, these devices can achieve social continence without the risks of bladder catheterization. A phallus of adequate size is required to support a condom catheter; however, even boys with small, retractile penises can use pubic pressure devices. When using a pubic pressure device, careful measurements are taken to ensure that it is the proper size. The device must be applied properly to minimize leakage. Children confined to a wheelchair or who are especially active should have the placement of the device checked frequently. Periodic evaluation is also important as the child grows. In addition, the collection bag needs to be emptied at regular intervals, usually every two hours, to avoid dislodging the penile sheath. The device is removed at night to allow the skin to air dry to prevent skin breakdown. Any area of redness or skin breakdown underneath the collecting device precludes wearing it. Clothes should be kept loose-fitting and comfortable. Jogging or sweat pants are preferable to tight jeans that might occlude the urinary drainage. To prevent odor, the device is cleaned nightly with cool water and baby shampoo and then allowed to dry. Components of the device may need to be replaced every 6 to 12 months. Young boys can easily learn to empty their "bag" but may need assistance in applying the bag or checking its placement. The most common reasons for discontinuing use of this type of device include problems with fit and leakage, boys wanting to wear shorts in the summer or wishing to participate in sports, and embarrassment.

Clean Intermittent Catheterization

Clean intermittent catheterization (CIC) is the preferred intervention to achieve social continence in all girls and in boys for whom an external collection device is ineffective or an undesired option. The rationale for use must first be explained to the child and family. Although many parents are interested in having their children stay dry, some parents do not mind their child's incontinence and see little reason to change their family routine. The social implications of an incontinent child in a peer setting need to be discussed, including the effects of incontinence on a child's self-esteem. Initiating catheterizations for social continence depends upon the motivation of the child and family, rather than a true medical need. If there is no medical urgency to proceed, catheterization instruction should be postponed when either the child or parent is depressed or outwardly resistant or if there is sufficient family stress to make the nurse doubt the efficacy of the intervention at that time. If self-esteem and level of motivation are low, attempts to initiate a new therapy as complex and intensive as CIC will be futile.

When CIC is chosen as a method of reducing urinary incontinence, the nurse must assess the child's developmental readiness to learn self-catheterization. Such an assessment takes into account the child's cognitive level, fine motor abilities, maturity, cooperation, and motivation. Further evaluation of the child's abilities by a psychologist and an occupational or physical therapist may assist the nurse in making this assessment. Impaired hand function and tactile dysfunction has been demonstrated in children who have meningomyelocele with hydrocephalus (Grimm, 1976). Knowledge of hand function for a particular child is crucial before expecting her or him to perform catheterizations, a skill that requires a fair amount of manual dexterity. Therapists can offer creative suggestions for modifying catheterization technique or can initiate therapeutic measures to prepare children for learning catheterization.

Cognitive level alone does not dictate whether or not a child will be successful at self-catheterization. Some mildly retarded children can catheterize themselves with ease whereas other children with higher cognitive functioning need constant supervision. Other factors, including parental attitudes and involvement, emotional stress, and perceived results, influence the rate of compliance with the CIC program. In general, children of normal to borderline intelligence are capable of self-catheterization around age seven to eight years. Some children as young as five years of age will be able to catheterize themselves but often do not really understand the rationale or maintain clean technique at that age.

Instruction in self-catheterization should be a gradual process that evolves naturally over time. Children as young as two to three years of age can be taught to wash their hands before and after catheterization and to assemble and help clean up supplies. They are told this is their way of "going potty" and can be encouraged to "catheterize" their dolls or stuffed animals. If a medication is administered as a bladder instillation, children can learn to push the syringe plunger. They can be gradually encouraged to accomplish each step of the procedure until they have mastered the whole catheterization. The most difficult step of the procedure, particularly for girls, is the actual insertion of the catheter. A small portable makeup mirror can be used to help girls visualize their genitalia and learn where to insert the catheter. Some parents are comfortable teaching their children self-catheterization at home, whereas others prefer professional assistance. If appropriate facilities are available, a child can be admitted to a hospital or rehabilitation setting for the purpose of learning self-catheterization. Simple anatomy and physiology of the urinary tract need to be reviewed, using pictures or diagrams. The child should be taught the rationale for catheterization, how to do the procedure, how to care for supplies and equipment, signs and symptoms of urinary tract infection, and how to record urine volumes and wet/dry states. An inpatient setting gives the nurse an opportunity to directly observe technique, experiment with various positions, manipulate the catheterization schedule and observe the results of a medication trial. An evaluation form is helpful in documenting competencies (Fig. 23–3).

When self-catheterization is initiated, it is important to assess environmental factors both at home and at school to assist children in maximizing their independence. Children need uninterrupted bathroom time for 15 minutes four times a day. If the family is large, mornings can be very hectic with several family members preparing for work and school simultaneously, which may rush the catheterization. The bathroom at home should be arranged so that the child can have easy access to necessary supplies, which will allow for independence in CIC. Physical facilities also should be evaluated at school. Children require a private place to catheterize, a schedule that provides the

Name _____ Date _____

Age _____ Evaluator _____

Understands verbal instructions: yes _____ no _____

Able to retain verbal instructions: yes _____ no _____

Laterality: right _____ left _____

Walks: independently _____ with aid _____

Uses wheelchair _____

Ability to do transfers: independently _____ with assistance _____

Ability to sit: unsupported _____ with support _____

Ability to visualize perineal area _____ with visual aid _____

Ability to grasp and release small objects: yes _____ no _____

Assembling of equipment:
  cotton balls/washcloth   _____

  catheter   _____

  lubricant   _____

  catch basin   _____

  soap solution   _____

Understanding of and ability to wash hands thoroughly: yes _____ no _____

Type of equipment used _____

_____

_____

_____

_____

Figure 23–3. Self-catheterization evaluation. (From the Nursing Department, Division of Developmental Disabilities, University Hospital School, University of Iowa.)

least amount of interference with academic time, and an adult who can assist or supervise the child.

Total urinary continence is seldom achieved by catheterization only four times a day. If a child remains wet between catheterizations, a fifth catheterization time is added. Some children are so motivated to stay dry that they will catheterize every two hours if needed. Such a frequent schedule of catheterization is usually incompatible with a family or school schedule, and medications may be introduced to achieve dryness. An anticholinergic medication such as oxybutynin is the first drug of choice to increase bladder capacity by inhibiting bladder contractions. Children with poor resistance to outflow of urine may also require an alpha-adrenegic medication such as phenylpropanolamine. Parents and children need to learn the expected actions of these medications as well as their potential side effects. Side effects often occur in the first two weeks of use and then may subside spontaneously. Common side effects include dry mouth, flushing of the face with circumoral pallor, and blurred vision. Parents, school nurses, and older children are encouraged to document wet/dry status and urine volumes. This information assists the nurse and physician in altering doses and times of administration for medications. The goal of using these medications is to achieve maximal dryness with minimal side effects. The nurse can make suggestions to lessen side effects such as having a child with a dry mouth suck on sugarless hard candy or gum. This relieves the symptoms without increasing overall fluid intake, which could contribute to incontinence.

Although many children who are maintained on a program of intermittent catheterizations plus anticholinergic or alpha-adrenergic medications can achieve relative dryness, they may have occasional periods of dampness. Increased fluid intake, consumption of caffeinated beverages, late or missed medications, and increased activity level can all result in increased wetness.

Commercially available incontinence

products can help the child feel more secure. Girls may find that an adhesive-backed mini- or maxipad is sufficient protection to prevent embarrassment. A portion of a disposable diaper can be inserted into a boy's undershorts. Both male and female patients can use commercially available incontinence pants with diaper inserts. Children should be encouraged to catheterize immediately before and after engaging in any activity that increases intra-abdominal pressure, such as recess, gym class, and even playing a musical instrument.

It is essential that the nurse be available by telephone to assist families in assessing problems that occur with catheterizations. In addition to concerns related to the character of the urine, occasionally there are mechanical problems with catheter insertion, particularly among boys. Coudé-tipped or curved-tipped catheters are helpful to adolescent boys who have difficulty inserting a straight, more pliable catheter. If a boy does not obtain urine during a routine catheterization, he should stop and attempt another catheterization an hour later since catheters can sometimes coil up within a "blind pouch" in the urethra. Injecting a water-soluble lubricant directly into the urethra prior to inserting the catheter assists the catheter to "float" into the bladder. If repeated catheterizations are unsuccessful, medical attention should be sought to rule out a urethral stricture or large blind pouch. At no point should a catheter be forcefully pushed past an obstruction. Bladder spasms may also increase resistance to catheterization among male and female children.

The most frequent problem seen in catheterizing children is adherence to the planned regime. Reasons for noncompliance are multifaceted and cannot be discussed in detail in this chapter. Nurses, however, are in an excellent position to problem-solve with the child and parents in order to increase compliance with the therapeutic regimen. Although children at any age may use improper catheterization technique or simply not do their catheterizations, preadolescents and adolescents are at greatest risk for these behaviors. Such behaviors may be either covert, such as when a child spends 15 minutes in the bathroom five times a day but does not catheterize, or overt, such as frequent "forgetting" to catheterize.

Noncompliance can be frustrating to parents who fear renal deterioration yet respect the need for their child's independence in self-care. Opportunities for both parents and children to verbalize their feelings are crucial. Children often resent having to miss parts of class, recess, or other play activities to catheterize, a procedure that only accentuates their being different from peers. Similarly, children who use excellent catheterization technique when supervised may use poor technique when on their own to "speed things up." If social continence has not been achieved through catheterization, children have little motivation to continue this practice. Reasons for these behaviors need to be explored before interventions are begun. Children's feelings need to be validated, yet they must understand what is expected of them. A catheterization schedule chart helps children remember catheterization times. Behavior modification programs are useful to give the child added incentive for compliance. In many cases, direct observation and supervision of catheterizations by an adult are needed on an ongoing basis to insure compliance with medical recommendations, particularly if urinary tract infections have occurred. These are difficult problems not specific to catheterizations but inherent in the developmental stage of adolescence.

Artificial Urinary Sphincter

Certain children with spina bifida are unable to achieve social continence with intermittent catheterizations and medication. Some of these children may be candidates for an artificial sphincter. Although such a device restores sphincter control, it does not induce bladder contracture. Therefore, artificial sphincters are used only in clients in whom the bladder contracts spontaneously or in conjunction with catheterization. Children with meningomyelocele who receive an artificial sphincter must catheterize routinely. Failure to open the sphincter periodically can result in urinary tract infections and, in some cases, erosion of the urethra.

Nurses can assist in determining what children are appropriate candidates for an artificial sphincter. Candidates must be carefully selected to minimize complications. The child and parents should be well motivated to achieve dryness, since compliance is critical to avoid serious complications.

Past patterns of compliance can be reviewed when making this assessment. The child and parents must be informed about the expectations for this type of management and the associated risks.

Once the artificial sphincter is in place, frequent telephone contact and regular outpatient follow-up are established to answer questions, provide support to the child and family, and intercept problems. A "Medic-Alert" bracelet should be worn that states, "Artificial Sphincter: Do Not Catheterize." The parents and child should be told never to catheterize when the cuff is inflated. They need to learn to insist on suprapubic bladder drainage rather than catheterization if acute urinary retention results from cuff failure. Finally, they should be taught the signs of urethral erosion: pain, swelling, urine retention, and incontinence.

Urinary Diversion

Since the advent of CIC for routine urological management, few children have undergone urinary diversion for neurogenic bladders. There remains, however, a sizable number of clients with urinary diversions who are now adolescents and young adults. Nurses working with this population need to periodically inspect the stoma, looking for evidence of erythema, edema, bleeding and hyperkeratosis. The fit of the appliance should be checked; no more than $1/16$- to $1/8$-inch should exist between the stoma and face-plate. If leakage occurs, a new appliance needs to be considered. The appliance should be changed every five to seven days and sometimes more frequently, especially in summer. The bag needs to be emptied every two to three hours during the daytime; a drainage bag is recommended overnight, which is often unacceptable to adolescents and young adults for social reasons. In particular, college students living in dormitories often refuse to use night drainage systems. Instead, they can be encouraged to use extension tubing and a leg bag to allow for urine drainage away from the stoma.

Education is provided for the child, parents, and siblings. They are instructed in changing the appliance, emptying the appliance, inspecting the skin and stoma, caring for the equipment, and skin care. The child's level of independence in managing urinary diversion can be evaluated and recorded on

a form available upon request from the authors. Fine motor difficulties or obesity may interfere with independent application of an ostomy appliance. Consultation with an occupational therapist or ostomy nurse specialist may be useful in planning intervention.

EVALUATION

Criteria for evaluating the effectiveness of interventions are established prior to implementing elimination control. Following actions to decrease constipation, children will demonstrate improved bowel elimination, characterized by soft regular stools, and will not develop a bowel impaction. Further, children and their parents will be able to describe the therapeutic bowel regimen, explain the rationale for intervention, and modify the bowel routine as needed. After intervening to control bowel incontinence, the child will demonstrate improved social continence characterized by fewer bowel accidents. In addition, children and/or parents will be able to describe the therapeutic bowel regimen, explain the rationale for intervention, and modify the bowel routine as needed.

Defining characteristics of urinary retention include residual urine on catheterization immediately following voluntary voiding or Credé of bladder, distended bladder, vesicoureteral reflux, and hydronephrosis. A urinary tract infection is characterized by pyuria and bacteriuria on urinalysis and greater than 50,000 CFU per ml of an isolated organism on urine culture. Urinary incontinence can be defined as involuntary urination characterized by damp or wet diapers or underwear after the developmental age of five years.

Following strategies to reduce urinary retention, there will be no urinary tract infections, as evidenced by an absence of bacteriuria and pyuria on a sterile catheterized urine specimen or less than 50,000 colonies of a single microorganism on urine culture. Also, children and parents will demonstrate proper clean intermittent catheterization technique. Similarly, they will also be able to describe the therapeutic bladder program, explain the rationale for intervention, describe the signs and symptoms of a urinary tract infection, and modify the bladder program as needed. After taking steps to control urinary incontinence, improved social continence will be demonstrated by fewer incontinent episodes each day. If applicable, the child will apply and empty an external collection device or ostomy appliance independently or with assistance. Finally, the child or parent will be able to describe the therapeutic bladder program, explain the rationale for intervention, and modify the bladder program as needed.

Case Study

Jason is a ten year old boy who has meningomyelocele at the S1–S2 sensory-motor level, hydrocephalus with a ventriculoperitoneal shunt, and a neurogenic bowel and bladder. He ambulates independently without braces. Although Jason has normal intelligence, he also has learning disabilities that are resulting in academic difficulties at school, where he is in a regular fourth grade class. Jason is an only child and resides with his divorced mother who works full-time.

Bowel management began when Jason was one year old; he was placed on a stool softener to prevent constipation. Scheduled toileting was initiated at the age of 2½ years, but no consistent regimen was followed due to his mother's work schedule and a variety of substitute caretakers. At the age of five years, Jason's mother expressed a concern about social continence, and Jason began to use an external urinary collection device (EUD). Over the next few years, there were increasing problems with bowel and bladder management despite a variety of interventions.

There were problems with leakage when the EUD was worn, and it was finally discarded because Jason was having frequent bowel accidents. These accidents were creating significant problems at school—the health aide did not have enough time to change his diapers, and Jason's peers were avoiding him because of the odor. During this period, Jason's school performance began to deteriorate and behavior problems were reported.

A hospitalization occurred when Jason was nine years old for the purpose of (1) improving bowel management, (2) initiating self-catheterization, (3) achieving a degree of social continence, and (4) evaluating behavior problems and academic status. During this admission Jason was able to avoid bowel accidents by using a combination of a stool softener, suppositories, and scheduled toileting. Jason learned to catheterize himself five times a day but, because of attention and motor problems, continued to require adult supervision during catheterizations. He remained dry between catheterizations when placed on anticholinergic and alpha-adrenergic medications. He expressed great pleasure in being able

to wear regular underwear at the time of discharge. Recommendations for educational programming and behavior management were also made to the school.

Problems in bowel and bladder management have again occurred. Jason's mother expressed frustration in managing Jason's behavior and his noncompliance with the bowel and bladder program. She appeared passive and depressed; there was obvious tension between her and Jason. Jason was once again wearing diapers due to bowel and bladder accidents. Although he continued to take his stool softener, he refused to sit on the toilet at regular intervals and therefore was having bowel movements in his diapers. Oxybutynin tablets have been found discarded behind the refrigerator at home, and he is almost always wet between catheterizations. Unless supervised, Jason will not do his catheterizations. Even with supervision his catheterization technique is poor as he often "forgets" to wash his hands and penis during the procedure. Jason stated that catheterizations interfere with his activities, and he preferred being in diapers. He had one urinary tract infection. The health aide at school reported that she watches every catheterization, since Jason is not trustworthy. However, there were not enough personnel at school to allow her to supervise his scheduled toileting and his medication administration. He is expected to be independent in these activities as "he is old enough to take care of himself." Although Jason denied problems with friends, he was frequently observed alone on the playground at recess. Jason was readmitted to the hospital.

The nursing diagnoses, expected outcomes, and nursing interventions for this hospitalization are summarized in Table 23–2.

Following this hospitalization, Jason was having regular bowel movements without accidents. He responded well to a behavior management approach that rewarded him for independent toileting, taking medications, and having clean pants. He continued to require some supervision during catheterizations but was remaining mostly dry during the day. Jason seemed to be joining in more peer activities at school. Some conflict remained between Jason and his mother at home, but she had begun counseling and was feeling less stressed. She had recently registered Jason for summer camp, about which he was very excited.

RESEARCH IMPLICATIONS

Despite the importance of bowel and bladder maintenance and the prevalence of bowel and bladder problems among physically disabled children, little nursing research has been done in this area. Decisions

Table 23–2. CASE STUDY

Diagnosis	Intervention	Outcome
1. *Bowel elimination, alteration in: Constipation*	1. Teaching: Explain etiology of problem and rationale for interventions. 2. Dietary counseling: Encourage increased fluids and fiber in diet. 3. Initiate use of stool softener. Explain dose, method of administration, and side effects. 4. Monitor character and consistency of stool.	1. Jason will have soft, formed bowel movements daily. 2. Jason and his mother can explain why he is constipated, can state the purpose of interventions, and can list high-fiber foods. 3. Jason will receive stool softener on a regular basis. 4. Jason will have a soft, formed stool every day or every other day.
2. *Bowel elimination, alteration in: Incontinence*	1. Teaching: (a) discuss neurogenic bowel as etiology of incontinence; (b) explain importance of regular bowel evacuations; (c) instruct parent in use of suppository. 2. Initiate use of suppositories. Re-evaluate and change type of suppository depending on stool patterns. 3. Initiate scheduled toileting every two hours, then after every meal. Encourage child to increase abdominal pressure while sitting. 4. Monitor and record patterns of bowel elimination.	1. Jason will sit on the toilet and do the Valsalva maneuver at least three times a day. 2. Jason will not have bowel accidents or fecal smearing. 3. Jason and his mother can explain why he is incontinent and can state the purpose of interventions.
3. *Urinary elimination, alterations in patterns of: Related to incontinence*	1. Discuss concept of social continence and options for achieving this. 2. Review CIC with parent and child, including rationale, supplies, procedure, and care of equipment. 3. Encourage parent/child to record times of catheterization, urine volumes, and wet/dry status. 4. Explain action, dose, method of administration, and side effects of medication to keep child dry.	1. Jason and his mother will state rationale for doing CIC. 2. Jason and his mother will demonstrate CIC, using clean techniques, and perform CIC five times a day. 3. Jason and his mother will record times of catheterizations, urine volumes, and wet/dry status. 4. Jason will remain dry between catheterizations.
4. *Self-care toileting deficit*	1. Assist Jason with self-catheterization. 2. Encourage Jason to sit on toilet and perform the Valsalva maneuver every two hours/after meals.	1. Jason will catheterize himself five times a day with supervision, using proper technique. 2. Jason will sit on toilet and do the Valsalva maneuver every two hours/after meals.
5. *Social isolation*	1. Teach bowel and bladder maintenance to achieve social continence. 2. Discuss with Jason social effects of wearing dirty diapers. 3. Encourage school personnel to facilitate Jason's involvement in playground activities. 4. Encourage participation in group activities outside of school (i.e., Boy Scouts). 5. Rehearse mock situations with Jason to (a) explain his disability to others, and (b) increase social skills (i.e., making friends).	1. Jason will be able to wear underwear and stay continent. 2. Jason will stay clean and free of odor. 3. Jason will have more positive peer relationships at school and outside of school. 4. Jason will have positive self-image.

Table 23–2. CASE STUDY *Continued*

Diagnosis	Intervention	Outcome
6. *Noncompliance with bowel and bladder management program*	1. Listen to Jason's feelings about bowel and bladder management. 2. Listen to mother's concerns about noncompliance and behavior management, and her feelings about the expected therapeutic regimen. 3. Encourage supervision of all catheterizations and medications. 4. Encourage mother and school personnel to remind Jason to go to bathroom. 5. Initiate system of positive reinforcement for compliant behavior (i.e., sticker chart; favorite activity if compliant all week, etc.). 6. Initiate referral to school psychologist if needed. 7. Invite Jason to join support group of children with meningomyelocele.	1. Jason will take medications as prescribed. 2. Jason will catheterize himself five times a day using clean technique. 3. Jason will sit on toilet and do the Valsalva maneuver after every meal.
7. *Urinary elimination, alterations in patterns of: Retention resulting in urinary tract infection*	1. Observe for breaks in Jason's catheterization technique. 2. Review catheterization schedule, technique, and care of equipment with Jason and mother and make modifications as needed. 3. Determine whether UTI was properly treated with antibiotics and obtain repeat urinalysis. 4. Discuss UTI with urologist to determine whether radiographic studies are necessary.	1. Jason will have a negative urinalysis and/or urine culture. 2. Jason will maintain a nighttime interval between catheterizations of less than 12 hours. 3. Catheterization supplies and equipment will be cared for and stored in recommended way. 4. Catheterizations will be done using proper clean technique.
8. *Alteration in family process related to developmental transition: Childhood*	1. Discuss Jason's behavior with mother, explaining it as normal reaction of school-aged child with health impairment. 2. Encourage mother to seek counseling to work through her feelings and learn behavior management strategies. 3. Provide a private place for Jason to catheterize at home and at school. 4. Encourage Jason to be independent in toileting and catheterizing. 5. Suggest list of leisure activities for Jason to foster his sense of competency. 6. Encourage mother to spend one evening a week sharing a mutually enjoyable activity with Jason.	1. Jason's mother will understand the developmental normality of Jason's actions. 2. The mother's frustration level and depression will be decreased. She will develop effective coping strategies. 3. Jason will have privacy when managing his elimination needs. 4. Jason will become more independent in toileting himself and doing self-catheterization. 5. Jason will feel competent and have a positive self-concept. 6. Jason and his mother will have more positive interactions.
9. *Knowledge deficit of school personnel resulting in inappropriate expectations*	1. Discuss rationale for scheduled toileting, regular CIC, and medications with school personnel. 2. Explain that Jason has learning problems that interfere with his ability to be independent in self-care. 3. Discuss concept of noncompliance in chronically ill school-aged children with school personnel. 4. Encourage supervision at school and use of positive reinforcement system.	1. School personnel will not expect Jason to be totally independent in self-care. 2. Health aide will supervise CIC, scheduled toileting, and administration of medication. 3. Regular telephone contact will be maintained between school and clinic.

Abbreviations: CIC, Clean intermittent catheterization; UTI, urinary tract infection.

regarding appropriate nursing interventions, for the most part, are based on experience and anecdotal information. Controlled research studies are needed to better document the effectiveness of nursing interventions.

Recommendations on laxative use and dietary modifications are often made by nurses, but the effects of these are seldom evaluated systematically. Comparisons of laxative use among physically disabled children or a comparison of laxative versus diet therapy for constipation would be useful.

Incontinence has been presumed to have deleterious effects on a child's social relationships, hence the importance attributed to "social continence." Unfortunately, few research data are available to substantiate this conclusion. Studies are needed to document the negative effects of incontinence and positive changes caused by increased continence. Children's self-esteem could be measured, using a standardized instrument, before and after social continence is achieved. It would be helpful to know whether children feel differently about bladder versus bowel incontinence. Similarly, information about the effects of various types of activity on continence would assist in planning interventions.

Further research is needed to provide more information on the response of children and parents to clean intermittent catheterizations. Different approaches to teaching CIC could be examined, as well as the feasibility of teaching CIC to preschool-aged children. The cultural attitudes toward CIC would be useful information for health professionals working with Hispanic, Southeast Asian, or other ethnic groups.

Nurses are continually challenged by noncompliant children or parents, particularly in the area of bowel and bladder management. Compliance enhancement is perhaps the single most significant void in current research. Nurses need to know what strategies can maximize patient compliance. First, research is needed to examine the attitudes of parents and children toward regimens, such as CIC or bowel management. Theoretical frameworks such as the health belief model provide concepts on which to formulate hypotheses. Factors influencing compliance with CIC at home and at school need to be explored. In addition, interventions such as peer support groups can be evaluated in terms of their impact on compliance

with CIC. A longitudinal study is needed to look at child and parent satisfaction and the side effects of particular therapies, such as CIC, ileal conduit, artificial sphincter, and the external collection device, over time.

As more nursing research is done in the area of bowel and bladder maintenance, more scientific data will become available on which to base nursing interventions. These data will provide information to enable nurses to make significant contributions that will have an impact upon the quality of life for many physically disabled children.

References

Action Committee on Myelodysplasia, Section on Urology. Current approaches to evaluation and management of children with myelomeningocele. Pediatrics, 63:663–667, 1979.

Barrett, D, and Furlow, W. The management of severe urinary incontinence in patients with myelodysplasia by implantation of the AS 791/792 urinary sphincter device. Journal of Urology, 128:484–486, 1982.

Becker, M (Ed.). The health belief model and personal health behavior. Thorofare, N.J.: Charles B. Slack, 1974.

Becker, M, Maiman, L, Kirscht, J, Haefner, D, and Drachman, R. The health belief model and prediction of dietary compliance: A field experiment. Journal of Health and Social Behavior, 18:348–365, 1977.

Brem, A, Martin, D, Callaghan, J, and Maynard, J. Long-term renal risk factors in children with meningomyelocele. The Journal of Pediatrics, 110:51–55, 1987.

Brunner, L, and Suddarth, D (Eds.). The Lippincott manual of nursing practice (4th ed.). Philadelphia: JB Lippincott, 1986.

Crooks, K, and Enrile, B. Comparison of the ileal conduit and clean intermittent catheterization for myelomeningocele. Pediatrics, 72:203–205, 1983.

Duespohl, TA. Nursing diagnosis manual for the well and ill client. Philadelphia: WB Saunders Co, 1986.

Ehrlich, O, and Brem, A. A prospective comparison of urinary tract infections in patients treated with either clean intermittent catheterization or urinary diversion. Pediatrics, 70:665–669, 1982.

Faller, N, and Vinson, R. The artificial urinary sphincter. Journal of Enterostomal Therapy, 12:7–14, 1985.

Gonzales, R, and Sheldon, C. Artificial sphincters in children with neurogenic bladders: Long-term results. Journal of Urology, 128:1270–1272, 1982.

Grimm, RA. Hand function and tactile perception in a sample of children with meningomyelocele. American Journal of Occupational Therapy, 30:234–240, 1976.

Hannigan, K. Teaching intermittent self-catheterization to young children with myelodysplasia. Developmental Medicine and Child Neurology, 21:365–368, 1979.

Hardy, D, Melick, W, Gregory, V, and Schoenberg, H. Intermittent catheterization in children. Urology, 5:206–208, 1975.

Henderson, M, and Synhorst, D. Bladder and bowel management in the child with myelomeningocele. Pediatric Nursing, 3:24–31, 1977.

Hendry, V, and Geddes, N. Living with congenital anomaly: How nurses can help the parents of children born with spina bifida to develop lasting patterns of creative caring. The Canadian Nurse, 74:29–33, 1978.

Hesz, N, and Wolraich, M. Myelodysplasia. In Wolraich, M (Ed.), The practical assessment and management of children with disorders of development and learning. Chicago: Year Book Medical Publishers, 1987, pp. 194–221.

Hunt, G. Spina bifida: Implications for 100 children at school. Developmental Medicine and Child Neurology, 23:160–172, 1981.

Lapides, J, Diokno, A, Silber, S, and Lowe, B. Clean intermittent self-catheterization in the treatment of urinary tract disease. Journal of Urology, 107:458, 1972.

Lyon, R, Scott, M, and Marshall, S. Intermittent catheterization rather than urinary diversion in children with meningomyelocele. Journal of Urology, 113:409–417, 1975.

McNeal, D, Hawtrey, C, Wolraich, M, and Mapel, J. Symptomatic neurogenic bladder in a cerebral-palsied population. Developmental Medicine and Child Neurology, 25:612–616, 1983.

Moore, K. Urinary incontinence and the artificial sphincter. The Canadian Nurse, 81:32–35, 1985.

Mulcahy, J, and James, H. Management of neurogenic bladder in infancy and childhood. Urology, 13:235–240, 1979.

Mulcahy, J, James, H, and McRoberts, J. Oxybutynin chloride combined with intermittent clean catheterization in the treatment of myelomeningocele patients. Journal of Urology, 118:95–96, 1977.

Richardson, K, Campbell, MA, Brown, M, Masiulis, B, and Liptak, G. Biofeedback therapy for managing bowel incontinence caused by meningomyelocele. MCN: American Journal of Maternal Child Nursing, 10:388–392, 1985.

Schott, CM. A study of the effectiveness of a selected method for eliminating swimming pool bacterial contamination due to bowel incontinence of spina bifida participants. Unpublished master's degree thesis. Iowa City, The University of Iowa, July, 1978.

Shurtleff, DB. Myelodysplasia: Management and treatment. Current Problems in Pediatrics, 10:1–98, 1980.

Stauffer, D. Catheterization—A health procedure schools must be prepared to provide. Journal of School Health, 54:37–38, 1984.

Sullivan-Bolyai, S, Swanson, M, and Shurtleff, D. Toilet training the child with neurogenic impairment of bowel and bladder function. Issues in Comprehensive Pediatric Nursing, 7:33–43, 1984.

Wald, A. Use of biofeedback in treatment of fecal incontinence in patients with meningomyelocele. Pediatrics, 68:45–49, 1981.

White, J, and Shaker, I. The management of neurological fecal incontinence. In Freeman, J (Ed.), Practical management of meningomyelocele. Baltimore: University Park Press, 1974, pp. 198–217.

Whitehead, W, Parker, L, Masek, B, Cataldo, M, and Freeman, J. Biofeedback treatment of fecal incontinence in patients with myelomeningocele. Developmental Medicine and Child Neurology, 23:313–322, 1981.

Wolraich, M, Hawtrey, C, Mapel, J, and Henderson, M. Results of clean intermittent catheterization for children with neurogenic bladder. Urology, 22:479–482, 1983.

CHAPTER 24

SUMMARY
The Future

MARTHA J. CRAFT, Ph.D., R.N.

As noted in the Introduction, the interventions chosen for this book are those that place nature in the best condition to act. They represent a beginning upon which to add for the next and future editions.

The first series of interventions develop strong coping abilities in the infant, child, and family. The interventions are designed to promote attachment, fathering, sibling support, family integrity, and anticipatory guidance. These coping abilities are necessary to handle effectively life experiences that children face. Normal coping challenges are presented to children by school, interacting with playmates, and dealing with family moves to new residences. However, some coping challenges may be greater, such as parental divorce, or illness or death of a

family member. If illness occurs, the entire family unit is affected.

The childhood life event that is the focus of this book is altered health status or illness. During this life event children and their families need help to maximize their coping in order to contain or minimize any negative emotional sequela resulting from the experience. It is the responsibility of nurses to work toward the return of family and child coping to baseline level or an enhanced level following an illness episode.

It is important to realize that effective coping also affects biophysical responses. The 11 interventions offered to facilitate coping include preparation, play, drawings, touch, behavior management, intracultural communication, support, friends, loss man-

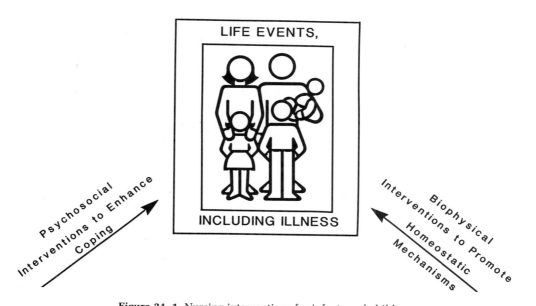

Figure 24–1. Nursing interventions for infants and children.

agement, self-care, and home care. Effective coping resulting from these interventions will affect sleeping, eating, the immune response, and reaction to illness diagnosis and management, such as pain. Interventions to further assist homeostatic mechanisms and alter biophysical responses are environmental manipulation, vestibular stimulation, sleep promotion, pain management, nutritional support, cerebral edema management, and bowel and bladder management. The global goals of these interventions are to promote biophysical and psychosocial functioning in children and families, and provide nursing care that maximizes functional status and improves quality of life.

While we recognize that many stresses are catastrophic and that the outcomes or prognoses may be unfavorable, at the same time nursing has the opportunity and challenge to enhance family strengths, mobilize resources and support systems, and work with families to facilitate coping with their life situation. Through carefully planned nurs-

ing interventions, these goals can be realized.

The conceptualization for interventions selected for this book is summarized in Figure 24–1. Please notice that there are many blank spaces in the drawing, which are meant to highlight the beginning nature of this intervention collection. It is the hope of the editors that you will add to this collection through identification and testing of nursing interventions for infants and children.

The editors close by offering a statement by Virginia Henderson, which synthesizes our beliefs regarding the importance of interventions:

When nurses' sensitivity to human needs (their intuition) is joined with the ability to find and use expert opinion, and the ability to find reported research and apply it to their practice, and, when they themselves use the scientific method of investigation, there is no limit to the influence they might have on health care worldwide.

INDEX

Note: Numbers in *italics* refer to illustrations; numbers followed by *t* indicate tables.